MW01471175

Spectacles and Other Vision Aids

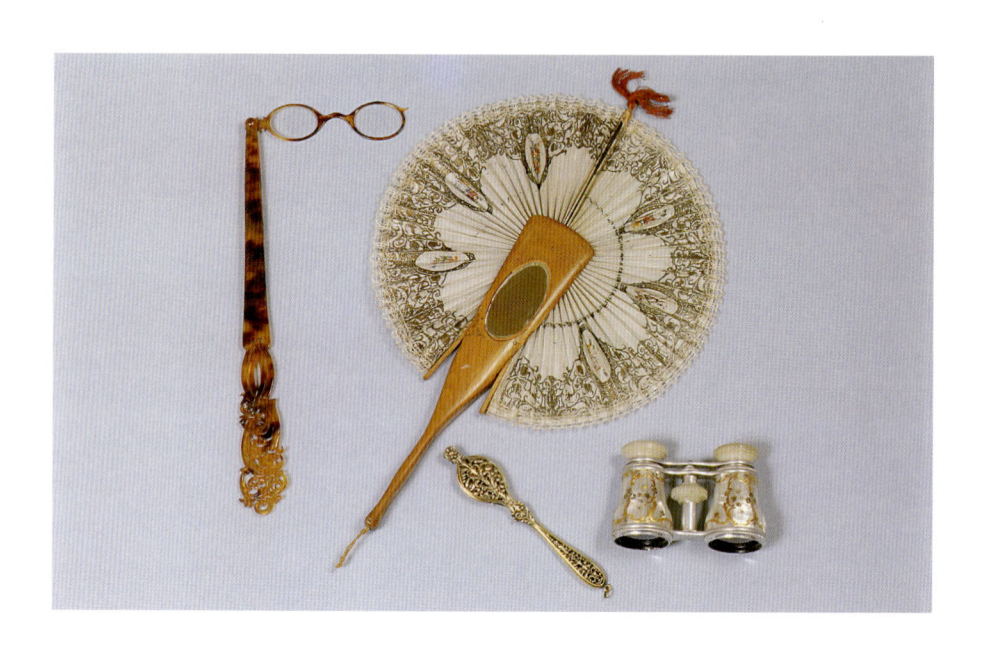

Spectacles and Other Vision Aids

A History and Guide to Collecting

J. William Rosenthal
M.D.

With Forewords by
Daniel M. Albert, M.D.
Frederick Allison Davis Professor and
Chair, Department of Ophthalmology,
University of Wisconsin Medical
School, Madison, Wisconsin
and
Joseph L. Bruneni, Optician
President of the Vision Consultants,
Inc., of Torrance, California and
Special Consultant to the Optical
Laboratories Association

Norman Publishing   San Francisco   1996

Copyright ©1996 by J. William Rosenthal, M.D.

All rights reserved. No part of this publication may be reproduced, stored in a retrieval system, or transmitted, in any form or by any means, electronic, mechanical, photocopying, recording, or otherwise, without the prior written approval of the publishers, except in the case of brief quotations embodied in critical articles and reviews.

Library of Congress Cataloging-in-Publication Data

Rosenthal, J. William
Spectacles and other vision aids : a history and guide to collecting / by J. William Rosenthal.
p.   cm.
Includes bibliographical references and index.
ISBN 0-939405-71-4 (alk. paper)
1. Eyeglasses—History. 2. Eyeglasses—Collectors and collecting.
I. Title
RE976.R665 1995–1996
617.7'522'09—dc20
95–16408   CIP

This book is printed on acid-free paper and its binding materials have been chosen for strength and durability.

Manufactured in Hong Kong.

Copies may be ordered from:
NORMAN PUBLISHING
720 Market Street
San Francisco, CA 94102–2502
Phone: USA and Canada: 1–800–544–9359
        Outside USA and Canada: (415) 781–6402
FAX: 415–781–5507
e-mail: orders@jnorman.com
Frontispiece, clockwise from left: tortoiseshell lorgnette, eventail cocarde fan, American gold lorgnette circa 1895, sea snail opera glasses.

Jacket images:
Front cover: enameled diamond gold lorgnette
Back cover: Top, clockwise from left: inlaid lacquer Chinese spectacles case; mid
             nineteenth-century Chinese tortoiseshell spectacles with dark tea-stone
             lenses; tortoiseshell Chinese spectacles case
             Center: Abalone opera glasses
             Bottom: English leather eyeglasses circa 1500

To Harriet

Contents

Foreword *Daniel M. Albert, M.D.*   xi

Foreword *Joseph L. Bruneni*   xiii

Preface   xv

Acknowledgments   xvii

Introduction   xix

Chapter 1   How to Manage a Collection   1

Chapter 2   The Detailed Examination of Historical Artifacts   5

Chapter 3   A Short History of Glass and Some of Its Applications   17

Chapter 4   The Development of Optical Quality Lenses   24

Chapter 5   A Review of the History of Spectacles   35

Chapter 6   Optical Manufacturing in the United States   50

Chapter 7   Development of Chinese Spectacles   62

Chapter 8   Ancient Chinese Eyeglass Cases   78

Chapter 9   Japanese Spectacles   96

Chapter 10   Steel Spectacles and Cases   99

Chapter 11	Martin's Margins 106
Chapter 12	Wig Spectacles 111
Chapter 13	Scissors Glasses 115
Chapter 14	Lorgnettes 118
Chapter 15	Monoculars (Spyglasses) (1603–1830) 138

Chapter 16	Opera Glasses 149
	J. Wm. Rosenthal, M.D.
	James H. Cohen, A.S.A.
	  History
	  Demand
	  Embellishments
	  Oddities
	  Handles
	  Cost
	  Indentification
	  Protective Cases
	  Cardboard Boxes for Initial Sales
	  What's in a Name?
	  Opera Glass Collection
	  Insignias
	  New Orleans Opera Glasses
	  Retailers
	  Cases in J. Wm. Rosenthal's Collection
	  Appendix

Chapter 17	Quizzing Glasses 220
Chapter 18	Optical Uses of Fans 224
Chapter 19	The Story of the Monocle 230
Chapter 20	Pince-Nez 236
Chapter 21	Bifocals 258
Chapter 22	Eyeshades for Invalids 266
Chapter 23	Lenses for Sun, Glare, and Related Eye Protection 270
Chapter 24	Eskimo Shades 278

Chapter 25	Industrial and Protective Goggles and Spectacles	284
Chapter 26	Shooting Glasses	295
Chapter 27	Specialized Spectacles	300
Chapter 28	Makeup Spectacles	306
Chapter 29	Trial Lenses and Frames	308
Chapter 30	Telescopic Operating Loupes	316
Chapter 31	Spectacles Cases	320
Chapter 32	The Evolution of Chatelaine Eyeglass Cases	332
Chapter 33	Magnifying Glasses	338
Chapter 34	Votive Offerings	344
Chapter 35	Miniatures	349
Chapter 36	Catalogs	354
Chapter 37	Spectacles in Art, Pictures, and Prints	358
Chapter 38	The Development of Contact Lenses 369 *Edward J. Fisher, M.A., D.Sc., F.A.A.O.*	
Chapter 39	Modern Frames	384
Appendix 1	Landmarks in Optical History	389
Appendix 2	English Translation of D. M. Manni's Book about Salvino Armati	395
Appendix 3	Alphabetical List of (Mostly) United States Spectacles Makers from 1700–1850	429
Appendix 4	History and Bibliography of Astigmatism: Original Work by Emile Javal	433
Appendix 5	Listing of Art and Illustrations Demonstrating the Use of Spectacles	437
Appendix 6	Great Ophthalmological Collections of Visual Aids around the World	465

Appendix 7	Concise Instruction in Grinding Lenses and Fitting Telescopes by Gottlieb Christian Hilscher	467
Appendix 8	Outline on the Early History of Spectacles	489
	Bibliography	496
	Name Index	503
	Subject Index	514

Foreword

Daniel M. Albert, MD

Among the 100,000 genes a human possesses, there undoubtedly exist a pair associated with *collecting*. Although many different varieties of this gene may exist, undoubtedly the most desirable prototype are the *collecting* genes possessed by J. William Rosenthal. Having had the privilege of serving with Bill for a number of years on the American Academy of Ophthalmology Foundation Museum, I know first-hand the energy, commitment, sophistication and intelligence that Bill brings to his collection of spectacles and other vision aides. His annual presentations to the Cogan Ophthalmology History Society have demonstrated the scope of his knowledge as well as his ability to provide historically useful and relevant information from theses artifacts.

Bill is now the author of the present history and guide to collecting of spectacles and other visual aides. This work is illustrated with nearly eight hundred photographs of spectacles primarily from Bill's collection. It provides knowledge of these fascinating artifacts to ophthalmologists, optometrists, opticians, visual scientists and other individuals with an interest and appreciation of this field. The book includes a commentary of the history and significance of these items in thirty-nine chapters, and eight appendices, and the field of spectacle and vision-aid development and collecting is discussed in a comprehensive and beautifully illustrated manner. Both in style and content this book fills an important niche in the history of the development of vision care and vision aids.

Bill Rosenthal is an alumnus of Tulane University and Tulane Medical School. He received advance training at the University of Pennsylvania culminating in his D.Sc. degree in 1956. Bill is a fellow of the American College of Surgeons, the International College of Surgeons, the Royal Society of Medicine (United Kingdom), and the French Ophthalmological Society. He is also a fellow of the American Academy of Ophthalmology and served as Chief Curator of Spectacles for the American Academy of Ophthalmology Foundation Museum in San Francisco. Bill is an ophthalmic consultant to the Smithsonian Institute, a member of the Board of Trustees of the American Optical Company Museum in Southbridge, Massachusetts, and founder and curator of the Jonas W. Rosenthal, M.D., Memorial Ophthalmology Museum at Tulane University.

Bill Rosenthal is a distinguished and busy practicing ophthalmologist. He is the author of more than sixty professional articles, and is editor of three ophthalmic books and various chapters in other works. It is to his credit that he has found the time to build such an outstanding collection, write this book, and make his many other contributions regarding the spectacle and vision-aid collecting in spite of a busy schedule. His charming wife Harriet Stern Rosenthal, an expert on antiques in her own right, has supported Bill thoroughly in this undertaking. Bill and Harriet's generosity in donating valuable parts of their collection to the American Academy of Ophthalmology Foundation Museum and other public collections deserves praise.

In summary, I believe this book is the culmination of an outstanding career of an astute ophthalmic collector of spectacles and other vision aids, and is consistent with Bill's goal of sharing his treasures and knowledge with others who possess the *collecting* genes.

Foreword

Joseph L. Bruneni

During the process of researching data for a recently published book on the history of the American ophthalmic industry, several things soon became apparent. The first was the limited scope of published information regarding vision aids, particularly frames and lenses, my primary interest at the time. As it turned out, I discovered the most effective information, both visual and written, was only available through the laborious process of searching out early catalogs, price lists, and published advertising. Dr. Rosenthal was a primary source for much of the frame information appearing in this published history.

During the research process, I discovered how many people have a deep interest in vision aids and their evolution through the years. Somewhat to my surprise, I discovered collectors of antique vision aids in almost every country, many having little or no direct connection with the optical industry or the ophthalmic professions.

For all these people, Dr. Rosenthal has produced what will surely become the final authority for collectors of vision aids. His curiosity and wide-ranging interest has produced a remarkable assortment of detailed information on an extensive variety of vision aids ranging far beyond lenses and frames. He even includes information for neophyte collectors with his personal advice on the best way to start a collection.

Dr. Rosenthal's book is an extraordinary work that will be a primary reference source for anyone interested in the optical industry or the ophthalmic professions. Better yet, his work will provide invaluable assistance to all those collectors of vision aids, whether they are world-class museums or individual collectors about to purchase their first piece.

Preface

Ophthalmic history has been examined and described by a number of authors in its four or five thousand years of development. Although book publication on the subject has increased in number in recent years, descriptions of vision aids have been only factual. This book intends to present not only artifacts previously discovered but also many not otherwise described. Nuances of life and the use of objects, as well as the reasons for their existence and the meanings of their decorations, will be unveiled.

Raw materials used in the manufacture of vision aids have not until now been really appreciated. For instance, what is described as mother-of-pearl by many in books, catalogues, and everyday life is actually the shell of the sea snail. Additionally, we have tended to subconsciously belittle transportation and commerce in the past few hundred years. Thus, we are surprised to learn that Brazilian pebbles were used in the grinding of European lenses in the last century.

As the author has devoted much of his life to this subject and has procured a large vision aid collection over the years, he has provided information to aid the collector—in addition to addressing the history of the subject. In short, this offering is a tribute to our ancestors—their abilities, their resourcefulness, their sciences, and their humanity.

Acknowledgments

Many minds and hands have gone into play during development of this book. The authors of previous histories deserve credit for their originality and research. Their names make up my bibliographies.

My wife, Harriet, has not only endured my "trashing her home" with collectibles and manuscripts, but has also joyously joined me in antique stores and flea markets in search of artifacts. Our son, Paul, and daughter, Susan Farrell, have also been thoughtful and helpful in collecting. Susan went so far as to marry an ophthalmologist, Dr. James Farrell. Paul went so far as to go into the antiques business (among other things).

Of course, the founders of this dynasty are my father, Dr. Jonas W. Rosenthal, an ophthalmologist, and my father-in-law, Henry Stern, an antiques dealer.

In preparation of the manuscript, a huge ton of thanks goes to Richard Cardoni for translating Manni's book on Armati from the Italian. Margaret Beveridge was also extremely helpful in her translation of the Latin in the same book.

Professor E. J. Fisher's chapter on the history of contact lenses speaks for itself and his multiple abilities. He has my heartfelt thanks.

Mildred Covert was not only a skilled typist but as an author in her own right gave advice and corrections on the use of language.

It has been delightful working with Ms. Deborah Noto Soler as the editorial "brake" on my usual informal enthusiasm of expression. Whereas oral presentations are usually filled with personal anecdotes, we have "kept to the facts" by her efforts. Additionally, she has added a point of view that has influenced the direction and rationale of the book. Because of this, and her fine composition abilities, I owe her a debt of thanks.

Robert Balkan, MD, and Mr. Brian Eschette (deceased) deserve appropriate credit for the time, energy, and expertise demonstrated in their beautiful photographs. Jeff Strout also contributed.

There are many friends and acquaintances interested in ophthalmic history who joined me in memberships in organizations studying the subject. Some, however, have been outstanding in their encouragement of my authorship. I would be remiss if I did not mention the names of Fred Blodi, MD; Robert McMaster; Andrew Ferry, MD; and Daniel Albert, MD.

And last with rousing appreciation, let me express my joy to the whole collecting melange of conferees, dealers, and associates. The Ocular Heritage Society members, The David Cogan Ophthalmological History Group, and the American Academy of Ophthalmology Foundation Museum staff and curators have been especially supportive. David Noonan,

Susan Cronenwett, Licia Wells, and John Handley should be named representing the museum. The Smithsonian Institution's Ophthalmological Curatorial staff was additionally helpful.

The spirit of camaraderie is exemplified when my receptionist tells me, "Sylvia Sze is on the phone from Hong Kong. She wants to know if her dad can send you some Chinese spectacles." Or—David Gladwell from Virginia calls to tell me that a spectacle collection is being sold in Oregon. Or—Bob McMaster writes from Sturbridge, MA, that he has some interesting artifacts.

This motley group is a true fraternity. Although there are some commercial aspects, we all share one basic interest—putting history together, piece by piece. We thank each other.

J. William Rosenthal, MD
New Orleans, Louisiana

INTRODUCTION

Starting a Collection

Throughout this book, you will find history on various vision aids. While this information is useful for a variety of purposes, it is especially useful to the collector. It provides background information essential to a good purchase. However, whether you're accumulating vision aids or other collectibles, this section will help you get started.

Often I am asked by a noncollector how and why I started collecting. Of course one needs to have an interest in a certain subject and an "accumulator" propensity to support this interest. Besides these basic "urges," there is usually a trigger mechanism. My edged weapon collection started when I lost a marbles game in grade school and I traded my marbles for a knife. To date, this collection is still growing. My interest in ophthalmic history began when my father, an ophthalmologist, passed away. I could not throw out all those old instruments, and the like, even though they were beyond their time. Meanwhile, I had joined a History of Medicine Society at Tulane University Medical School and married the daughter of an antiques dealer. All of these things played a part in my interest in collecting.

My wife and I did not have a houseful of antiques early on during our marriage. We learned how to be patient and to pick and choose fine old pieces in good condition to furnish our home. The same technique can be used in collecting: Start the collection with common, ordinary, and less expensive pieces. Then add older, more rare, and more expensive pieces as they come along and can be afforded.

Meanwhile, you, the collector, should gain as much knowledge as possible about your particular interest. Find books, magazines, and articles on the targeted subject. Join local or national organizations. Attend conventions and other meetings as well as local and nationally sponsored shows. All of these can lead to information not otherwise available.

Other sources of information are the many dealers who buy and sell objects that you desire to collect. Some are knowledgeable, and some are only interested in a sale. Antique stores, flea markets, and garage sales are all places where your treasures might be found. Always ask the seller for information regarding the object of interest. What is the age? Manufacturer? Condition? Where was it purchased? Who owned it? In other words, what is the provenance?

You might also gain additional information by simply finding others in your community who share the same interest. An advertisement in a local newspaper for those interested can bring surprising results. Many collectors might enjoy an evening of discussion on the subject, and this could lead to the formation of a collectors club. Endless hints are traded at this type of meeting.

While collecting requires time and effort, knowledge, and persistence, it should be enjoyable as well. Making the effort a family affair or outing is rewarding. Different aspects of the subject can thus be covered, and older family members can be helpful with information and lore. Talk to your friends and see whether they are interested in collecting. Their interests may differ from yours, but going out in a group for an afternoon of searching, garage sale hopping, or flea marketing is a lot of fun. Besides, more eyes are available for artifact searching when you work together.

After a few months of activity, your subject and collecting interest will become known. Local dealers will call to tell you of a piece they have acquired and thus will stimulate your acquisitiveness. Friends and other collectors will direct you to stores where you might find a prime object. Eventually, out-of-town dealers will write you to buy things they have acquired or send you lists or photographs. This will show that you are an accepted, knowledgeable collector, and it will not be long before other collectors will seek out your expertise.

1

How to Manage a Collection

Purpose

Determining the purpose of a collection may be difficult at first. Once you realize that you have the beginnings of a small collection, it is best to decide what you will do with it as it grows. Personal gratification is understood, of course, but will the collection be decorative (in the home, office, or other location)? Will it complement other collections, such as those found in a library, museum, or school? Do these institutions want such a collection? Are others doing the same thing? (Do not reinvent the wheel.) Definition of purpose, then, will aid in later decisions of about such things as scope and costs.

Scope of the Collection

How many times have I heard: "I should have limited my collection to. . . ." We all get interested in the subject at hand; and in the spirit of learning, in the heat of an auction, or when observing a beautiful specimen, we deviate from our original purpose and purchase something out of the range of our original aims. We really must be militant and manage ourselves harshly to keep the collection within bounds.

When we start a collection, we are neophytes and do not realize what a large subject we are choosing. Later, we may even have to cut down on the scope of the collection as originally envisioned. For instance, if you decide to collect knives, should you collect hunting knives, pocketknives, swords, or others? If pocketknives, should they be made by only one company such as Case or Imperial? Should you collect knives with only stag handles? Should you collect only whittlers? Barlows? Knives made between 1950 and 1980? Antique? Custom-made?

Perhaps this demonstrates the consideration and decisions regarding the scope of the collection that must be made at the start!! It is always easier to expand a collection than to restrict it, so start small and learn what interests you and what you can handle.

Housing and Protecting the Collection

If you live in an apartment, it would be folly to start a collection of antique automobiles without preparation to house them adequately. Even small objects, such as thimbles or spoons, need to have an adequate repository if they are to be treated appropriately. Available space, the proper furniture, shelves needed, and other factors, must all be considered.

Many collectibles are best housed in closed, locked cabinets, which protect against dust, breakage, pilferage, and the like. Care should be taken to avoid placing the cabinet in direct sunlight. The heat so engendered will deteriorate some materials, and light itself will cause fading of colors on some pictures and instruments. The lack of humidity will cause ivory to crack. Cabinets should be inspected so that rodents and insects, such as roaches, cannot reach delicate objects. Some animals are prone to attack such things as tortoiseshell spectacles and cases. It is amazing the number of tortoiseshell frames and wooden cases I have seen with gouges from rat teeth.

Most vision aids, as described in this book, can be accommodated in a drawer. Ideally, a drawer about three inches (7.5 centimeters) high is satisfactory. Lining the drawers can be tricky. Do not use modern foam as it can react chemically with several materials, mostly plastics. Cotton-based felt is great, and some materials (Pacific cloth) can be used with silver items to discourage oxidation and tarnishing. Also, 3M Company puts out a strip for the same purpose. The area should be enclosed, such as in a cabinet.

Dust can play havoc with instruments such as ophthalmoscopes, so they should be protected. Plastic film wrapping can be used if open shelves are the only space available, but closed cabinets are best for these instruments.

In the case of books, prints, or other paper objects, professional advice is needed. Suffice it to say that acid-free paper and specially constructed boxes should be used to preserve ancient tomes. Leather objects, such as spectacles and cases, take particular care, and instructions should be followed to prevent disintegration.

For completeness' sake, I will mention the following for obvious reasons: Do not house your valuables in an unheated or uncooled attic. Place rare, valuable objects such as jewel-encrusted lorgnettes, in a bank safety deposit box. Take appropriate measures to house your collection if you live in an area where natural disaster is likely to occur (tornado, flood, fire). Consider fire, smoke, and burglar alarms for added protection.

Exhibiting and Lighting

Permanent exhibits of artifacts are best done commercially to be fully appreciated. Their arrangement must be pleasing, labeling literate and legible, and lighting adequate. Artificial light is easier to use, as it can be turned on only when viewing is required. Lights inside a cabinet may produce too much heat, so ceiling lights, though expensive, should be considered. A less desirable solution is to vent the cabinet and place a glass of water inside.

If objects are kept in drawers, lights above them or good general lighting is needed. Drawers should be labeled as to content.

Certain flat articles, prints, and pictures, can be framed and hung on the wall. Some small items are adequately viewed in shadow boxes, while some objects look attractive when exhibited under a glass dome. A coffee table/vitrine arrangement makes a pleasant repository for viewing.

Insurance

When a collection is valuable enough, appropriate insurance is a must. Consult an agent to determine the best and most affordable coverage. Some home or business insurance policies will cover many collections without further policies. Other collections are so valuable that they must be itemized on existing policies or covered separately.

In addition to breakage, pilferage and burglary, natural events such as fire, wind, and flood should be covered.

To substantiate a claim, present the adjusters with a catalog, pictures, and prices of the missing or damaged artifacts. Prices, particularly, should be backed up by invoices, checks, or evidence of recent sales of similar objects. Perhaps a professional appraisal might be considered.

Catalogs and Labeling

It is a good idea to start off correctly by giving all artifacts an accession number (see museum publications for the various types), date, description, and price, as well as provenance and name of donor or store where purchased. The number should be placed on the artifact in a way that will not harm it but will remain for indefinite (but removable) identification. Similar objects should be stored together for comparison's sake but need not have consecutive numbers.

A less attractive alternative to catalog use is labeling. Tags and stickers may be inscribed with the above-mentioned information. It is more difficult to keep track of the collection with tags, and one might purchase duplicates, being unaware that an example had previously been part of the collection.

Dealers use codes to denote prices on tagged objects, and it may please you to use a code on your tags or in your catalog. Do not neglect to tell some family member, a trusted employee, or your lawyer how to solve your code.

Pricing of Artifacts

A beginner should be instructed by friends on the basic price of standard objects to put into a collection. Naturally, the older a piece, the more expensive. Also, we pay more for rare pieces, pristine (mint condition) pieces, complete pieces, and those made or owned by famous persons.

A gold lorgnette is more valuable than one that is gold-filled. Spectacles made by William Beecher should be worth more than similar ones without a provenance. While prices on some objects are fairly stable, some will rise in response to the increasing popularity, say of an artist. Later, the price may fall.

Certain parts of the world bring higher prices than others. For example, objects found in large cities ordinarily cost more than those found in the surrounding countryside.

Certain dealers see each piece of stock as a treasure, and consequently ask a fortune for it. They may, of course, run an expensive operation in a high-rent district with numerous employees, fine decorations, and thick vellum stationery. You pay for that. However, these dealers did not become successful overnight and usually have the knowledge, organization, contacts, and stock to furnish first-class artifacts. Therefore, they earn their price.

Rare objects produced are difficult to price. How high is high? One's own purse is limitation enough, and some things we might really desire have to be left in the store because of the high price. Such objects do not usually sell rapidly. Therefore, if you inquire again sometime later, the price may have come down or terms might be arranged, so keep in touch.

This does not mean you cannot find a "treasure" in a third-class flea market. Such an event is not too likely, but it is certainly possible, as we have all done so. Some fine dealers may have an object in stock but have expertise in another line, thereby pricing that artifact you want too low. Never pass an object you desire without asking its price.

You will find that after you have been a customer of a dealer and he feels comfortable with you, the dealer will give you good prices, write or call you if he finds something you want, or give you other perks. It is to your advantage, then, to help him or her in any way that you can.

Your catalog tells you what you paid for an artifact. The updated price would be good to note also. If you got a bargain, mark it up. If you did not notice a defect on purchase, your flawed object should be marked down. Current pricing has many facets and should be done periodically.

Sales and Swaps

When your collection has grown, duplicates will appear. There is no reason they should not be sold or traded to other collectors or dealers. They may be placed in a flea market or garage sale. You should be just as fair to others regarding your pieces as you would want them to be with you. Do not hide defects, but do show off the good points. Remember that a dealer must make money. He can buy wholesale from others, and that means about half your price. Unless he really needs your duplicates, his offer may be less than what you paid for the piece.

It is fun to swap pieces with another collector. Nothing gives me greater pleasure than to furnish a friend with an artifact he needs to complete a collection. It is also nice to be able to donate an artifact to a museum when it is needed for an exhibit.

Loans

Many hospitals, museums, schools, and sundry institutions have temporary exhibits for several months or a year at a time. Your collection may be tapped to provide artifacts. You should be proud that such a request is made and honored by the signs acknowledging your largesse.

However, some places may be less than businesslike. You should insist that the institution pay for the transport of the objects (you'd better do the packing) as well as for the insurance to cover transport and exhibition. To prevent damage, be sure the outside exhibiting agency does not put your artifacts in excessive light or heat. The area should be locked during off-hours and prying hands kept away by appropriate cover.

Describe and number the pieces (with a tag or sticker) and record this information on a list of loaned objects. Always count the number of pieces returned against the number loaned.

Literature

The stark presence of an object has fewer attributes than one backed up by research and understanding of the reason for existence, area of production, and the materials used. I have a certain carved wooden Chinese eyeglass case that is beautiful. The case took on a whole new meaning, however, when I found that the carving represents one of the events in an ancient Chinese novel: "Treading through the snow in pursuit of the plum flower." This, I discovered only after seeing the same figures in the carving placed on a Chinese snuff bottle.[1,2] Research brought me to a book that told the story.

It is therefore important to learn as much as possible about your purchase. Inquire with the dealer in detail about the provenance. Procure as much information as possible on the country of origin, as it is much more difficult to do so later, with time and distance separation. Also, try to obtain literature that is translated into your native language, though book translations can be a tedious (perhaps expensive) process. Such knowledge not only will add to your enjoyment of the subject but also will make you sought after to give lectures and share your knowledge.

Reference books are always good to own. One cannot remember everything, and others will ask questions you must answer. Knowing where to find the answer is almost as good as having it verbatim.

Restoration

Antiques by definition are old and must have been used. Many have been misused and should be repaired. However, because it is old is no reason it should be dirty—so clean it!! But clean it properly so that the object will be enhanced and not destroyed. When shining an object, do not ruin its patina—just remove the dirt.

I cannot improve on a small book by Ronald J. S. MacGregor entitled *Restoring Ophthalmic Antiques* and published by the Ophthalmic Antiques International Collectors' Club.[3] Before you begin to repair your artifact, please read the instructions. MacGregor's book includes information on restoring books, leather, metal, tortoiseshell—the lot!

Conclusion

"Buy what you like" is a good basic rule. Using good light and a magnifier ensures that the object is what you thought it was originally. If you do find something you like and can afford it, buy it immediately. Later, it may be gone.

Notes

1. Raymond Li, *A Glossary of Chinese Snuff Bottle Rebus* (Hong Kong: Nine Dragons Publishers, 1976).
2. C. A. S. Williams, *Outlines of Chinese Symbolism and Art Motives* (New York: Dover Publishers, 1976).
3. R. J. S. MacGregor, *Restoring Ophthalmic Antiques* (United Kingdom: Ophthalmic Antiques International Collectors' Club, 1990). See also *Collecting Ophthalmic Antiques* (United Kingdom: Ophthalmic Antiques International Collectors' Club, 1992).

2

The Detailed Examination of Historical Artifacts

The principles involved in examining vision aids are the same as those used to evaluate other antique and historical artifacts. For instance, hallmarks found on British silver spectacles are the same as those found on other British silver objects (Figure 1). Therefore, a general knowledge of silver hallmarks is helpful in determining the age, maker, place of manufacture, and quality of silver spectacles as well as of other silver products. The same reasoning can apply to porcelain, glass, tortoiseshell, and other materials.

Presented here are areas of concentration where knowledge is essential to the collector. Numerous specific examples are provided, as well as information on literature available for reference.

History

Knowledge of the history of certain artifacts is necessary to identify the place and approximate year of origin. For example, the history of Chinese exports of porcelains helps us to determine whether a Chinese bowl bearing a figure was done in China (Figure 2) or whether it was done, say, in southern France, where chinoiserie was quite popular. On minute examination, the Chinese painted scenes reveal that the human figures have Chinese-shaped eyes.

Prior to the Industrial Revolution (1832), decoration of porcelain, lacquer, and other materials was done by hand by true artists. It was most certainly fine work. Later, the process of transferring was used: A design or a previously made or machine-made figure was placed on the object (Figure 3). Transferring compares with putting a decal on a window and is not a particularly fine way to decorate. Some transfers were actually put on articles with a little paint smeared around to make them look as if they were done by hand (Figure 4). These, of course, were not done by artisans and are identified as inferior.

It is helpful to know that around 1750, the Meissen factory in Germany produced a series of figures, "The Criers of Paris." This series depicts local salespersons. Amongst them is the figure of the old eyeglass peddler (Figure 5). The gentleman here is seen with a tray of eyeglasses in front of him that he is presenting to the public. The crossed swords on the bottom of the figure tells us that it was done in Meissen and is German. A later series was also produced (Figure 6).

The author has in his collection a religious figure (St. Lucy) carved in wood from Brazil (Figure 7). St. Lucy is standing with a plate in her hand, and ostensibly, her two eyes are lying on the plate. In the story of St. Lucy, she plucked her eyes

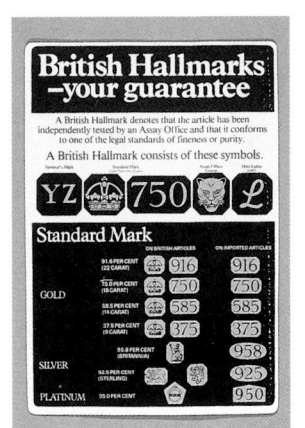

Figure 1. Table of British hallmarks.

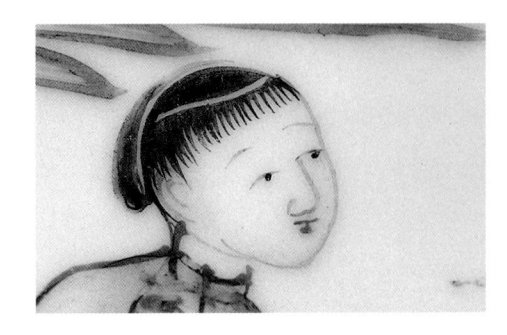

Figure 2. Figure on porcelain showing Chinese eyes.

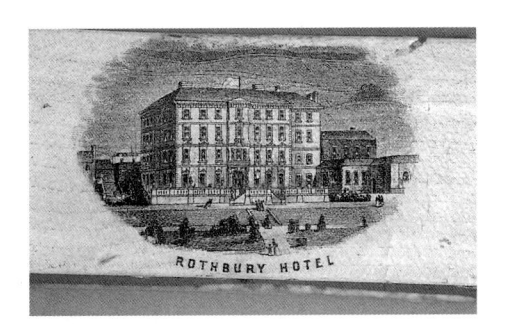

Figure 3. Transfer decoration.

Figure 4. Augmented transfer decoration.

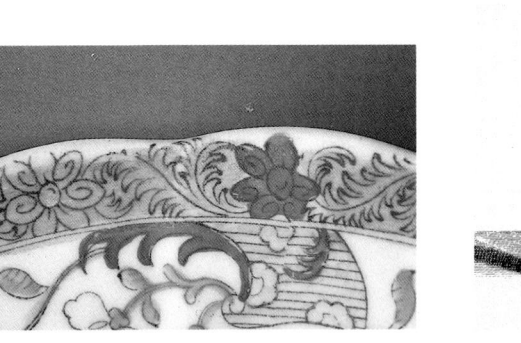

Figure 5. *The Old Eyeglass Peddler.*

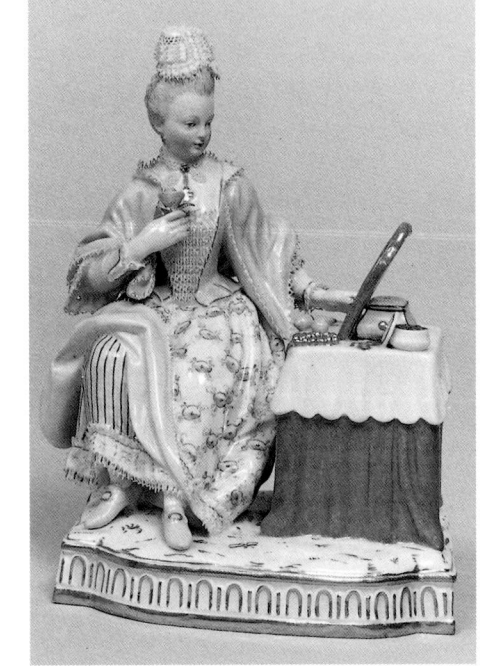

Figure 6. Meissen statue of one of the five senses, *Sight*, circa 1850.

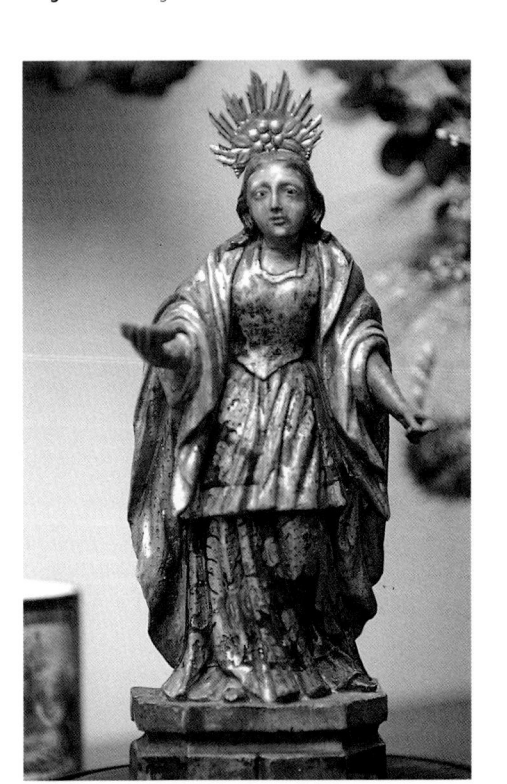

Figure 7. Wooden statue of St. Lucy.

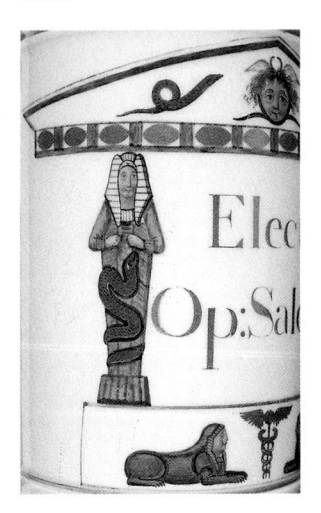

Figure 8. Egyptian figure on French apothecary jar.

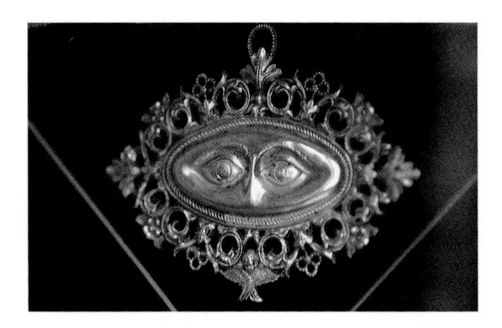

Figure 9. Baroque ex-voto.

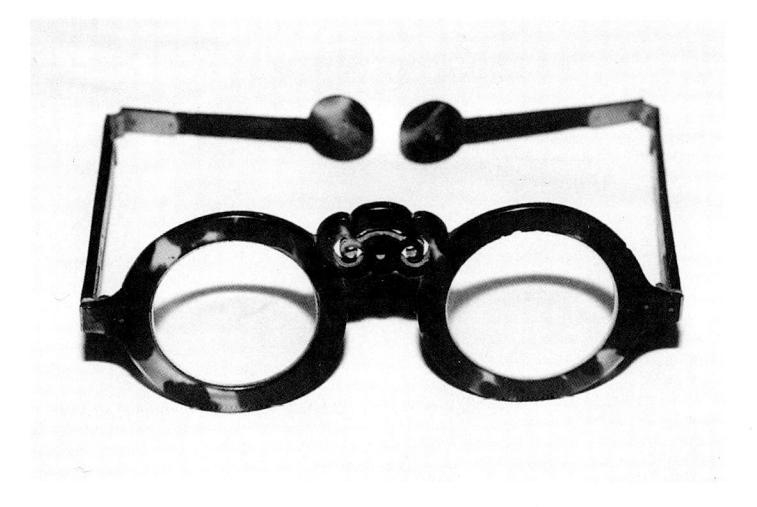

Figure 10. Glass lenses in Chinese tortoiseshell frames.

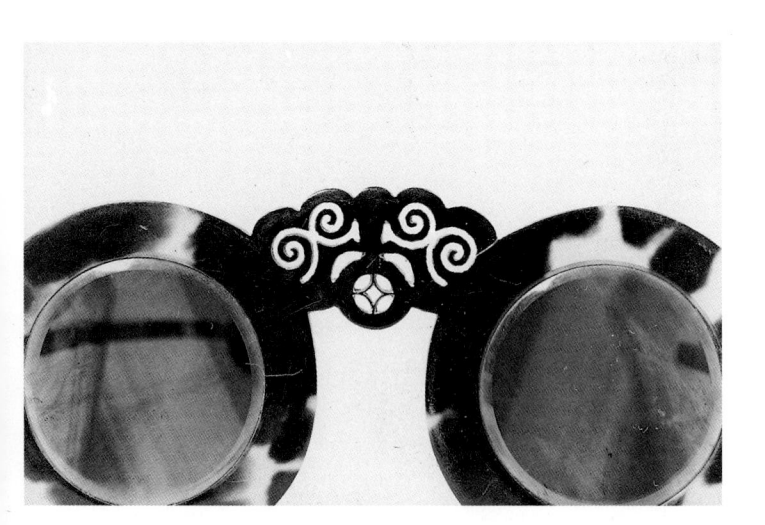

Figure 11. Chinese spectacles with teastone lenses.

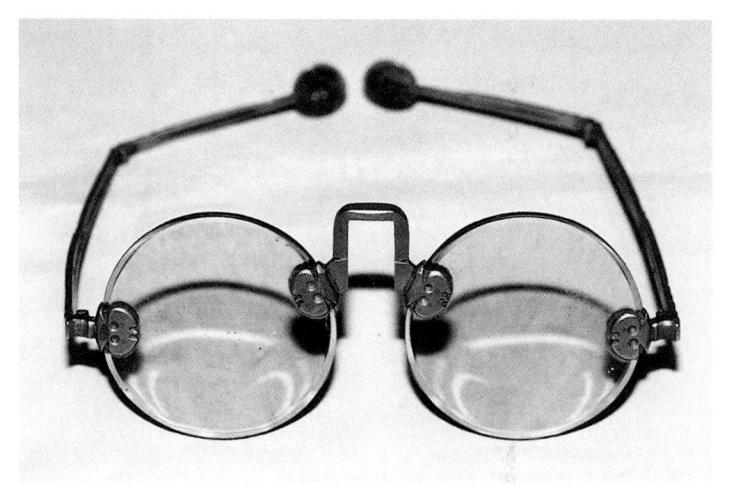

Figure 12. Chinese spectacles with glass lenses circa 1800.

from her head when about to be violated and subsequently presented them to her tormentor. Knowing this story allows identification of the figure.

An understanding of the conquering armies of Napoleon and their relation to the Egyptian campaign also helps in noting that the Egyptian motif (Figure 8) is present in many French antiquities (furniture, apothecary bottles, scissors glasses). Therefore, these French articles date to the Napoleonic era.

Amulets of silver or pressed iron plate were used on the doorposts of houses in southern Europe to "protect" the houses from the ravages of eye disease. This information can be used to identify these peculiar looking faces. They are called "ex votos" (Figure 9) and are found throughout southern Europe. Some are small enough to be carried on the person or hung from the neck, much as people currently wear religious medals.

Familiarity with the dating of Chinese eyeglasses is useful in determining whether the lenses were made of real glass (Figure 10); teastone *ai tai* (Figure 11), which was used in the 1200s; or glass made in later years around 1800 (Figure 12). An important fact is that early glass—soda glass—was not crystal clear and had imperfections. It was not until the time of Charles II (1660s) that a man by the name of Ravenscroft (about 1665) in England discovered that adding flint to the glass made it crystal clear, or crystalline (like crystal). Clear

EXAMINATION OF ARTIFACTS

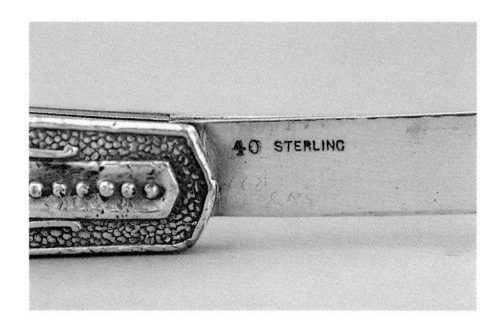

Figure 13. Sterling stamp on knife blade.

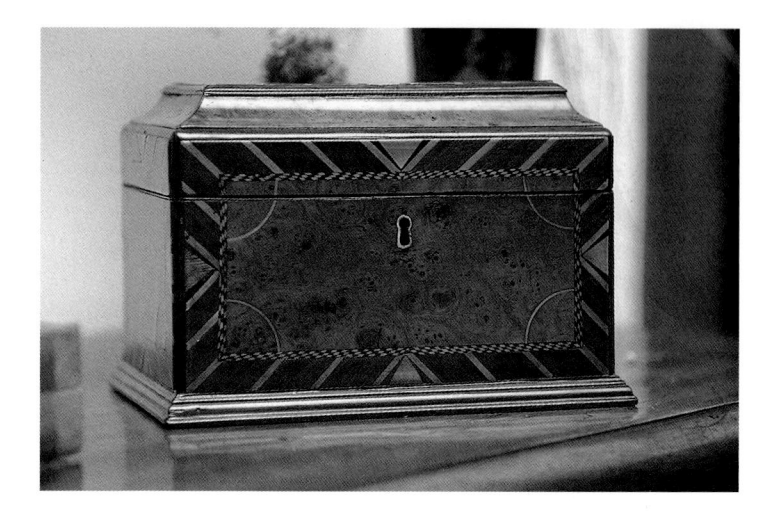

Figure 14. English inlaid wooden tea caddy.

quartz was mined from the caves of Siberia and Brazil and was up to that time the clearest known substitute for glass.

While history often aids us in identifying artifacts, it can sometimes act as a double-edged sword. The author was offered a very fine pair of spectacles dating around 1400. The spectacles appeared to be authentic as the glass was old. However, after putting them under the lensometer, it was found that each lens measured exactly two diopters. Since the diopter was not invented until 1876, this precise number suggested that the glasses had been recently ground and that the pair may have been altered. The purchase was declined. Later, an old catalog on eyeglasses revealed a comparison of the relative strength of the diopter with the previously used increment—the pouce. Looking down the list, it was found that two diopters equaled exactly twenty pouces. Therefore, the lensometer actually revealed a 20-pouce lens and a perfectly ground pair of antique spectacles! Unfortunately, this wonderful purchase opportunity was missed.

Literature

Knowing which literature is available on various subjects is certainly helpful. One obvious book that comes to mind contains the listing of the hallmarks of various silver and gold objects. These hallmarks denote certain countries, meaningful words, and numbers. For example, the word *sterling* (Figure 13) was mandatorily placed on silver objects in the United States starting in 1865. However, certain silver articles made in England were also stamped "sterling" when being exported to the United States. Coin silver is also a useful term: The silver in the object being viewed was the same amount as was placed in the coin of the realm of that time.[1]

Literature on dating certain objects is available. That which pertains to spectacles, of course, can be found in our modern books as well as in books and catalogs that are out of print. Many books on numismatics and philately contain the desired information.

It is a good idea to have the catalog of collections available to find literature on the identification of various objects. The line of spectacles, for instance, has the Library of Congress, the Becker Collection in St. Louis, James Leeds, American Optometric society, the Wellcome Collection in London, and many others.

It is a pity that we, as Americans, are not more fluent in foreign languages. It would enable us to better realize what a rich heritage we have, and it would allow us to use that heritage in researching our historical documents. Unfortunately, many books are out of print. Many others are in foreign libraries, where either they are unavailable or must be translated.

Materials

A background on materials is helpful in identifying various artifacts. For instance, the color, weight, and grain of wood are important (Figure 14). However, examining the surface, edges, and lines of a wooden object will determine whether the object was made with primitive tools before the Industrial Revolution in 1832 or with mechanical tools after that date. A dowel (Figure 15) with wavy lines, for example, dates before 1832, because the lathe on which it was turned was foot powered and thus had an irregular type of cutting power. This

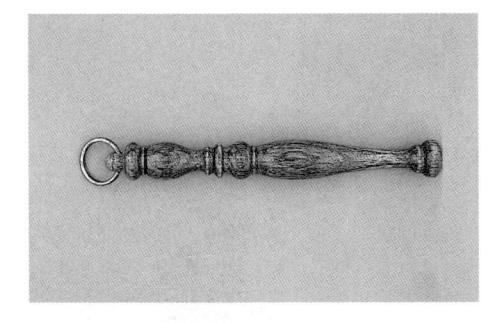

Figure 15. Handmade dowel.

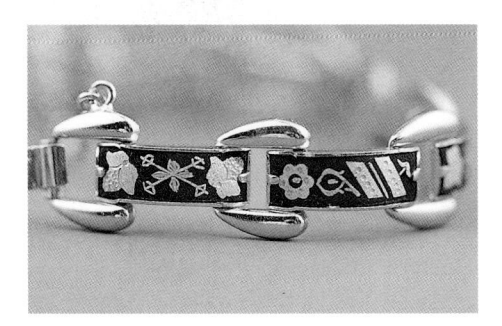

Figure 16. Damascene bracelet.

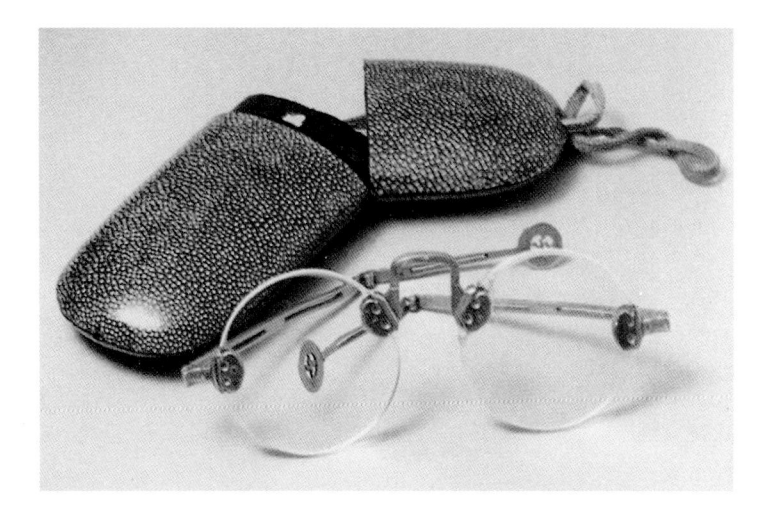

Figure 17. Chinese shagreen spectacle case.

was reflected in the final product. A certain wave can be felt on antique furniture, particularly on flat surfaces, that is not present on wood cut with a mechanical saw and sandpapered. Also helpful is familiarity with the types and origins of wood. Padouk wood comes mostly from Goa on the Indian Ocean. There are several types of mahogany: Central American is different from South American. There are also many types of reeds found in different parts of the world. Of these, Tonbridgeware, from Tonbridge, England, is used to make eyeglass cases as well as boxes and other decorative articles. The origin, therefore, is easily determined.

One must also be familiar with where and when certain processes were used. Damascene (Figure 16), for instance, originated in Damascus and was used around the Middle Ages. However, Damascene is no longer made in Damascus but is now made in Kyoto, Japan, and Toledo, Spain. Therefore, these objects could be either quite old or modern. They can, however, be dated easily, and their point of origin can then be ascertained.

Shagreen   For many centuries, cultures around the world have used shagreen (sharkskin or ray skin) as an exotic decorative covering for many type objects. Because of its original pebbled surface, its name is from the Turkish *saghri*. In France, it is known as *galuchat*.

After stripping the skin from the animal, a 16-step process is used. This includes bleaching, drying, filing the surface nubs flat, and dyeing—usually green, with the aid of copper acetate. Other colors seen are natural (tan), red, and black. The central parts of each scale do not usually take the stain, resulting in a pleasing pattern (Figure 17). The spaces between the scales can be filled with a colored mastic. The treated and dyed skin is then secured to a cardboard or wooden base with a water-soluble glue.

Samurai sword handles, eyeglass cases from England and China, French etuis, clock cases, and purses have all been covered with this beautiful material.

Cetorhinus (Small Variety of Shark)   Cetorhinus is used to make small shagreen cases where a smaller sized scale is more appropriate. It looks much like lizard skin.

Roussette   Roussette is a type of shark with a dark brown-red colored skin. It is also used in making cases. Therefore, we have a most durable and attractive case for telescopes, chatelaines, and scientific or practical instruments.

Plastics   Although cellulose nitrate (celluloid, xylonite) was first produced in 1855, it was used internationally in the first part of the twentieth century.[2] This substance decomposes slowly, can be dissolved in acetone, and, when scrubbed, smells like camphor. It is highly flammable.

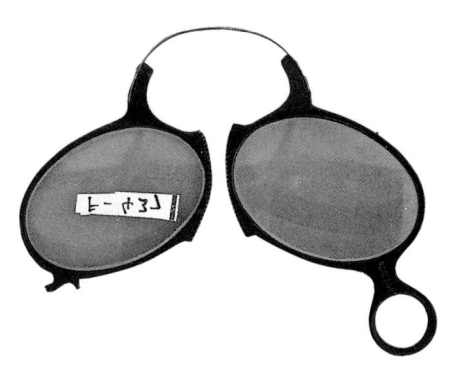

Figure 18. Hard rubber pince-nez frame.

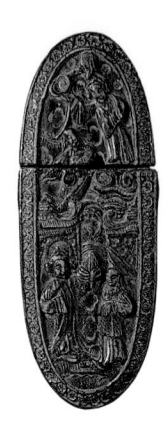

Figure 19. Chinese gutta percha spectacle case.

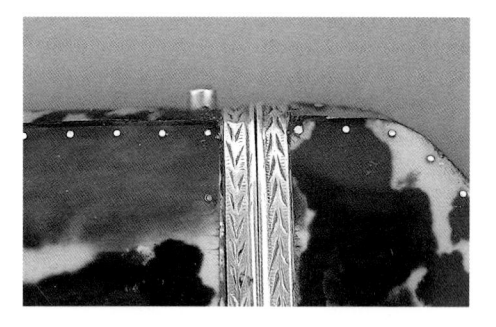

Figure 20. English tortoiseshell spectacle case with engraved silver banding.

Figure 21. Horn cover for English lens set.

Because of the latter danger, cellulose acetate (casein) became a substitute material around 1925. Although it does dissolve in acetone, it does not burn easily. Other plastics, such as perspex, optyl, and nylon, were not used for optical purposes until 1945. Therefore, these newer plastics will not be found as the base material for older spectacle frames and the like.

Hard Rubber   Though latex rubber has been collected for centuries from trees in Brazil, it did not reach England until 1774. It was altered in various ways and used for such things as erasers, automobile tires, raincoats, and tubing. When it is vulcanized with 25 percent to 50 percent sulfur, it becomes very hard and is known as vulcanite or ebonite (Figure 18). John J. Bauch first used it for spectacle frames in 1861 in Rochester, New York.

Gutta Percha   This natural material is a hard substance scraped from palaquium trees in Borneo, Sumatra, and Malaysia. It becomes a malleable paste when softened in hot water. It can be moulded and carved, and its hardness and resistance to chemicals and electricity, among other things, made it quite useful in many fields. Eyeglass cases were made from this material, including some Chinese cases (Figure 19).

Tortoiseshell   Tortoiseshell (Figure 20), actually the shell of the sea turtle (hawksbill), can be identified by using the same tests as those used for plastics. When tortoiseshell burns, it smells like singed hair. Unlike plastic, it has surface whorls. This rippling is due to the annual growth of the plates. The natural shell can be heated in water and softened, and the plates separated by thickness or flattened and cut to shape.

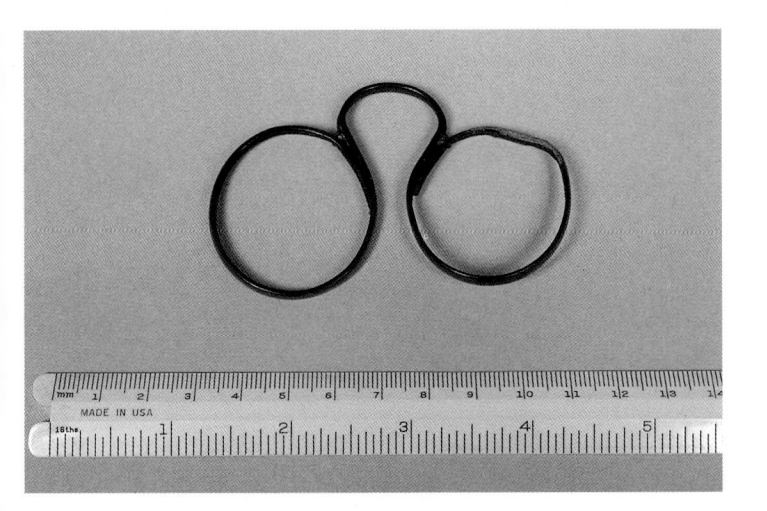

Figure 22. Baleen spectacles circa 1550.

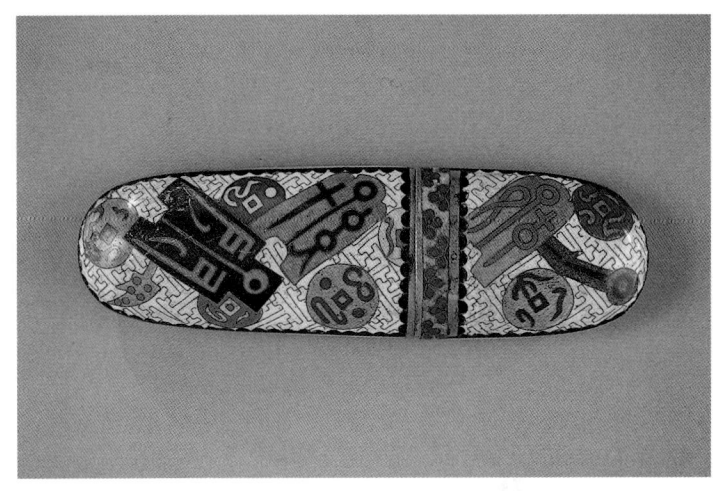

Figure 23. Cloisonne Chinese spectacle case.

Unlike horn or plastic, when sections of tortoiseshell are heated and pressed together, they will adhere. This is true even in old worked pieces and is useful in spectacle repair.[3]

Horn   This animal product, a keratinized protein, has been worked by man for centuries (Figure 21). The source in organized societies was usually cow, but ox and water buffalo were also used. Baleen (Figure 22), another hornlike substance, is from the jaw of the whale and is used to make many objects.

Originally horn was heated, split, and shaped. It can also be ground and compressed into molds. The Chinese used it as rims on folding spectacles. Eskimos used baleen for their slit-shaped snow goggles. Europeans also used baleen in a more sophisticated manner to fashion spectacle frames.

The following description of horn preparation is offered by Gary Kelley:[4]

> PREPARATION OF ANIMAL
> HORN FOR USE IN SPECTACLE FRAMES
> Unless a colonial hornsmith wanted to use horn in its natural shape—such as for a powder horn, a blowing horn or fog horn—he would first saw off both ends. After soaking the horn for several days he would boil, or roast, it until it was soft. Then he would slit it from end to end, open it out and flatten it between heated iron plates in a powerful screw-type press. He tempered the flattened pieces by plunging them, while still hot, in cold water. This way the horn held its shape after being removed from the press, or mold. The resulting wedge-shaped horn blanks were sold to other craftsmen for knife handles, combs, eyeglass frames and even lanterns.

Cloisonne   Cloisonne is a mode of decoration seldom seen in relation to eyeglasses, but the Chinese did use it in producing an occasional unusual eyeglass case (Figure 23). The desired design is produced by braising the edges of flat strips, usually brass, to a flat base. Then various colored and/or textured enamels are poured into the spaces, allowed to dry, and then polished. When done well, very fine detail can be accomplished.

Vermeil   Used before electroplating and chemical plating, vermeil is a process that places a thin layer of gold (gilding) on a silver or brass base (Figure 24). The base is then heated to burn off the mercury, leaving a very thin but well-attached layer of gold on the base. Unfortunately, it took a while for people to realize that the burned-off mercury was being inhaled by the workers. These workers lived only about three to five years in this business. Interesting to note is that the original formula to prepare the base consisted of a liquid composed of arnotto, gambage, dragon's blood, salt of tartar, and saffron—boiled in water.

Rolled Gold 1850–1900   Rolled gold is a film of gold joined to a backing of another metal by rolling. It was used to make spectacle frames.

Gold-Filled   Gold-filled objects are made of metals filled with a base metal over which a thick covering of gold is laid (Figure 25).

Gold-Plated   Gold-plated objects are metals coated with a thin layer of gold, generally using an electrical apparatus to attract the gold molecules.

Pinchbeck   Pinchbeck is an alloy of copper, zinc, and tin forming a cheap imitation of gold. It was produced by Christopher Pinchbeck (England, 1732).

Repousse   Repousse is the art of fashioning designs on metal sheets by hammering them from the back surface (Figure 26). Reverse molds were sometimes used. Some eyeglass cases were fashioned in this manner rather than using embossing.

Papier Mache   Papier mache is a method of fashioning objects and was patented in 1772 by Henry Clay in Birmingham, England. Cellulose pulp from ground paper or wood was mixed with animal glue or gum arabic, pressed into a mold, and heated in an oven until dry. After being removed from the mold, the object was finished by discarding the excess, sanding, polishing, and decorating. Embellishment could be made by painting, transfer (decal), or inlay (mother-of-pearl or other shells) (Figure 27). A final process of lacquering or japanning finished the job.

An alternate technique consisted of shaping layers of wet paper pulp over a mold. The pulp was then dried and

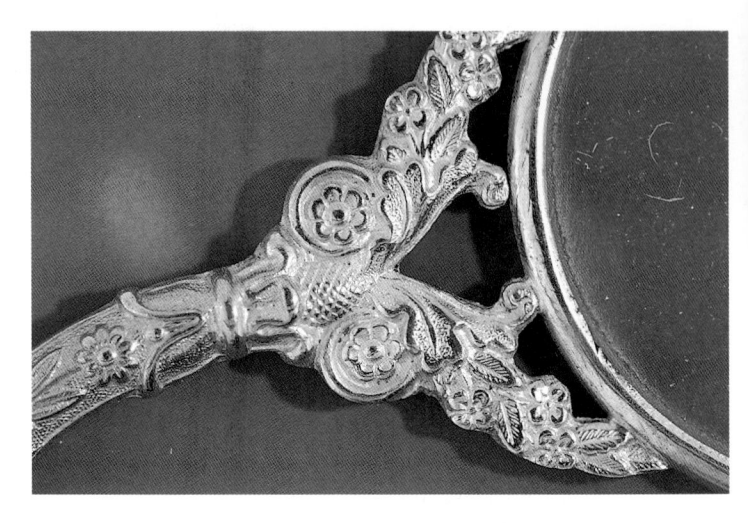

Figure 24. Vermeil French scissors glasses.

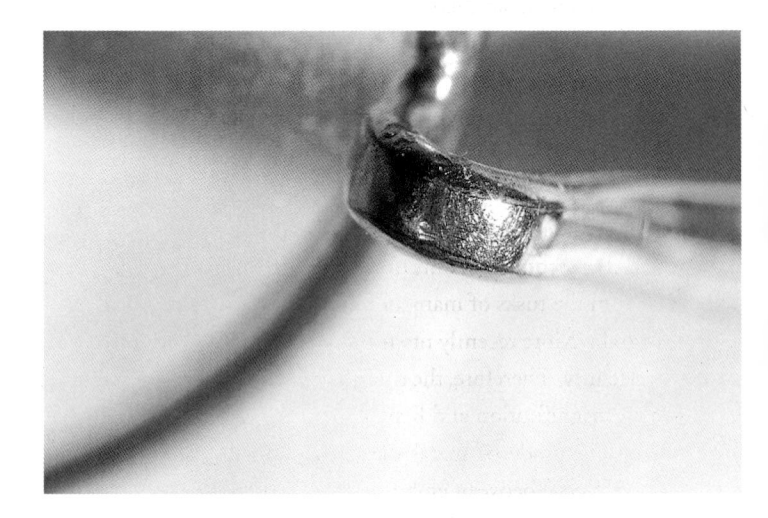

Figure 25. Spectacle bridge showing wear on gold filling.

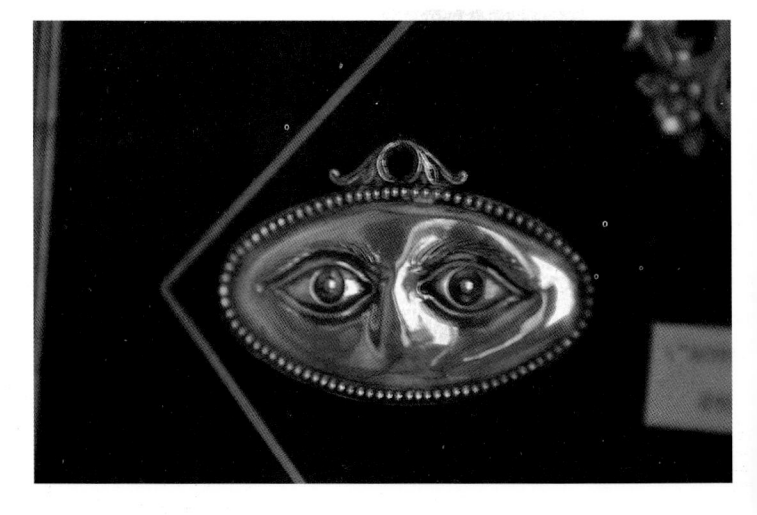

Figure 26. Repousse ex-voto.

decorated. Sometimes silver wire inlay was used. Many spectacle cases have been made of papier mache.

Detailed Examination of Objects with Adequate Light and Magnification

The examination of objects with adequate light and magnification allows identification otherwise not possible. An example of this, of course, would be the magnified examination of a faceted gemstone. With such an examination, we can determine the stone's gross dimensions and proportion, the quality and age of the faceting, and whether or not the stone is broken. We can also determine whether or not the stone contains any flaws and whether these flaws are of sufficient amount to decrease the value of the stone. This, of course, applies to all artifacts.

When confronted with an object possibly containing a crack, exposed edge, or missing piece, one should examine the area with a magnifying glass. Evidence of repairs may not be visible to the naked eye. Porcelains should be examined with an ultraviolet light to check for repairs, and the edges of bowls should be tapped with a fingernail to help locate cracks.

Ivory comes not only from the elephant (Figure 28) but also from the tusks of many other animals. Each has a particular grain. More recently made pieces of ivory may be difficult to identify. Therefore, the true grain is best revealed with the use of magnification and light.

The grade of metal pieces is partly determined by the difference between embossing (Figure 29) and engraving. In

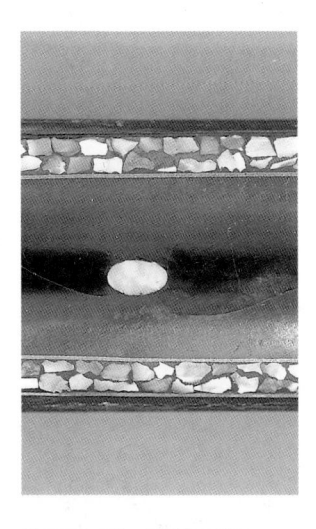

Figure 27. English papier mache spectacle case inlaid with mother-of-pearl.

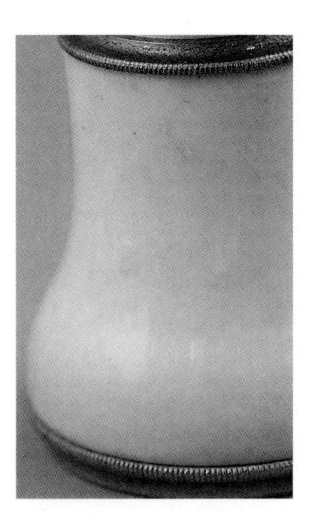

Figure 28. Ivory barrel on English monocular.

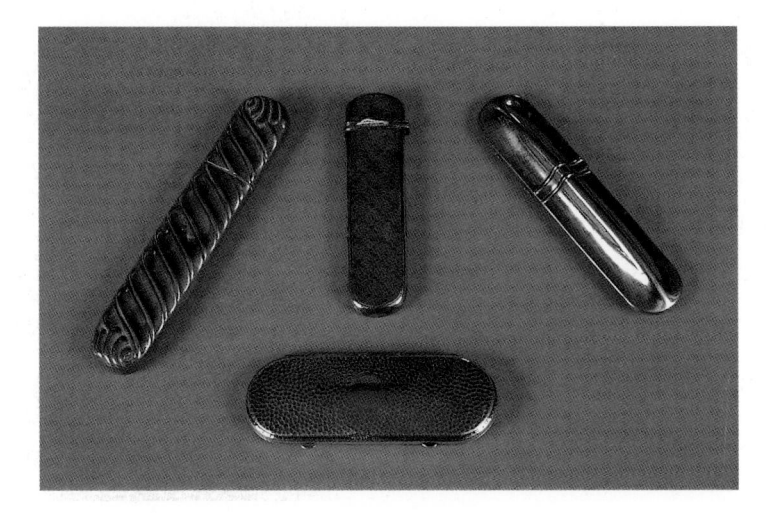

Figure 29. Case on left is embossed, case in center is engraved, case on right is pressed, case on bottom is hammered.

EXAMINATION OF ARTIFACTS

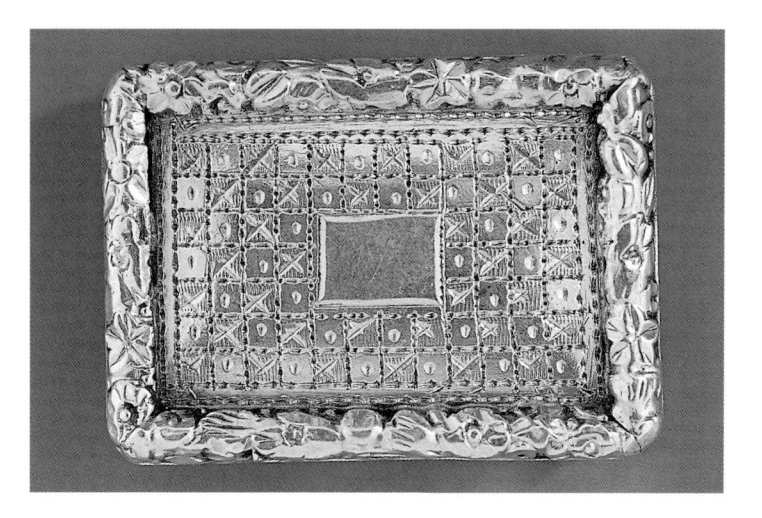

Figure 30. Engraved English vinaigrette.

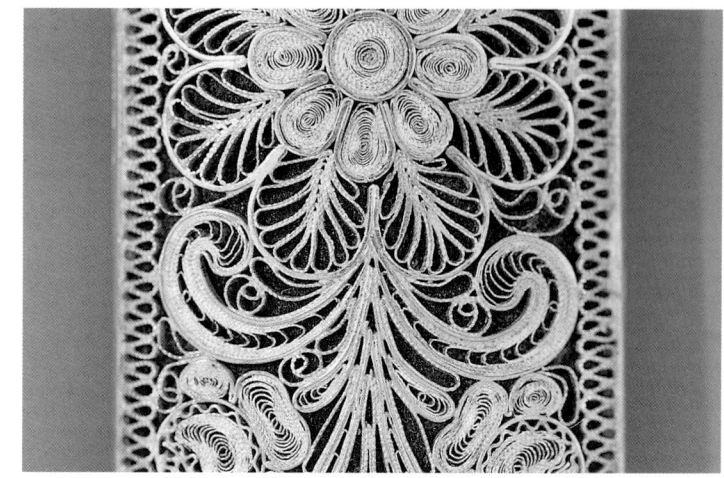

Figure 31. Silver filigree.

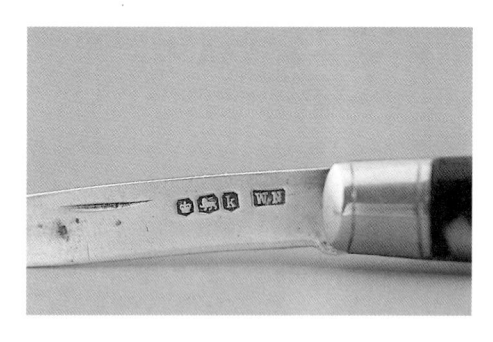

Figure 32. English hallmarks on silver knife blade.

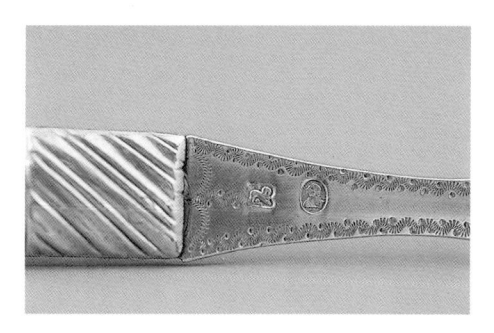

Figure 33. Head of King George and *lion passant* on English silver fork.

the former case, a piece of metal or other materials are simply impressed with a design through pressure of a machine. Engraving (Figure 30), however, is done by hand, with tools that cut into the metal or other material. This method produces a much finer piece and can be identified through magnification.

Silver filigree (Figure 31) is made only in certain parts of the world, particularly in the Philippines. Thus, it can be identified. Simple detection of iron or steel can be accomplished by the use of a small magnet.

Useful information is that of the touchmarks of the French against the hallmarks of the English and the mark of sterling on American objects. German and Russian hallmarks are different, and essential to know is the amount of silver and gold usually used in metal objects from these countries. For instance, American fine silver is .999 but usually is .925 (sterling). German is usually .820, and Russian is .810. English is .951, and French is .905. The French have unorganized marks—each principality being different.

If the head of Queen Victoria is present on English silver, the piece was made between 1837 and 1901, the years of her reign. An anchor tells us that it was made in Birmingham, England. A crown represents Sheffield, while a head with a crown or *lion passant* is from London (Figure 32). Additionally, a head of a male is usually that of King George (Figure 33). George I (1714–1727) faces left, and George II (1727–1760) faces

14   CHAPTER 2

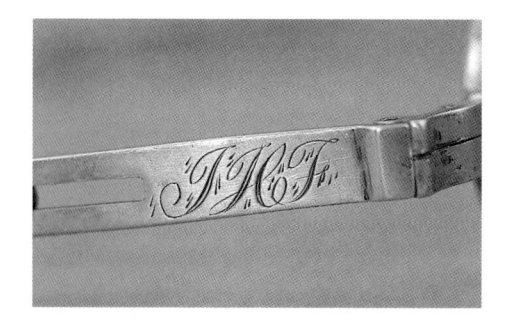

Figure 34. Personal monogram on English silver spectacle temple.

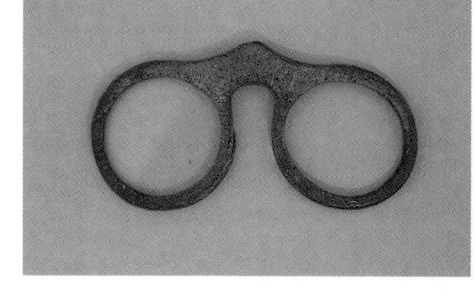

Figure 35. English leather eyeglass frames circa 1500.

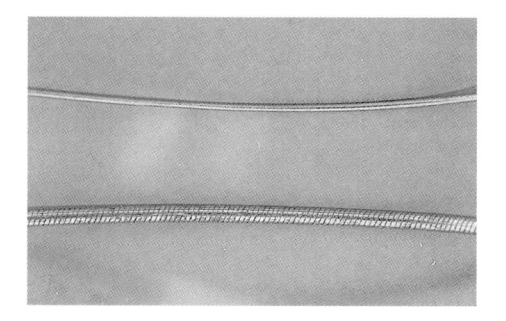

Figure 36. American temples showing wire and cable temples.

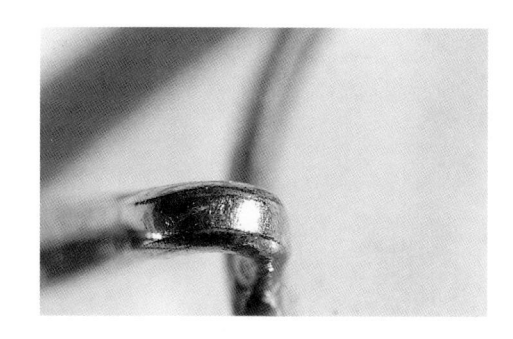

Figure 37. Gold plating worn off spectacle bridge.

right. William IV (1830–1837) preceded Queen Victoria. These figures are revealed through magnification, and books carrying these listings are available.

Regarding spectacles, one must be aware of where and how to look. Most eyeglasses are identified on the bridge or temple. The country and, many times, the date can be found in these areas. The manufacturer, type of material, hallmark, etc. can be found there as well. A personal monogram (Figure 34) or focal mark, however, can be misleading.

Detailed examination of spectacles often aids in determining the date and condition of the piece. In one instance, tears in the surface of a pair of spectacle frames were found through magnification. This revealed that the frame was made of leather and dated approximately 1500 (Figure 35). Magnification also aids in establishing whether the temple of a glass frame is wire or one with a wire core wrapped with other flat wire (cable temple). The conclusion will help date the pair of spectacles: Wire temples were generally used between 1875 and 1900 roughly, whereas cable temples came after 1900 (Figure 36). Because cable temples worked better, they were then used almost exclusively.

Many pieces are sold as solid gold. However, the use of magnification aids in examining worn areas of metal objects. For instance, areas of spectacles near the nose piece and the end of the ear piece become worn. Proper light and magnification reveal where the gold layer has worn off, thereby exposing the base metal (Figure 37). Therefore, this piece is not solid gold but gold-plated or gold-filled.

Magnifying a lens surface reveals whether the lens was perfectly ground or carries imperfections found in hand grinding. In this manner, the author was able to identify old lenses by their edging. This can also be accomplished with the use of reflected light. Using light from another source to reflect on the surface of the lens will reveal whether or not there is perfection in the curve. The lensometer determines whether or not there is perfection in the dioptric power by examining the lens at its various parts. One might take the trouble to use a small flashlight and look inside of eyeglass cases or under linings. The author recently acquired a quizzing glass and attributed it to a German origin after finding German script inside its case.

Conclusion

Provided here is a sample of helpful hints to aid the collector. The most important aid in purchasing an antique is *information*. Knowledge on the history of the artifact, the material of which it was made, and the condition of the artifact is essential in assuring a good buy.

Notes

1. Seymour Wyler, *Old Silver* (New York: Crown Publishers, 1937).
2. Sylvia Katz, *Early Plastics* (Aylesbury, Bucks U.K: Shire Publishers, Ltd. Cromwell House, 1986).
3. R. J. S. MacGregor, *Restoring Ophthalmic Antiques*.
4. Gary Kelly, "Hornucopia," *Blade* August 1993, 12.

3

A Short History of Glass and Some of Its Applications

In attempting to raise the ubiquitous mist of antiquity from the Eastern shores of the Mediterranean about 4500 years ago, we find that Pliny records a tradition of the discovery of glass in Syria. A group of Phoenicians, we are told, cooked their meals in pots resting on blocks of natron. The sand under these blocks had turned to glass when the pots were cooled and removed. Natron, being an impure form of sodium carbonate, probably melted and combined with the sand to form a silicate of soda. This, though not a permanent glass, is enough like it to suggest the possibility of creating a permanent transparent substance. Pliny further describes the production of a permanent glass: It was obtained by adding magnesium limestone to the mixture of sand and sodium carbonate, which then fused and produced a true glass. Supposedly, this occurred on the river Belus, close to Mount Carmel, where all of these raw materials could be found. Lumps of glass are still being dug up in this general location.

Some historians, however, think that Pliny was mistaken, as it is impossible to make glass in the open air. Other technicians state that the high temperature necessary would not be produced by the heat under cooking pots.

Egypt

Although Egypt was well supplied with raw materials for the making of glass and had experience with vitreous glazing and the use of various colors, no trace of glass has been discovered there in its primitive form. Glass beads that date sometime after the Sixth Dynasty (after 2500 B.C.) have been found in Egypt. A green glass rod that possibly dated 2600 B.C. was found at Eshnuna in Babylonia. Also, a small piece of blue glass was found at Eridu, dating before 2200 B.C.[1]

In a tomb of a pharaoh of Thebes is a wall painting depicting men blowing glass using much the same tools as are used today. Thutmose II, who reigned about 1500 B.C., had a piece of glass placed in his tomb. Old Egyptian mosaic glass beads contained designs found hundreds of years later in the canes of old glass paperweights. From that time forward, glass objects were found in the palace sites of Thebes and many other Egyptian rulers. Possibly, some of the glass objects found in Egypt were the production of captive Syrian glassblowers who were carried to Egypt after wars of conquest.

Middle East

Little is known of the glass made during the period immediately after 1000 B.C.. in Mesopotamia. However, Nineveh tablets and the remains of glass in various forms excavated by M.E.L. Mallowan at Nimrud were practically certain proof that glassmaking was carried on there from the eighth to the sixth centuries B.C.

Greece

Glass was made in Greece in Mycenaean times, usually in the form of small molded architectural details. From the sixth century B.C., however, glass began to appear in great quantities, particularly on the Greek inhabited isles of the Aegean and of Greece itself. The same is true for Italy, Sicily, and even farther west. This profusion of specimens contrasts with the paucity of findings of glass on Egyptian soil.

Ceylon

In pre–sixth-century B.C., there is a record of "mirrors of glittering glass" being carried in a procession in India. Ceylon is thought to be the source of this glass.

The Roman Empire

Alexandria seems to have come to the fore of glassmaking in the crucial period around the first century B.C., which saw the beginnings of glass as it is known today. The use of sand core techniques in the manipulation of colored glass rods to make composite canes is the same as that used in later times (mid-1800s) in the French Bacharac, Clichy, and St. Louis factories. It is also the same as in the modern Scottish glass factories in Perthshire today that produce paperweights.

A mold-pressing process was developed and was a most important antecedent to the innovation of glass manufacture called blowing. A lump of glass on the end of a hollow tube was found to be as easily blown into a mold as it was to be poured. Never before the Roman era was glass so widely used in the production of luxury vessels.

Glass was also used in thin plates to coat walls, pave, and decorate as well as to make windows, tableware, urns, jugs, etc.

The Romans produced opaque and transparent colored glass. The latter came in the following colors; blue, green, purple, amber, brown, and rose. Opaque glass colors made were white, black, yellow, green, orange, blue, and red.

There is some question as to whether the Syrians were the actual originators of glassblowing, as their type of glass was especially apt for this purpose. Again, the Romans may have captured Syrians and brought them back to ply their trade at the Roman centers.

China

In 140 B.C., the annals of the Hun Dynasty of China recorded the establishment of a glass plant under the direction of Wu-Ti. The plant made an opaque substance called *lieou-li*, which was made into small beads and rods for various uses. There is no record to determine whether this was an original discovery or whether it was knowledge spread from other areas.

As early as the third century A.D., glass objects were brought to China from the West. However, there have been finds of small glass objects of typical Chinese shape dating from the Hun Dynasty. This suggests that even if the materials were brought from the West, they could have been worked on the spot to conform to Chinese usage. These were probably regarded as cheap substitutes for jade. The Chinese themselves do not claim to have made glass before the fifth century A.D. Even then, it is doubtful whether they knew more than how to make beads and other small objects. Vessels of glass occasionally found in burials of the Tang Dynasty (A.D. 618–906) may be assumed to have been imported. In making porcelain, however, the Chinese ground petuntze (a form of feldspar) with kaolin to create a base. During the years 1723–1796, the emphasis on blown glass forms of China was subordinate to the desire to make glass a substitute for natural stones. The glass is often found to have been fashioned as though cut from stone in a lapidary type of treatment. We frequently find soda glass seals crimped on the ribbons of Chinese eyeglass cases from the mid-1700s (Figure 38).

Optical glass was used in China at that time (Figure 39), but as we know, the crystal stone (a quartz) called *ai tai* (Figure 40) was used for making spectacles in the earliest times in China. It was mined from the caves of Mongolia and was found in clear to dark colors. It was not until the Chien Lung period (about 1736) that glass was used for optical purposes.

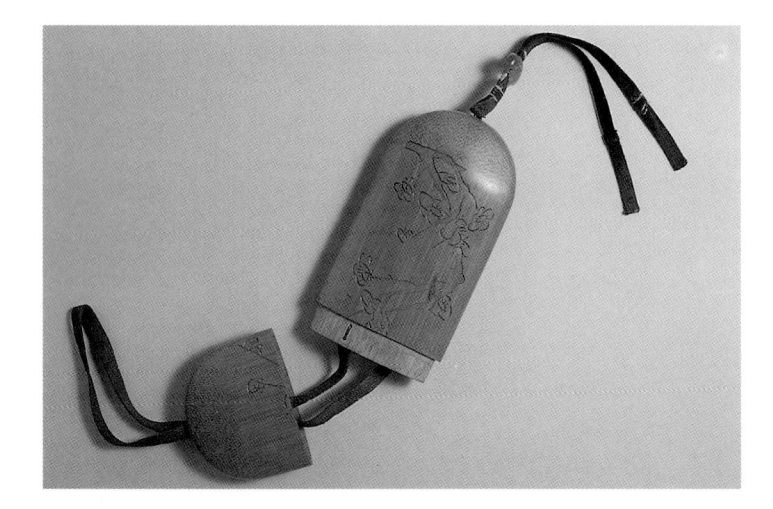

Figure 38. Chinese eyeglass case circa 1750.

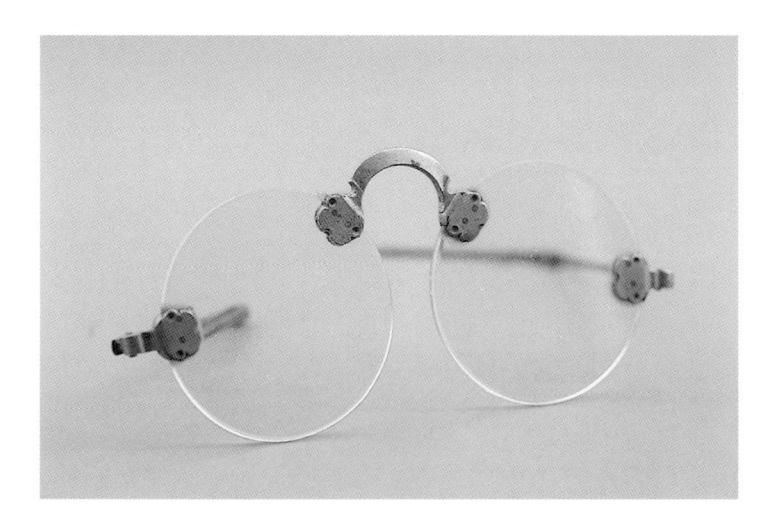

Figure 39. Chinese spectacles with glass lenses.

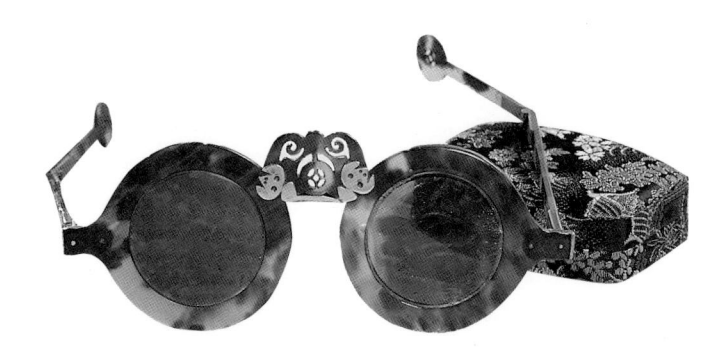

Figure 40. Chinese spectacles with tea-stone lenses.

HISTORY OF GLASS 19

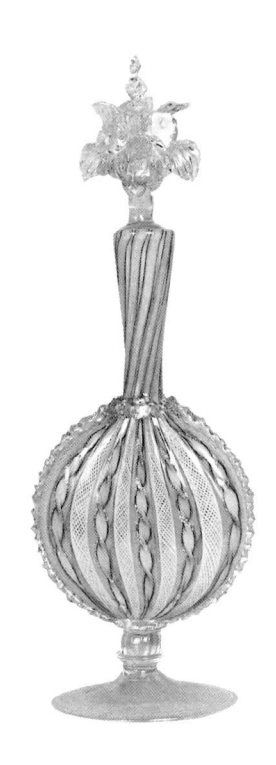

Figure 41. Venetian glass perfume bottle.

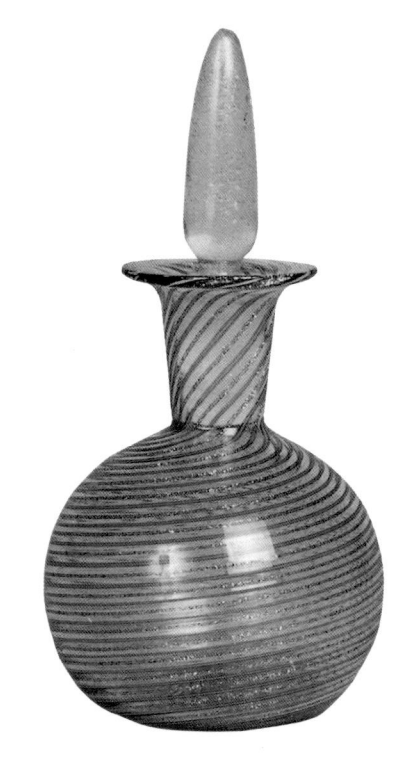

Figure 42. Glass flask made in Murano circa 1983.

Venetian Glass

Glassmaking in Venice started around the fifth century A.D. (Figure 41). By the twelfth century, glass factories were so numerous in Venice that they were considered to be fire hazards. That may be one reason for moving them to the Island of Murano (Figure 42). Commercial intentions may have been another. Venetian glass was so sought after that the rulers of the country confined the skilled workers to the island. The workers were given nobility status as well as excellent living and working conditions. Unfortunately, they were still held as captives so that their secrets could not be revealed.

Eventually, the glassmakers guild at Altare hired out workers to Bohemia, France, England, and finally the United States. Caspar Lehmann, a Bohemian glassworker, invented the process of engraving on glass. He used a rotating copper disc saw which, of course, was rather soft. This tool resulted in slightly wavy cuts, which are one way to distinguish the old glass engraving from the new.

Diamond cutting of glass was used in the sixteenth century. The author found two optical lens edgers from that period in the French Alps, and both used diamonds for their edge cutting ability. One of these edgers is in the Smithsonian Institution's collection, and the other belongs to the American Academy of Ophthalmology Foundation Museum.

England

The first glass in England was made during the Roman occupation. The remains of a Roman glass plant of considerable size have been discovered near the Manchester ship canal at Warrington. This glassmaking declined with the fall of the Roman Empire. It wasn't until the thirteenth century that glass making was revived—first in France and then in England. There are records of deeds granted to three different glass producers in the parish of Chiddingfold, Surrey, England.

It was not until the sixteenth century that glass was produced in any quantity in England, France, or Germany. The soda glass being used at that time in Europe was cloudy and contained many bubbles. Lead glass (or flint glass) was discovered by Ravenscroft in England in 1560.[2] The clarity of this glass was identical to the mined crystals used previously for optical purposes. This new glass was called crystalline (like crystal). Today, of course, we term this clear glass *crystal*. James Aycough refers to this glass in his monograph of 1754.

The Americas

It is of interest to note that as early as 1535, glass was being made at Puebla de los Angeles in Mexico. In 1592, a glass house was located in the territory of Rio de la Plata in the town of Cordova del Tucuman, Argentina.

The United States

Although it seems unlikely, it has been written that the London Company of Virginia set up a glass house in Jamestown in 1608 for the manufacture of "glasses and beads." Although this colony starved to death during the winter of 1608 (probably as a result of poor business), the company tried to establish a glass house in 1621. This, too, failed. For more than a century after Jamestown, there was little American glass to speak of. The American colonists' early successful glass house was started in 1739 by Casper Wistar. He made only utilitarian vessels and window panes. Henry W. Stiegel established a glass house in 1763 at Manheim, Pennsylvania.

Although several other glassworks were founded, few survived the Revolution. It was not until about 1830 that American glass houses produced fine lead glass and used the full-size, incised mold. Finally, also, came the pressing machine.

The Bausch and Lomb Optical Company started making fine optical glass in 1915. This was a happy event for the United States, since during World War I, its supply of glass from European centers was cut off. Bausch and Lomb produced most of the United States' glass during those war years. (Details of this company's undertakings are covered in Chapter 6.)

Later Products

We should acknowledge the fact that fine glass was made after 1850 in Great Britain, the United States, Czechoslovakia, Austria, Germany, France, and the Scandinavian countries. Belgium and the Netherlands produced the Val St. Lambert types. Italy delivered the Venetian and Murano products. Even Spain and Argentina contributed from works in the Balearic Islands.

Optical Glass

Optical glass became a commercial necessity after the invention of spectacles in 1280 and the printing press around 1500. The achromatic telescope objective by Galileo in 1609 also spurred on this activity, as the ordinary soda glass of this period was so lacking in homogeneity that it was almost useless for optical purposes. The terms *flint* and *crown* as applied to optical glass, were the first to be needed and used. The term *crown* applies to the thick glass used for window panes. Flint is glass with increased lead content, as invented by Ravenscroft to make the glass clearer. Plate glass was first rolled in 1688 at St. Gobain in France, but it was not until 1807 that P. L. Guinaud & Son operated the first successful optical glass factory. This glass was developed by Fraunhofer, although Dollond used flint and crown glass to make achromatic lenses in 1757.[3]

It is interesting to note that by the end of the eighteenth century, Guinaud, a Swiss, attempted to overcome the lack of homogeneity in glass by stirring the molten glass with a cylinder of fire clay. Later, he went to Bavaria and Munich and continued his experiments in conjunction with Ulz Schneider. He also did investigations with Fraunhofer, who was his pupil. He was the originator of the specification of refraction and dispersion of glass in terms of a certain line of the spectrum, designated now as the "Fraunhofer Lines." Guinaud's process was further developed in France.

In England in 1824 the Royal Astronomical Society of London appointed a committee, including Farriday, to do experimental work. The committee produced several new kinds of glass for optical use. In 1848, Bontemps went to England and instituted the manufacture of optical glass at the Champs Glass Works near Birmingham. In France, zinc crown glass of optical quality was produced in 1851, and Lamy produced a dense thallium glass in 1867. Boric acid use in glass manufacture was investigated by Stokes.

The most distinctive advance in optical glass manufacture was in Jena, Germany, in 1876, with the interest and collaboration of Dr. Schott, who founded the Institute of Schott and Genossen. The Institute produced newer glasses that contained a much wider variety of chemical substances than the older crown and flint glass. Most important of these additions were the oxides of barium, magnesium, aluminum, and zinc.

One problem was to produce glass that was comparably free from color and numerous bubbles. Another was the tarnishing of the surfaces of crown lenses. We attribute the optical industry of the present and the advanced state of optical lenses and instruments to the excellent research done at the Schott and Genossen Institute glass plant.

Pebble

Pebble, a naturally occurring stone in Brazil, was used in the eighteenth and nineteenth century to make optical lenses in Europe and the United States. Although the mineral is as clear as flint glass, not all specimens were suitable for lenses. Great care was taken to weed out the smoky pieces and those full of imperfections. The brown color in some however, could be removed by gradual heating, as in the sun.

The following comments on pebble are quoted from J. T. Hudson, Chapter III:

> When the very best is selected, suitable for spectacles, an operation requiring the greatest care, and occupying a considerable portion of time; it is slit or cut by the lapidary into little pieces or slabs, about the size of a spectacle lens.
>
> This slitting of pebble can only be accomplished by the aid of diamond dust, the pebble being so hard that nothing else will cut it as well. A small, soft iron, circular saw, is used, about seven inches in diameter, which is fixed horizontally in a lathe, and then rubbed or charged with the diamond dust, and lubricated with Oil of Brique.
>
> The diamond dust used is the small pieces broken off the larger diamonds, and pulverized in a hardened steel mortar, made to fit the pestle exactly, which is about four inches long, of cylindrical shape, and half an inch in diameter.
>
> The slabs thus cut off are then given to the optical lens-grinder, who grinds them, twelve or fourteen pieces together, in a brass or iron tool of the required convexity or concavity, with emery of several degrees of fineness, diluted with water.
>
> This is a work of great labour and skill, especially when they are polished, which is done on a similar tool of the same curve, covered with a coarse woolen cloth, water and putty powder (a polishing material well known) being all that is used in this operation.
>
> The lenses are now ready to fit into the spectacle frames, which is done by shivering or breaking the edges with a small pair of nippers or plyers to the shape of the frame, and then grinding them on the edges with a small Bilston grindstone, till they fit into the eye of the frame exactly; care being taken that all roughness be ground off the edges, or it will be seen in the frames, when they are finished. That all this is very fatiguing and laborious, I need not remind the reader, and the use of diamond dust, renders the operation one of great expense.
>
> Pebbles have one advantage, when compared with glass lenses; they are much harder, and will cut glass so deep as to resemble the cut of a diamond, nor do they so easily scratch by continual wear of wiping, as glasses.
>
> For this reason they are useful in spectacles that are likely to be used roughly, or without a case; as the dust or grit gives glasses, after a short wear, the appearance of being rough ground on the surfaces, or semi-transparent, especially towards the centers of those that are very convex. Pebbles may be ground thinner than glasses, and are not so liable to break with a slight blow or accident.
>
> In other respects, I believe, the best glasses answer the purposes of vision as well, or even better than pebbles. Some persons consider that pebbles are colder to the eyes than glasses: they are certainly colder, because they are denser in their natural state; but I believe they imbibe the heat from the body, just the same as glass, only that they retain it for a longer period; they cannot, therefore, have any advantage in this respect.
>
> Pebble grows in layers, or laminae, which are linear: therefore, when the edges of these layers appear on the surface, as in the case of a convex pebble lens; consequently they do not possess the even surface requisite for transmitting equally the different rays of light, which a well-fused glass lens will do much better.
>
> Their density, and consequent refractive power, is unequal; hence pebbles cannot be used in the object-glasses of telescopes or opera-glasses . . . where correctness is required.[4]

Conclusion

The history of glass, its development and its use in commercial and particularly optical products is fascinating. The results of glassmaking are extremely beautiful as well as practical. Collections of all types of glass products are historically significant. This is expressed in no greater form than modern imitations of old glass products, including goblets, vessels, and even several supposed ancient Chinese spectacles, made with 1992 plastic lenses.

Notes

1. Theo E. Obrig, *Modern Ophthalmic Lenses and Optical Glass* (New York: The Chilton Co., 1935), 1–11.
2. Henry Stern, , personal communication, 1990.
3. J. T. Hudson, "On the Best Materials for Spectacle Lenses," in *Useful Remarks upon Spectacles, Lenses, and Opera-Glasses; with Hints to Spectacle Wearers and Others. . .* (London: Joseph Thomas, Finch-Lane, Cornhill, 1840), 16–17.
4. Ibid, Chapter III.

4

The Development of Optical Quality Lenses

Amazingly, amidst all of today's modern technology, we actually are now and have all along been using methods of lens grinding developed hundreds of years ago. The progressive changes in methodology are represented solely by the use of new plastics, molds, and fully automated assembly lines. For the ophthalmologist who may have pondered on the evolution of lenses, a brief history is presented here. For those who desire to delve further into the intricacies of this subject, numerous references are noted.

Lenses in Antiquity

Optical quality lenses have been discovered in caves of Crete dating from the Miocene period.[1]

As early as 2283 B.C., a Chinese emperor was supposed to have used lenses made of rock crystal (teastone or quartz) or topaz to observe the stars.[2]

Sir Arthur Evans found lenses in the Palace of Knossos and in the nearby Mavro Spelio Cemetery. These date from 1400 B.C. Other (undated) rock crystal lenses have been found in Anatolia, Cyprus, Ephesos (Temple of Artemis), Troy, and other places in the Middle East.

A report by Caius Plinius (Pliny A.D. 23–79) noted that Nero viewed the fights of the gladiators using an emerald. Perhaps the jewel was used as a sun shade or a mirror (to protect against attacks from the rear).

Following is a series of quotes by professors, scientists, and others who have studied the literature available to them regarding the history of lenses. An insight into the history of spectacles is presented in *Katalog Einer Bilderausstellung Zur Geschichte Der Brille*, by Professor Dr. Greeff:

> It may be looked upon as certain that the ancient Egyptians, Jews, Greeks, and Romans did not know any kind of optic glasses, either in the form of spectacles or magnifying-glasses, or as telescopes. In the rich literature on medicine and natural science of those days we do not find anything about them. The Romans were only acquainted with the magnifying action of a glass sphere filled with water but did not ascribe the magnification to the curved planes but to the water. (Seneca Jr. 4 B.C. –A.D. 65). On the other hand Roman authors (Cicero, Cornelius Nepos, Suetonius), already wrote about the fact that in old age the eyesight became weak, and that all the remedies of the doctors were no good against this, so that there was nothing left for it but to have oneself read to by a slave. If there had been pocket-lenses or spectacle-glasses at the time these famous Roman authors would certainly have known about them and have procured them.
>
> In classical places (e.g. in Nineveh, Tyre, Troy, Crete and Egypt) lens-shaped, transparent bodies have been excavated many a time which were rashly looked upon as the oldest

magnifying-lenses. They are made of glass or rock-crystal, are ground convex on one side and level on the other. Grinding is a very old art indeed. These objects never served optical purposes, however, but were just show-pieces, badges, ornaments on girdles, or were used as buttons on clothes. Sometimes traces of a mounting are found on the back.[3]

Theo. E. Obrig provides us with the following:

Before going into the subject of ophthalmic lenses, it will be of interest to trace the steps which have led to their development. The first lenses produced were no doubt burning glasses and the first recorded description of them was given in 424 B.C. by Aristophanes, who mentions in his "Comedy of the Clouds," Act 2, saying "That fine transparent stone with which fires are kindled, by which placing myself in the sun, I will, though at a distance, melt all the writing on the summons," referring to the waxen tablets used at that time for writing.

The ancient Greeks and Romans are not known to have produced lenses of long focus. Those lenses contained in the collections of European museums are all convex lenses of short focus made of glass or of rock crystal.

There was found in a grave in Nola, a plano convex piece of glass about 45 millimeters in diameter mounted in gold; in Mayence, one of 55 millimeters in diameter; a similar one in Pompeii; a double convex lens in England. The oldest lens existent is plano convex, ground from rock crystal, slightly oval in shape, about 35 × 45 millimeters, and about 5 millimeters thick, with a refractive power of + 10.D. The fact that lenses have been so seldom found and that one was mounted in gold, leads to the assumption that they were rare possessions of wealthy and prominent people.[4]

(Note the early method of lens grinding in Figure 43.)

Similarly, in writings by George Sines and Yannis A. Sakellarakis, the following is noted:

A recent find in the Idaean Cave in Crete of two rock crystal lenses of unusually good optical quality led to an investigation of other lenses from antiquity. The evidence indicates that the use of lenses was widespread throughout the Middle

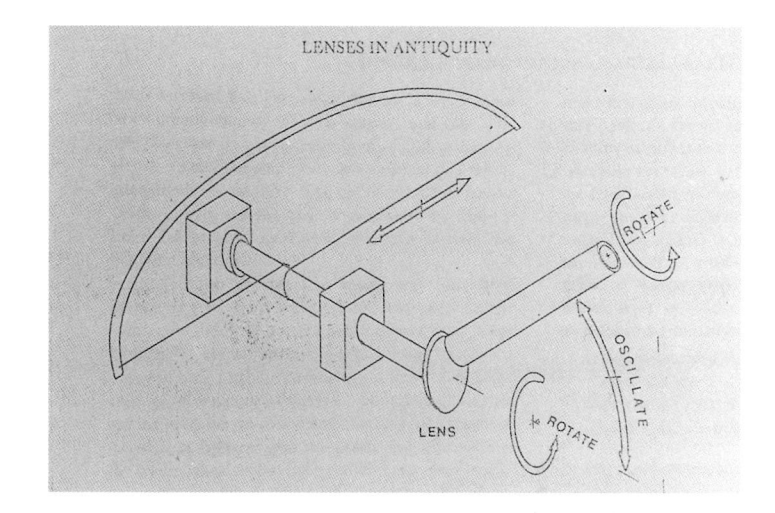

Figure 43. Primitive method of lens grinding.

East and the Mediterranean basin over several millennia. The quality of some of these lenses was sufficient to permit their use as magnifying glasses. The use of lenses as burning glasses in Classical Greece is noted, as is the need for magnifying lenses to authenticate seal impressions. The probability that magnifying lenses were used by gem carvers and seal engravers is discussed. The fine detail of Roman gold-glass portrait medallions and the discovery of a lens in the house of an engraver in Pompeii and another in the house of an artist in Tanis are presented as evidence for the use of the lenses for magnifying purposes. Methods of producing optical quality lenses by simple procedures are also presented.[5]

Figure 44 illustrates some early grinding and drilling tools.

Otto Durham Rasmussen wrote the following in his *Chinese Eyesight and Spectacles*:

> Historically considered, available data leaves little doubt that spectacles, holding plain, colored crystals, were used for sunglare and as a remedial agent in the time of Confucius (551–479 B.C.), but there is no evidence that they were used for old sight, or presbyopia, earlier than the thirteenth century A.D., and no evidence as yet, except the overwhelming testimony of abuse of sight and its manifestations, when they constructed a concave lens for short-sightedness. The first authentic reference to the use of reading spectacles is attributed to Marco Polo, whose 17-year sojourn in China was at the court of Kublai Khan, of the Mongol dynasty (1260–1368 A.D.). He reported that old people used lenses with which to read fine print. Nothing more. He did not say what sort of lenses they were, or even if they were in spectacle form, but from the term "fine" we can assume they were for purposes of magnification. Concave lenses could have existed without his knowledge, because he lived at the court and etiquette would have forbidden their "obvious" use. The same etiquette would have kept them out of sight as his important cortege traveled back and forth from Peking. But that is purely an inference.
>
> The next reference appears in texts of the Ming dynasty (1368–1644 A.D.) when it was mentioned that a Chinese gentleman gave a fine white horse for a pair of spectacles.
>
> There are no references in literature to the manufacture of lenses, cutting of tortoiseshell, or the grinding of quartz crystal.[6]

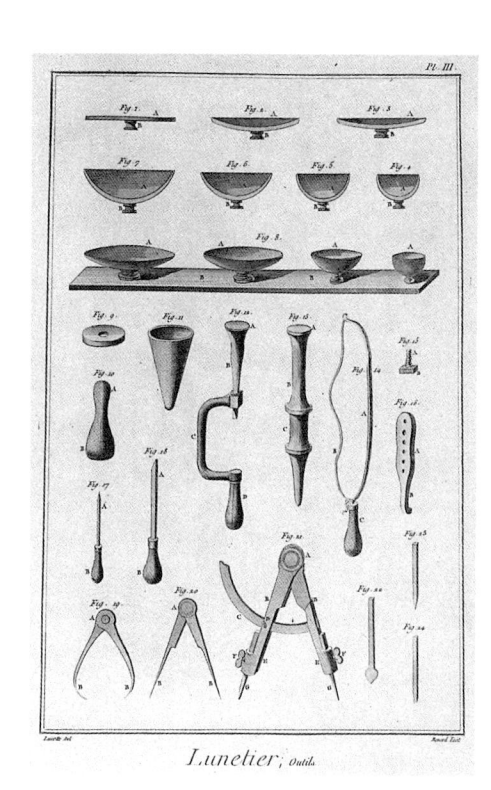

Figure 44. Grinding and drilling tools.

Julius Hirschberg provides an enlightening view in his second volume of *The History of Ophthalmology*. This volume addresses the sixteenth and seventeenth centuries and was translated by Frederick C. Blodi, M.D., Professor of Ophthalmology, University of Iowa.

> 1. First of all I would like to re-emphasize that the Old Greeks and Romans did not know anything about ground lenses of glass or transparent stone which could be used to improve visual acuity for near or for the distance. They knew, however, about the magnifying power of a sphere (103). They knew about presbyopia, asthenopia (atonia) and

myopia (compare preceding volume), but they knew nothing about spectacle lenses. They prescribed for these conditions ointments which should strengthen the eyes. They prescribed these also to workers who needed fine, detailed vision. To assume that these people used magnifying lenses is an error.

2. We find in the complete and well preserved Arabian textbook of ophthalmology by Ali B. Isa not the slightest hint of any convex or concave lenses. This book was written after an exhaustive study of all the old, i.e. Greek, authors. A patient who sees well at distance but not at near (an affection which usually occurs in old patients) should keep a healthy lifestyle and should put styptic medication into his eye. A patient who sees well at near but not at distance should take liquid food and should sometimes use a salving medication into his eye. (Remarkable is also that the Old Testament mentions mirrors, cutting of precious stones and the preparation of glass, but nowhere does it mention spectacles. The same is true for the Talmud though it also mentions artificial teeth.)

I also asked the greatest authority in this area Professor Fr. Hirth, now at the Columbia University in New York, who wrote me on June 26, 1906 the following: "The Chinese ground, already centuries before Christ, possibly even during the 12th century B.C., concave mirrors of bronze (to make fire) and convex mirrors (for rituals and make-ups). It is, however, unproved that they made lenses of glass or crystal before the Europeans invented them.[7]

We must temper the preceding quotes by noting that all existing literature was destroyed by edict in China in the second century B.C.

Evidence of Scientific Work on Lenses

Just before the first century A.D., the Phoenicians learned the art of glassmaking.[8] They discovered that nitre mixed with sand had melted into a coarse glass by the heat of the sun. The oldest known lens made of rock crystal was found in the ruins of Nineveh (Iraq). It is 1 ½ inches in diameter, with a 4 ½-inch focal length. As it could not possibly be used before the eyes, it was probably used as a burning glass to erase writing on wax, as a burning parchment, or for cauterizing wounds (Pliny).

Seneca from Cordoba in A.D. 3 noted that objects appeared larger and clearer when viewed through a glass full of water. He did not further develop that observation. Lucius Annaeus Seneca (The Younger) 4 B.C.–A.D. 65, noted, "Thin, muddled writing looks larger and clearer through a bag full of water."[9]

Claudius Ptolemy, a second-century astronomer, was familiar with the principle of magnification, but lenses available then were not suitable for his use.

About A.D. 1000, Arabian physicians and mathematicians were well acquainted with planoconvex lenses used resting on a page while biconvex lenses were held in the hand.

Alhazen (A.D. 956–1040), the astronomer, formulated theories about light, vision, and refraction in his *Optical Thesaurus*.[10] He stated that a segment of a crystal sphere caused objects to appear larger. He did not use his observation to produce usable lenses.

Roger Bacon, the Englishman, in his *Opus Magnus* wrote of extolling the magnifying powers of planoconvex lenses for use in reading.

In 1618, a textbook on optics by Sirturus of Milan advocated the grading of lenses by their radii of curvature rather than the age of the person being fitted. He criticized the quality of Roman and Venetian spectacle lenses both in the grind and in the glass itself.

Bryden and Simms

Bryden and Simms have reviewed and researched the discoveries and use of lens-grinding improvements of optician John Marshall of London. Their excellent thirty-two-page monograph not only is scholarly and descriptive but also (at times) whimsically explores issues of science, commerce, advertising and the use of the Royal Society of that time. Although we do not actually know the details of Marshall's lens-grinding process, the article by Bryden and Simms (written in 1993) suggests that techniques have not changed radically for 300 years:

> The letter sent by the Royal Society to the London optician, John Marshall, in 1694, commending his new method of grinding, has been reprinted, and referred to, in recent years. However, there has been no comprehensive analysis of the method itself, the letter and the circumstances in which it was written, nor the consequences for trade practices. The significance of the approval by the Royal Society of this innovation and the use of that approbation by John

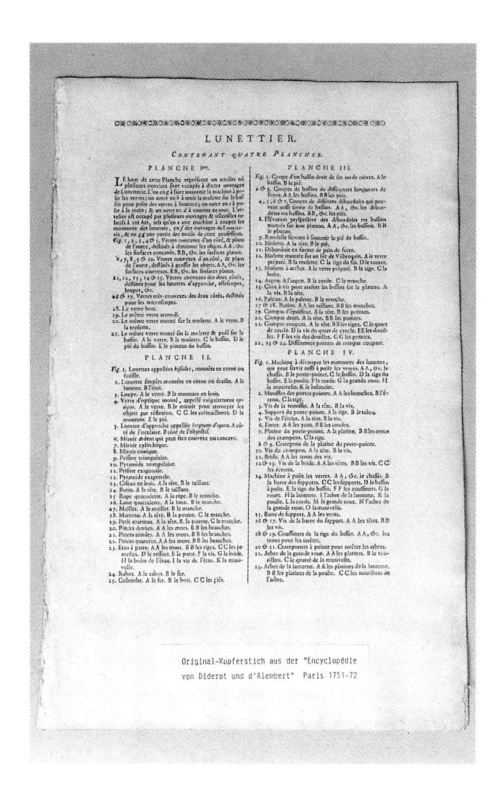

Figure 45. Descriptive page.

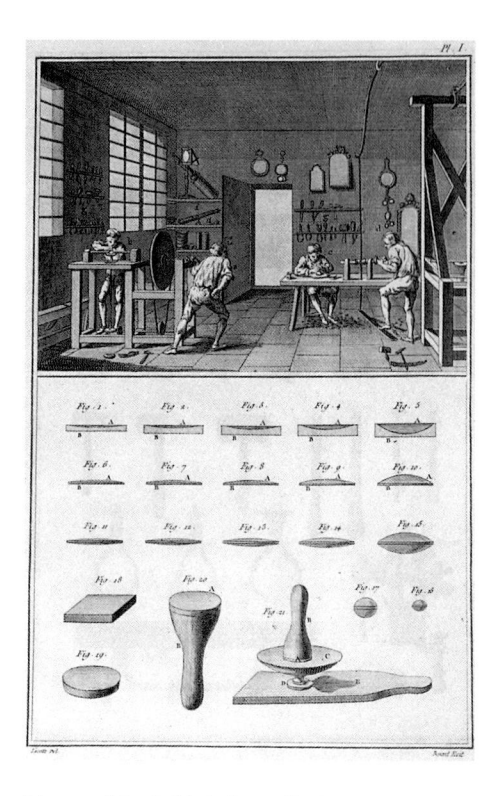

Figure 46. Optician's shop and tools.

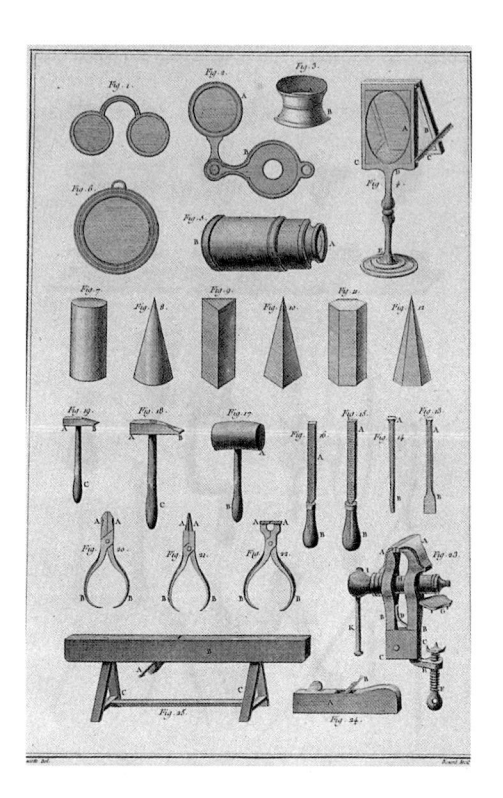

Figure 47. Lenses and tools.

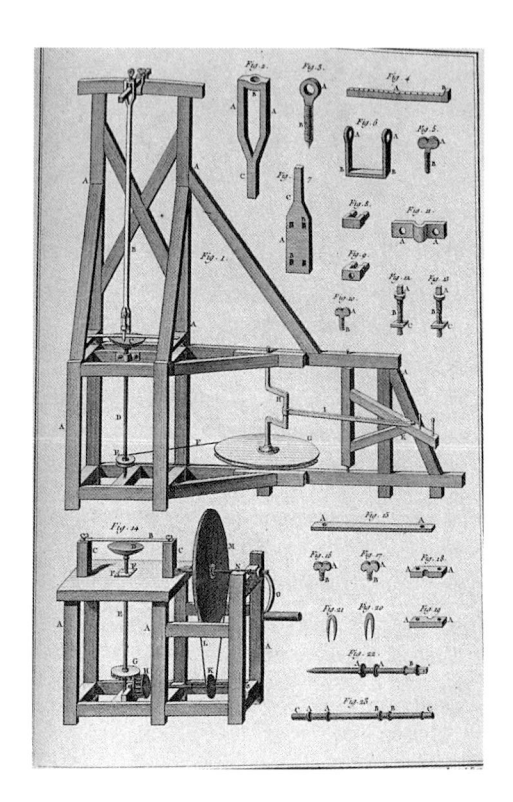

Figure 48. Cutting and grinding machines.

28 CHAPTER 4

Marshall and other practitioners are examined. Gaps in existing accounts of Marshall's method are partly remedied by supplementing surviving written materials with accounts of contemporary, and present-day, trade practices based on his method. The reasons why Marshall and his contemporaries failed to record his method and specify his improvements are discussed. The reactions of the Spectacle Makers' Company and its more prominent members, both to the innovation itself and to the Royal Society's letter, are analyzed. The impact of the new technique on contemporary and later opticians is described.[11]

The basic, unfortunate fact is that Marshall's technique, although quickly adopted by opticians of the period, was never actually described in writing. It formed the basis of lens grinding well into the twentieth century. One only needs to see the hundreds of idle lens grinders at the old American Optical Company buildings in Southbridge, Massachusetts, to realize how useful Marshall's invention had been. It was used for over 200 years in industrial practice!! Only with the invention of new optical substances, plastics, injection molding and the like has the method been superseded.

Because of the in-depth analysis afforded by Bryden and Simms and the availability of their work, the reader is respectfully referred to the original for satisfying details. Appreciation is due Mr. Trevor Waterman of London for calling the author's attention to this fine work.

Further Development The German mathematician Hertel recommended use of the meniscus lens in 1716. Gottlieb Christian Hilscher, a German manufacturer, wrote *Concise Instruction in Grinding Lenses and Fitting Telescopes* in 1741. (Appendix 7 contains the translation of the pertinent portions of his book.)

Original illustrations cut from the *Encyclopedie von Diderot und d'Alembert* indicate the machines, instruments and techniques used to grind lenses in Paris in 1751–1772 (Figures 45–48).

In 1750, an English optician, Dollond, invented the achromatic lens, adopted for spectacle use by Addison Smith. In 1784, Benjamin Franklin, an American, designed the first bifocal glasses. (This development is detailed in Chapter 21.) In 1804, W. H. Wollaston (English) (Figure 49) advocated the

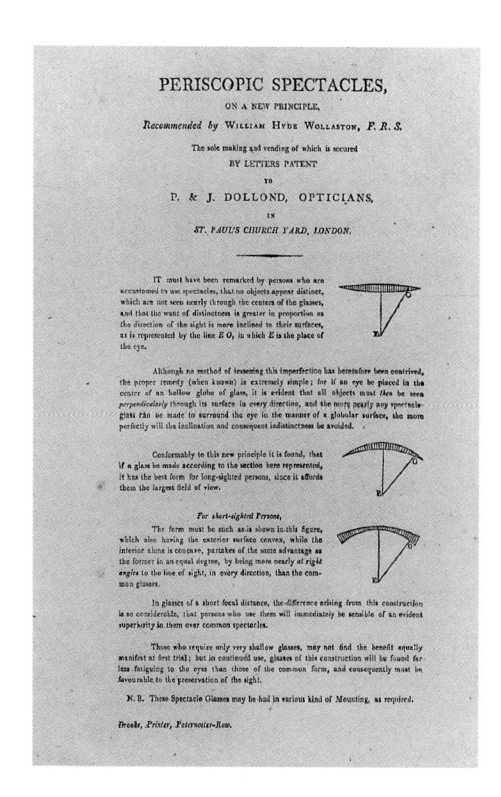

Figure 49. Wollaston's flyer.

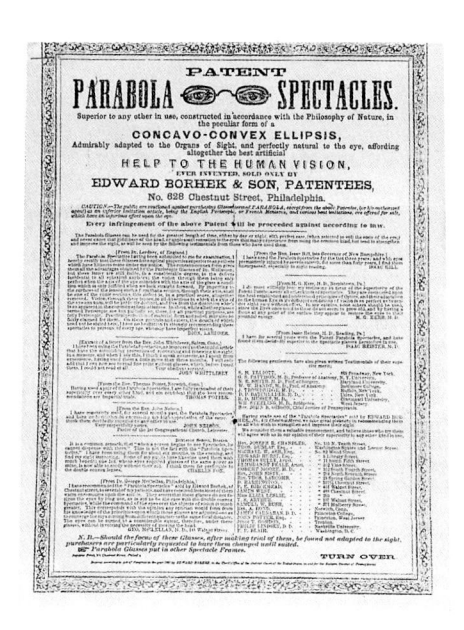

Figure 50. Advertisement for meniscus lenses in Philadelphia, PA.

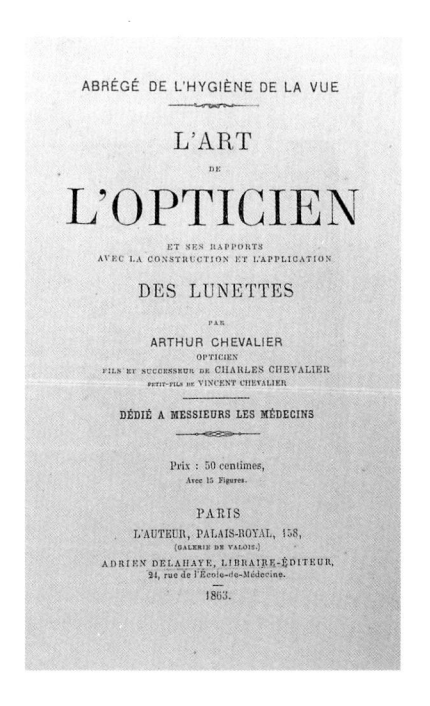

Figure 51. Title page of *L'Art de l'opticien*.

use of meniscus lenses instead of the plano convex, plano concave, or double convex lenses then in use. He called them periscopic lenses because of the concave surface being nearest to the eye. He secured the sole making and vending of these lenses by letters of patent to P. & J. Dollond opticians. Whereas the periscopic lens had been produced with various base curves dependent on the lens strength, it was standardized around 1880 using a −1.25 base curve (Figure 508) Also in the early 1800s, lenticular lenses were designed to reduce the weight of what would be, in ordinary form, very heavy lenses, as in high degrees of myopia and hyperopia (especially in aphakic eyes). Convex lenticular lenses are made by cementing the requisite scale on the center of a plano or planocylinder.

In 1863, Arthur Chevalier wrote an interesting book, *L'Art de l'opticien*, which illustrated the typical optician's work (manufacturing) area of the era (Figures 51–53).

Astigmatism   In 1801, Thomas Young demonstrated the condition of astigmatism in his own eye.[12] The same year, Young also discovered color vision (trichromatism). In 1827, an optician named Fuller, of Ipswich, made Airy's spherocylindrical lens, the first glass for the correction of astigmatism. McAllister also did this in Philadelphia the following year. Suspice of Rome used toric lenses for the correction of astigmatism in 1844. Emile Javal has outlined the history of astigmatism in his article, "History and Bibliography of Astigmatism"(this can be found in Appendix 4).

Prisms   Following is an excerpt from *The American Encyclopedia and Dictionary of Ophthalmology* by Casey Wood.

> In 1844, Charles Chevalier, of Paris, recommended glasses for the correction of squint. It is possible that he meant prisms, for at that time there was no appreciation of the relationship between errors of refraction and squint, and no practice of the refinements of refraction with the aid of cycloplegics as understood today. In 1865, Dyer called attention to the value of prisms for gymnastic exercise of weak ocular muscles. For the past fifty years prisms have been widely used. Accuracy in refraction has in itself so righted muscular imbalance that prisms are no longer used extensively as part of the correcting lenses; but as instru-

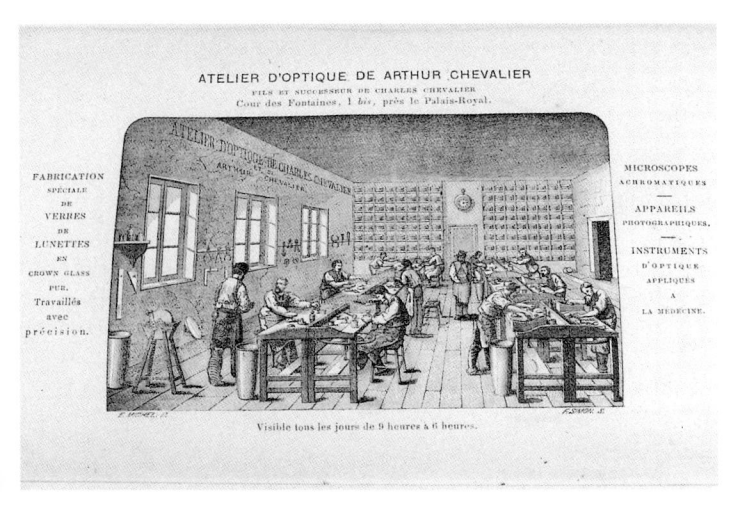

Figure 52. General view of optical shop.

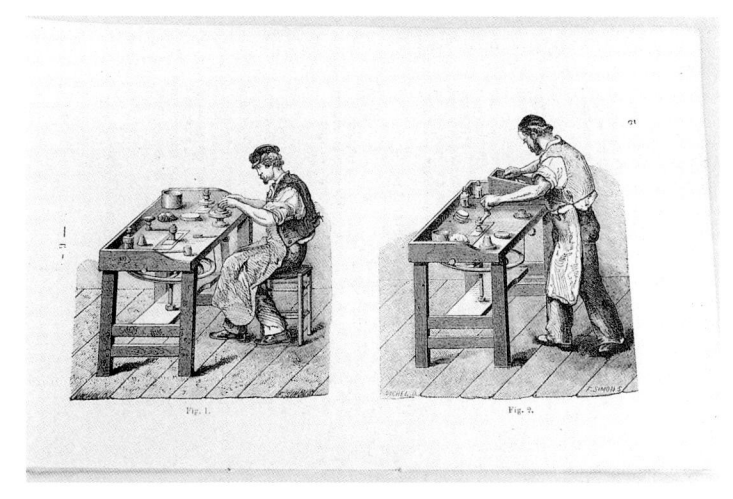

Figure 53. Individual manufacturing benches.

ments for gymnastic exercises, as tests for malingering, to measure the power of the several extraocular muscles, and to relieve diplopia they have a large place in ophthalmic practice.[13]

Dr. Jules Sichel   In 1848, Dr. Sichel covered subjects from the following chapter headings in his book *Les Lunettes*:

1. The way of vision.
2. The accommodation factor in the different distances.
3. General causes that determine how to see.
4. Presbyopia and myopia in general.
5. The glasses in general and the strength of the glasses.
6. The shape and the frame of the glasses and how they are worn, etc.
7. The influence of accommodation on the adequate comfort of the presbyope and myope.
8. Precautions of hygiene in eyes.
9. Degree of lighting needed in presbyopia.[14]

Dr. Sichel's clinical examinations were significant and indicated the changing thought toward ophthalmic examination and refraction. Still further ophthalmic discoveries followed as evidenced by (a) the ophthalmoscope (Helmholz 1851), (b) refraction of the eye (Donders 1864), (c) the retinoscope (Cuignet 1871), and (d) the ophthalmometer (Javal 1882).

Lenses for the correction of astigmatism (the condition discovered by Thomas Young in 1801) were not commonplace until the latter of these inventions—the ophthalmometer—came into more general use in 1882.

The toric lens, with a shallower base curve than the periscopic lens, was first ground in America by Anton Wagner in 1885. Another outstanding contribution to ophthalmic science was made in 1888 by C. F. Prentice, who proposed the generally accepted designation of "prism diopters" to show the amount of bending of a light ray by a certain strength prism. His further, original work resulted in the redesigning of lenses for vertex refraction.

Upon recommendations by Ostwalt, Tscherning, and Percival during the period of 1889–1904, improvements in lens design occurred, resulting in the six base meniscus and toric lenses.

Lens Power Designation   The first recorded method of indicating lens strength was that of the Jesuit Father, Franciscus Maurolycus (1494–1575).[15] At the age of 60 (according to Abelstrom), Father Maurolycus wrote that he remembered, "Master spectacle makers used to stamp numbers on spectacles which indicated the age at which they should be worn."

Several decades later, the Italian monk Tomaso Garzoni (1549–1589) wrote that spectacle makers surfaced glass with a curvature marked in degrees, numbered from ½ to 15. Certain lenses were to be used for certain ages, such as 30 to 40, or 40 to 50, up to 100 years. Lenses designed for cataract extraction patients had a power of 8 degrees.

We must sympathize with opticians of that day, as not only was there no universal lens strength designation, but grinding tools were inaccurate. Glass was of poor quality, and it varied from country to country.

In 1623 Daca de Valdes stated: "Both the convex and concave glasses were made in specific powers or grades. These grades are sections of a sphere, the largest being two 'vara' (i.e., Spanish ells) (one vara equals 840 millimeters) in diameter. Other spheres were smaller and smaller until the smallest was no bigger than the opening of the eye. This smallest sphere correspond to 30 grades and the largest to 1 grade."[16]

If lenses of that time had an index as today's (n = 1.5), then a 1 grade lens would be about a 0.6 D lens in a planospherical configuration. Despite the fact that this numbering system facilitated sale of spectacles to people of various ages, de Valdes still insisted that the lenses chosen be those that gave the best vision to the individual.

The law of refraction was discovered by the Dutchman Willebord Snell (1591–1626) but was not published until the 1660s. This law was true of all kinds of glass and all strengths. Therefore lenses of the same strength but different glass densities had different focal lengths.

Christian Gottlieb Hertel (1683–1743) classified lenses according to the radii of their grinding tools. Under the circumstances, this was not very accurate.

Lens Strength Measurements   At the beginning of the seventeenth century, a collaboration of Edward Scarlett and his son, along with John Hadley (1682–1744), taught the opticians the precise methods used by scientists in measuring lenses. By labeling a lens with a number showing its focus, its strength, precise use, and ability were indicated. Scarlett stamped the focus marks on the spectacle frame. This was not ideal, as lenses became broken and were replaced.

In the 1820s and 1830s, opticians marked the lens focal power on the lens itself by engraving close to the edge on the hinged side. In Sweden, this was called "the number of the glass," and patients demanded lenses so marked until the 1920s.

Later (1850), focal lengths of lenses were marked (usually on the temples of spectacles) in inches by English and American opticians. The French used focal lengths in pouces in the early nineteenth century. The French royal pouce is longer than the English inch (13 English inches equal 12 French royal pouces—see Bull scale, Figure 54).

Diopters   A great step forward was marked in optical science when, in 1875, the international scale of measurement of diopters (D = 1/M) was adopted. This was first suggested in 1866 by Nagel. The term *diopter*, proposed by a Frenchman named Monoyer, is now universally used and designates the dioptric or refractive power of a lens of one meter focal length.

Information on the Best Materials for
Spectacle Lenses in the Nineteenth Century

In the early nineteenth century, there was no optical glass house in England. Opticians needed to take plate glass and use it for spectacles, although it was not good for other optical purposes (such as telescopes). J. T. Hudson, an optician, stated that a variety of experiments were made using other substances for spectacle lenses. Solids and liquids, precious stones, gums, resins, etc., were all rejected.[17]

According to Hudson in 1810, crystal (or pebble) was a beautiful, natural, transparent stone ideal for spectacle lenses. It was imported from Brazil and possibly sometimes from Czechoslovakia. Never was Scottish pebble used, as it was not transparent. In Brazil, pebble was carried on mules in great quantities from the interior to the sea and then sent to England. Much of the stone had to be rejected for spectacle use, as it was full of feathers and trash, and some was brown or smoky. The brown color could be removed by heat, especially if left in the sun.

The stone was slit by a lapidary, using diamond dust, into pieces the size of spectacle lenses. The pieces were cut using an iron circular saw with "oil of brique" as lubrication for the diamond dust. (This author's personal purchase of lens edgers in the Southern Alps revealed the use of diamonds as cutting edges.)

The slabs of pebble were then ground to the correct convexity or concavity using emery in a brass or iron tool. Polishing was accomplished with cloth, water, and putty powder. The edges of the lenses were fit into the spectacle frame by nipping them, shivering or breaking the edges with pliers to the proper shape. They were smoothed with a grind stone.

Though difficult to realize, according to Bull, rock crystal was still being used to make spectacle lenses as late as 1889.[18] Frequently, the temples of frames containing crystal lenses were marked "PEBBLE." The best grade was as clear as glass, could be ground to prescription, and was harder to scratch than glass lenses.

Rock crystal was also used by the Chinese, whose supply came from Mongolian sources. The best glass, however, was Venetian (Murano) and was called mirror crystal. These pieces had higher indices of refraction than German glass, which was softer and easier to work.

Conclusion

Although the "original" lens was probably a clear quartz found in a stream bed after tumbling to approximate optical quality, it did not take long (only a few hundred years) to develop the geometry and mechanics to produce lenses of optical quality for use as burning stones, magnifiers, spectacles, telescopes, and the like. Furthermore, findings of eyeglass frames and lenses from China circa 1720 with optical corrections and thinness of one to two millimeters certainly contradict the current concept of the "new" thin grind!!

Notes

1. Theo E. Obrig, *Modern Ophthalmic Lenses and Optical Glass* (New York: The Chilton Co., 1935).
2. O. D. Rasmussen, *Chinese Eyesight and Spectacles* (Tonbridge, Kent, England: Tonbridge Free Press Ltd., circa 1950).
3. Prof. Dr. Greeff (Berlin) *Katalog Einer Bilderausstellung Zur Geschichte Der Brille* (Amsterdam, 1929).
4. Obrig, op.cit.
5. G. Sines and Y. A. Sakellarakis, "Lenses in Antiquity," *American Journal of Archaeology* 91(1987):191.

Table de concordance entre les numéros en dioptries et les numéros en pouces.

Numéros en DIOPTRIES		Numéros en POUCES
0,25	=	144
0,5	=	72
0,75	=	48
1,	=	40
1,25	=	30
1,5	=	26
1,75	=	24
2,	=	20
2,25	=	18
2,5	=	16
2,75	=	14
3,	=	13
3,25	=	12
3,5	=	11
4,	=	10
4,5	=	9
5,	=	8
6,	=	7
7,	=	6
8,	=	5
9,	=	4 ½
10,	=	4
11,	=	3 ½
12,	=	3 ¼
13,	=	3
14,	=	2 ¾
16,	=	2 ½
18,	=	2 ¼
20,	=	2

Figure 54. Table of pouces and diopters — Dr. Geo. Bull.

6. Rasmussen, op. cit.
7. Julius Hirschberg, *History of Ophthalmology* Vol. 2 (Bonn: Wayenborgh, 1985), 266–273.
8. Obrig, op.cit.
9. Sines and Sakellarakis, op. cit.
10. Hirschberg, op. cit.
11. D. J. Bryden and D. L. Simms, "Spectacles Improved to Perfection and Approved of by the Royal Society," *Annals of Science* 50 (1993): 1–32.
12. Obrig, op. cit.
13. Casey A. Wood, M.D., *The American Encyclopedia and Dictionary of Ophthalmology* (Chicago: Cleveland Press, 1915).
14. Dr. Jules Sichel, *Les Lunettes* (Paris, 1848).
15. G. J. Bull, M.D., *Lunettes et Pince Nez* (Paris: G. Masson, ed., 1889).
16. T. Tato-Guerra, "Benito Daca de Valdes," *J.A.O.A.*, February 1961, 541.
17. J. T. Hudson, *Lenses and Opera Glasses* (London: Joseph Thomas, Finch-Lane, Cornhill, 1840).
18. Bull, op.cit.

Other Sources Consulted for Chapter 4

1. M. Chamblant, *Nouveaux verres d'optique, surfaces de cylindre*. Brevet pour l'exécution, rue Basse-porte-St. Denis, No. 26, Paris.
2. J. Monnerel, *Le Lunetier-Opticien*. 2d. ed. L. Eyrolles, editor. Paris, 1890.

5

A Review of the History of Spectacles

One of the oldest pair of glasses in preservation is in the Nuremberg Museum. They were donated by the antiquarian Jacques Rosenthal, of Munich, who found them in an old volume of the latter part of the fifteenth century. They are primitive, round-rimmed eyeglasses with a solid bow joining the rims. They are made of leather, lacking lenses. They predate 1470 (Figure 55).

Despite superb finds, as the one just mentioned and as shown in Figures 56 and 57, tracing the exact history of spectacles is quite another matter. The further we reach in time and distance from the origins of truth, the more varieties, shadows, and utter falsifications, for many human reasons, we find. And so it is with the history of spectacles. Numerous versions of the origin of spectacles exist, a few of which follow.

The ancient Chinese, we believe, used spectacles that were not ground to correct vision but were used as sunglasses (Figure 58). The lenses were said to contain a spirit (the *yoh shui*) that was believed to help the wearer's vision and enhance the wearer's importance.[1]

A teacher of the Church, Sofronuis Eusebius Hieronymus (A.D. 340–420) is frequently credited with the invention of spectacles because he has often been represented with three insignia—a lion, a skull, and spectacles.[2] He has been regarded as the patron saint of spectacle makers. Saint Fridolin, who lived about A.D. 500, has also been regarded as the inventor of spectacles and was later considered the patron saint of people with visual defects. St. Lucy was likewise afforded this consideration.

A Florentine, Amato degli Armati, has a tombstone stating that he was the inventor of spectacles. Appendix 2 contains details of this falsification.

Consider also Roger Bacon, who is actually credited by some with the invention of spectacles. He was unable to produce even one useful pair. He did, however, note in his *Opus Major* that lenses "will prove to be a most useful instrument for old persons and all those having weak eyes, as they can see in this manner the small letters. . . ." His book dates 1267.

In 1271, on his first voyage to China, Marco Polo noted persons wearing spectacles.[3] (A dissenting opinion of this observation is detailed in Hirschberg, volume 2.)

Ironically, fourteenth- through seventeenth-century artists portrayed Moses, the apostles, and other biblical personalities wearing spectacles. Artists modernized their subjects by surrounding them with the fashionable accessories of the time. The earliest of these portraits is that painted at Treviso in 1352 by Tommaso da Modena. It portrays Hugh of St. Cher Cardinal Ugone wearing riveted spectacles on his nose and was done a century after his death. As with the biblical figures, the invention of spectacles came long after Hugh's lifetime.

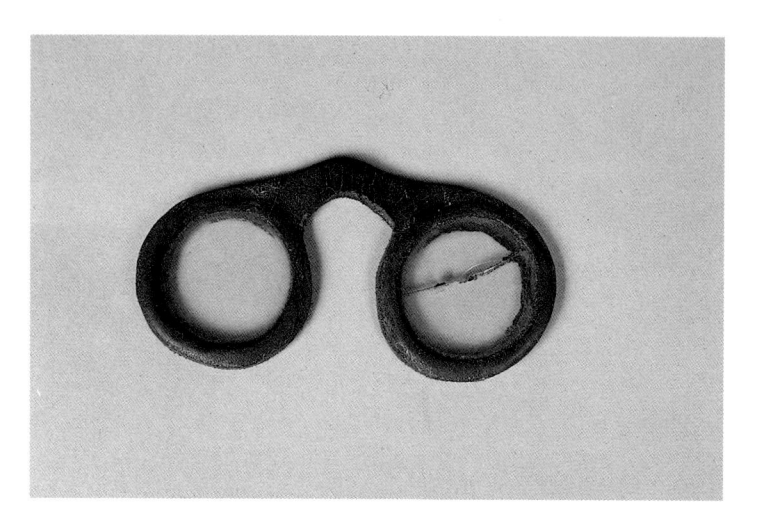

Figure 55. Leather spectacles, similar to Nuremberg pair.

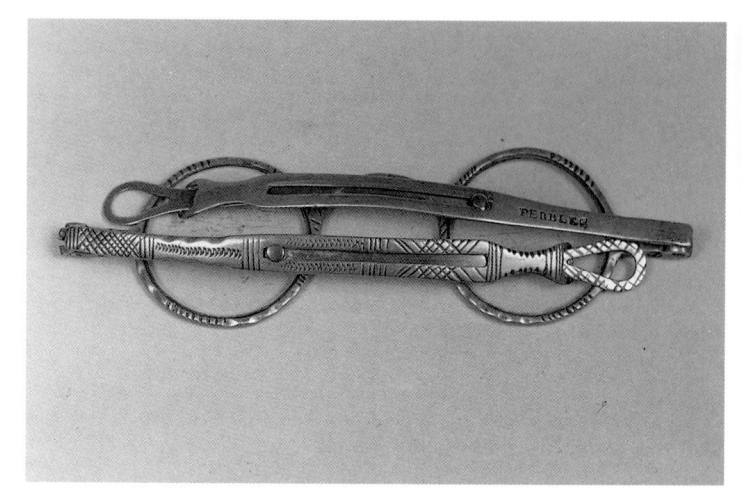

Figure 56. Spectacles made in India for the British trade. (Very unusual. The author has seen only three or four pairs in his lifetime.)

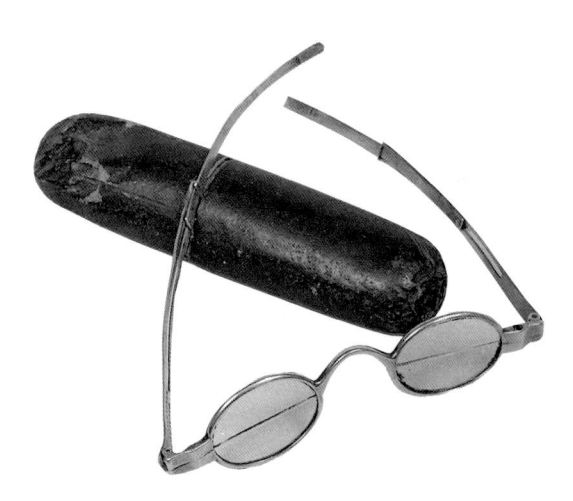

Figure 57A. Spectacles made by McAllister circa 1790 with "M.W" on the temple.

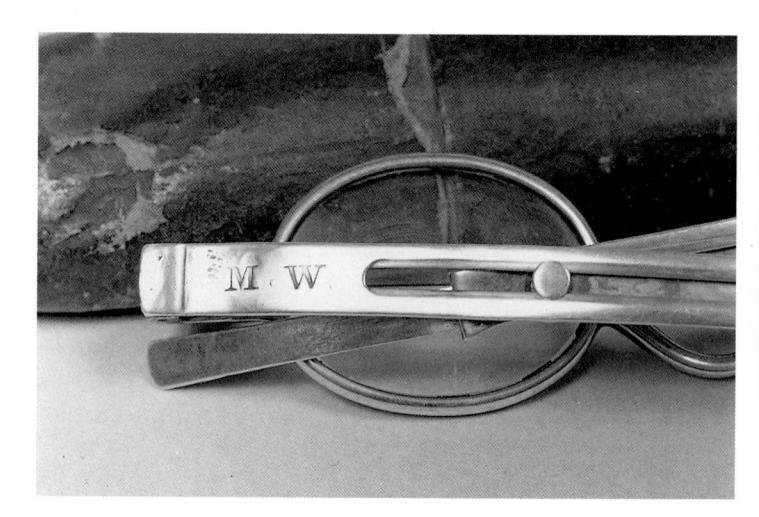

Figure 57B. Close-up of spectacles in 57A. (Could these be for Martha Washington?)

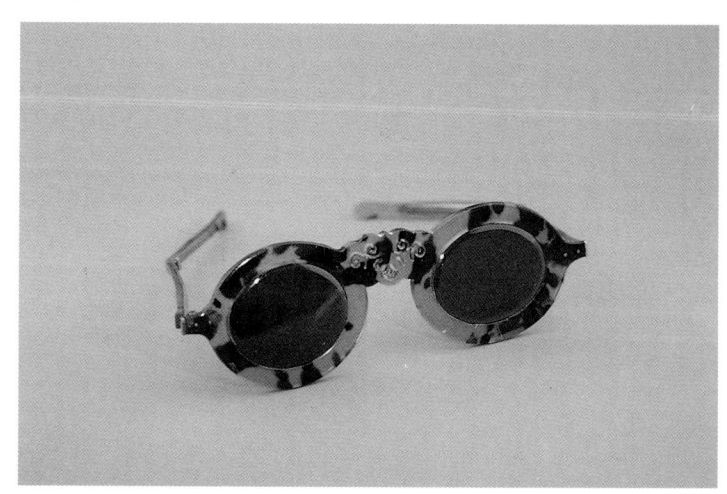

Figure 58. Carved tortoiseshell spectacles circa 1700.

Following is an excerpt from the second volume of *The History of Ophthalmology* by Julius Hirschberg, regarding the inconsistencies in the literature on the history of spectacles:

When carefully following the history of ophthalmology during the Middle Ages we may come to the conclusion that no major advance had been made during that time. However, we have to discuss now one invention which had been absolutely unknown during classical antiquity as well as among Arabians. These are the spectacles without which a modern ophthalmologist could not practice anymore.

The invention of the spectacles is still shrouded in darkness.

It is possible that the Europeans imported the first spectacles from China. Such ideas have recently been put forward by Scrini and Fortin in Paris who said: We know, on the other hand, that when Marco Polo traveled to China he learned that the inhabitants of China had for a long time already used spectacles. This contention is absolutely unproved.

I have carefully screened the German translation of the book by Marco Polo (2nd edition, Leipzig 1855) and also the original text (*le livre de Marco Polo* by Pauthier, Paris 1865, two volumes): they do not contain a single word about spectacles in China. The highly respected sinologist Professor Grube was kind enough to screen for me the English edition (by Yule, London 1875) and came to the same negative result.

This sentence by Scrini and Fortin has therefore to be erased and should not reappear in the literature.

The following is quoted in the giant encyclopedia "T'u-schu-tsi-tsch'ong," Section 32, Chapter 228: *ai-tai-king* (literally "cloudy mirror or lens"), "old men who cannot read fine script anymore put it in front of their eyes so that the writing becomes clear."

It is explicitly added that this device was imported from the country Mau-la-kia—i.e. Malakka.

In the Chinese texts Malakka appeared only after the beginning of the 15th century B.C. I therefore have to presume that the first spectacles were there imported from Europe and then traded to China.

Parenthetically I would like to note that I asked two scholarly Chinese in Berlin about this question and they both declared that spectacles were known in China for a long time as the Emperor Kang-hsi had been given a most precious pair of spectacles. But Kang-hsi reigned from 1662–1723 A.D., i.e. 400 years after spectacles had become known in Europe and at a time when French and English traders were already allowed to enter China.

All claims that spectacles had been known in Europe before the year 1270 A.D. are in error. The famous historian Wilhelm Wattenbach says the following: "Weakness of the eyes was alleviated with spectacles. We find already in the dictionary of Alfric (page 38 in Wright) the words: *specularis, thurshyne stan*; already in the 'Life of Wilfrid of York' (died 709) which was written in the 10th century by Fridegod we find (Mab. Actt. III, 1, 195): *Protinus admisso micuit syntagma berillo*. The meaning is not quite clear and as long as it was thought that the magnification is a property of beryllium itself the use must have been quite limited."

The scholarly Abbot Aelfric lived around the year 1000. However, *specular* or *speculare* means a bull's eye window of glass or transparent stone (mica). This can be deduced from Martialis (VII, Epig. XIV), Pliny the younger (Epist. II), and from Cael. Aurelian, Siccens. lib. 2 acutorum cap. 37 and from S. Hieronym. in cap. 41 Ezech: These windows were made in such a way that instead of transparent (*speculari*) stone or glass pieces interrupted pieces of wood (which could be shut) were used.

As far as the verse from "The Life of Saint Wilfrid" is concerned we should not translate it as: "Immediately after the spectacles have been put on, the scripture becomes clear." *Admisso* does not fit into this sentence, *micuit* means actually "glistened, sparkled" and *syntagma* does not stand for the scripture, but means a roll of a text.

The verse has to be interpreted in context. The entire text is reprinted in:

Acta Sanctorum Ordinis S. Benedict... edited by J. Mabillon III, 1,

Paris 1672,—

Apparently only one manuscript was used for this print and even that one was defective. The text stops in the middle of a sentence and the editor adds: Other parts are also missing in this manuscript. The editor informs us about the author and the manuscript:

Several authors have celebrated Wilfridum, the abbot and bishop... after Heddium followed Fridegodus, then Odo, the bishop and then arrived the Vvillemus. The poem has been written by Fridegodus.

In the XLVII chapter of this heroic poem (which is not characterized by clarity) we find on the margin a note concerning the contents. It was probably added by the editor. Wilfrid was removed from his bishop seat and went to Rome in order to await the decision by the Pope. He was reinstalled.

The three first verses of this chapter deal with their English opponents, verse 4 and 5 describe the judicial or advisory college of the Roman fathers.

In verse 6 and the following St. Wilfrid has audience with the Pope: "Wilfrid was admitted immediately and in his hand there was a document which because of the beryllium glistened vividly. This appeared like a special reflex. Wilfrid showed a document which appeared like gold and had a brilliant shine. . . ."

We have to deduce therefore that he is not speaking here about spectacles but is alluding to a beryllium which like an ornament was used to close the document. The Romans already used beryllium for ornaments (We only have to look into the Latin-German Dictionary by Georges. We find there in *Juvenal, Satir. V,* 38: *inaequales berillo phialas,* i.e. cups which are embellished by beryllium.) It is well known that this kind of ornament of various objects continued to be used in the Middle Ages.

I therefore think that these two references to spectacles have been clearly explained and do not need to cloud the literature on this topic in the future.

The European physicians of the Middle Ages used up to 1300 only collyria and not spectacles for the correction of refraction. Even Arnaldo de Villanova (294) recommends against weakness of vision in old age only fennel. The extensive literature of the Catholic clergy mentions the use of spectacles for the Mass not before 1660 (Manni, 4, page 37).[4]

Obviously, there are numerous versions of who invented spectacles and/or where they originated. However, the strongest documentation comes from Italy—leading us to the true account of the invention of spectacles.

Friar Giordano of Pisa delivered a sermon in February 1306 in which he spoke of the invention of eyeglasses twenty years previously. He noted that he had seen and spoken to the inventor, but did not name him. *Thus, we can conclude that about 1287 spectacles were invented in Northern Italy.* Although simultaneous use in China or other parts of Asia cannot be ruled out, the Italian documentation is the strongest.

Further support is found at a monastery in Pisa recording the death (in 1313) of a Dominican monk, Alessandro della Spina, who could reproduce any object he had seen with his own eyes. This monk had seen spectacles made by an unnamed person who wished to keep the invention for his own benefit. Della Spina, however, realized their potential and made many copies, which he distributed with a "cheerful and benevolent heart."[5]*

The First Spectacles

The first spectacles—riveted nail spectacles—were simply two magnifying glass handles riveted together at the end and hung on the nose (Figure 59). The lenses were made of pebble (quartz) or beryl, a sea green stone of beryllium aluminum silicate (thus the German word for spectacles *brille*). Emerald and aquamarine are examples of beryl.

As riveted spectacles were so difficult to maintain in place, alternate ways of securing them were tried.[6] They included hooking them to a hat brim, attaching them to a plate over the forehead, and holding the spectacles against the eye with a handle while attaching them with a string around the ears. Other methods of fixing frames before the eyes were clamping on the temples, fixing in the hair, and putting spatula-like extensions under the hat. Soon, rigid bridges were developed with frames made mostly of leather, but some of metal and bone.

The sturdiest spectacles and most comfortable for continuous wear were those with lenses mounted in horn. The horn attached to a flat leather band (like a goggle) that tied to the back of the head. Some frames were made of bone with tiered (slit) bridges for elasticity (Figures 60 & 61).

While riveted spectacles had to be held from above, the so-called scissors glasses, having longer curved handles, had to be held from below (Figure 62). They first appeared in Italy in the fifteenth century and had handles that grasped the bridge of the nose with a scissorlike action.[7] (Chapter 13 details these glasses).

---

* Regarding the *Ghent Bird*, this scholarly and erudite dissertation, well researched and thought out to the terminus of painful minutia is, from this author's vantage point, illogically based on the fact that this creature is wearing spectacles. I think not.

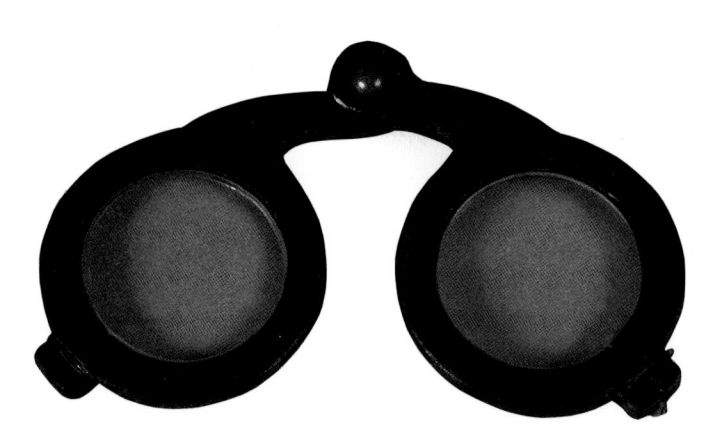

Figure 59. Replica of riveted spectacles.

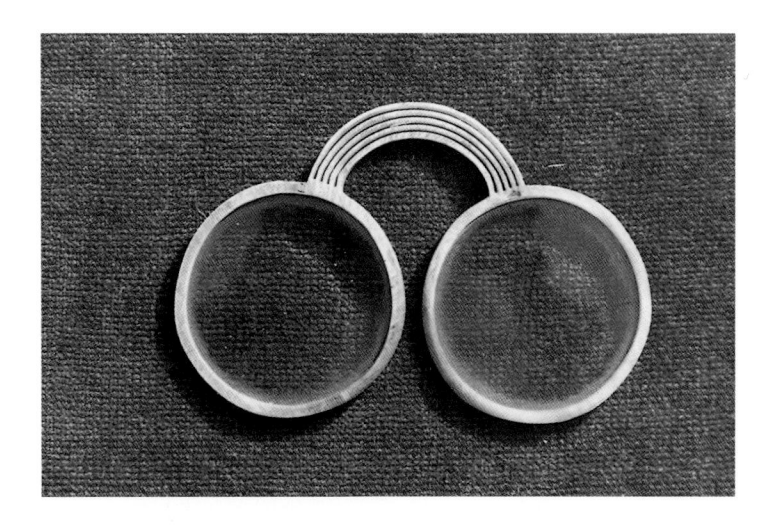

Figure 60. Bone slit bridge spectacles circa 1600.

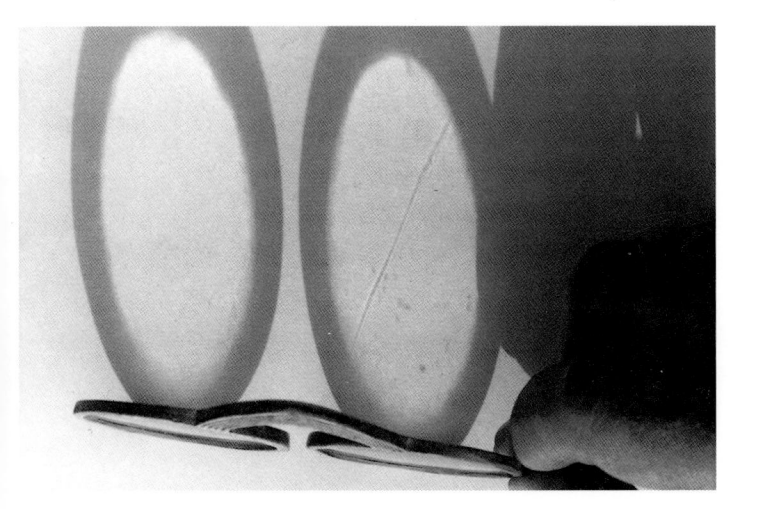

Figure 61. Bone slit bridge spectacles, showing frontal curve of bridge and lens defects (circa 1600).

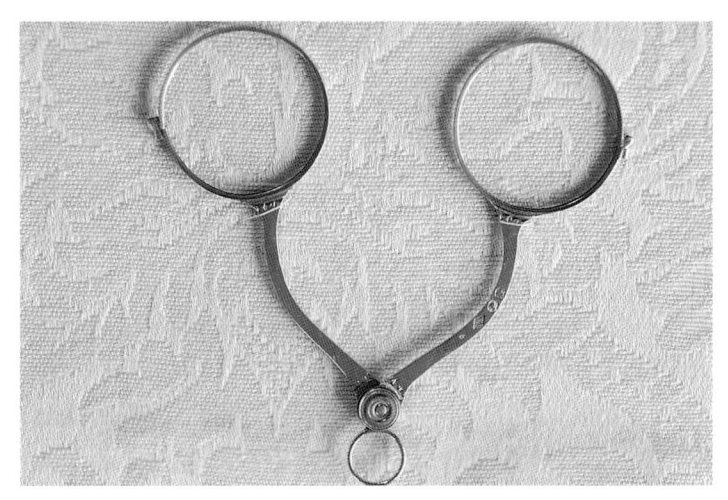

Figure 62. Scissors glasses circa 1790.

As printed books proliferated, so did the demand for spectacles. Mass production methods were instituted, and sweatshops (in Nuremberg, for instance) turned out dozens of pairs daily (Figure 63). All of the products were primitive and of poor quality. Therefore, in 1465, the Spectacle Makers' Guild reviewed merchants before the French king. In this way, spectacle makers were recognized and were separated from other glassworkers so that quality could be improved.

In the middle of the sixteenth century, leather was commonly used in spectacle making. However, it was a very tedious process. Following is the technique (from Waterer, 1956) described: "Pieces of leather must be boiled in wax

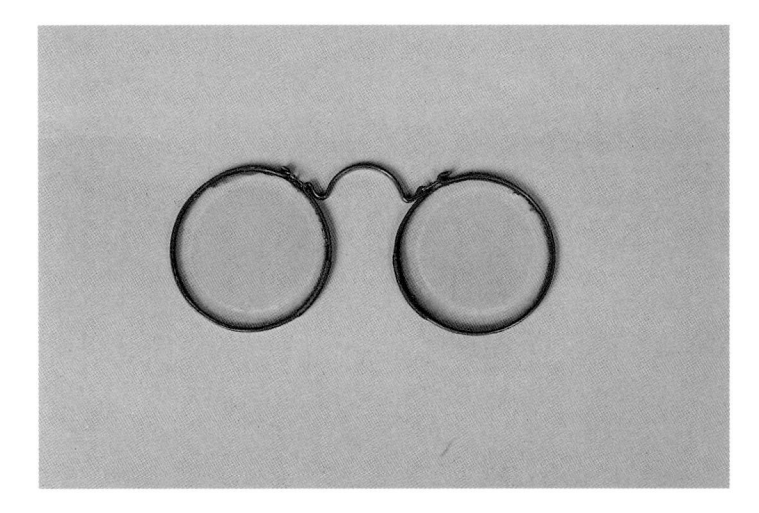

Figure 63. Nuremberg spectacles.

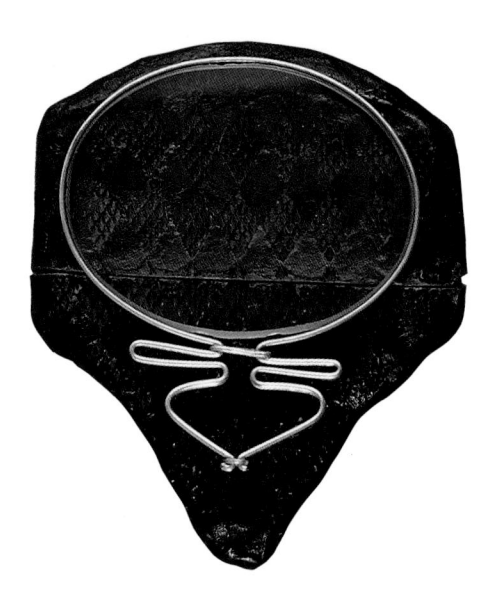

Figure 64. Seventeenth-century single glass and case.

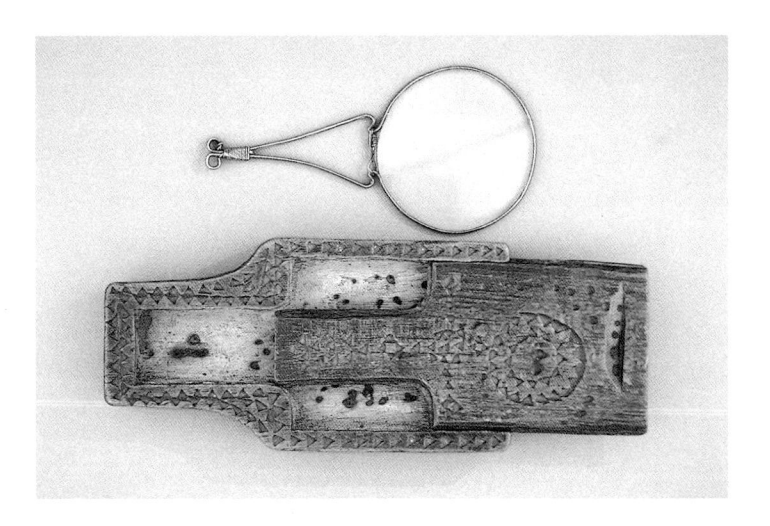

Figure 65. Seventeenth-century magnifier, carved wooden case.

mixed with resin and glue. Once boiled in this manner the leather preserves whilst it is moist, sufficient pliability to enable it to be molded and when it is dry it possesses a hardness and rigidity nearly equal to that of wood to which it is preferable by reason of its lightness." Lenses that have been edged to size can be fitted into the wet frame, which contracts as it dries and holds the lenses firmly. Court and Von Rohr (1928–29) described frames with leather rims to which a steel rim had been riveted (circa 1750). Teunissen (1983) dates a similar pair 1730.

Literature

In 1623, Benito Daca de Valdes, (1591–1634), a Jacobin friar and notary of the Spanish Inquisition, wrote a book printed in Seville entitled *Uso de los Antoios* (*Use of Spectacles*) (see Figure 699 in Chapter 36).[7] It is probably the first book on spectacles and comprises three parts:

1) This section deals with the anatomy of the eye, improvements in vision due to proper fitting glasses, and shortsightedness.

2) This section deals with convex, concave, and plano lenses. It also contains a chapter on the size and measurement of convex and concave lenses, as well as several illustrations.

3) This section contains four dialogues on the subject, with rules, opinions, and animated anecdotes.

Apparently the book is still available, as the author was recently offered a copy at $14,200.

Though still essential in the seventeenth century, spectacles were out of fashion for the upper classes in Europe.[9] Rather than use spectacles with their peculiar attachment problems, they preferred to use the single (distance) glass hung around the neck (Figures 64 & 65). These were called perspective glasses. Other alternatives to spectacles were used as well. Also called lorgnettes by the French, the term *prospect glass* at times is further confused with the perspective or prospective glass. The prospect glass is a small hand telescope adopted by both women and men to use for daily observation of their neighbors. It was also used at the theater so as not to miss any social event. We enlarge on their use separately in the chapter on monoculars. The only common use of spectacles in the upper class at that time was for protection from sun and glare—

glasses with lenses colored red, yellow, blue, and green. Chapter 23 is devoted to sun and glare protection.

During these years, the Chinese increased their use of spectacles.[10] Frames were made of brass, tortoiseshell, and silver. Occasionally, horn, and even reed, were used.[11] A full discussion of Chinese spectacles is offered in Chapter 7.

The Eighteenth and Nineteenth Centuries

Corson states:

> The 18th century brought a number of striking developments in eyeglasses, the most significant being a practical means of keeping them on. Unfortunately these glasses were evidently too utilitarian in appearance to be considered fashionable. The more decorative and stylish forms of glasses were mercilessly ridiculed by the satirists as affectations. As usual, those at whom the satire was directed paid no attention and continued to carry their fancy eyeglasses whether they needed them or not.[12]

By the latter part of the seventeenth century in Europe and the beginning of the eighteenth century in America, there were many opticians' stores. Few reputable opticians succeeded prior to the scientific concern of refraction by the medical profession. Among these notable opticians' firms were the firms of Nuremberg, where the most valuable collection of old glasses is found.

By this time, steel was being made, and its springlike quality was utilized in the manufacture of eyeglass frames. A semicircular-shaped spring acted as a bridge. The same spring was embedded in baleen and leather (Figure 66).[13]

In 1727, Edward Scarlett, a London optician, offered spectacles with temple pieces of rigid steel.[14] These ended in large rings which many times were padded (Figure 67). The optician Thomin of Paris advertised "branches" of steel or silver that did not obstruct respiration. Later they were extended posteriorly, hinged, and looped around the ears.

Sliding extensions were offered as well (Figure 68). Besides steel, they were made of gold, silver, brass, horn, and tortoiseshell.

James Ayscough experimented with spectacles, and in 1752, he advertised his frames with double-hinged side pieces. They

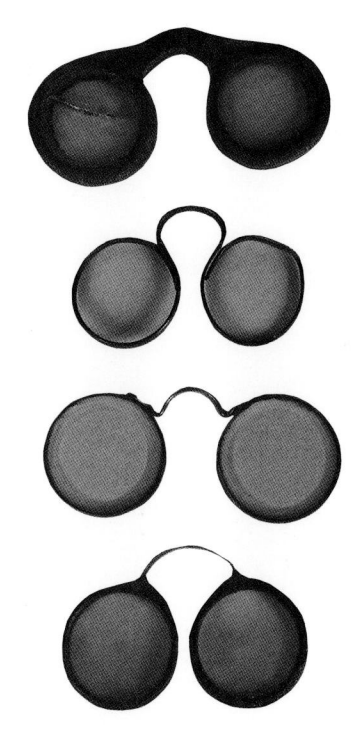

Figure 66. Eighteenth-century glasses: leather, baleen, Nuremberg and leather with hinged-spring bridge.

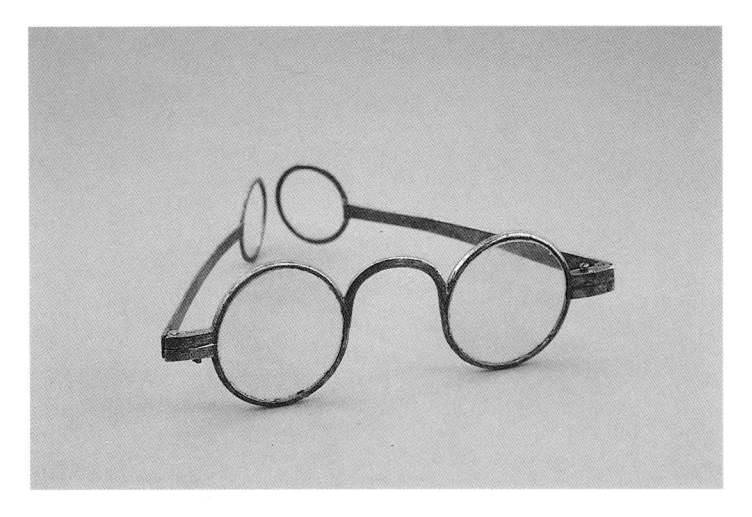

Figure 67. Steel spectacles, ring temples.

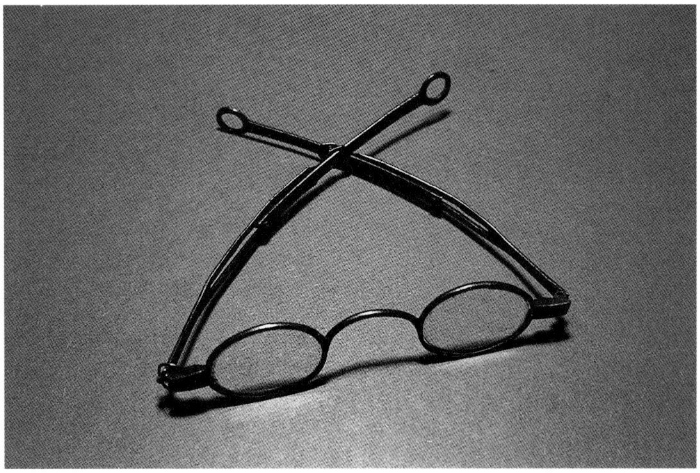

Figure 68. Sliding steel temples.

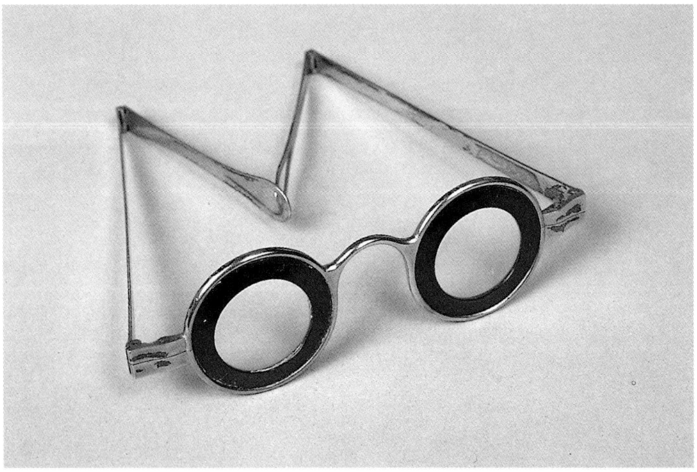

Figure 69. Gold Martin's Margins.

became extremely popular. Not so sought after, however, was the new glass with a greenish cast that he espoused. Rock crystal and Brazilian pebble were in vogue at the time.

About this time (1760), Benjamin Martin emerged on the scene with "Martin's Margins" (Figure 69). Chapter 11 is devoted to his story. An article in the September 1982 issue of the *Ophthalmic Antiques International Collectors' Club Magazine* provided some information on syllepsis glasses:

> The Optical Historian, Prof. von Rhor, said that William Storer of Gt. Marlborough St., London, advertised in 1783 that he made small Syllepsis Glasses. I have a silver pair in my collection. It has two pairs of eyes the outer or distance pair are glazed R&L +2.00 bi-cx glass, inset in "Martins Margins" the size is 30×23m/m. The second pair are glazed in a silver bevel rim 23×18m/mR&L +3.00 bi-cx glass, an idea developed by A. Smith. The PD is 50m/m and DBL 20m/m crank bridge 12m/m up and flush. The sides are 90m/m long and 5m/m thick halfway along the side and tapered to the end and serrated. Storer claims in his patent—"New and Peculiar Method of Preparing and Making of Optick Instruments in General, reading glasses and spectacles."[15]

In 1785, the Spectacle Makers' Guild was abolished, making way for peddlers to open shop again. Spectacles were sold at stalls on the street and in markets.[15] They were peddled by street hawkers in towns, villages, and farms. These spectacles were made of oxhorn and leather. Some had frames made of a continuous ribbon of brass or copper with mildly flexible bridges. These were made by the "Musierwelle," whereby a round wire was pressed and a groove was put into one side.[17] Also offered were small telescopes made of cardboard tubes.

Although most of the spectacles used were mass produced and inexpensive, those of higher quality and price were also available. Frames were made of gold and silver, embellished with armorials and other trappings of state and position. Lenses could be ordered from as far away as Venice, if necessary.

Turn-pin temples were seen about 1770. In 1771, George Adams described extendable bows that could be placed behind the back of the head. A modern type of spectacles with

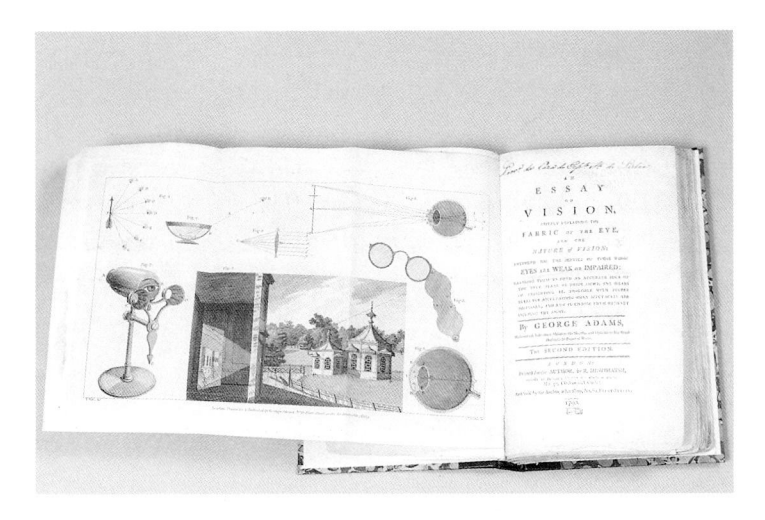

Figure 70. Frontispiece from Adams's *Essay on Vision*.

temples that curve behind the ears appeared only after 1850.[18] In his *Essay on Vision* (Figure 70), Adams gave his opinions on the use of spectacles. He listed available types of spectacles in his shop (Table 1). "Riding bow" temples originated in England as "riding spectacles." Regarding eyeglass springs, Casey Wood—in *The American Encyclopedia and Dictionary of Ophthalmology*—stated:

> In the matter of eyeglass springs very little advance over the crude medieval models is noted until the nineteenth century. In England as late as 1825 the bridge was heavy and there was no flexibility at the ends. In France in 1839 the coiled springs were used and the bridge portion was of light weight. Further improvement came from America where Cadman, in 1872, made a horizontal band-spring with pads projecting backwards against the sides of the nose. In 1880 Hopkins, of New York, devised a horizontal projection from the eyeglass to be attached to a vertical spring. E. B. Meyrowitz, in 1886, made a spring to slant forwards escaping contact with the brow; this was called the "tilting spring." In 1888, Edward Fox and D.V. Brown, of Philadelphia, made the "Grecian Curve" spring. Martin, of Philadelphia, in 1889, used a wire spring with coils near the ends; and another saddle-shaped band spring, like that of Meyrowitz, but fitting close to the nose.[19]

TABLE 1.
OPTICAL INSTRUMENTS SOLD BY GEORGE ADAMS

Type	£.	s.	d.
The best double-jointed silver spectacles, with glasses	1	1	0
The best ditto, with Brazil pebbles	1	16	0
Single-joint silver spectacles, with glasses	0	15	0
Ditto, with Brazil pebbles	1	10	0
Double-joint steel ditto, with glasses	0	7	6
Best single-joint spectacles	0	5	0
Ditto, inferior frames, from 2s. 6d. to	0	3	0
Nose spectacles, mounted in silver	0	7	6
Ditto in tortoise shell and silver	0	4	0
Ditto in horn ans steel	0	1	0
Spectacles for couched eyes	Spectacles		
Spectacles with shades			
Concave glasses in horn boxes, for short-sighted eyes			
Ditto, mounted in tortoiseshell and silver, pearl and silver, in various manners, and at different prices			
Reading glasses, from 2s. 6d. to	2	2	0
Opera glasses, from 10s. 6d. to	2	2	0
Ditto on an improved construction, 1l. 7s. and	1	11	6
Ditto to be used at sea by night	1	1	0
Diagonal operas of a new construction	1	1	0
Telescopes of various lengths, sizes, and prices			
Acromatic telescopes, portable and convenient for the pocket, the sliding tubes are of brass, and therefore not subject to the inconveniencies of those that are made with vellum drawers, from 1l. 11s. 6d. to	8	8	0
Telescopes to be used at sea by night			
Acromatic perspective glasses for the pocket, from 10s. 6d. to	2	12	6
An optical vade mecum, or portable acromatic telescope and microscope, from 3l. 13s. 6d. to	4	14	6
A thirty-inch acromatic telescope, with different eye-pieces for terrestrial and celestial objects; made for general purpofes, from 8l. 8s to	11	11	0
An acromatic telescope, about three feet and an half long, with different eye-pieces	18	18	0
A three-feet reflecting telescope, with four magnifying powers, with rack work	36	15	0
A ditto, two-feet long, with ditto	21	0	0

A two-feet reflecting telescope, with two powers	12	12	0
An eighteen-inch ditto	8	8	0
A twelve-inch ditto	5	5	0
Adams's LUCERNAL MICROSCOPE, for opake and transparent objects; it does not fatigue the eye, is in all cases a proper substitute for the solar microscope, and on many occasions superior to it	21	0	0
A small double-reflecting microscope	2	12	6
A larger ditto	3	13	6
An improved universal double microscope	6	6	0
Ditto fitted up in a different form, from 8l.8s. to	14	14	0
Ellis's aquatic microscope	2	2	0
Ditto with an adjusting screw	2	12	6
Withering's and other botanical microscopes, from 10s. 6d. to	3 Small	3	0
Small pocket microscopes, from 6s to	3	13	6
Solar microscopes	5	5	0
Ditto	6	6	0
Solar microscopes for opake and transparent objects, from 1l. 16s. to	21	0	0
A microscope and lanthorn to imitate the solar microscope			
Curious collections of objects for the microscope, either opake or transparent			
Collections fo salts, properly prepared for the microscope			
Magnifying glasses for botanical, anatomical, and other purposes, from s. to	1	11	6
Small magic lanthorns, with the sliders better painted			
Large ditto, from 1l. 5s. to	1	11	6
Optical machines for viewing perspective prints, from 18s. to	1	16	0
Scioptric balls	0	10	6
Small camera obscuras, from 10s. 6d. to	3	3	0
Book and pyramidical camera obscuras, from 3l. 3s. to	7	7	0
An artificial eye for illustrating the principles of vision			
Prisms, mounted in various manners			
Concave and convex mirrors, from 7s. 6d. to	18	18	0
Cylindrical ditto, from 1l. 1s. to	13	13	0

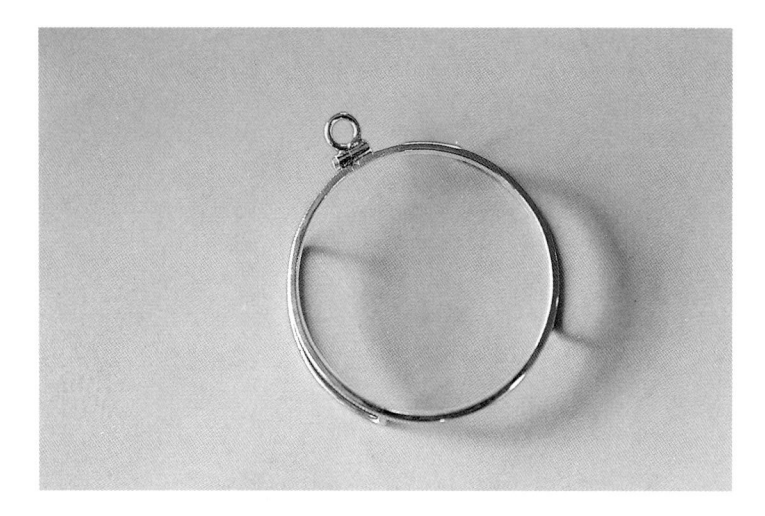

Figure 71. Gold monocle.

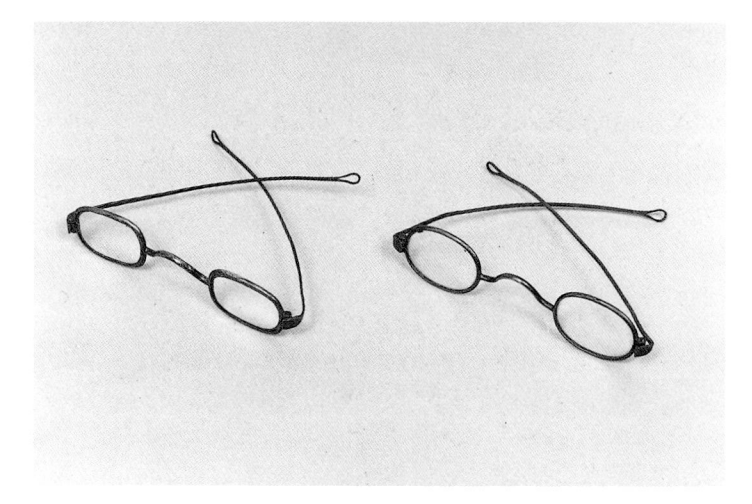

Figure 72. The crank bridge.

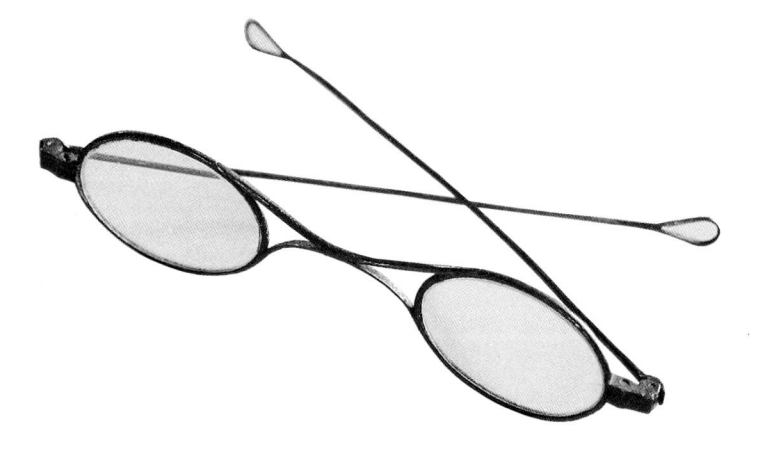

Figure 73. The X-bridge.

The monocle as we know it today was developed by the German Baron Philip Von Stosch (1691–1757) (Figure 71).[20] Its use spread throughout the European countries in the following centuries, finally falling into disrepute after World War I. Chapter 19 details the account. The lorgnette, according to R. Greeff, was first constructed by the English optician George Adams (1780). This subject, as well, is covered in Chapter 14.

Bridges

Of course the original bridge was on the riveted spectacles. The leather bridge was next, followed by an elastic type of construction of brass, copper, and slit bone.

In the last quarter of the 19th century, the "crank" bridge appeared—also known as the English style (Figure 72). The cheapest frames were made using a bridge attached to the eye wires with a weld holding the notched ends of the bridge.[21] Another inexpensive method of production included the use of a retaining ring at the bridge to hold the ends of the eye wire. More expensive bridges sported a scroll on the ends of the bridge. Steel bridges were usually C-shaped, but more sophisticated shapes were the saddle bridge, the X-bridge (Figure 73) and the K-bridge. Pads were added to the sides of the eye wires both separately and intimately. Regarding the saddle bridge: With the substitution of the saddle bridge for the older C-bridge, which was used with the straight temples, and the riding bows already described, spectacles had reached the present highly perfected form. The saddle bridge distributes pressure widely and evenly over the bridge of the nose, being capable of infinite variation in angle according to the shape of the nose. It also allows the use of larger lenses than were possible with the C-bridge without altering the interpupillary distance.

Bridges of pince-nez originally secured spectacles by the elasticity of the slit bridge. Then, it was accomplished by the silk thread wrapped around the eye wires in the Nuremberg types. Later, with more sophisticated designs, cork was used, as well as horn and tortoiseshell for pads. Some were plain, and others were ribbed for friction. These included bar-spring and finger-piece. Smooth alloys and gold were popular.

Prior to the manufacture of gold filled frames, the public had a choice practically limited to steel, gold, and some of base metal.²² The greater part of the business around 1890 was of the blued steel spectacle frames (Figure 74) The post–Civil War period of expansion in this country gave the jewelry business the innovation of rolled gold plate. The individual craftsman no longer made gold plate to his individual needs by hammer and anvil, because gold plate could be rolled by applying gold in correct proportion to the base metal and rolling it out to the required thinness by power. For wire, the sheets of gold were soldered around cores of base metal, usually brass, and pulled through drawplates into wire of the desired size. But with the invention of seamless gold-filled wire, the jewelers of Attleboro and vicinity were the first to avail themselves of the new opportunities for using this economical plating of gold in a thoroughly practical way. This enabled Peter Nerney and Mace Short, partners in the jewelry business since 1862, to produce frames of standards that we now think of as gold-filled.

It was not until about 1875 that empty frames became available. Edged lenses were being fitted to them after trial by the individual patient.

Rimless Spectacles

Although some rimless spectacles appeared in 1825, it was not until 1840, when a Viennese optician, Waldstein,²³ made his version, that they were popularized. The lenses and bridge were made from one piece of glass. Despite the fact that they were inconspicuous and light, they broke frequently and lasted only until mid-century. They were also produced by Voigtlander. Few are seen today, even in large collections.

Rimless pince-nez were popular in the decades before and after 1900. They were protected from breakage by attaching them with small chains to the ear, hair, and clothing (Figure 75).²⁴

Other Vision Aids

Several variations of spectacles, as well as alternatives to them, have been mentioned throughout this chapter. Other vision arrangements, such as quizzing glasses, bifocals, and specialized spectacles, are each fully described in Chapters 17, 21, and 27, respectively.

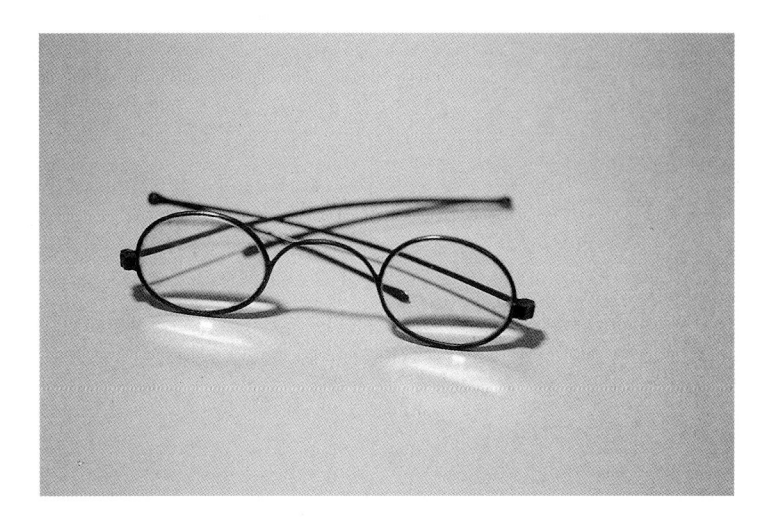

Figure 74. Blued steel frame, U.S., circa 1880.

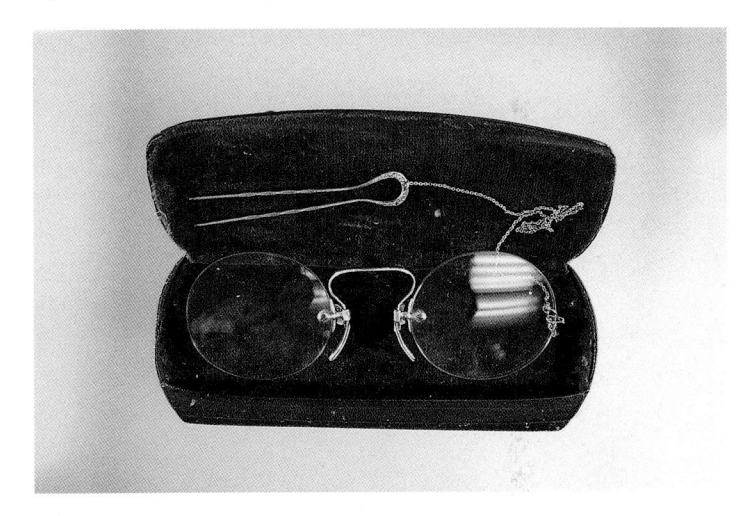

Figure 75. Rimless pince-nez in case with chain and hair pin, circa 1890.

Conclusion

A short review of the history of spectacles is offered, temporally touching the highlights of this fascinating story. History is still being made. Twentieth-century advances have hardly been acknowledged in this chapter. Perhaps, "What is past is prologue."

Notes

1. C. P. Rakusen, *Chinese Medical Journal*, 53:3(1938): 379–390, Peking.
2. H. W. Holtmann, *A Short History of Spectacles*, in Hirschberg, *History of Ophthalmology* (Bonn: Wayenborgh, 1982).
3. Richard Corson, *Fashions in Eyeglasses* (London: Peter Owen, Ltd., 1980).
4. Julius Hirschberg, *History of Ophthalmology*, vol. 2 (Bonn: Wayenborgh, 1985), 266–273.
5. Corson, op. cit., 20.
6. Corson, op. cit.
7. W. Poulet, *Atlas on the History of Spectacles*, trans. Frederick Blodi, M.D. (Badgodesberg, Germany: Wayenborgh Publishers, 1978).
8. Daza (Daca) de Valdes, *Uso de los Antoios* (Seville, 1623).
9. Carson, op. cit.
10. Rakusen, op. cit.
11. E. J. Rosen, *J. Hist. Med.* 11(1956): 13–46, 183–218.
12. Corson, op. cit.
13. Rosen, op. cit.
14. Otto Ahlstrom, "Edward Scarlett's Focus Marks," *The Optician*, July 15, 1951.
15. *Ophthalmic Antiques International Collectors' Club Magazine*, September 1982, 8.
16. Corson, op. cit.
17. Poulet, op. cit.
18. Rosen, op. cit.
19. Casey A. Wood, M.D., *The American Encyclopedia and Dictionary of Ophthalmology* (Chicago: Cleveland Press, 1915).
20. Corson, op. cit.
21. Rosen, op. cit.
22. American Optical Company, *The Story in a Pair of Spectacles*. Reprinted from *The Book of Wonders*, 2d. ed. (London: Hatton Gordon, 1921).
23. Corson, op. cit.
24. Rosen, op. cit.

Other Sources Consulted for Chapter 5

1. Rishi Kumar Agarwal, *The Optician*, September 14, 1962, p. 250; November 20, 1964, p. 512.
2. *American Optical News* Vol. 5, No. 5, 1968.
3. Anonymous, *Amer. J. Ophthal.* 32(1949):1064.
4. Anonymous, *The Optician*, December 30, 1960.
5. Anonymous, *The Optician*, July 15, 1960, p. 3.
6. Anonymous, *Minerva Med., Tor.* 48(1957):82:1648–1653 (It.).
7. Anonymous, *Policlinico* (Prat) 67(1960):1425–1426 (It.).
8. Anonymous, *The Optician* 142(1961):611–616.
9. Horst Appuhn, *Spectacles* (Oberkochen/Wurtt.: Carl Zeiss,) No. 27, p. 1.
10. Arrington. *A History of Ophthalmology* (New York, 1959).
11. C. Barck, *The Optician* 139(1960):457–463 (Reprinted from *Open Court*, 21[1907]:206–226).
12. Edward C. Bull, O.D., American Optometric Association. (San Francisco, 1926).
13. G. J. Bull, *Lunettes et pince-nez* (Paris: S. Masson, 1889).
14. G. T. W. Cashell, "A Short History of Spectacles," *Proc. Royal Soc. Med.*, 64 (October 1971).
15. Chiu Kai Ming, *Harvard Journal of Asiatic Studies,* July 1936, pp. 186–193.
16. Leonardo da Vinci, *Leonardo on the Eye* (New York, 1979).
17. Frank Devlyn, "The History of Eyewear in Mexico," *Ophthalmic Antiques International Collectors' Club Newsletter*, October 1994.
18. G. Ten Doesschate, *Brit. J. Ophthal.* 30(1946):660–664.
19. P. and J. Dollond, *Periscopic Spectacles* (London, 1804).
20. Donders, F. C. *On the Anomalies and Accommodations and Refraction of the Eye* (London, 1864).
21. S. Drake, *Isis* 52(1961):95–96.
22. Samuel L. Fox, *Highlights in the History of Spectacles* (Baltimore, MD).
23. Benjamin Franklin, *Survey Ophthal.* 4(1959):683–686.
24. M. Freedman, *Ophthal. Optician* 2(1962):435–436, 445.
25. G. J. Fukushima, *Clin. Ophthal.* 16(1962):730–732 (Tokyo).
26. Fred A. Gannon, *Optical Journal Review,* January 15, 1941, p. 180.
27. Tomaso Garzoni, *La Piazza Universale* (Venice, 1585).
28. Walter Gasson, *The Optician,* April 23, 1971, p. 14.
29. A. E. Glancey, *Amer. J. Physiol. Optics* 6(1925):393–402.
30. George Gorin (Wilmington, Dela.: Publish or Perish, Inc., 1982).

31. T. Grossmann, *Klin. Mol. Augenh.* 129(4)(1956):559–561 (Ger.).
32. S. Gyorffy, *Transactions of the International Ophthalmic Optical Congress. (1961)* (London: C. Crosby Lockwood & Son, Ltd., 1962), 266–267.
33. G. Hakushima, *Amer. J. Ophthal.* 55(1963):612–613.
34. S. Hardy, *The Optician* 148(1964):566.
35. Christian G. Hertel, *Vollstandize Anweisung zum Glas* (Schleiffen, 1716).
36. Emory Hill, *American Encyclopedia of Ophthalmology,* Vol. 7 (Chicago: Cleveland Press, 1915), 4894–4953.
37. G. D. Hunt, F.S.M.C., *The Optician,* February 22, 1963, p. 168.
38. Edward Jackson, *Amer. J. Ophthal.* 10(1927):606.
39. Emile Javal, *Annales d'oculistique.* Volume 55, 9th pub., Volume 5, 3d & 4th issues, March 31 & April 30, 1966. Translated by Mrs. Linda L. McDonald in the December 10, 1970, issue of *Optometric Weekly,* p. 23.
40. Robert T. Jordan, *Stechert-Hafner Book News* 18(8) (1964):97–100; (9):113–117.
41. J. H. Jugler, *Bibliothaecae Ophthalmicae* (Hamburg, 1783). (The first bibliography and history of ophthalmology.)
42. H. Kirsch, *Klin. Mol. Augenh.* 115(1949):109–111 (Ger.).
43. Henry A. Knoll, *J. Amer. Optom. Assn.* 38(1967):946–948.
44. F. W. Law, *Ann. oculist.* 199(1966):143–154. (Fr.).
45. Ralph I. Lloyd, *Guildcraft.* 16(1): June/July, 1942, pp. 34–50.
46. Maddox, *The Clinical Use of Prisms* (London, 1893).
47. Pierre Marley, *Spectacles and Spyglasses* (Paris: Hoebeke, 1988).
48. T. G. Martens, *Proc. Mayo Clin.* 35(1960):217–222.
49. Mauzini, *L'Occhiale all'occhio* (Bologna, 1660). (The second book on the making of spectacles.)
50. Francis W. McAllister, *The Optical Journal* March 15, 1917, p. 761.
51. Wm. Y. McAllister, *Optical Catalogue* (Philadelphia, 1870).
52. K. Mueller, *Klin. Mol. Augenh.* 137(1960):104–107 (Ger.).
53. J. F. C. Muggeridge, "The Discovery of Spectacles," *Royal Soc. Health J.,* August 1982.
54. N. J. T. M. Needham, *Science and Civilization in China,* Vol. 4, Part 1 (Cambridge, 1962), 118–122.
55. George Nerney, "Developments in Metal Frame and Mounting Manufacture," *Optical Journal Review,* January 15, 1941.
56. I. Newton, *Opticks* (London, 1704).
57. Henri Obstfeld, *Int'l. Coll. Club Newsletter,* October 1991.
58. G. H. Oliver, *Brit. Med. J.* October 25, 1913, pp. 1049–1054.
59. Lyle S. Powell, *The Eye Ear Nose and Throat Monthly,* Lawrence, Kansas, March 1930.
60. Justine Randers-Pehrson, Notes to accompany an exhibit on the early history of spectacles at the Armed Forces Medical Library/Reference Section—Washington, July–August 1956.
61. O. D. Rasmussen, *The Optician* 139(1960):569–570.
62. C. J. Robb, *The Optician* 141(1961):526.
63. Von Rohr, *Eyes and Spectacles* (London, 1912).
64. E. Rosen, *Isis* (Cambridge, Mass.) June 1953, pp. 135–36:4–10.
65. E. Rosen, *Arch. int. d'histoire des sciences* 7(1954):1–15.
66. J. Wm. Rosenthal, *A History of Spectacles.* AAO Museum Pamphlet, 1991.
67. C. W. Rucker, *Proc. Mayo Clin.* 35(1960):209–216.
68. C. W. Rucker, *Curr. Med. Digest* 29(1962):51–57.
69. W. F. Scott, *The Optician* 140(1960):269–272.
70. Scrini & Fortin, *Manuel pratique pour le choix des verres de lunettes et l'examen de la vision* (Paris, 1906). First Edition.
71. Thomas Shastid, *Encyclopedia of Ophthalmology* (Casey Wood) "History of Ophthalmology," p. 8525.
72. Dr. Jules Sichel, *Spectacles* (Boston, 1850).
73. E. T. Smith, *Med. J. Australia* 2(1928):578–587.
74. C. Snyder, *Arch. Ophthal.* 55(1956):397–407.
75. Arnold Sorsby, *A Short History of Ophthalmology* (London and New York, 1948).
76. J. Strajduhr, *Lijecnicki Vjesnik.* March–April 1952, pp. 70–71 (Zagret, Yugoslavia).
77. C. J. S. Thompson, *The Connoisseur.* 94(1934):231–239 (London).
78. P. D. Trevor-Roper, *Med. Illust. Lond.* 6(7)(1952):359–368.
79. G. L. E. Turner, *A Spectacle of Spectacles* (London, 1988).
80. Edwin P. Wells, *The Optical Journal,* p. 26.
81. H. A. William, *Aesthet. Med.* 13(1964):1–15, 1964 (Berlin).
82. W. H. Wollaston, *Periscopic Spectacles* (London, 1804).
83. Shi-hwan Won, *History of Eyeglasses in Korea* (Seoul, Korea: Opticians Association of Korea, 1986).

6

Optical Manufacturing in the United States

While new inventions in the optical arena sparked attention and hope in the afflicted, making these aids available to the general public through mass production was another matter. Prior to the Industrial Revolution, production of optical goods was done almost solely by hand. New machinery in the years following changed the face of optical manufacturing.

Following is an article on the history of lens grinding in America by Deborah Jean Warner of the National Museum of American History.

> The first American optician who has yet come to light was a woman. In 1753 the widow of Balthasar Sommer advertised in the New York Gazette that she was a "grinder of all sorts of optic glasses." Forty years later John Benson, a lapidary from London, announced in the New York Daily Advertiser that he "polished scratch'd glasses." The one other early American optician we know of is David Rittenhouse, whose ability to make and use instruments for astronomy and surveying was justly famous. By 1780 Rittenhouse was sending to Europe for good optical glass to grind into telescope lenses. In 1783 he ground spectacle lenses for George Washington. A search through eighteenth century newspapers might uncover a bit more information about Mrs. Sommer and Mr. Benson, and evidence of a few more people like them. But I doubt there would be much.

American demand for optical goods was simply too small to support a local industry. And because optical lenses are high-value, low-bulk durable goods, they were easily imported from low-cost production centers in Europe.

In addition to questions of supply and demand, the very nature of the optical business ensured that it would not easily take root in American soil. The optical business is, of course, really two businesses. At one end of the spectrum is the production of spectacle lenses which, even in the eighteenth century, had long been industrialized and mechanized, and required little in the way of either training or artistry. At the other end the grinding and polishing of lenses, mirrors and prisms for scientific or military purposes was a difficult and demanding task. There was very little business in the middle, the area in which colonial craftsmen in other fields excelled. As the nineteenth century unfolded Americans began to develop an optical capability, yet we continued to import the bulk of our optical goods. By the Civil War some Americans were making precision lenses that compared favorably with those made in Europe, but owing in large measure to the high cost of American labor, we never developed a strong, independent industry. American spectacle lenses did not hold their own until, toward the end of the century, the establishment of integrated and mechanized factories were protected by a high tariff.

The War of 1812, which disrupted commerce with England stimulated the development of a number of American industries. I suspect it was a factor in McAllister's [see Appendix 3] decision to manufacture spectacle frames. It seems, however, to have had little impact on the optical business. The only American I've found who did optical work was Thomas Whitney of Philadelphia—and that for two years only. In 1817 Whitney added to his standard advertisement for surveying compasses the notice, "also makes optical glasses, glasses for spectacles, &c." While Whitney could do optical work, he was not primarily an optician. When English lenses again became available he dropped this line of work.

When the American optical business got underway in the 1820's, it was composed of two types of people: German immigrants who had learned their trade through apprenticeships in Europe, and native-born Americans of English descent, who were largely self taught. The first of the Germans was Isaac Schnaitman [see Appendix 3] who arrived in Philadelphia in 1824, announcing his presence by entering "lenses and spectacle glasses" in the Franklin Institute Fair. The judges, who were in good position to know the scientific resources in Philadelphia, expressed unusual exuberance over his work. In bestowing his award they hoped "that he will find encouragement in his business, as it is a branch of industry deserving the patronage of the Institute." The following year found their ardor undiminished: "The principal merit of this Artist's work lies in the grinding and polishing of the glasses which are prepared by him. The execution of these was very good; their form true. It is desirable that Mr. Schnaitman should meet with sufficient encouragement to induce him to attend exclusively to this branch of business, which we believe, is not carried on by any other mechanic in this city." In 1836 Schnaitman obtained a patent for an improved bifocal. His invention involved grinding "each glass so as to have two focal centres," rather than cementing segments of different foci. I suspect it was moderately successful as he continued to advertise "Patent Double Focus Spectacle Glasses" for some twenty years.

During the 1830's and early 1840's several other German immigrant opticians followed Schnaitman's lead. By 1837 John George Wolfe was in New York advertising as "optician, manufactures all kinds of optical glass," and his "specimens of optical glass grinding" won a diploma at the American Institute Fair. Philip Bowers identified himself as a "glass grinder." Soon after he set up shop in New York, Leon Lewenberg was advertising a $400 five inch objective lens for a telescope. He also had a blank for a 12–14" lens but "from want of means cannot proceed with it." Lewenberg's example reminds us that optics, like so many small businesses in nineteenth century America, was at best precarious. Many opticians must have wanted to tackle large and complex jobs, but few had the necessary resources.

Frederic Hall [see Appendix 3], who settled in Cincinnati in the mid 1840's, advertised that he was prepared to manufacture "to order, on short notice, and of the best quality every description of Telescopes, Magic Lanterns, Dissolving Scenes, Thermometers, Barometers, &c. [and] the latest improved Daguerreotype Apparatus." Bruno Hasert, also of Cincinnati, made a six inch telescope for the Farmer's College in Ohio, and advertised others "from one to nine inches in diameter." Hasert was particularly proud of his microscopes, even going so far as to enter one in the London Crystal Palace Exhibition of 1851.

The political upheavals of 1848 which swelled the German immigration to the United States had a major impact on the American optical and scientific instrument business. Bausch and Lomb were notable optical 48-ers, as was the microscope maker, Joseph Zentmayer. I would like to call your attention to other men who, while not so famous, were perhaps more typical. One optical 48-er, Adolph Wirth by name, supplied lenses for surveyors' levels and transits made by America's foremost mathematical instrument maker. Another, Charles Usener, made lenses for the leading American camera manufacturers. Yet another was William Gerhardt. Together with E. Prussen, Gerhardt opened an "Optical Institute" in New York City where he gave "theoretical and practical instruction in optics, manufacturing achromatic telescopes, achromatic microscopes, single lenses, and Speaces' achromatic object glasses, speculums for telescopes, achromatic Signeri apparatus, magic lanterns in every style. Also, apparatus for the analyzation of light." Gerhardt later moved to Philadelphia, and there he met the young scientist-to-be, Elihu Thomson, who left for us a wonderful description of Gerhardt's workshop. It was "on the second floor of a small, two story dwelling and consisted of two rooms not more, perhaps than 12 × 12 feet in dimensions. His equipment was mainly a foot-lathe of ancient type, a work-bench, and a small coal-stove of ordinary type, in which he actually moulded and annealed fair sized pieces of optical glass, such as used for prisms." Here, Thomson continued, Gerhardt produced "some of the finest optical work I have ever seen."

The greatest concentration of German opticians was in New York, but many fanned out across the country, settling in communities in which they had little optical competition. In the antebellum period, German opticians settled in Albany, Brooklyn, Chicago, Cincinnati, Cleveland, Louisville, Memphis, New Haven, New Orleans, Rochester, St. Louis, San Francisco, Washington, D.C., and Worcester, as well as New York and Philadelphia.

As might have been expected, the demand for precision optics was not great in these fairly new and raw towns. Most opticians paid their rent by selling a variety of mathematical, philosophical and optical instruments, most of which they did not make. Several, to distinguish themselves from the competition, advertised their connections with leading optical houses in Europe. M. Hassler & Co. of Philadelphia advertised "the New Conservation Convex and Concave Glasses of Kriegsman Brothers, Opticians at the Prussian Court, whose only agents in the United States, we are." Edward Scholetzer in Rochester boasted "the exclusive right of sale of those spectacles ground at the Optic-Oculistic Institute, Leipsig, which are so celebrated for their spherical accuracy." As the nineteenth century advanced, the import business remained strong, becoming the primary occupation for many immigrant opticians.

Most of the immigrant opticians came from Germany, but not all. John Roach was an immigrant from Ireland who advertised "lenses ground to any curve required" and "object glasses of various sizes, ground to order and warranted achromatic." Other lens grinders, whose country or origin is as yet unknown, were John Smith [see Appendix 3], who identified himself as a "manufacturer of lenses," and Abraham Prince whose Stanhope lenses, exhibited in 1844, were believed to be the first ever made in this country.

While European opticians learned their trade through apprenticeships and other on-the-job training programs, most would-be American opticians had to learn on their own how to grind and polish lenses and mirrors. What is surprising is that so many tried. The impetus for their endeavors seems to have been the growing popular and professional interest in science and education, which began around 1830, and which led to a growing demand for telescopes and microscopes. In an 1830 article "On the Improvement in the Microscope" Edward Thomas mentioned achromatic instruments recently constructed by his friend Alden Allen and himself. Thomas died soon thereafter, and nothing else is known of Allen, or of the John Boggs who exhibited a "compound microscope" at the Franklin Institute Fair of 1833.

The first important microscope maker in America was Charles A. Spencer of Canastota, N.Y. His biographer termed him a "genius." Unlike the typical American entrepreneur, Spencer was more interested in excellence than income. Fortunately he was able to keep going long enough to develop and produce some very wonderful instruments. Spencer issued his first circular around 1838. Within ten years his microscopes were acclaimed as good as, and sometimes superior to, the best European ones. Americans took special pride in the fact that this achievement had been by a backwoodsman. Spencer was succeeded by his sons, and that business was eventually bought by the American Optical Company.

The American telescope business also began around 1830 when Amasa Holcomb, a surveyor in what is now Southwick, Mass., began making Newtonian reflectors on simple mounts. To promote his wares Holcomb took a telescope to Yale where Professor Benjamin Silliman was an enthusiastic proponent of the American instrument industry. In the *American Journal of Science* which he edited, Silliman inserted notices of Holcomb's telescopes, adding that "It gives us pleasure to aid in making known an artist, self taught, and as, we believe, worthy of patronage and encouragement." Holcomb also found encouragement from the Franklin Institute, which examined several of his telescopes, pronouncing them reasonably good, and cheaper than European imports. Holcomb managed to sell perhaps a dozen or two telescopes, but he was soon overtaken by younger and more accomplished men.

In 1844 Josiah Bennett Allen, an optician of Springfield, Mass., showed a reflecting telescope at the Massachusetts Charitable Mechanics Association Fair. The telescope probably wasn't very good but the judges awarded it a diploma, stating that "The first early efforts to establish this manufacture among us ought to be encouraged."

The following year, in 1845, Henry Fitz of New York won a gold medal at the American Institute Fair for a six inch telescope, "the first good American achromatic ever heard of." Fitz was a locksmith by training, and a pioneer photographer—he is reputed to have been the first in the world to take a daguerreotype self portrait. Fitz was undoubtedly proud of his telescopes, but he was also keen to make a living. Accordingly, he took steps to industrialize the process, devising machines for grinding and polishing the lenses, and hiring cheap labor to operate them. Yankee girls were best, he said. They had the necessary skills, their wages were low, and they were unlikely to learn the business and strike out on their own.

The other important antebellum telescope maker was Alvan Clark, a portrait painter in Boston who began to figure lenses around 1846. Like Spencer, Clark aimed for quality, and by the time of the Civil War had gained recognition in Europe as well as across the United States. Fitz died young. Clark, on the other hand, lived into his 80's. Together with his equally accomplished sons he made all the large refracting telescopes in the United States, and many medium sized ones too, as well as several important ones for European observatories.

Soon after Daguerre's announcement of his photographic process several Americans were including Daguerreotype apparatus among the optical instruments they were prepared to manufacture. The first American to specialize in photographic optics was Charles C. Harrison of New York. By 1850 he was advertising as a "manufacturer of cameras, and camera lenses, of all sizes and the latest improvements." His globular lens, patented in 1862, won high commendations from many quarters.

City directories and census reports list a great many other opticians and spectacle makers but, as far as I've been able to tell, almost all of these opticians simply sold optical goods, while the spectacle makers made the frames. In addition to Charles Schnaitman whom I've already mentioned, I've found only a few other antebellum Americans who actually figured spectacle lenses. M. Hassler & Co. boasted a "superior stock of spectacle glasses, of their own manufacture," while Louis Shrisheim advertised spectacles "ground by him . . . warranted superior in quality, polish and finish to any made in this country."

In 1804 the English scientist, William Hyde Wollaston, obtained a patent for a meniscus lens for spectacles which gave a wider field of view than did the ordinary biconvex or biconcave. These periscopic lenses were illustrated and described in Sir David Brewster's book on Optics published at London in 1833, and reprinted that same year in Philadelphia. I have not, however, found any American ads for meniscus lenses until 1844–45. After that date such ads were common. Many probably referred to imported lenses, but at least two American opticians—John Burt and Henry M. Paine—made lenses of this sort.

Burt's listing in the Hartford city directories for 1844–47 is "optic glasses" or "meniscus optic glasses." By 1851 he was sufficiently confident of his product to hire William Willard, a jeweler in Syracuse, to be his agent. Willard advertised "J. BURT'S periscopic, Gold and Silver Spectacles—the best glass ever yet discovered. The glass is ground upon scientific principles, which not only strengthens the eyes, but give a larger field of vision than any other glass used . . . the name 'J. BURT' is stamped upon the frames. . . ." In 1859 Burt and Willard obtained a patent for a spectacle frame held to the head by cups. However curious this frame, Burt remained in business as a spectacle manufacturer throughout the 1860's.

H.M. Paine brought out his perifocal spectacles in 1843, showing them at the Franklin Institute Fair accompanied by testimonials from physicians pronouncing their superiority to all others in use. These lenses, reputedly different from the French meniscus or the English periscopic, were touted as "Solely of American invention." They were manufactured at the Optical Works in North Oxford, Mass., said to be the only establishment of the kind on this continent. How these lenses were actually figured is not yet known. In 1846, however, Paine obtained a patent for heating a biconvex lens and letting it melt into a meniscus. Henry M. Paine was not primarily an optician, but he had several relatives who were. John P. Paine, also of Worcester, invented an instrument "whereby the exact focal distance of each eye is measured with mathematical precision" in 1847, and four years later he patented an improved spectacle frame. Charles M. Paine, a Boston optician for some fifty years, showed 'one case of perifocal spectacles' at the Massachusetts Charitable Mechanics Association Fair of 1847. After this showing Paine's perifocals disappeared for two decades, reemerging in 1866, in Newark, where Henry M. Paine was then living, manufactured and sold by Henry's brother George. Henry M. Paine, the originator of the perifocals, was a typical ingenious Yankee, fascinated by the workings of things, and eager to improve them all. In 1849 he patented a portable copying press; in 1852 he patented a system for ventilating railroad cars; and in later years he obtained more than a dozen patents for such things as steam generators and electromagnets.

By and large the patterns in the lens grinding business established by the time of the Civil War held for the next quarter century. The most important change in this latter period was the introduction of incorporated stock companies which provided the financial and managerial resources necessary for expanded production. The year 1867 saw the incorporation of the Boston Optical Works, formed expressly to enable Robert Tolles "to compete successfully by enlarged resources with the European Mfrs. & thus make the 'Hub' renowned for its superior telescopes." That same year the American Optical Company, capitalized at $150,000, was organized in New York to produce Harrison's camera lenses and other photographic apparatus. The American Optical Company of Southbridge, Mass. was incorporated in 1869. Although AO then made only spectacle frames, when, in 1883, it began to manufacture spectacle lenses, it was able to do so on a scale that was truly competitive with Europe.[1]

As you can see, numerous individuals played a part in the early history of optical development and manufacturing. Following is the history of optical manufacturing in one area of the United States—Southbridge, Massachussetts—the site of American Optical Company. The endeavors of a few families led to the development of this company—a major player in the history of optical manufacturing.

Early Spectacle Makers of Southbridge

ROBERT W. MCMASTER IN HIS SPEECH TO THE SOUTHBRIDGE HISTORICAL SOCIETY MAY 1983

It all started with a man named William Beecher who was born in Southbridge, Connecticut (near Danbury) in 1805. He learned the jewelry business in Providence. He and his brother Smith Beecher came to Southbridge in 1826. Smith Beecher was Mrs. Ruth (Beecher) Eaton's grandfather. William Beecher was 21 years old in 1826 when he set up his jewelry store at Hartwell's Corner with a Robert Cole as an apprentice at 14 years of age. We will hear more about him.

1827   William Beecher married Hanna Ammidown, a Southbridge girl, 2-20-1827.
(B. 1-18-06) (D. 3-28-61)
Three Children:
William Ammidown Beecher B. 7-10-1828 D. 7-9-1876 [see Appendix 3]
Hannah Jane B. 5-7-1832
Nancy Ellen B. 7-5-1836 D. 1-14-1871
Son William married Hester Billings Thacher in Boston, 10-12-1853. (Died 10-22-1853) A tragedy—no information on it.
Remarried Ester Ann Stridiron 10-7-1869 at St. Croix in Danish West Indies where he was in business (now Virgin Islands).
One daughter, Jane Elizabeth B. 1-14-1871.
Daughter Hannah Jane married Reverend Oakman Stearns who later became Dr. Stearns, Professor of Biblical Literature at Newton Theological School from which he graduated.

1831   William Beecher was Town Clerk 1831–32. He built the house at 185 Main Street which was torn down by Credit Union a few years ago and was known to most of us as the Robert H. Cole residence.

1833   Started making spectacles. [Cited as the start of the American Optical Company.]

1853   Member of Board of Selectmen.

1860   Member of State Legislature from the Dudley-Southbridge District.

1861   His wife Hanna died 3-28-1861.

1862   Retired from spectacle manufacturing. Moved to Boston and Newton, Mass. Retained his suffrage in Southbridge and visited often.

1892   Died in Newton at age of 87. Buried in Oakridge.

[William Beecher] brought a new trade and skill to town in 1826. He started to make silver spectacles [Figure 76], because the imports were scarce and expensive. He apparently was a skillful mechanic and inventor as he developed means of producing thin steel spectacles which were immediately in big demand.

From [Beecher's] small beginning at Hartwell's Corner, the manufacturing of spectacles in this town grew on and on. At the time of his death in 1892, Southbridge was producing approximately two million pairs of spectacles and eyeglasses and approximately one million pairs of lenses per year.

I will now review the early optical companies of Southbridge. The main figures were William Beecher, Robert Cole, Holdridge Ammidown, and [Ammidown's] son Lucius.

Beecher married Holdridge's sister.
Cole married Holdridge's daughter.
So Beecher and Holdridge Ammidown were brothers-in-law.
Cole and Lucius Ammidown were brothers-in-law.
So there were close family ties in the early companies.

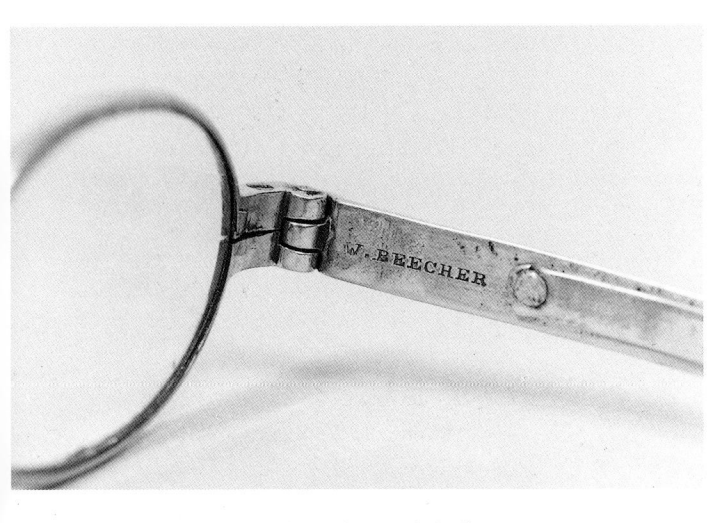

Figure 76. W. Beecher-made spectacles in silver.

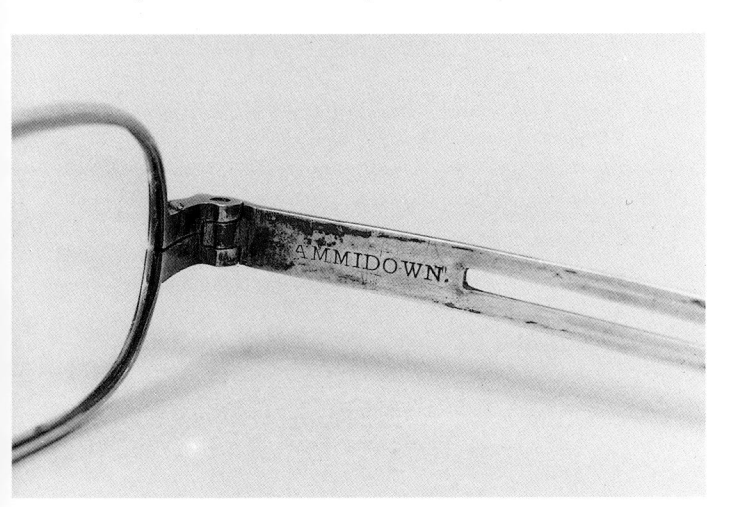

Figure 77. Ammidown-made spectacles in silver.

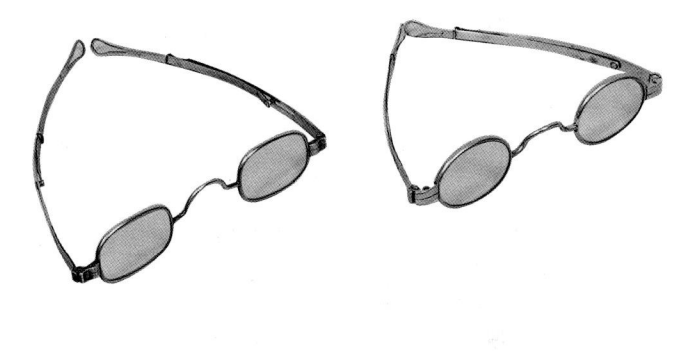

Figure 78. Ammidown (left) and Beecher (right) spectacles.

A list of the early spectacle makers follows:

	Co. Name	Location	Owners
1833	William Beecher	Hartwell's Corner	William Beecher was the sole owner. Age 28.
1840	Ammidown & Putney	Lower Main St.	H. Ammidown and J. Putney
1842	Ammidown & Son	Lower Main St. [see Appendix 3]	H. Ammidown & his son Lucius
1850	Ammidown & Co.	Lower Main St. [Figures 77 & 78]	Lucius & his brother-in-law Robert H. Cole. Lucius died 1853.
1860	Beecher & Cole	Lower Main St. [Figures 78, 79, & 80]	William Beecher married H. Ammidown's daughter. Robert Cole married H. Ammidown's daughter.

OPTICAL MANUFACTURING IN U.S. 55

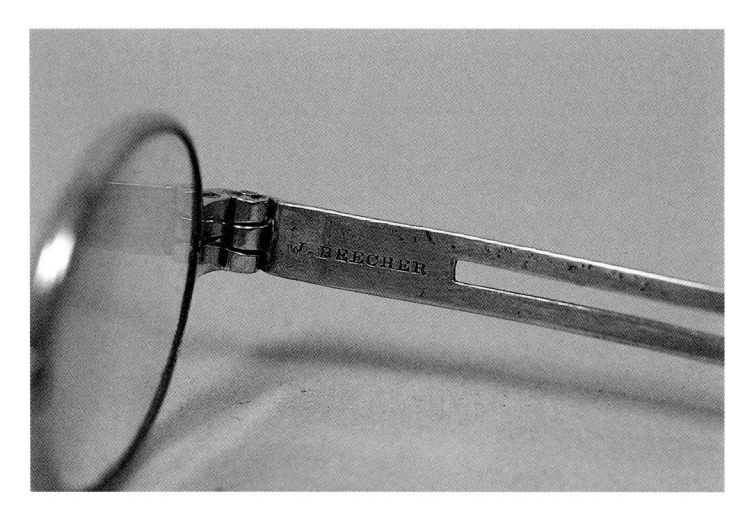

Figure 79. W. Beecher-made spectacles in silver.

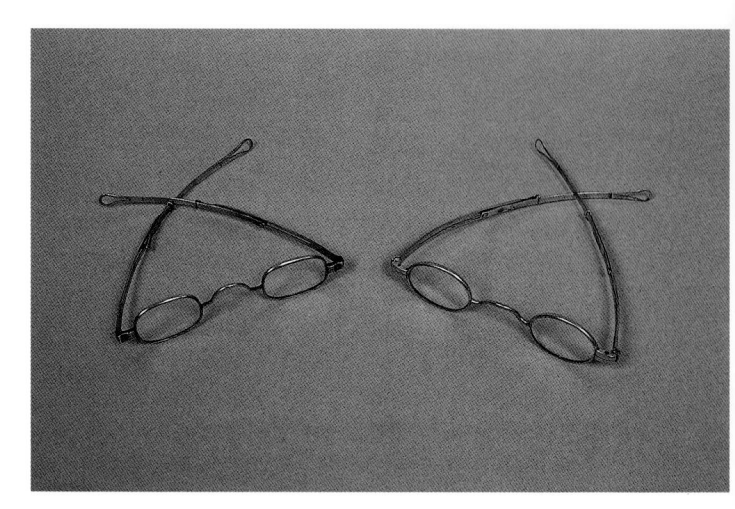

Figure 80. W. Beecher-made spectacles in silver.

1862	Robert H. Cole & Co.	Lower Main St.	Robert H. Cole* and his brother E. Merritt Cole
1865	E. Edmonds & Son	Mechanic & Main	E. Edmonds & his son C.S. Edmonds
1868	H.C. Ammidown & Co.	Mechanic & Main	Henry C. Ammidown & C.S. Edmonds
1869	H.C. Ammidown & Co.	Mechanic & Main	G.W. Wells* & H.C. Wells

*Cole and Wells merged to form American Optical Company [AO]. The original 1869 stockholders of the AO were:

President	Robert H. Cole (Age 61)	150 shares
Treasurer	E.M. Cole (Brother of Robert)	80 shares
	A.M. Cheney	50 shares
Clerk	G.W. Wells (Age 23)	40 shares
	Hiram Wells (Brother of G.W.W.)	50 shares
	C.S. Edmonds	30 shares
		400 shares

Robert H. Cole was probably the first employee of William Beecher in 1826. When William Beecher decided to give up the jewelry shop in 1833 and devote his efforts to making spectacles, Robert H. Cole bought the jewelry store and operated it until 1850. When he became a partner in Ammidown & Co., due to his brother-in-law's (Lucius) poor health, he participated in the merger of 1869 and became the first president of American Optical Company, a position that he held until 1891, when he resigned.

[Cole's] daughter Ella gave the town the area known as Cole Forest, which is adjacent to the Oak Ridge Cemetery. She also gave funds for the Cole Trade School, which is now part of the high school.

Through his association with William Beecher, [Cole]

was involved in spectacle making from 1833 to 1892 (59 years). G. W. Wells became treasurer in 1879 and president in 1891. His sons Channing, Albert, and Cheney all started to work in the 1890's. Then the third generation took part in the AO business, which included George B. Wells [son of Albert B. Wells], John, Turner, and McGregory [sons of Channing McGregory Wells]. Peak employment in Southbridge was reached in 1942 with 5,486 employees. There were also manufacturing facilities in Canada; Keene, New Hampshire; Brattleboro, Vermont; Cambridge, Massachusetts; Frederick, Maryland; Buffalo, New York; England, Germany, and Brazil and about 250 branch shops in the United States.

AO was sold to Warner-Lambert in 1967. It in turn sold most of the Southbridge facility to M&R Industries in 1982.

Through the years, AO has provided wages for countless numbers of people in this general area. American Optical Company and the Wells families have given funds to many local groups, including churches, the YMCA, and the Harrington Memorial Hospital. The G.W. Wells Foundation continues to give large amounts to area groups.

Albert Wells was a collector of artifacts, and in his lifetime he accumulated thousands of items. Albert, his brother Cheney, and his son George conceived the idea of a living museum to house all the items. Hence, Old Sturbridge Village was built, and it stands today as one of the greatest living museums in the United States.

LENSDALE

Let's return now to Lensdale, where I spent 40 years as an engineer, to give you a brief picture of the company

In the late 1800s, Lensdale made double convex and concave items and flat cylinders. Then it made periscopic lenses (first step towards deeper curves inside for better vision). By 1910, it was making the center series—spheres and toric lenses with much deeper inside curves. The following documents Lensdales's further activity:

1910	The Kryptok bifocal, the first fused bifocal
1915	The one-piece bifocal
1925	The Tillyer "D" bifocal, a fused bifocal, color corrected
About 1925	Tillyer Series, spheres and toric lenses corrected for marginal vision
1935	The Tillyer, a curved top bifocal
1940	The Tillyer Flat Top
1960	The Trifocal Executive, a one-piece with a wide field

OTHER SOUTHBRIDGE SPECTACLE MAKERS

Between 1869 and 1900, five other groups were organized to make spectacles in Southbridge. Most of these spectacle makers gained their experience at American Optical Company and started out on their own.

1. 1878   Vinton and Jacobs Spectacle Shop—very little information on this venture.
2. 1882   Southbridge Optical Company—sold to AO in 1901.
3. 1887   Dupaul Young Optical Company—sold to Shuron in 1924.
4. 1895   Blanchard Optical Company—very little information.
5. 1900   Central Optical Company—in business until 1951.

SOUTHBRIDGE OPTICAL COMPANY

This company was founded in 1882 and 1883. William C. Barnes was listed as president and treasurer. They started business in the old Spec Shop on lower Main Street. In 1885, Benajah V. Bugbee was president and general manager. In 1888, the company erected the wooden building on Marcy Street. Harrington Cutlery occupied the building for many years. Several additions were made to it, and in 1898 it was three stories × 25' × 150'.

After the death of B.V. Bugbee in 1898, the officers were his sons:
L.W. Bugbee, President
B.L. Bugbee, Treasurer and General Manager
C.B. McKinstry, Director
A.W. Wheeler, Director

The company manufactured spectacles and eyeglasses in gold, gold-filled, and steel and employed over 100 people in 1898. It was sold to American Optical Company in 1901.

L.W. Bugbee worked for AO as head of product development until 1918, when he moved to Indianapolis to manage Continental Optical Company, which later became Shuron Continental. He was an inventor and through the years had 86 patents granted to him.

B.L. Bugbee drowned in a canoe accident on the Quinebaug River in Sturbridge in 1907.

Much of the preceding information came from L.W. Bugbee's son, Willis Bugbee, who was born here and lived here [Southbridge] before going to MIT and Oxford University in England, where he majored in physics. Later he worked for several optical companies. He is now a patent lawyer in the Detroit area.

DUPAUL YOUNG OPTICAL COMPANY

This company was established in 1887 by Jos. M. DuPaul, Leon Young and J. A. Caron, all experienced spectacle and eyeglass makers. Mr. DuPaul started to work for E. Edmonds and Son in 1866 and was considered one of the veteran spectacle makers of Southbridge.

Both DuPaul and Young married sisters of J. A. Caron, so these men were brothers-in-law. In 1925, George DuPaul joined the company, which became DuPaul Central Optical Company. The company continued operation until 1951.

In 1887, the company started manufacturing in old Stephen Richards' shop on lower Elm Street. It was incorporated in 1892 with 65 employees. In 1896, it moved to the old Spec Shop on lower Main Street.

In 1896, the officers were:

Leon Young, President
J.A. Caron, Treasurer
F.H. Orr, Clerk (died in 1912)
J.M. DuPaul, Superintendent

In 1907, Felix Gatenaux built the brick building on Marcy Street and employed about 200 people in 1915. In 1918, he built a lens plant on DuPaul Street, which was called DuPaul Lockart. In 1924, he sold the business to Shuron Standard of Rochester. He operated the company as a division of Shuron. In 1927, the business moved to Rochester. Leon Caron, son of J. A., was the assistant treasurer from 1915 to 1927. The company made steel and gold-filled spectacles and eyeglasses.

BLANCHARD OPTICAL COMPANY

This company existed on lower Elm Street in about 1895. I've seen several references to it, and an advertisement for it appeared in an 1897 issue of the *Optical Journal.* Beyond this, I have no information.

CENTRAL OPTICAL COMPANY

This company was founded in 1900 with François Tetreault, president; Alfred Galipeau, vice president; P.N. LeClaire, treasurer; and E.D. Desroisier, secretary. It started manufacturing in the basement of Blanchard Optical Company on Elm Street and then moved to another building on the same street in 1901.

In 1910, the officers were:

Ronaldo Guilmette, President
Hector M. LeClaire, Treasurer
Edward LeClaire, Secretary

The company made goggles for shopworkers, mechanics, and motorists.

SMALL SOUTHBRIDGE OPTICAL MANUFACTURERS

The following is a list of small optical manufacturers in Southbridge that existed for short periods after 1900:

Eastern Optical Company, Crane Street, Alfred LaPierre, 1914
Quality Lens Co., Hartwell Street, Wilfrid Lavoie, 1916, Central Street, M. Ernest Decelles, in a small store of N.E. Putney, 1895
Southbridge Optical Supply Company, Central Street, M. Zepherin LePage, automobile goggles, 1914
Southbridge Toric Lens Company, Joseph Ouimet, 1919
Independent Optical Company
Southbridge Spectacle Manufacturing Company
Nomar Optical Company
Eccel Rest Guard Company
South Toric Lens Company
Optical Specialty Company
United States Optical Company.

American Optical Company Activities

Robert McMaster gave us the preceding history of the events that led to the establishment of American Optical Company. The following presents details of the company's undertakings.

In 1883, American Optical Company began manufacturing its own lenses. Prior to that, all of its lenses were imported. The first production-line type of lens, the Centex, came with the establishment of a system of interchangeability of sizes and a systemic standard of foci for its lenses. Previously, lenses were individually and painstakingly set into frames using hand edging. Uniform density, clarity, and centration were ignored.

The company's glass-molding operation saved time in "roughing out" for high power lenses, strong base curves, etc. The grinding room (485 feet long and 128 feet wide) held 108 machines. Each machine held 200 to 1,000 spindles, depending on the curvature of the lenses to be ground. Total grinding capacity was said to be 10,000 spindles. In this same building, lenses were cut and edged to the desired shape.

In addition to supplying white glass, American Optical Company supplied blue, smoked, amber, pink, amethyst, euphos (yellow-green) glass, and roentgen.

The following excerpt regarding American Optical Company was taken from an article by G. W. Wells in the *Quinebaug Historical Society Leaflets*:

> Until the year 1884, all spectacle lenses excepting a very few, manufactured by hand to fit special cases, were imported, and the growing demand upon the American Optical Company was such that is was practically impossible to get a proper and adequate supply, owing to the indifference of the foreign manufacturers to increase their factories as they could not believe that the demand from the United States was legitimate. It was also impossible to get goods of the proper quality and sure of focus. The orders were often a year in being filled, and in some cases, it was impossible for our company to fill orders for frames set with lenses, which was the usual way in which goods were then purchased, for the want of lenses to go into the frames.
>
> Under the date of February 15, 1871, the following is a report of the examination of imported lenses by George W. Wells (clerk of the American Optical Company at this time).

> "This unreliablity of the focus numbers in the packages as they were imported was an important feature in determining the American Optical Co. to enter the manufacture of lenses, so as to get something more reliable not only in quality but in focus."
>
> In 1883, the first steps were taken toward producing lenses in Southbridge. It was a mighty task; there were very few in this country who knew anything about the practical problems involved, and importers were prophesying failure.
>
> April 1, 1883, work was commenced in earnest in building machinery and getting in position to manufacture spherical lenses. In the fall of the same year, machinery was placed in the Mechanic Building, size 60 ft. by 30 ft., two stories and basement; and on January 18, 1884, the first finished lenses were produced. Much time, labor and money were spent on this venture with some failures and discouragements. All of the machinery produced was condemned in the fall of 1884 at which time there were 80 spindles running. At this time, an entirely new system of machinery was built to supplant the old wooden machinery. The first iron machinery in the world with the old English motion was installed in 1885.
>
> The manufacture of cylinder and compound lenses was commenced in 1893 and the dioptric system of measurement adopted.
>
> The company purchased and operated the Hardy-Delaney patents for grinding cylinder lenses which was a decided improvement over the old methods.[3]

Lens Grinding The following is from an article in *The Southbridge Journal*, dated February 15, 1884:

> It is well known that the American Optical Company has only made the frames of eyeglasses and spectacles, importing the lenses. For some time, they have been contemplating and preparing for the grinding of lenses themselves, and have finally got this department in running order, although not on a scale to supply the entire establishment with all the glass required.
>
> A brief description of the process will prove to be an interesting contribution to local reading. The business is carried on in a building near the "Spec Shop" which the company purchased from the Central Mills Company for this purpose. The glass used is the finest quality of plate glass, but for convenience and other reasons, it is imported

in small squares rather than the large sheets seen in store windows. When the glass is unpacked, it is taken by girls who break off the corners leaving it in oblong shaped pieces. Then boys place the pieces in rows, one deep on large concave shaped iron disks, and fill the interstices with fine sawdust. These disks are then heated by steam and partly filled with hot melted pitch.

A convex disk of similar size and curve is then placed inside the concave disk in the hot pitch. When cool, the disks are separated and the pieces of glass are all stuck by the pitch in the convex one, the spaces which were filled with sawdust being left vacant. This convex disk is placed on a standard so that it can be revolved. Upon this is placed a concave disk of smaller size; the smaller disk riding on one side of the larger like a boy with his cap on the side of his head, but being stationary.

The large glass-covered disk is slowly revolved and coarse emery powder sprinkled between the disks to grind down the edges of the glass. When this process is completed, the glass has the milky appearance known as a ground glass. The process is repeated a great many times, each time a finer emery being used till at last only a very fine rouge is needed to polish the lenses. When the disks are taken from the last grinders or polishers, the glass is ground on one side and perfectly clear and spotless. The whole process is then repeated so that the lenses may have the same convexity on both sides. The lenses are then focused, packed, and labeled and sent to the main shop.[4]

New Lens Machinery

The following is from an article in *The Southbridge Journal*, dated August 15, 1884:

> The new machinery can be best understood by saying that it reverses the operation. The under disc is concave and the glass is stuck to a convex disc which turns about, by an eccentric motion in the concave disc. By this process, the emery powder is retained on the concave disc and as none has to be applied after starting, the machine does not require such close attention as the old one, causing a savings in labor. The process of grinding by the new machines not only grinds the curve but reduces the fineness of the emery so that the discs do not have to be moved from one machine to another but receive all the needed grinding where they are first placed, again saving considerable time.[5]

Bausch and Lomb

In 1896, the Bausch and Lomb plant in New York began manufacturing meniscus lenses, followed by the toric form in 1898.[6]

Dr. Moritz von Rohr of Jena (Germany) introduced the Punktal lens in 1911.[7] This optically correct lens for compound lenses gave the required powers in the two meridians while still allowing equally distinct vision from center to margin. Bausch and Lomb Optical Company began producing these lenses for the American market in 1915, making the center thickness less and adding Kryptok and Ultex bifocals. Its Orthogon series of lenses followed. World War I unfortunately disrupted this cooperation on lens production. Therefore, Bausch and Lomb opened its own glass plant.

The following was taken from an article from Bausch and Lomb Optical Company, Rochester, N.Y., written in 1915:

> Glass is an amorphous, transparent or translucent mixture of silicates by definite chemical formulas. The essential materials for glass working are silica, an alkali and lime or lead. Part of the lime or lead may be replaced by oxides of other metals, also by certain borates and phosphates to replace a part of the silica especially in glass manufactured for optical purposes.
>
> COLORED GLASS
> Various colors used to moderate light entering the eye are found in spectacles. Blue is produced by adding cobalt oxide to melted glass; green by adding chrome oxide; ruby—gold oxide; yellow—silver oxide; violet—manganese oxide; smoke—by using several of the above oxides.[8]

Despite a "glass house" being established in Jamestown in the 1500s, the Bausch and Lomb glass plant was the only plant producing optical glass during World War I. The plant finally came out with the Nokrome lens—made of a dense, barium glass. Subsequently, Bausch and Lomb produced the Orthogon "D" bifocal—a color-free corrected lens. In 1930, the Panoptic lens emerged from the Hammon patent.

Amateurs

As late as 1938, individual production of lenses was so popular that a 231-page book by Orford and Lockett went through at least five editions, describing in detail how these products could be made.[9] The book covered grinding, finishing, setting, testing, and computing of lenses with tools that could be made at home. Making lenses was an interesting but time-consuming hobby, with the intended result being self-satisfaction.

Conclusion

Obviously, optical manufacturing has come a very long way since the first individuals began tinkering at the trade. It is now a flourishing industry answering the needs of a demanding public.

TABLE 2
OVERVIEW OF AMERICAN OPTICAL COMPANY DEVELOPMENT

1833–1840	William Beecher (sole owner)
1840–1842	Ammidown & Putney (Holdbridge Ammidown & Jairus Putney)
1842–1849	Ammidown & Son (Lucius Ammidown & Holdridge Ammidown)
1850–1851	Ammidown & Company (Lucius Ammidown & Robert H. Cole)
1851–1854	Ammidown & Company (Lucius Ammidown, Robert H. Cole, & William Beecher)
1854–1859	Ammidown & Company (Holdridge Ammidown, Robert H. Cole, & William Beecher)
1860–1862	Beecher & Cole (William Beecher, Robert H. Cole, & E. Merritt Cole)
1862–1866	Robert H. Cole & Company (Robert H. Cole & E. Merritt Cole)
1866–1869	Robert H. Cole & Company (Robert H. Cole, E. Merritt Cole, & A.M. Cheney)
1869–	American Optical Company (Robert H. Cole, president; George W. Wells, clerk; E. Merritt Cole, treasurer)

Source: American Optical Catalog #4258, 1912, p. 11.

Notes

1. Deborah Jean Warner, *OHS Proceedings*, Southbridge, 1984.
2. Robert McMaster, speech prepared from articles found: Old Sturbridge Village Library; Sturbridge American Optical Company Research Library; Southbridge Essex Institute, Salem, Massachusetts; *Fashions in Eyeglasses*, Richard Corson; London Ammidown History; Jacob Edwards Library; Southbridge American Optical Company History, QHS Leaflets.
3. G. W. Wells, *Quinebaug Historical Society Leaflets*, American Optical Co., Part 3, 191–92.
4. Ibid.
5. Ibid.
6. Bausch & Lomb Optical Company, *Ophthalmic Lenses* (Rochester, NY, 1935).
7. D. J. Bryden and D. L. Simms, "Spectacles Improved to Perfection and Approved of by the Royal Society," *Annals of Science* 50 (1993): 1–32.
8. Bausch and Lomb Optical Company, op. cit.
9. H. Orford and A. Lockett, *Lens-Work for Amateurs* (London: Pitman, 1938).

Other Sources Consulted in Chapter 6

1. American Optical Company, *Spectacles, Eyeglasses, Lenses* (Southbridge, MA, circa 1933).
2. R. B. Carter, *Good and Bad Eyesight* (Philadelphia: P. Blakiston & Co., 1882).
3. G. Hartridge, *The Refraction of the Eye* (Chicago: W.P. Deim & Co., 1895).
4. Stanley Newbold, *The Optician* 141 (3655) (April 1961).
5. Theo E. Obrig, *Modern Ophthalmic Lenses and Optical Glass.* (New York, 1935).
6. Ruth Dyer Wells, *The Wells Family* (Southbridge, MA: Privately printed, 1979).

7

Development of Chinese Spectacles

From the Caucasian standpoint, spectacles were invented by an unknown Italian in Northern Italy about A.D. 1287. The invention of spectacles in China probably predated that by a decade or two, but we are unable to record this precisely because of distance and language difficulties. The latter, as well as the lack of historical libraries, precludes the credit to any particular Asian inventor. The Japanese apparently obtained eyeglasses from the Chinese and were not involved in the origination process. In 1915, Rasmussen stated the following:

> To attempt to trace the exact genealogy of anything in China is a well-nigh hopeless task. China is a vast beginningless and endless symposium and is at once modern and antique. Things of antiquity are in present use while things of comparative modernity are relegated to equal acceptability with ancient modes and methods. This Oriental country with its revolutions and without its evolutions is the one great cyclical "Middle Kingdom" at the center of the earth's dominions, and to bear out her own metaphor, being at the center of the revolving elements, moves the least.
>
> The story of Chinese spectacles differs little from the usual Chinese stories and is equally illuminated with its fancies, superstitions, and tales. Eminent Orientalists do not usually take all that the old Chinese writers state very seriously, for with the evident absence of scientific knowledge the old historians could not very well be expected to approach matters of natural laws with more than a simple wondering attitude and a mind ready to believe in the mysterious, spirit-like origin of that which they could not understand.[1]

Unfortunately, contradictions appear in the numerous references made to the history of Chinese spectacles. W. H. Holtmann states the following in W. Poulet's book, *A History of Spectacles*:

> The Chinese used spectacles 2000 years ago (circa 22 B.C.)—but not to improve their vision. They used them with the thought that an imaginary force, the yoh shui—which was supposed to be present in the glass—would help visually deficient patients. According to Karl Richard, these spectacles were produced of tea-stone (Ai Tai), which comes in a light and in a dark color. Spectacles were also used as a protection against bright light.[2]

Chinese historians claim that eyeglasses came to China from Arabia around 1071. Two centuries later in 1271, on his first voyage to the Orient, Marco Polo found that eyeglasses were being used. He also found that reference to the importance of the use of eyeglasses was made in old Chinese encyclopedias and noticed that older people in China used lenses for reading. Rasmussen pointed out that for the use of glasses to have been established at the time of Marco Polo, they would have had to have been invented several decades earlier.[3] He assumes, therefore, that the invention of spectacles in China preceded that of the invention in Northern Italy.

The famous poet and scholar Chao I Ou Pei (1727–1814) did establish the existence of eyeglasses in Chapter 33 of his *Kai Yu Tsung Kao*. He referred to the book *Fang Chau Tsa Yen* by Chang Ching Chih from the era of the Ming Dynasty (1368–1615), where it is stated that the "first eyeglasses were brought into China from the West in the era of the Ming Dynasty which began in 1368."[4] The same book also contains the statement that Shuan Tsung (1399–1435) gave his father Tsung Po a pair of eyeglasses, described as follows: "the lenses are as big as coins; they are made of mica stone (tea-coloured quartz); the two lenses can be folded together. When an old man holds the glasses in front of his two eyes characters appear to be up to twice as large and are clearly seen."[5]

Additional information regarding the history of spectacles in China comes to us from an article by Eugene Chan and Winifred Mao:

> Chinese optic knowledge can be traced to as early as the Zhou Dynasty (1066–256 BC). In the "Book of Rites", fire was mentioned as being produced in two ways: rubbing wood against wood and reflecting the sun's rays with an object which looked like a mirror. Ice was carved into convex lenses to reflect the sun's rays and produce fire. This was mentioned by Liu An (179–122 BC) in the Han Dynasty. The bronze mirror is one of the oldest optical instruments in China. The mirrors were of both concave and convex types, so that the images could be enlarged or reduced.
>
> Mezi was credited with his achievements of knowledge about optics. Early in the period of the 'Warring States' (475–221 BC) he wrote the book "Classic Me", which consisted of 15 volumes, eight of which concerned optics: the definition of shadow and its formation; the relationship between light and shadow, the straight line character of light; reflection of light; the relationship between the light source, distance, and the size of the shadow; in the sixth to eighth parts, plane, concave and convex lenses as well as the relationship between an object and its shadow were discussed. The above principles are the same as stated in the theory of light in modern optics. In the Song Dynasty (960–1279 AD) Shen Kuo, a scientist, further discussed in "Notes in a Dream" the principles of image formation with concave and convex lenses and the phenomenon of inverted image.

THE HISTORY OF SPECTACLES

The lead eye shield in the Tang Dynasty (713–741 AD):
An ancient tomb but no longer with its usual memorial inscription stone was unearthed in 1967 in Turpan County, the Xinjiang Uygur Autonomous Region, northwest China. Based on the style of the tomb and the burial articles it was probably 713 to 741 AD. A lead eye shield which would be mainly of interest to ophthalmologists was found. It is of elliptical shape and measures 17 cm horizontally, 4 cm vertically and is 3 mm thick. There are many small perforations in the areas corresponding with the location of the eyes. Centrally, there are indentations for the nose. The margin of the shield is rimmed with 1 cm faded silk. This shield was found placed in front of the eyes. The eye [shield] bears resemblance to pinhole spectacles of modern times. Pinhole spectacles can improve vision of patients with presbyopia, irregular astigmatism, keratoconus, astigmatism and incipient cataract. Since this cultural relic was found in the Xinjiang Uygur Autonomous Region, a far remote northwest area of China, it may mean that even at that early time usage of pinhole spectacles to improve vision was very popular. There were also fragments of "Lun Yu", a book of conversations of Confucius and his disciples. According to the recent research work of Nie Chong Hou, it was recorded in the Song Dynasty that a judicial officer, Shih Hong, wore a crystal glass to improve his vision. It might be the world's first written record of using spectacles, about a half century earlier than that of Europe. Zhao Hsi Hou (the South Song Dynasty), in his book "Dong Tien Qing Lu", described: "Ai Dai (spectacles) can help the old to read small words; without it reading is not possible".

According to the research work of Toshisada Naba (Japan), there are different editions of the book of "Dong Tien Qing Lu". He himself has seen many editions, only one of which mentions Shih Hong and the words "Ai Dai". Kai Ming Chiu published an article in the proceedings of the Carnegie Institute of Harvard University which said that there were no records of "Ai Dai" in its earlier editions, and that it was probably added by others afterwards. Therefore the book "Dong Tien Qing Lu" may not be a reliable source for the spectacles of Shih Hong in the Song Dynasty. Zhu Mu, in his book "Fang Yu Sheng Lan", mentioned: "Ai Dai (spectacles) have come from "Man Ci Jia'" (Malacca, now in Malaysia) and therefore probably are introduced into China by foreign merchants during the Song Dynasty. The Italian trader Marco Polo visited China in the South Song Dynasty and mentioned in his travel notes the usage of spectacles.

Spectacles in the Ming Dynasty   The records of spectacles appeared more frequently in the Ming Dynasty. For instance, Zhao O Bei in his book "Hai Yu Cong Kao" wrote, "He has seen a pair of spectacles in the Capital. It consisted of two pieces, each one as large as a coin, with the color of mica. The lenses were very thin and mounted onto a metal frame. The two lenses could pivot at the bridge into one [Figure 81]. It could improve the poor vision of the old so that the words become clear". He observed a case in which a horse was exchanged for a pair of spectacles in a foreign country, "Man Ci Jia". There were also descriptions of spectacles in books such as "The Four Treasures of the Study" by Tu Long and "Qi Xiu Xu Gao" by Lang Ying. Further, there was a poem written by Zhao O Bei concerning spectacles:

It has been heard in the year "Xuan De",
The spectacles came by ship overseas,
Being a royal reward to an old official,
It is as precious as gold.

In conclusion, glass spectacles were rare and precious in the Ming Dynasty and most likely were brought into China from abroad.[6]

Development and Use of Spectacles in China after Marco Polo

Fortunately, the development and use of spectacles in China following the time of Marco Polo is somewhat easier to trace than the actual invention. In Europe in the year 1300, there was no printing, and very few people were able to read. Therefore, the use of eyeglasses was not accepted by the general public but was accepted only by certain scholars and monks. Since eyeglasses were also quite expensive, their use, manufacture, and appreciation took a long time to develop.

By the fifteenth and sixteenth centuries and beyond, it is

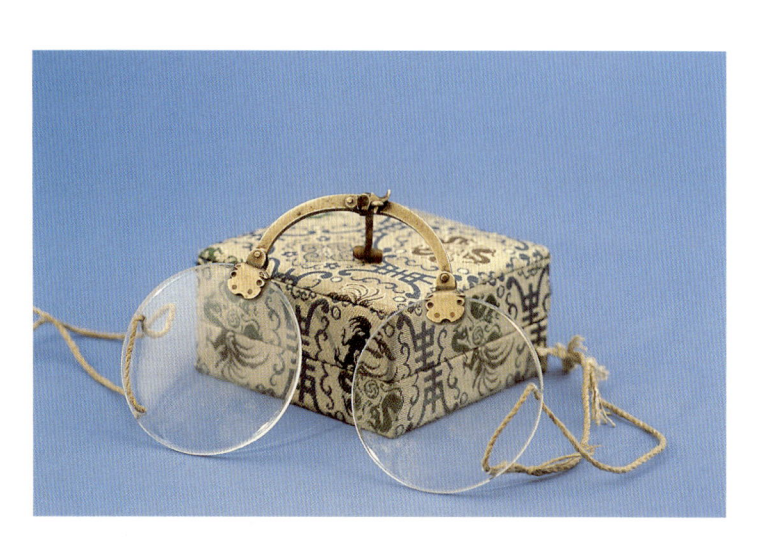

Figure 81. Rimless folding Chinese spectacles.

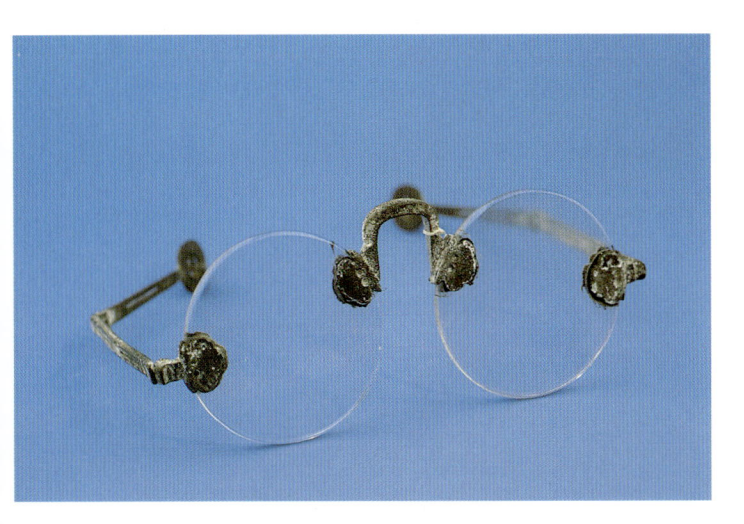

Figure 82. 5-centimeter round Chinese spectacles.

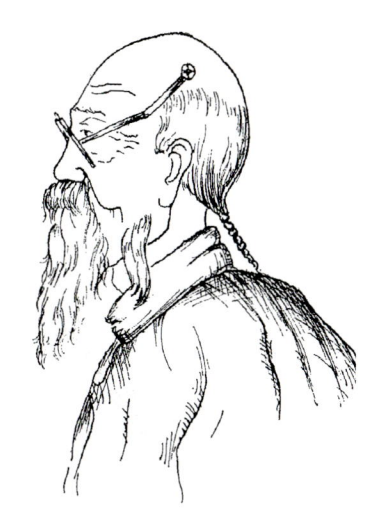

Figure 83. Technique of wearing Chinese spectacles.

safe to say that the development of spectacles in the Orient paralleled that of those in the Western world. We find, however, intriguing and amusing methods in their purchase and uses as well as in the curious customs associated with them. For instance, a Chinese dispenser of spectacles stated in a letter to American Optical Company in 1910: "Wearing spectacles in those ancient times was generally thought to establish the wearer as intelligent, affluent, and influential."[7] Spectacles, therefore, became a status symbol to the Chinese.

Furthermore, the larger the spectacles, the more intelligent the wearer was thought to be. This is why many of the early Chinese spectacles were so large (Figure 82) and predate our current large fashion eyewear by about 500 years. The dispenser commented, "The Chinese wearer of old spectacles cares nothing for comfort or fit. . . . I sometimes think the increase in size shows a decrease in mental capacity."[8]

Most lenses at that time were fairly large and circular and were thought of by many to have healing powers. The Chinese eyeglass dispenser stated, "The lenses are many times made of crystal which comes from secret places and is supposed to cure various diseases of the eye. I am frequently asked if my glasses have good medicine in them. . . . Some lenses are said to have power to enable to see at night and some to see into the earth to find hidden treasures, minerals, etc."[9]

In the sixteenth century, lenses were worn at a 45-degree angle (Figure 83), and the temples were always straight with a joint for folding.[10] A thread or string was also used as a temple piece to hold the frame to the face (Figure 84). The temples were

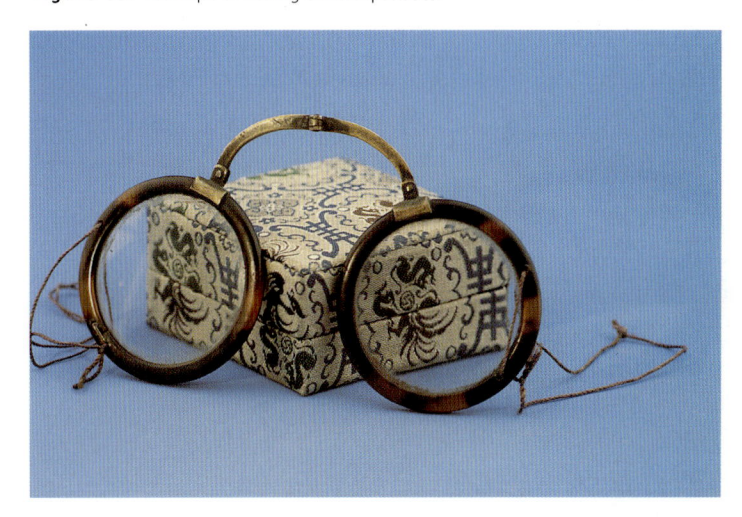

Figure 84. Chinese spectacles with temple strings.

CHINESE SPECTACLES   65

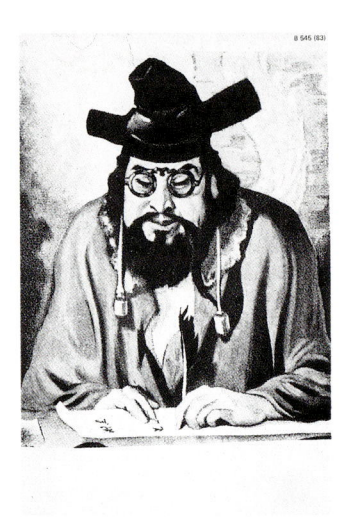

Figure 85. Technique of wearing Chinese spectacles with temple strings and weights.

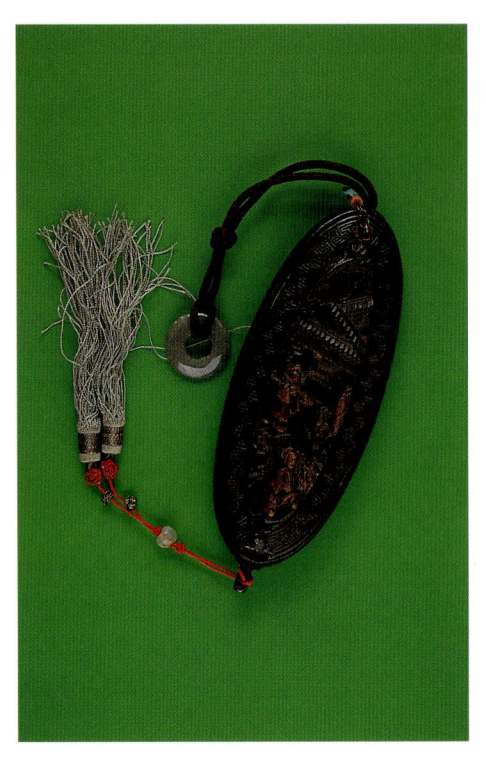

Figure 86. Chinese spectacle case with sash weight.

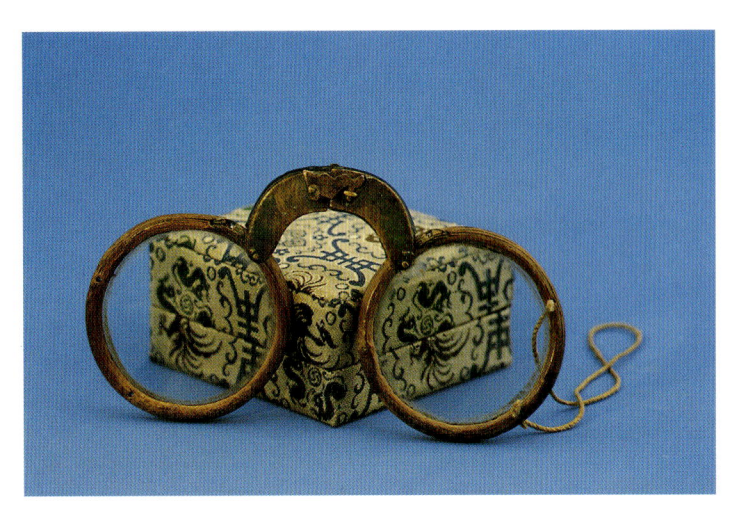

Figure 87. Chinese spectacles with raffia frame.

either tied behind the head or looped over the ears (Figure 85)—as did the Spanish, with a weight fastened to the end of the string and left to hang behind the ears.[11] The eyeglasses were usually carried in a case attached to the clothing or hanging over the arm (Figure 86).[12]

The author has a pair of folding spectacles in his collection, probably dating sixteenth century, with a raffia (reed) frame (Figure 87). Folding glasses not only were used with string temples but also had a horn pad to press against the forehead. They were kept in a small circular case of wood, leather, or shagreen (Figure 88). Some of the more ornate frames were made of carved tortoiseshell (Figure 89). The tortoise, a sacred animal to the Chinese, is believed to be endowed with the ability to bring good luck and long life. Therefore, the Chinese used it to make spectacles and other objects. (The decorative carving on the tortoiseshell frames had definite meaning, discussed at the end of this chapter.) Some frames carried clear lenses, where others had dark or tea-stone lenses.

66 CHAPTER 7

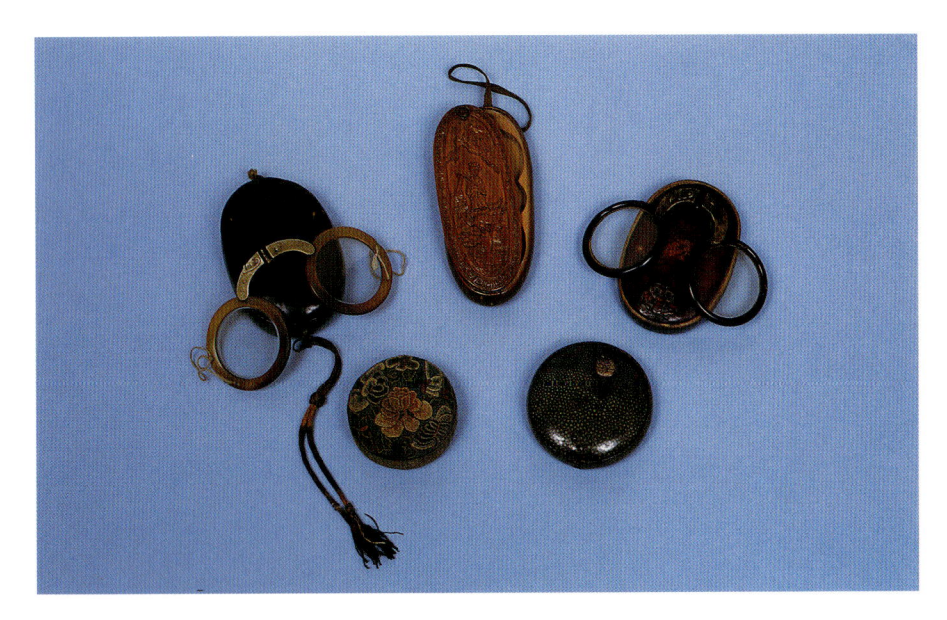

Figure 88. Selection of Chinese cases for folding spectacles.

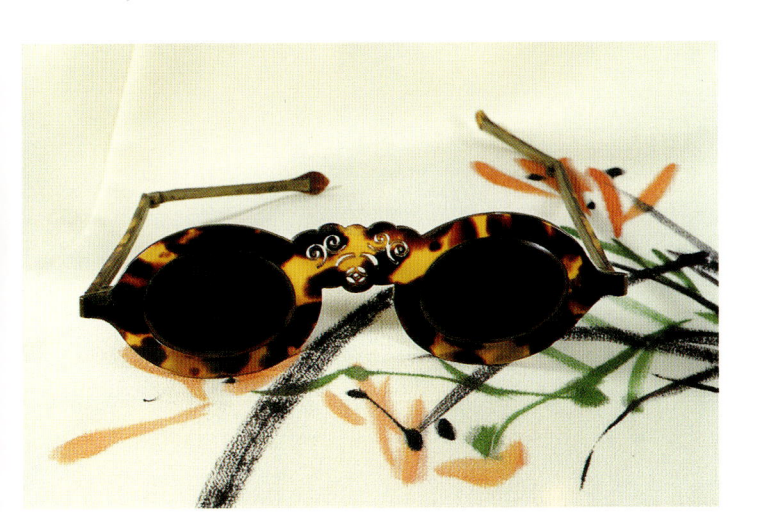

Figure 89. Carved tortoiseshell Chinese spectacles.

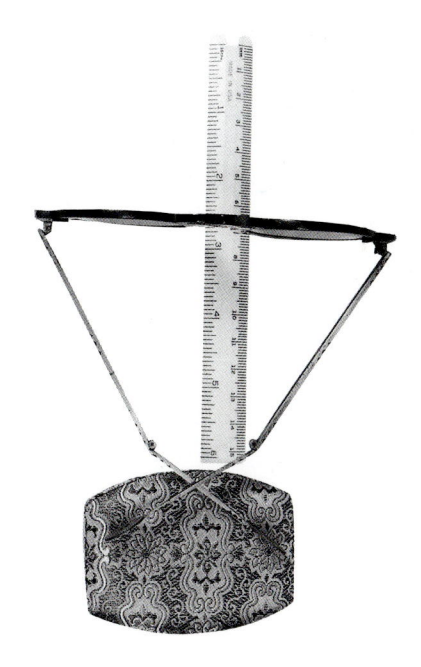

Figure 90. Top view of Chinese spectacle reveals thickness.

Many lenses were not only plano but also fairly myopic. Both glass and tea-stone lenses as well as frames were of a like thickness—most being very thin—about 2 millimeters (Figure 90). We find them very light in weight, affording comfort and the ability to remain on the face. So much for the "newly invented" thin grind!

Some old Chinese frames were constructed of horn and others of sandalwood. The "fronts" of the latter type were made in two sections (anterior and posterior) so that lenses

CHINESE SPECTACLES 67

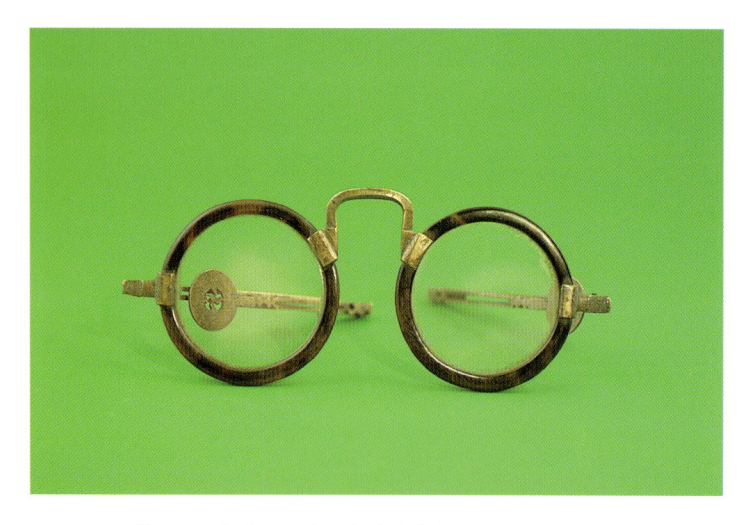

Figure 91. Brass and tortoiseshell Chinese spectacles.

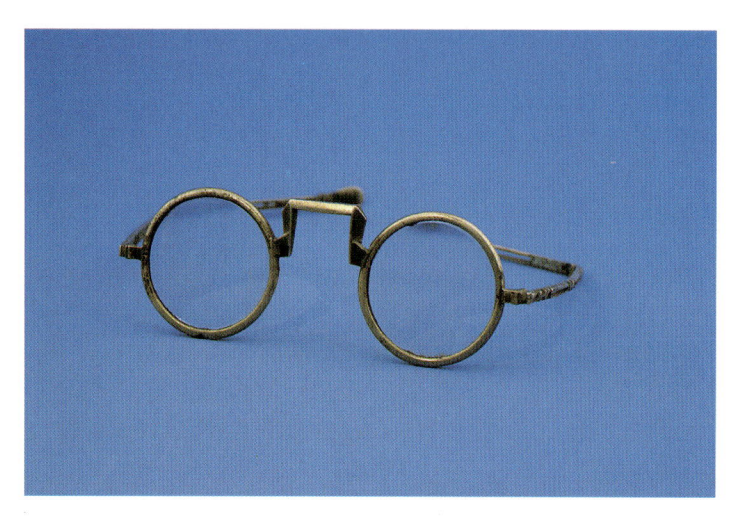

Figure 92. Brass and glass common Chinese spectacles.

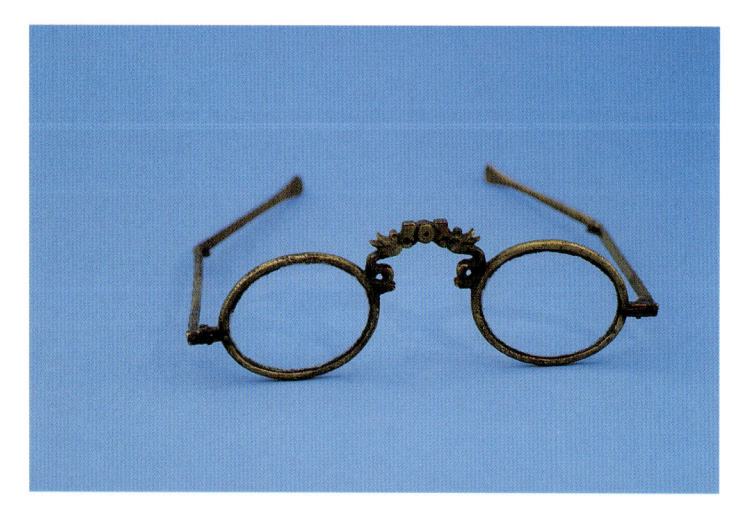

Figure 93. Brass and glass small-sized Chinese spectacles.

could be inserted and the whole glued together. Lacquer and horsehair were used for binding.

Besides the rock crystal lenses, topaz and amethyst were used.

Unusual types of Chinese glasses recorded but never seen by this author are the half-eye spectacles called *pan ching* and the monocle called *yuan ching*.

Spectacles then—and in later times—being considered marks of literary attainment were also used as props to show respect. It was always considered proper to remove the spectacles in China when in the presence of superiors, and even in the presence of inferiors or friends. Rasmussen said, "It is a grave sign of disrespect to the presiding judge to wear spectacles in his presence.... When passing a friend on the street, it is also courteous to remove one's spectacles immediately before the greeting."[13] This custom, coupled with the superstitions of the Chinese, sometimes held more weight than the obvious benefits of spectacles and medical treatment in later times. The dispenser of Chinese spectacles also stated in his letter to AOC in 1910: "The Chinese are also very subject to the most severe forms of eye disease and know nothing about the contagious nature of trachoma, etc."[14] Although he discussed numerous customs and superstitions in his letter, he as well addressed what he considered to be the real problems: "Myopia is much more common among Chinese than foreigners. I use frequently minus 10 to minus 15. One man in town, a writer in the American consulate, a man now nearly 60, wears a minus 24."[15]

Modern Developments

By the latter half of the nineteenth century and the early part of the twentieth century, spectacles in China were progressively made of more usable brass and alloy metals (Figure 91). Many of the more common frames were made completely of brass (Figure 92). The lenses were made of glass, not quartz, which could be ground to more exact specifications for nearsighted, farsighted, and presbyopic persons. Quite possibly by this time, at least some of the "customs" had faded, as the lenses were smaller in size (Figure 93). European influence contributed to the size reduction. The lenses were predominantly oval-shaped, approximately two by three centimeters. Although the lenses mimicked those found in occidental countries, the cases and frames still maintained an oriental flavor.

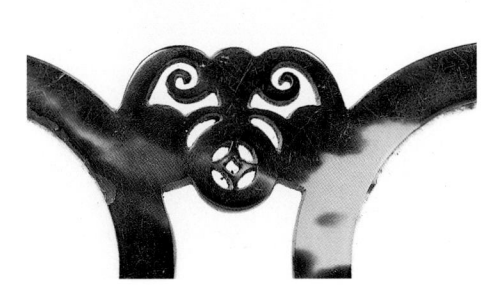

Figure 94. Carved Chinese tortoiseshell bridge showing sign of money (below).

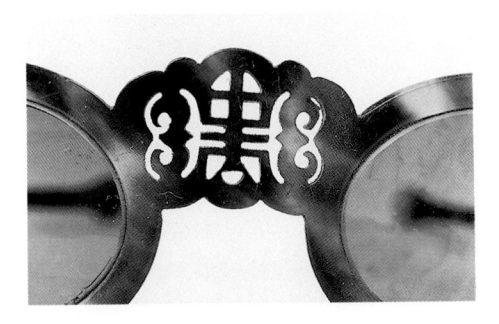

Figure 95. Carved Chinese tortoiseshell bridge showing sign of the bat (sides).

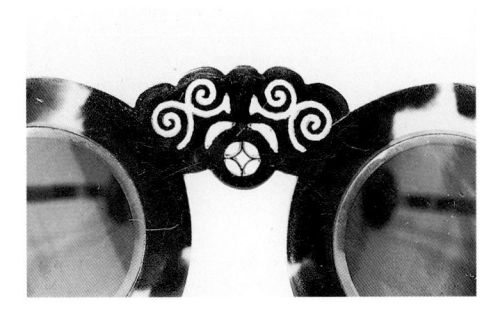

Figure 96. Carved Chinese tortoiseshell bridge showing sign of the butterfly (above).

Conclusion

Whereas current debate pits European versus Chinese origins of spectacles, the most definitive evidence we have indicates Northern Italian origins. Utilization of spectacles in China is evident pre-Marco Polo, but indicates Middle Eastern origins.

Significance of Carvings on Chinese Tortoiseshell Spectacles

Most Chinese tortoiseshell spectacles have ornately carved bridges. Many are similar, but the author has located at least nine different motifs. The significance of some may as well be similar, but as the carvings are done by various artisans, differences do exist.

The sign of money (Figure 94), of course, needs no explanation. The bat (Figure 95) is a sign of happiness and longevity. It is believed that certain types, if eaten, will ensure good sight.

A butterfly carving on the bridge (Figure 96) is a symbol of joy, of conjugal felicity—sort of a Chinese Cupid.

Where you find the most ornate carving, however, is the sign of freedom (Figure 97). Other types are illustrated in Figures 98–102.

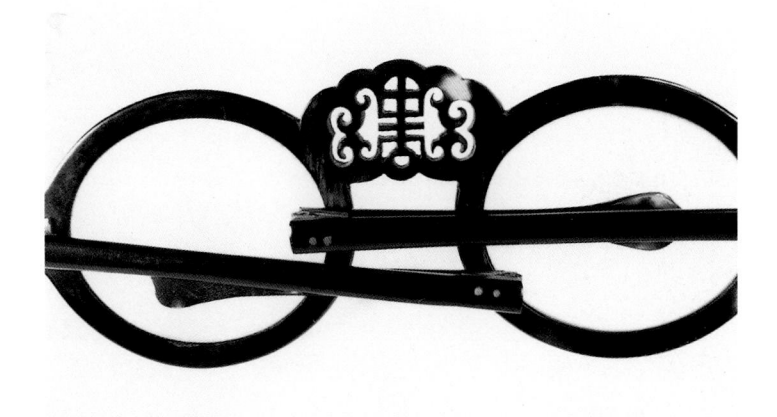

Figure 97. Carved Chinese tortoiseshell bridge showing the sign of freedom (center).

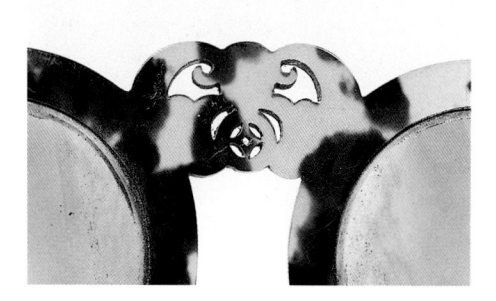

Figure 98. Carved Chinese tortoiseshell bridge showing sign of the bull.

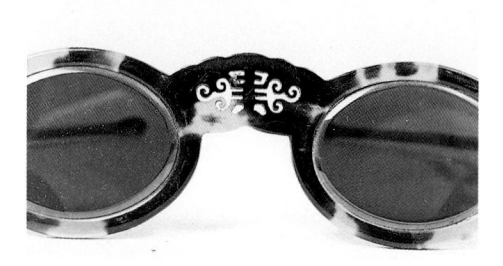

Figures 99–102. Variation of carved Chinese tortoiseshell bridges.

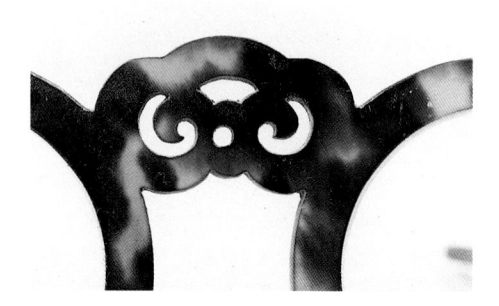

Figure 100.

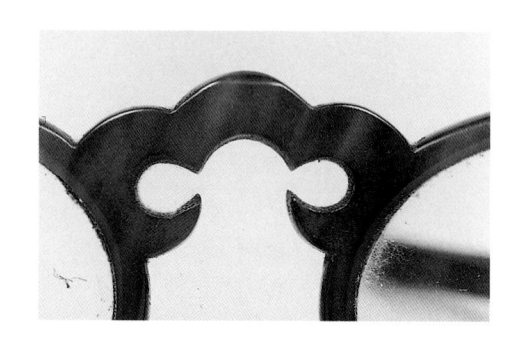

Figure 101.

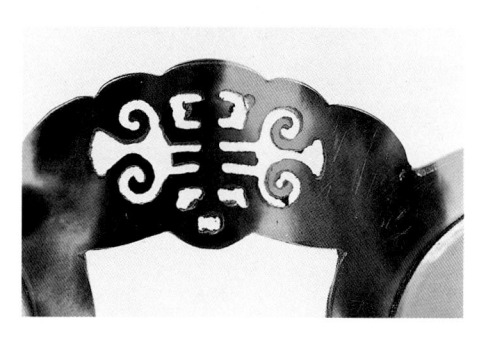

Figure 102.

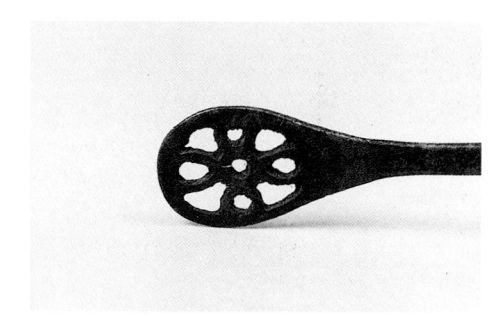

Figure 103. Reticulated temple piece.

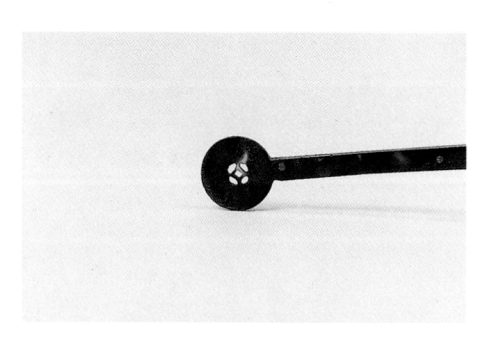

Figure 104. Carved Chinese tortoiseshell temple in the sign of money.

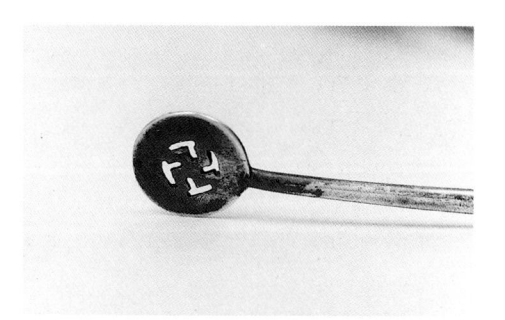

Figure 105. Cast brass Chinese temple end showing the sign of the swastika.

70   CHAPTER 7

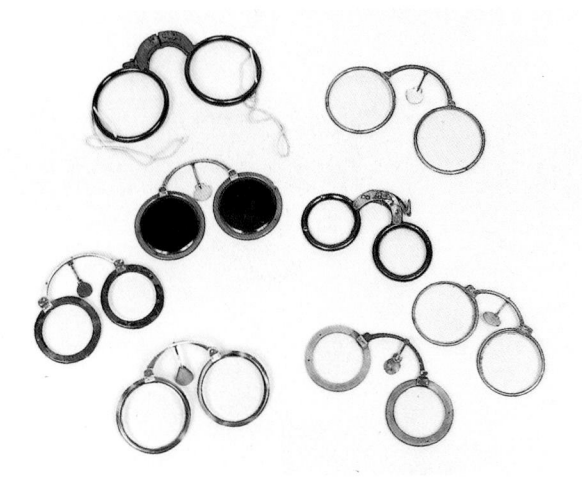

Figure 106. Various forms of folding Chinese spectacles.

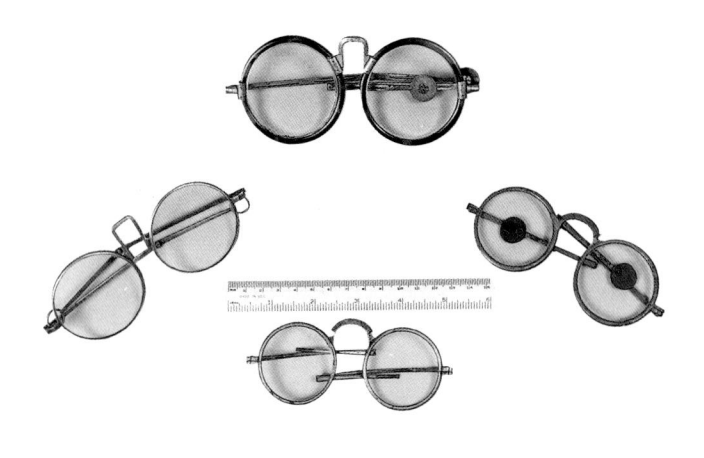

Figure 107. Large-sized Chinese spectacles.

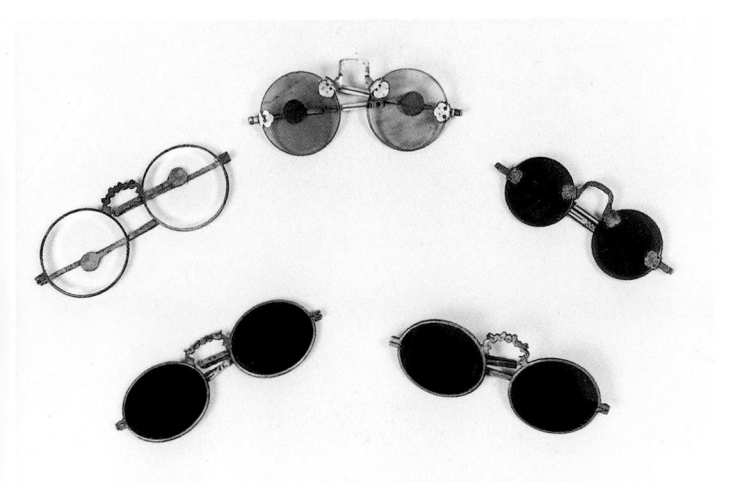

Figure 108. Bridge variations in Chinese spectacles.

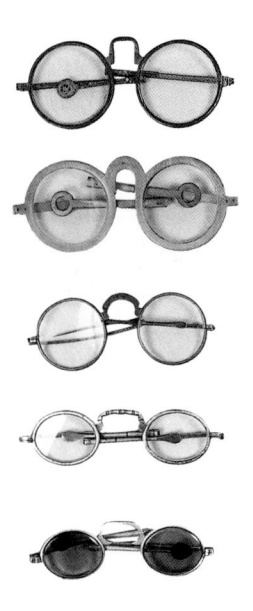

Figure 109. Materials used in Chinese spectacle frames (from above)—bronze, horn, brass, brass, alloy.

The ends of temple pieces are plain or carved (round or oblong) (Figure 103). However, some of the round examples have significant carvings. They are carved (sometimes cast in brass) in the sign of money (Figure 104), and some in the sign of the swastika (Figure 105). The latter is of great antiquity and is common to many countries: In India, it is the monogram of Vishnu and Siva. In Scandinavia and in Peruvian symbols, it is the battle-ax of Thor. It would appear to be a Buddhist importation in China and Japan.

As the erudite collector should be aware of the various forms of Chinese spectacles and their expression, the following illustrations are offered as demonstration (Figures 106–122).

CHINESE SPECTACLES 71

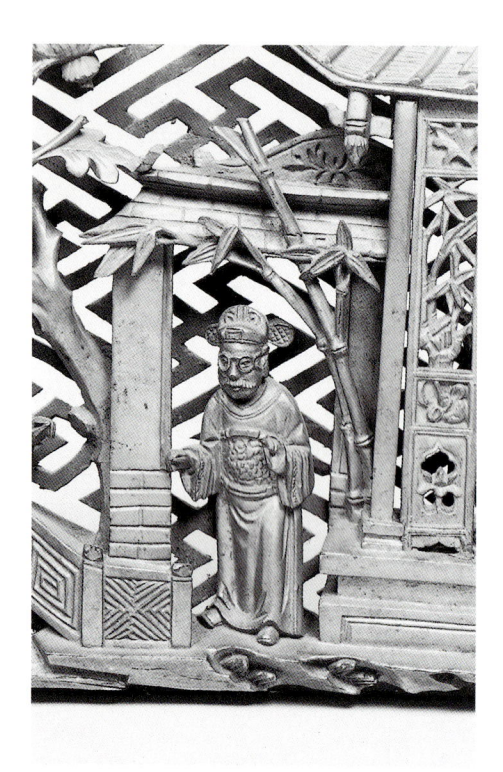

Figure 110. Wood carving showing man wearing spectacles.

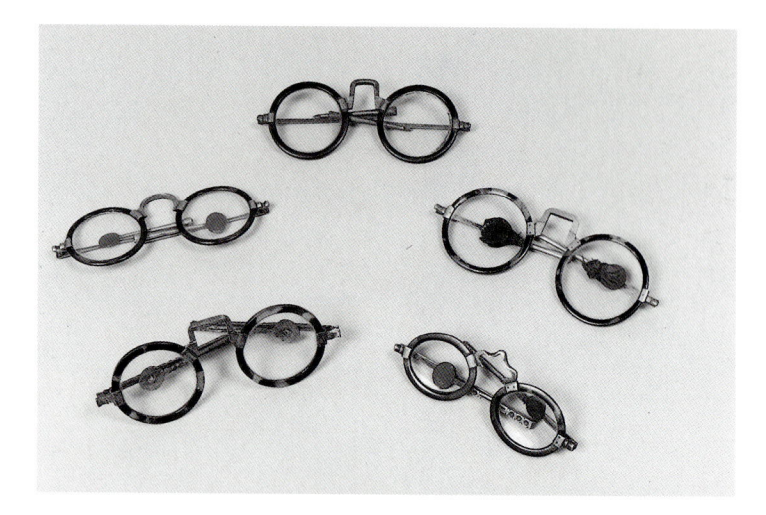

Figure 111. Variations in tortoiseshell Chinese frames.

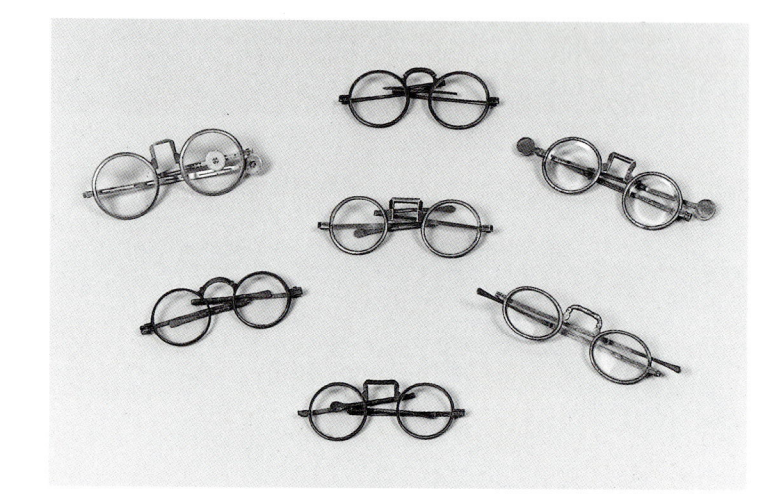

Figure 112. Various forms of nineteenth-century Chinese brass spectacle frames.

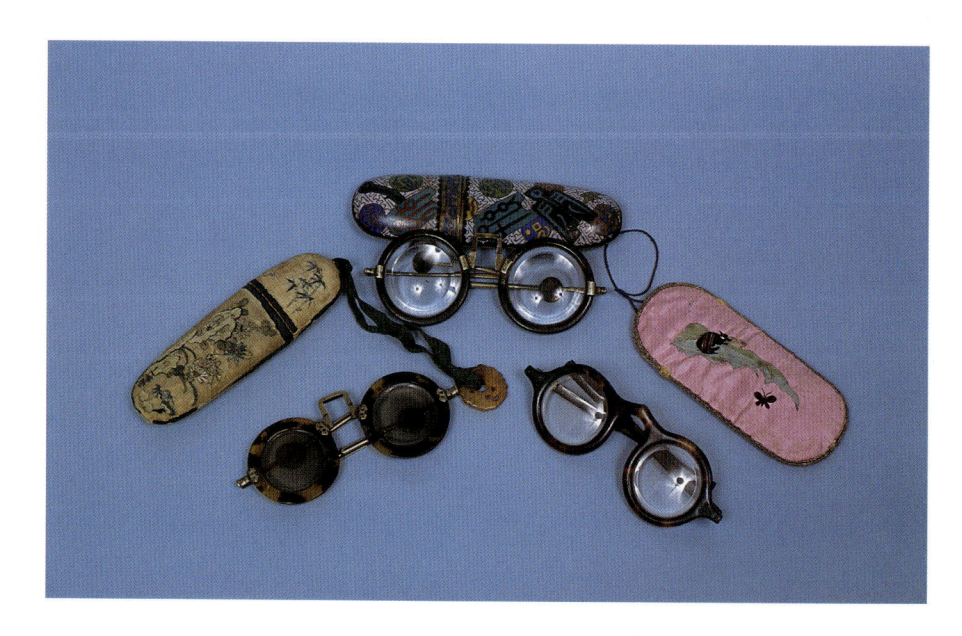

Figure 113. A selection of tortoiseshell frames and cases (top is cloissone).

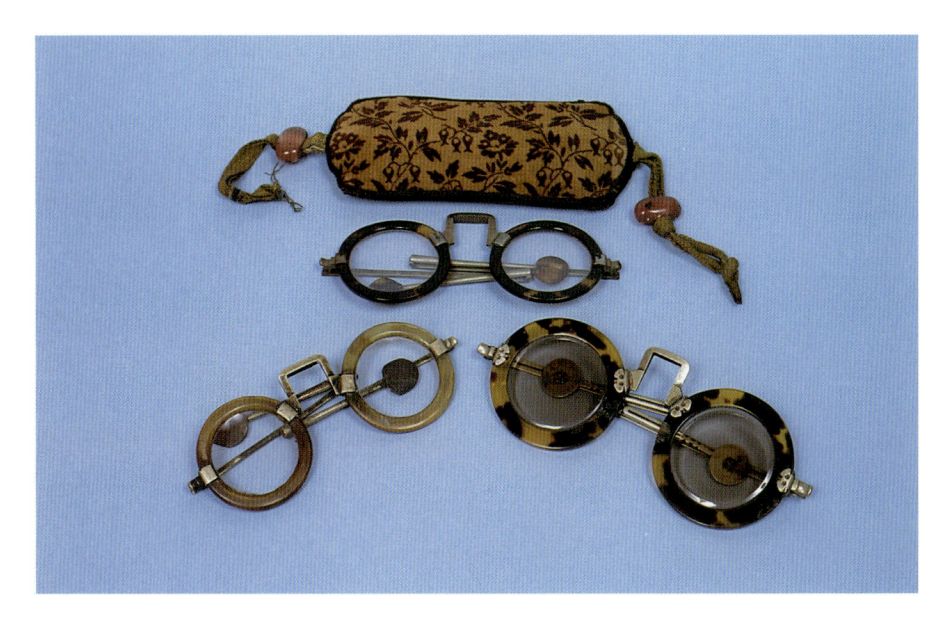

Figure 114. Tortoiseshell and horn-rimmed Chinese spectacles.

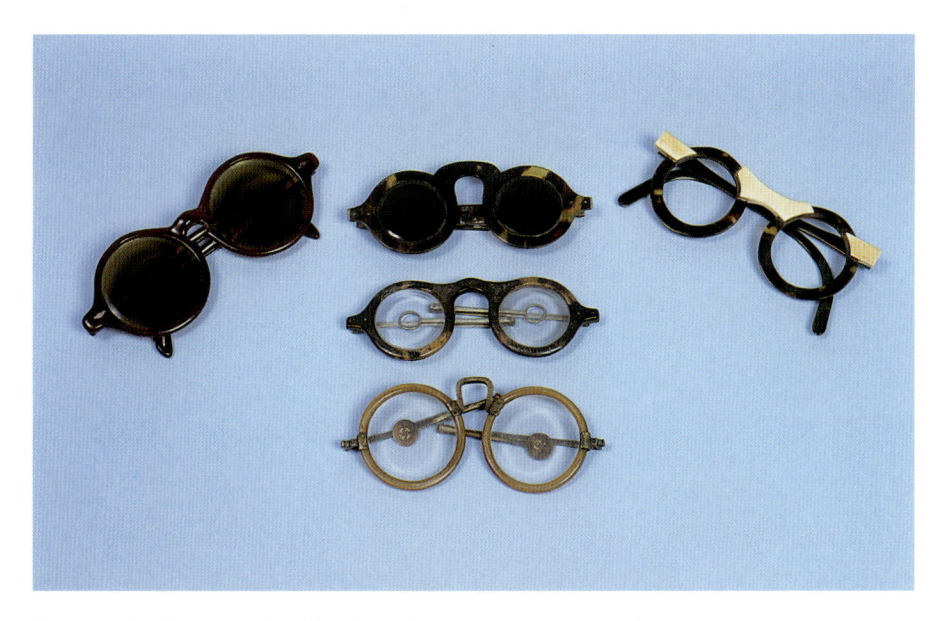

Figure 115. Chinese spectacles of the nineteenth century showing European influence.

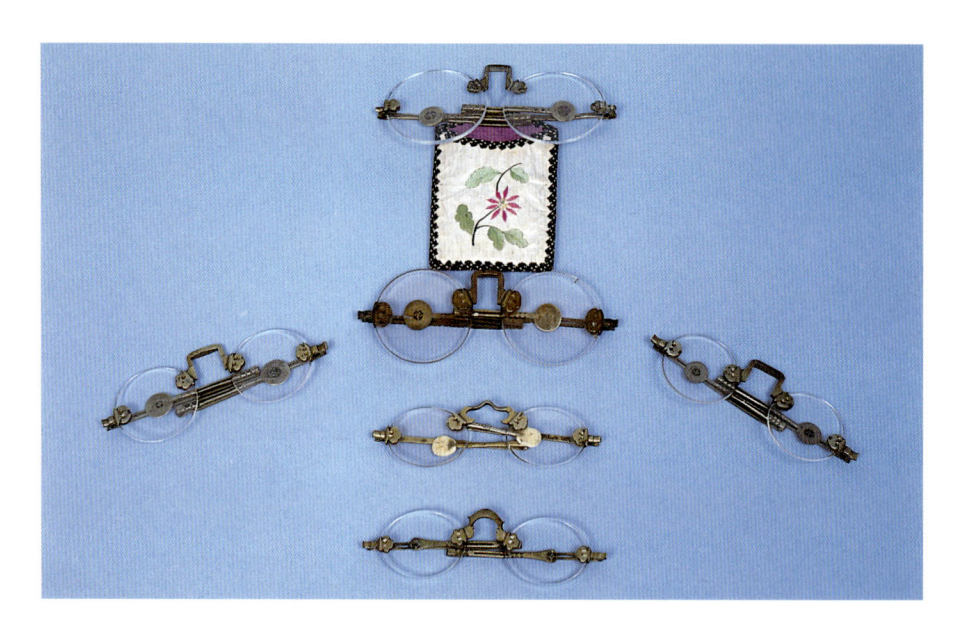

Figure 116. Forms of rimless Chinese spectacles.

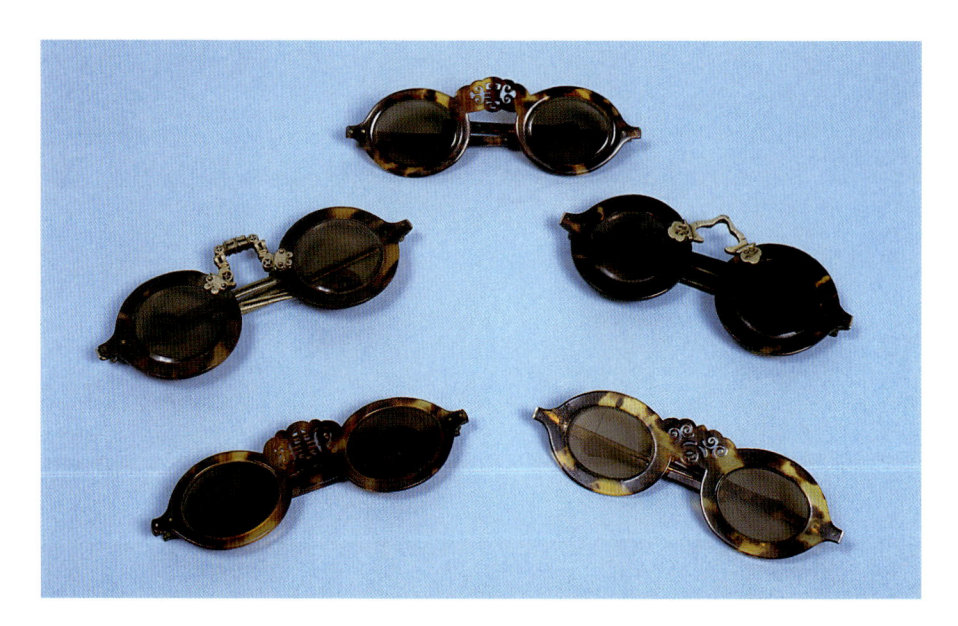

Figure 117. Mid nineteenth-century tortoiseshell spectacles with dark tea-stone lenses.

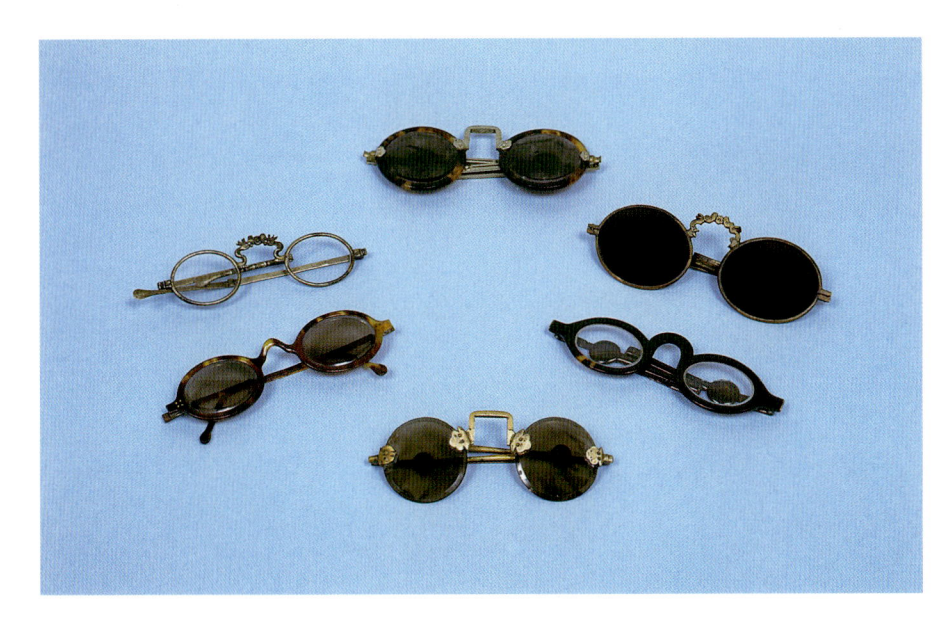

Figure 118. Forms of late nineteenth-century Chinese spectacles.

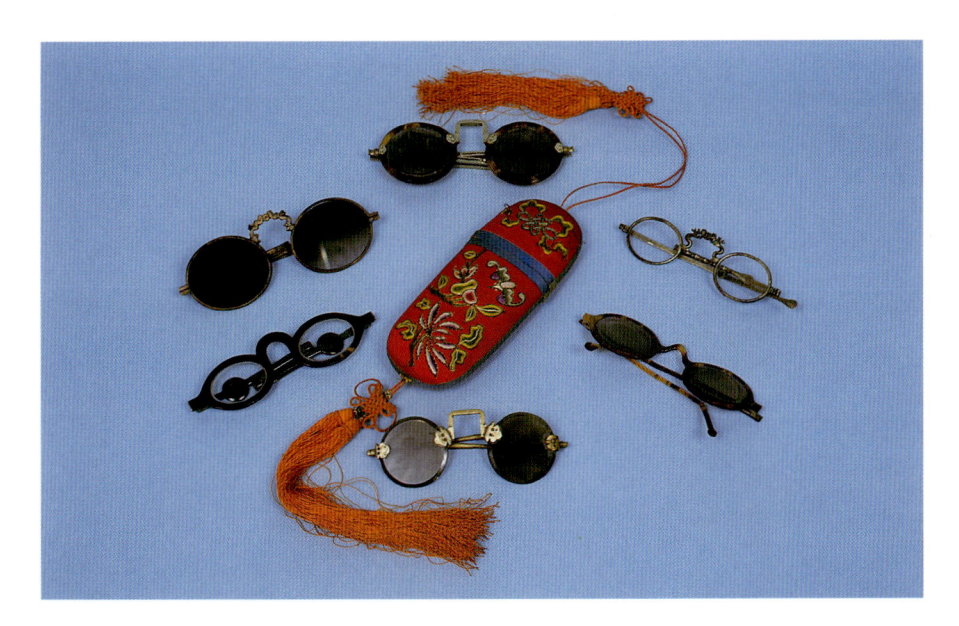

Figure 119. Nineteenth-century Chinese spectacles and case.

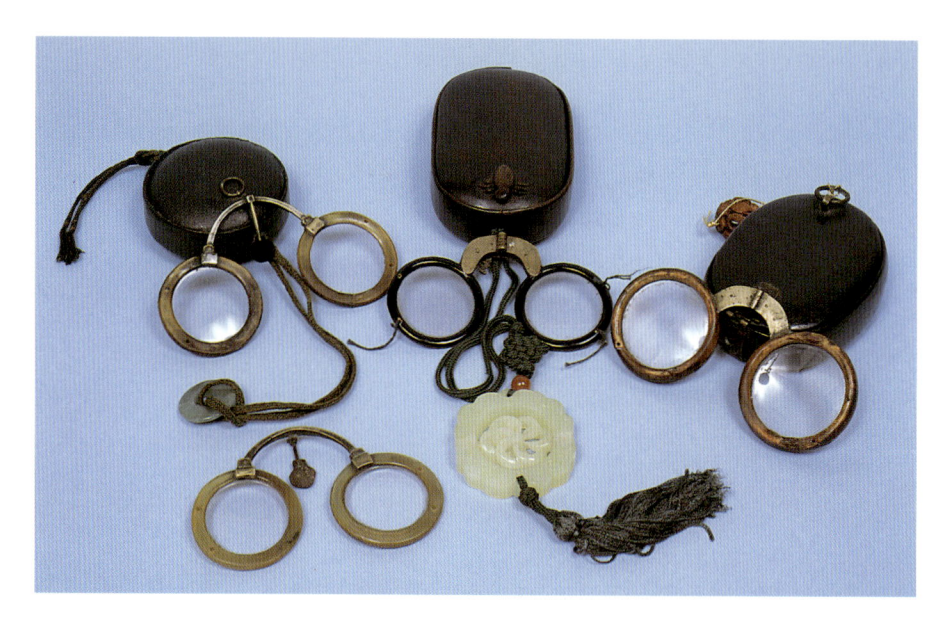

Figure 120. Reed, lacquer, and horn folding spectacles of the seventeenth and eighteenth centuries with cases.

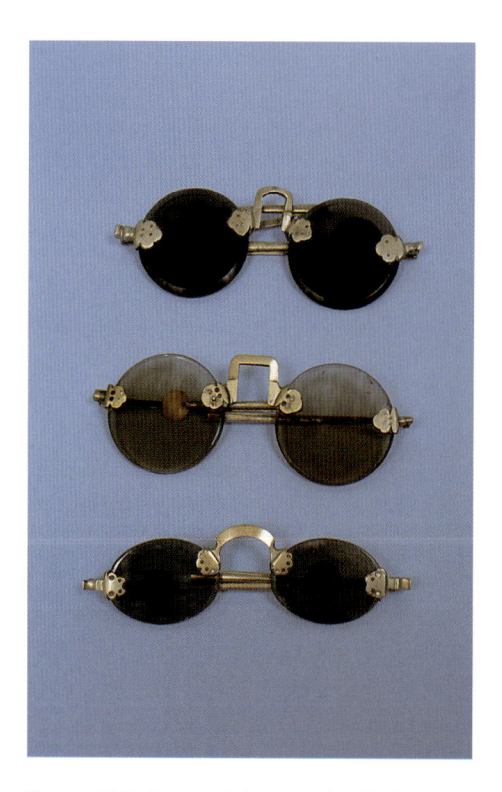

Figure 121. Tea-stone rimless spectacles with silver (above) and brass frames.

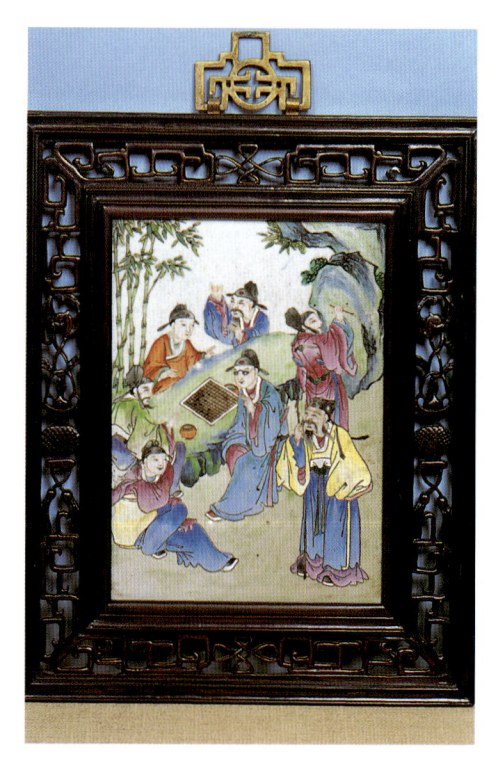

Figure 122. Chien Lung Period (A.D. 1736–1796) Famille rose painting on porcelain—seven scholars under the bamboo tree.

76   CHAPTER 7

Important Dates In Chinese History By Rasmussen

1. At the beginning of the second century B.C., Emperor Chin Shih ordered the destruction by fire of all existing Chinese literature. Some copies, of course, escaped.
2. Calligraphy started in A.D. 171.
3. Painting began in the fifth century A.D.
4. Porcelain came in the ninth century A.D.
5. About 1066, the Chinese invented moveable wooden type.
6. In 1403, they invented moveable metal type.
7. Cloissone began in the seventeenth century A.D.

Notes

1. O. D. Rasmussen, *History of Chinese Spectacles* (Hankow, China, 1915).
2. W. Poulet, *An Atlas on the History of Spectacles*, translated by F. Blodi (Badgodesberg, West Germany: Wayenborgh, 1978).
3. Rasmussen, op. cit.
4. Sekiya Shirayama, *Ophthalmic Antiques International Collectors' Club Newsletter*, July 1991.
5. Ibid.
6. Eugene Chan and Winifred Mao, "The History of Spectacles in China," *Proceedings of the XXVth International Congress of Ophthalmology*, Rome, May 4–10, 1986, 731–34.
7. Rasmussen, op. cit.
8. Ibid.
9. Ibid.
10. Richard Corson, *Fashions in Eyeglasses* (London: Peter Owen, Ltd., 1980).
11. Ibid.
12. Ibid.
13. Rasmussen, op. cit.
14. Ibid.
15. Ibid.

Other Sources Consulted for Chapter 7

1. Colin Fryer, *Ophthalmic Antiques Newsletter*, April 1995.
2. Raymond Li, *A Glossary of Chinese Snuff Bottles Rebus* (Kowloon, Hong Kong: Nine Dragons Publishers, 1976).
3. G. L. E. Turner, *A Spectacles of Spectacles* (London, 1988).
4. John M. Young, *The History of Eyewear*, Optical Heritage Museum, 1985, pp. 71–82.

8

Ancient Chinese Eyeglass Cases

The use of spectacles in ancient China was generally thought to establish the wearer as intelligent, affluent, and influential. Because of this, every scholar and fortune-teller needed to wear them. Couple this with the tradition that spectacles should be removed when passing a friend on the street, in the presence of both superiors and inferiors, and we recognize the importance of spectacle cases (Figure 123).

Changes in size of cases obviously paralleled those of the spectacles. Initially, the Chinese believed that the larger the frame (Figure 124), the more knowledgeable the wearer. Therefore, the cases that housed them were large. As time went on, the size of spectacles moderated (Figure 125), and in the latter half of the nineteenth century, Chinese frames tended to imitate imported European and American lens sizes (Figure 126), shapes, and construction. It is logical, then, to equate smaller lens and case sizes with those more recently manufactured. Those cases measuring 15 × 6 centimeters (approximately) are usually older (circa 1840) (Figure 127) than those measuring 13 × 5 centimeters (circa 1890) (Figure 128).

Early eyeglass cases to protect expensive, ancient purchases (Figure 129) were of a style and quality to enhance the aura. As these cases were closed with a cord, ending with a decorative carved stone, wood, or coin (Figure 130)—much like the Japanese *netsuke*—it was easy to carry them looped over a sash or belt or over the arm. In such an obvious position for casual observation, they would indeed impress friends and business associates.

The ancient Chinese, believing in the mysterious, spiritlike origin of many natural conditions, decorated their eyeglass cases with carvings and emblems of their fancies, superstitions, and tales (Figure 131). These are of enduring charm and beauty. On one such case (Figure 132), we could trace the carved imagery to find that it represents a famous story from the *Three Kingdoms* entitled "Treading Through the Snow in Pursuit of the Plum Flower."[1] Another is of sandalwood. The carving is on a background of peonies, which signify riches (Figure 133). In addition to this fenestrated style (Figure 134), various other styles made of wood have been found (Figures 135–139).

Besides carved wood, other materials such as gutta-percha (Figure 140), lacquer (Figure 141), papier mache (Figure 142), shagreen (Figure 143), bamboo (Figure 144), and ivory (Figure 145) were used. The author's example of a case for folding Chinese spectacles made of a dried tangerine skin is unique (Figure 146)! Later, as spectacles were more plentiful and reading skills were more widespread, cases were used to exhibit a favorite poem, saying, or fable (Figure 147). Sayings of good luck, goodwill, and good health prevailed as well. Later still, cases were used for advertising the optician (Figure 148).

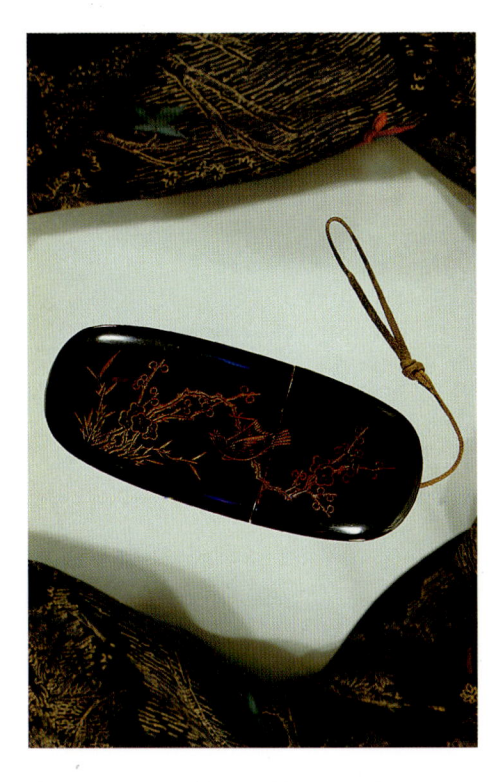

Figure 123. Carved lacquer Chinese spectacle case circa 1800.

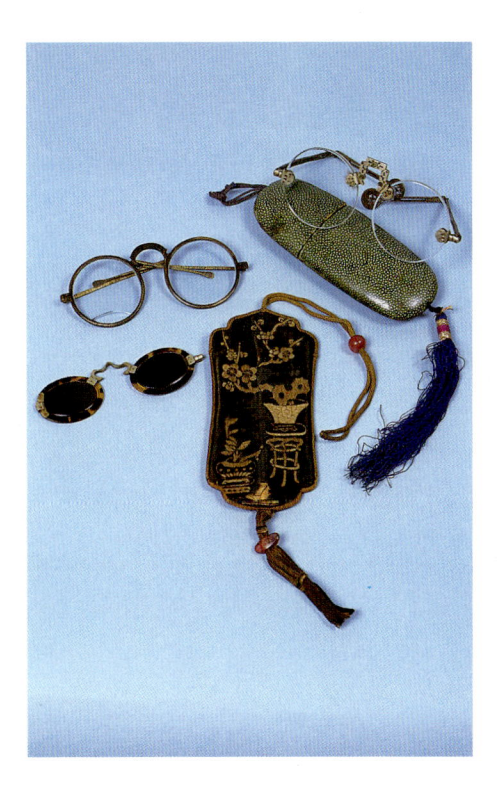

Figure 124. Large Chinese spectacles and cases circa 1750—size contrast circa 1880.

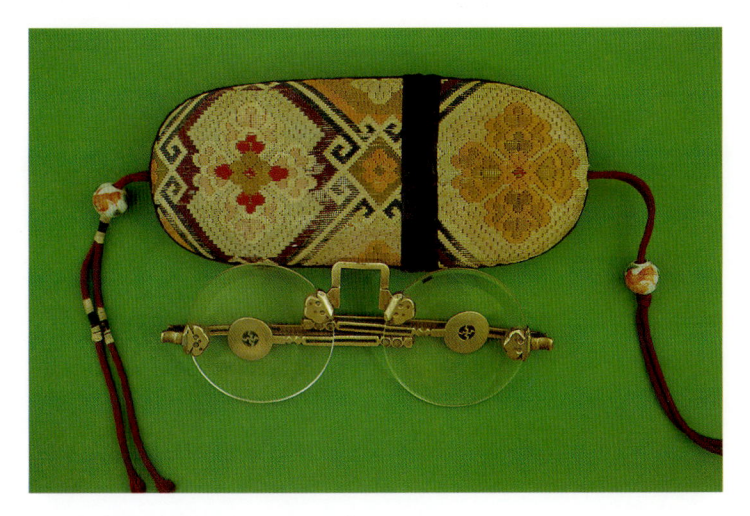

Figure 125. Chinese spectacles and case circa 1850.

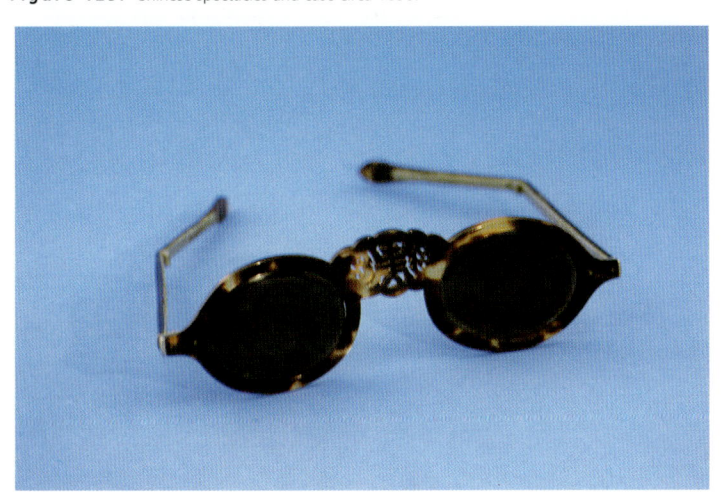

Figure 126. Tortoiseshell Chinese spectacles circa 1875.

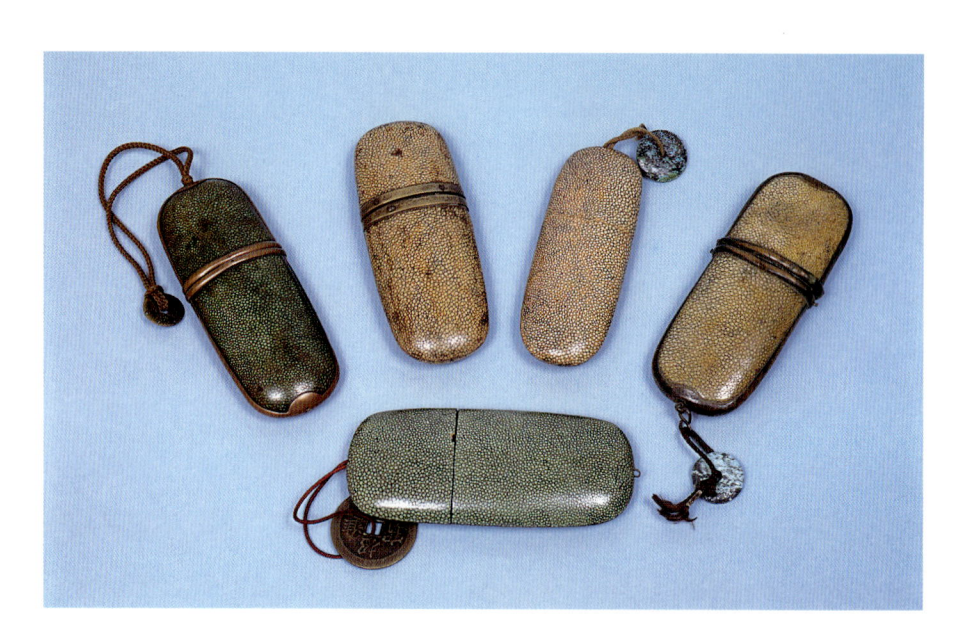

Figure 127. Shagreen Chinese spectacle cases circa 1840.

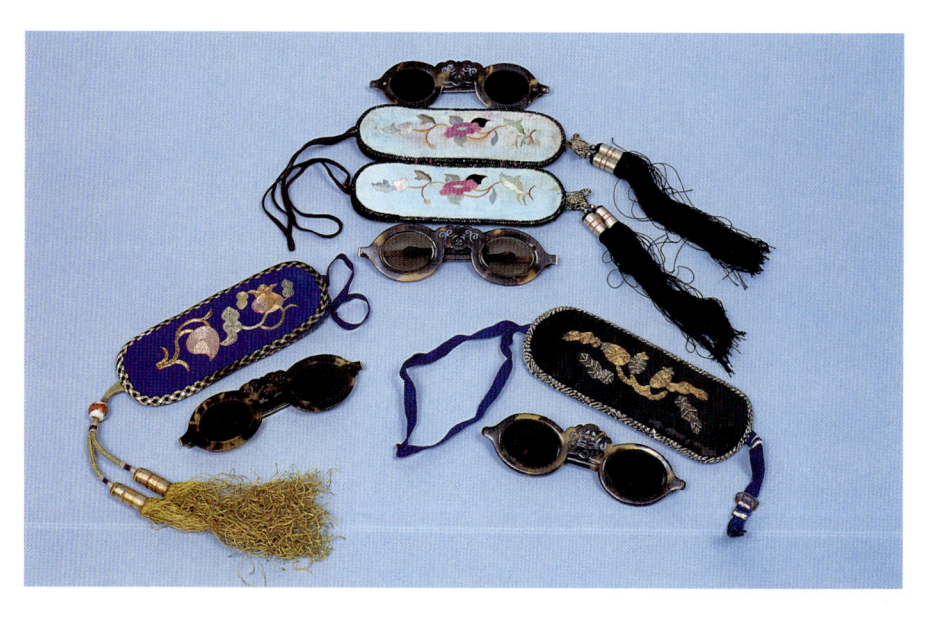

Figure 128. Silk Chinese spectacle cases circa 1890. Note double (above).

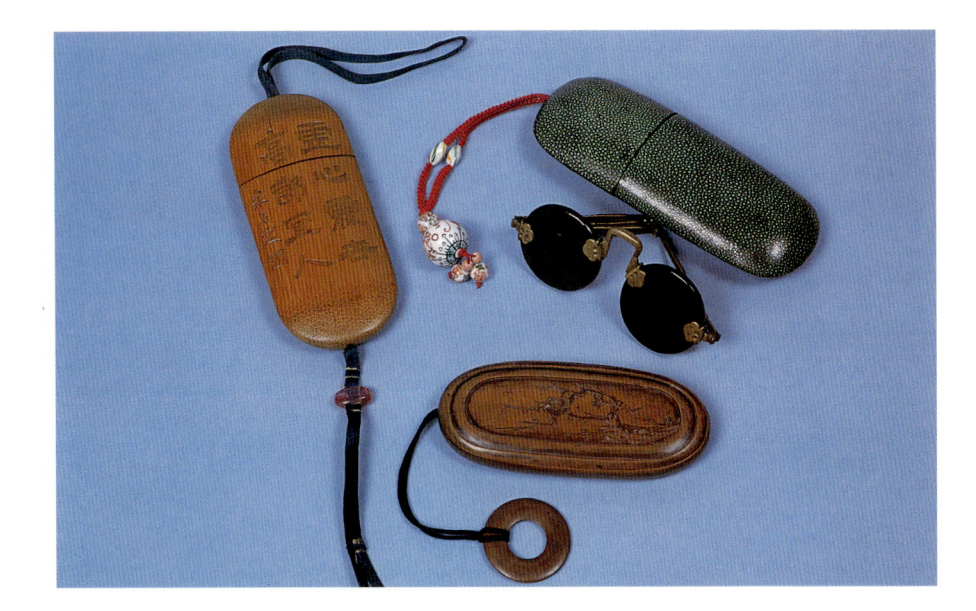

Figure 129. Chinese spectacle cases 1790–1830.

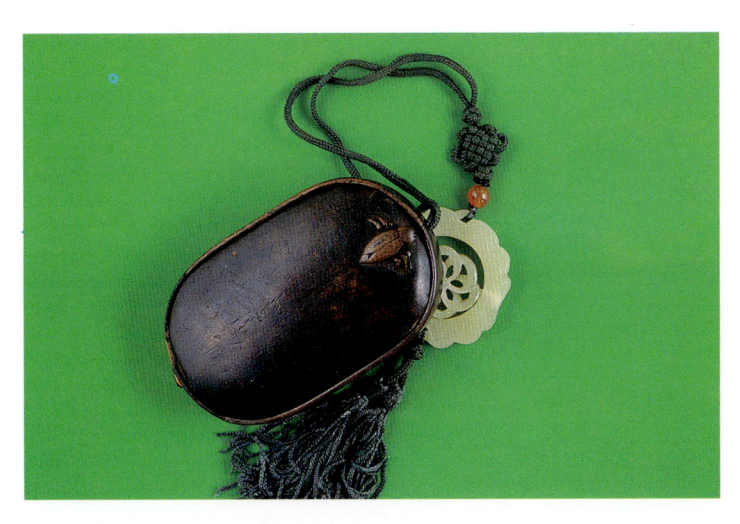

Figure 130. Wooden case for folding spectacles circa 1790.

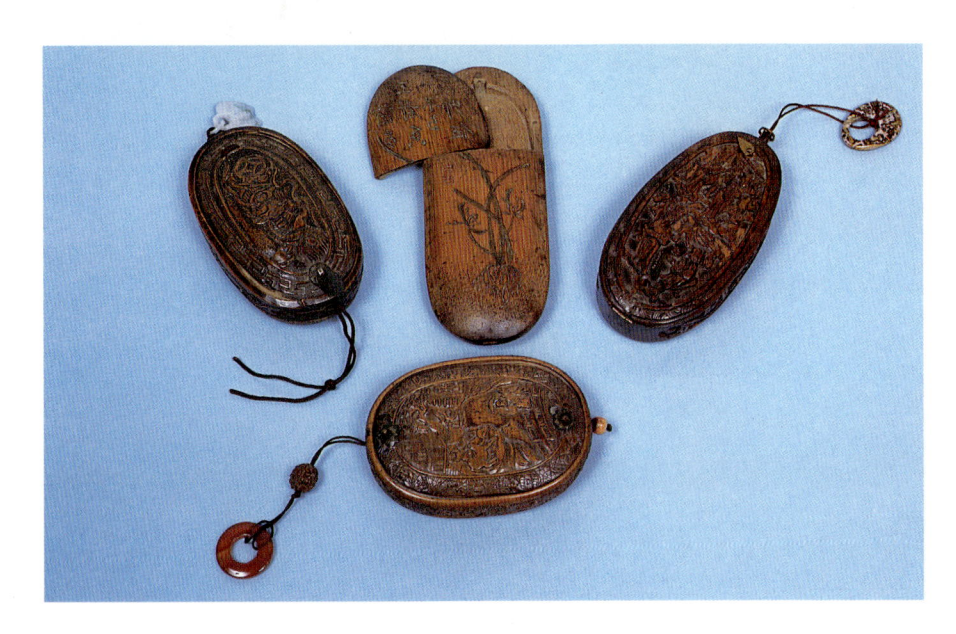

Figure 131. Various carved wooden spectacle cases circa 1720–1790.

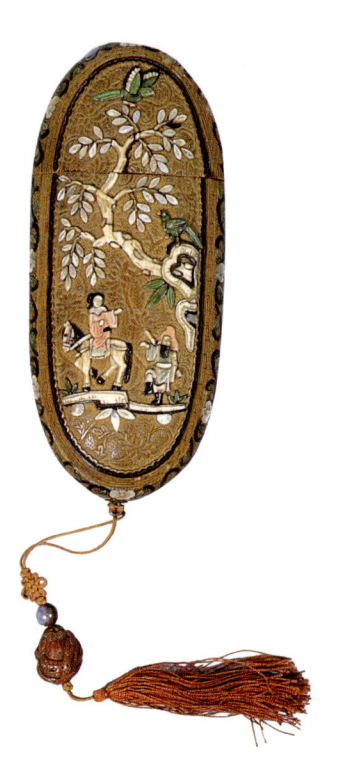

Figure 132. Carved spectacle case inlaid with semiprecious stones.

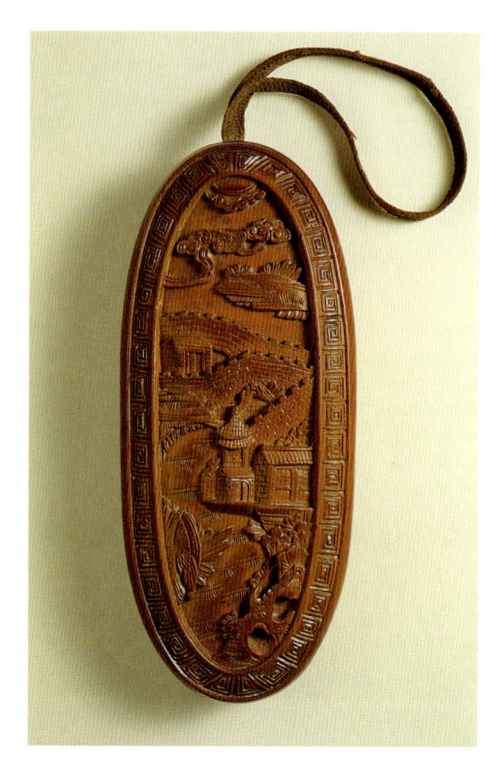

Figure 133. Sandalwood carved spectacle case.

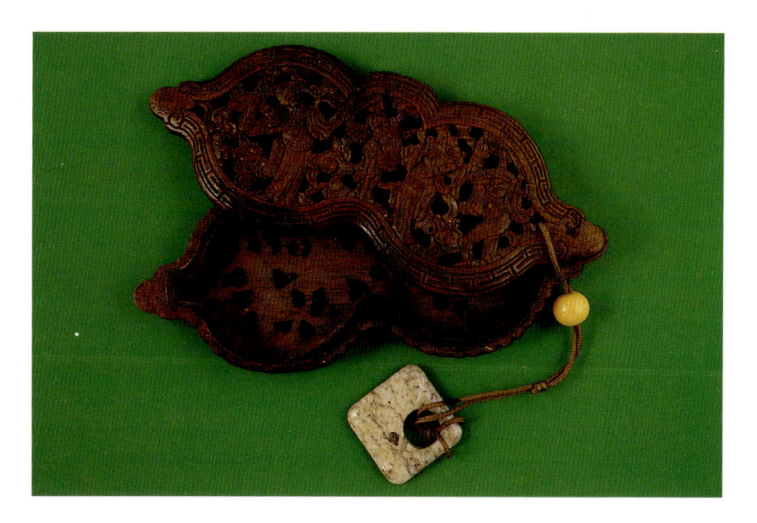

Figure 134. Fenestrated wooden Chinese spectacle case.

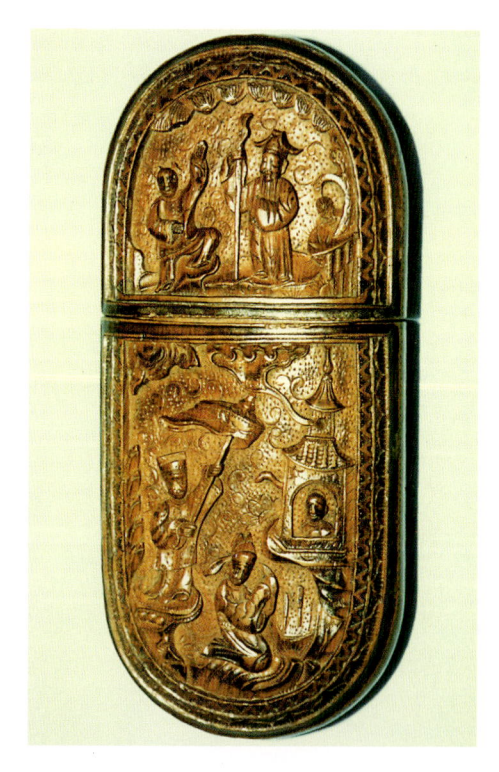

Figure 135. Carved wooden Chinese spectacle case.

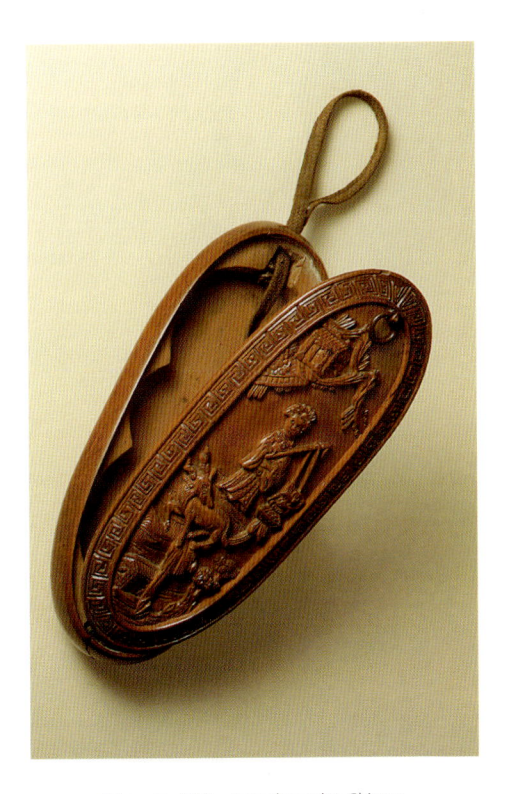

Figure 136. Carved wooden Chinese spectacle case.

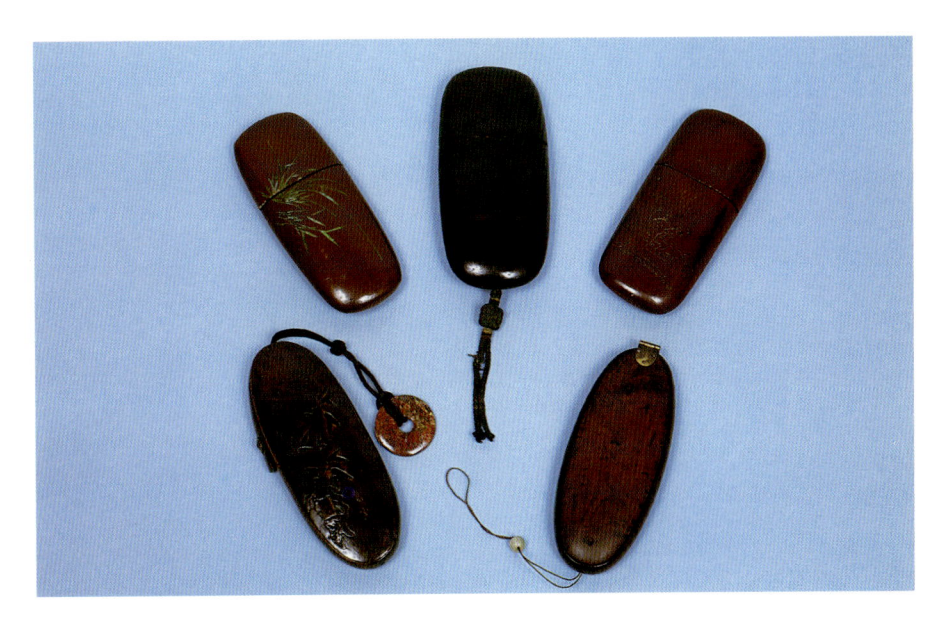

Figure 137. Carved spectacle cases.

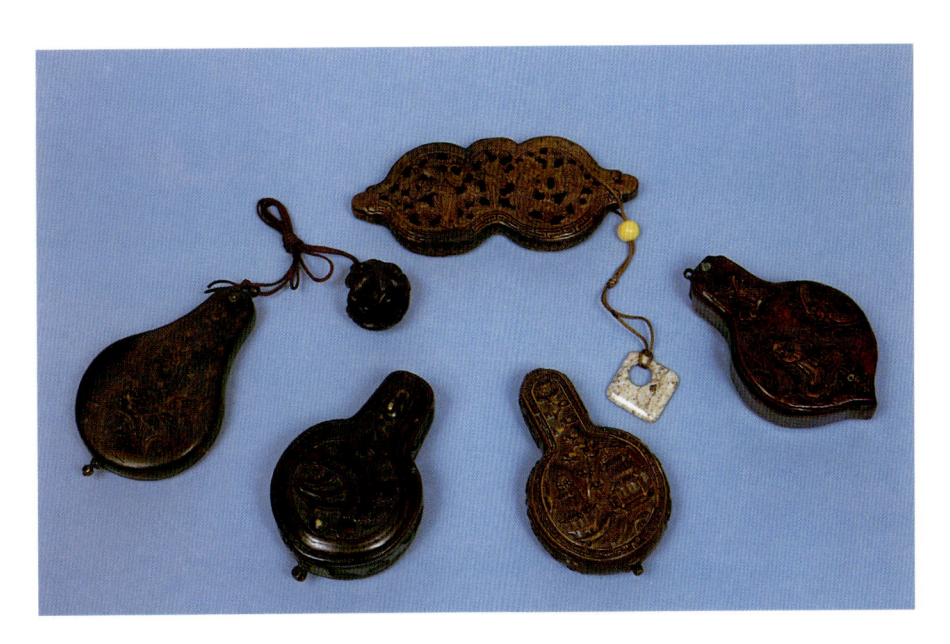

Figure 138. Carved Chinese spectacle cases for folding spectacles (below).

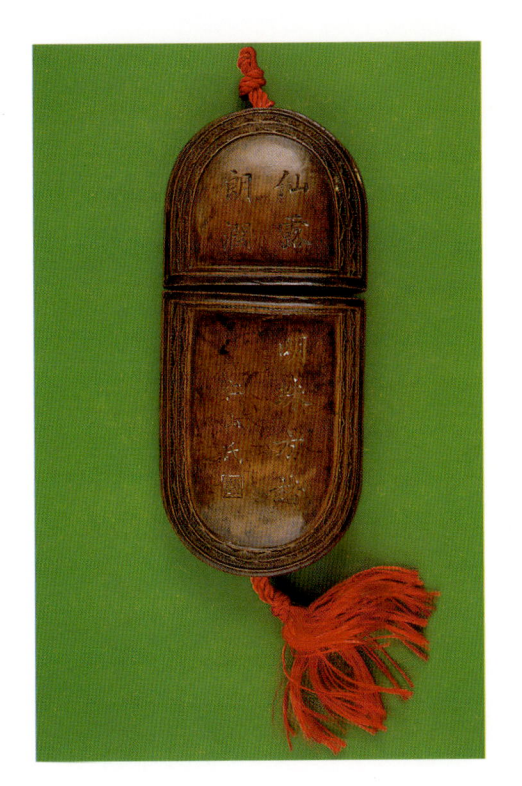

Figure 139. Carved Chinese spectacle case.

CHINESE EYEGLASS CASES **83**

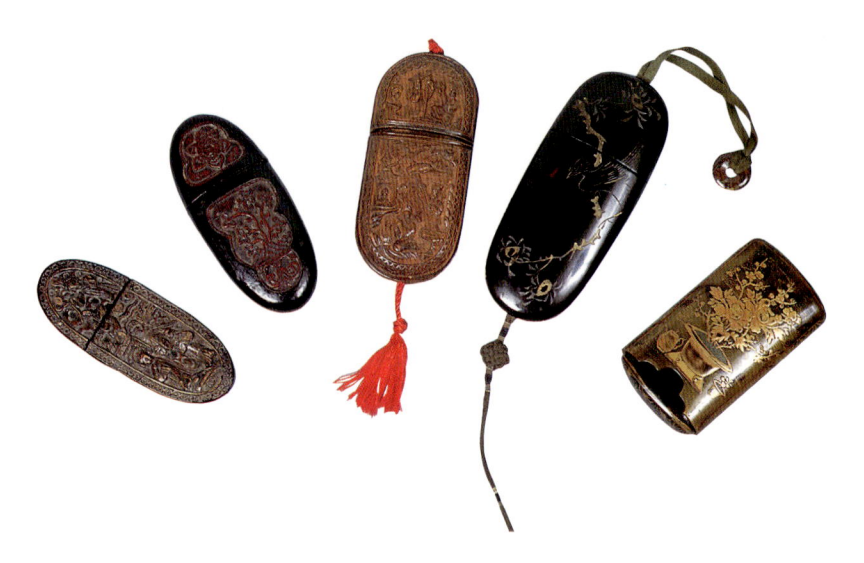

Figure 140. Carved gutta-percha spectacle case (left).

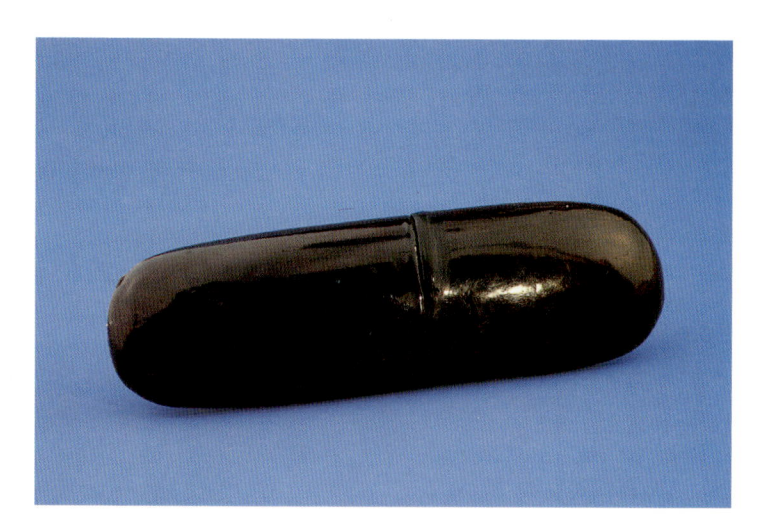

Figure 141. Black lacquer spectacle case.

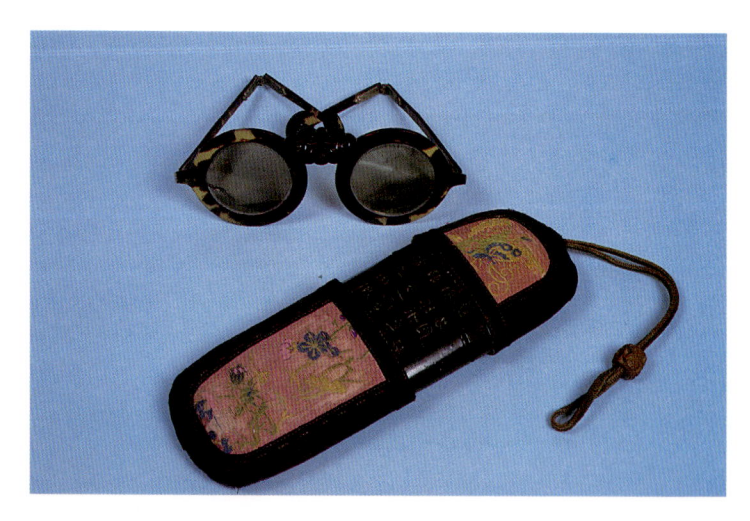

Figure 142. Papier mache incised spectacle case in separate cover.

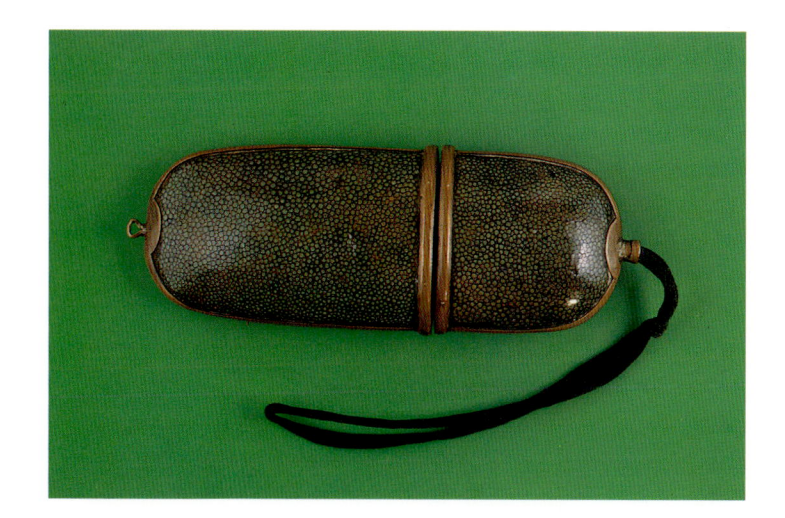

Figure 143. Shagreen spectacle case banded in copper.

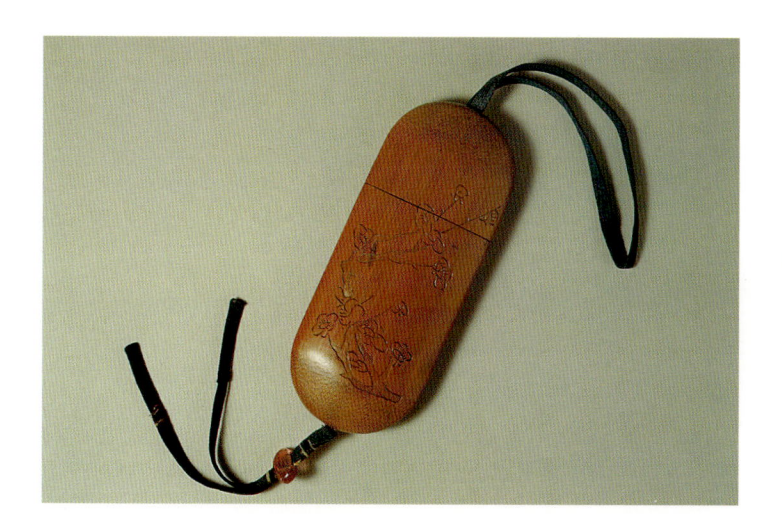

Figure 144. Incised bamboo spectacle case.

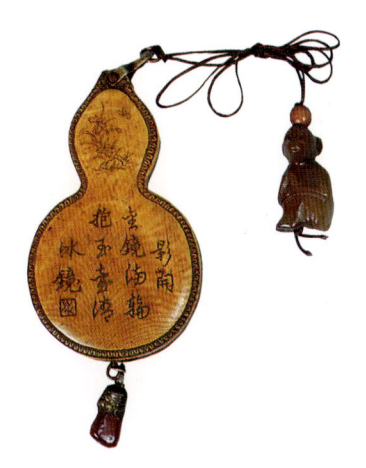

Figure 145. Ivory case for folding Chinese spectacles circa 1700.

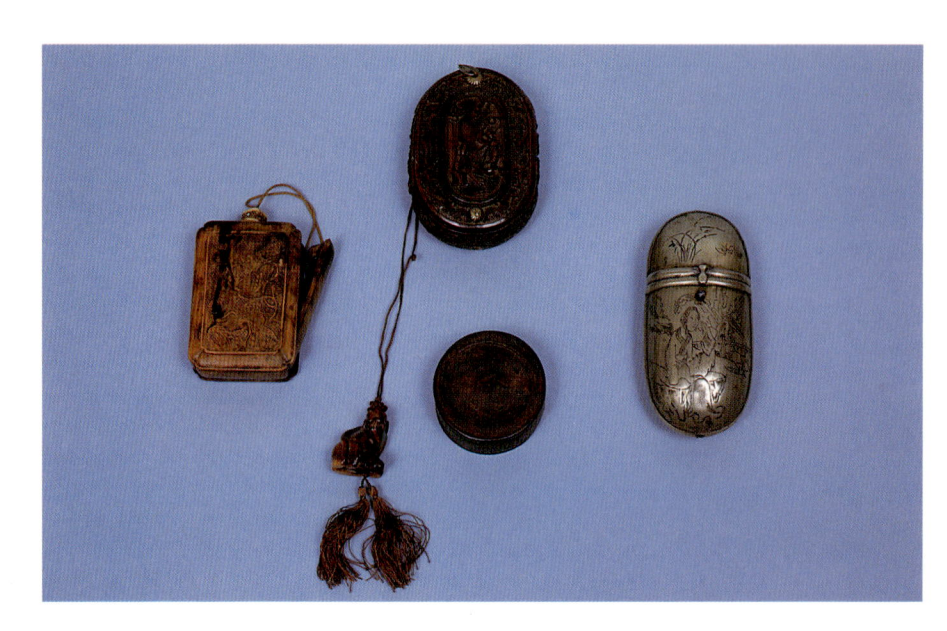

Figure 146. Tangerine-skin spectacle case (below, center) and *pai-tung* (right).

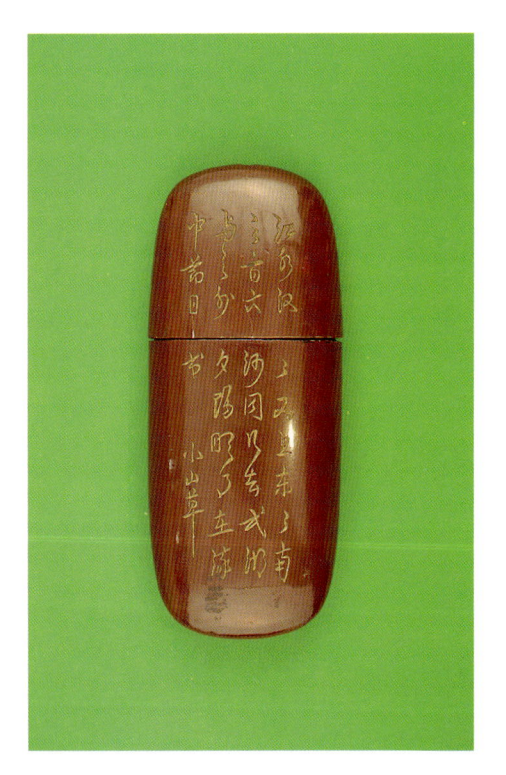

Figure 147. Spectacle case with Chinese saying.

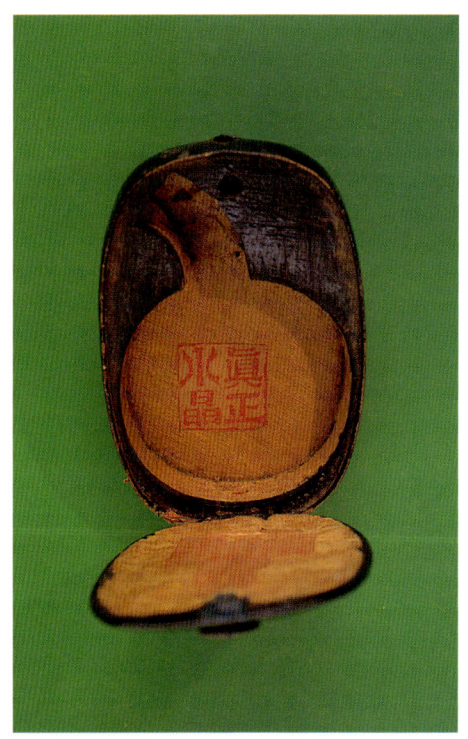

Figure 148. Folding spectacle case advertising the optician.

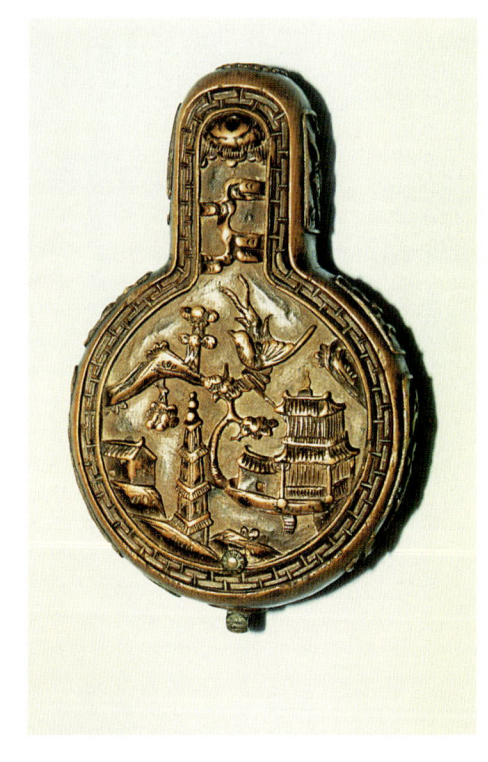

Figure 149. Carved spectacle case for folding spectacle—boxwood.

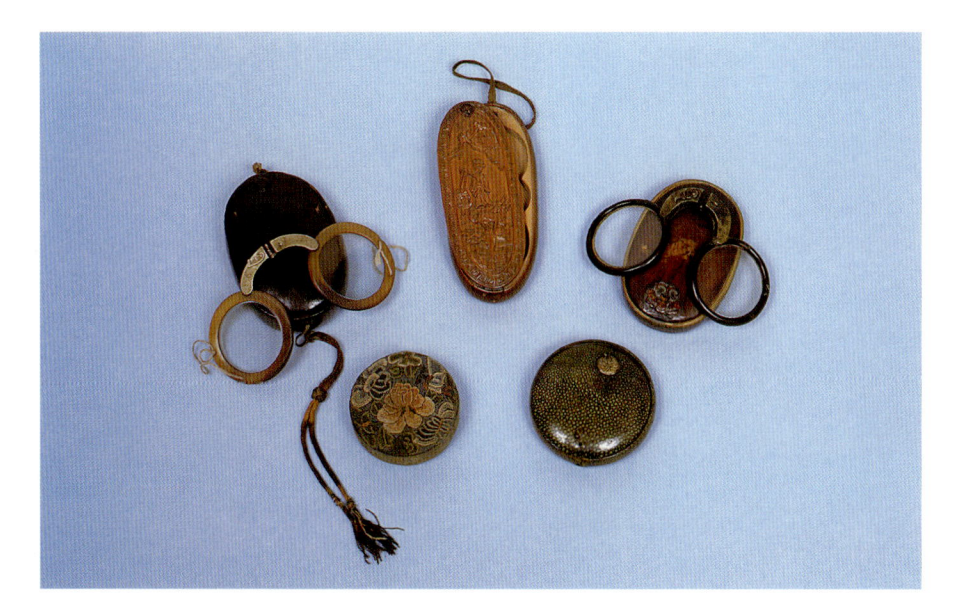

Figure 150. Types of spectacle cases available.

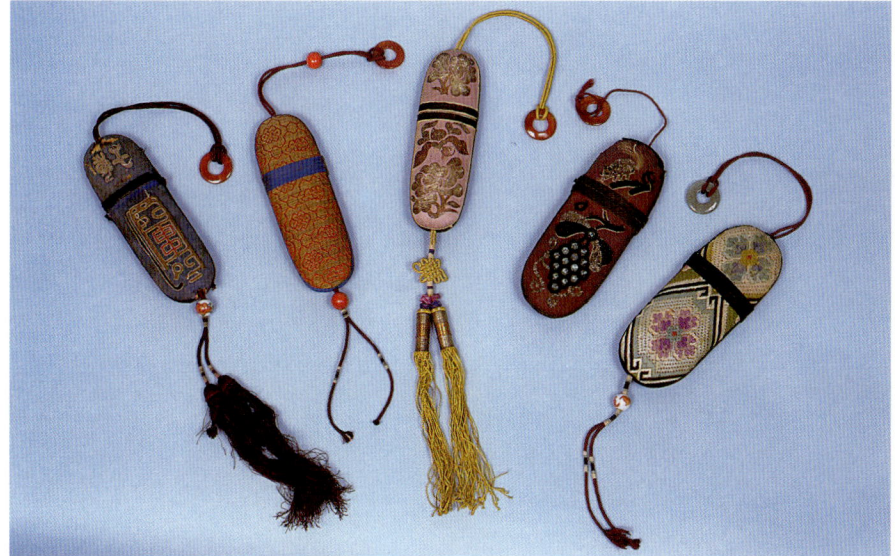

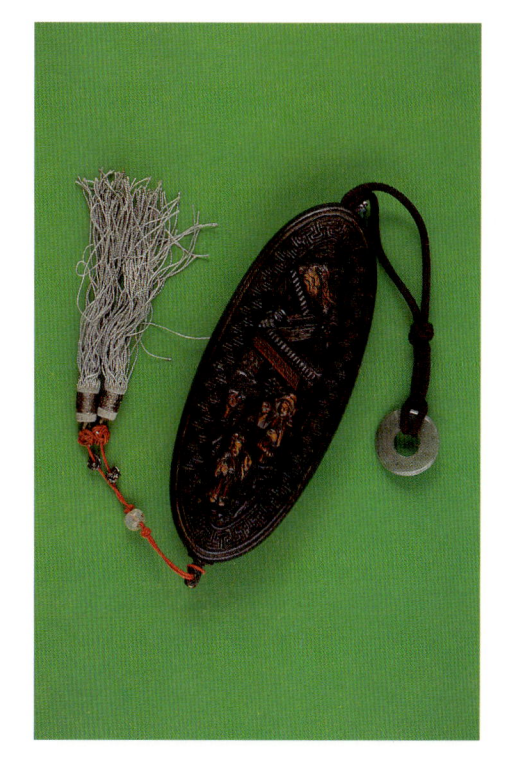

Figure 151. Clay over wood spectacle case.

Figure 152. Embroidered Chinese spectacle cases circa 1830.

When the folding variety of glasses was used (mostly in Northern China) (Figure 149), cases followed suit and their compactness was an advantage.[2] Even so, they were carved and decorated according to the whim of the purchaser. Still, we must remember that these persons were quite wealthy and could commission the type of case and carving they desired (Figure 150).

Rasmussen wrote that most of the spectacle cases were of a wooden base and then simply polished and stained.[3] Some were covered by carvings, and others by carved clay (Figure 151). Valuable cases were covered by embroidery (Figures 152 & 153) of various qualities. Rasmussen also stated that the most serviceable cases were covered with sharkskin (shagreen) (Figure 154).

CHINESE EYEGLASS CASES **87**

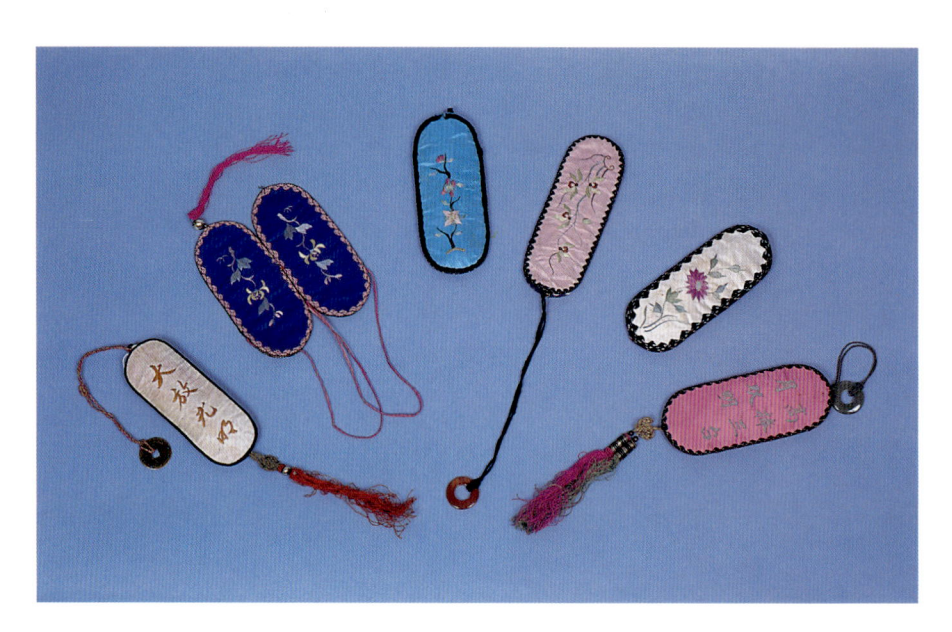

Figure 153. Embroidered spectacle cases circa 1880 (note double).

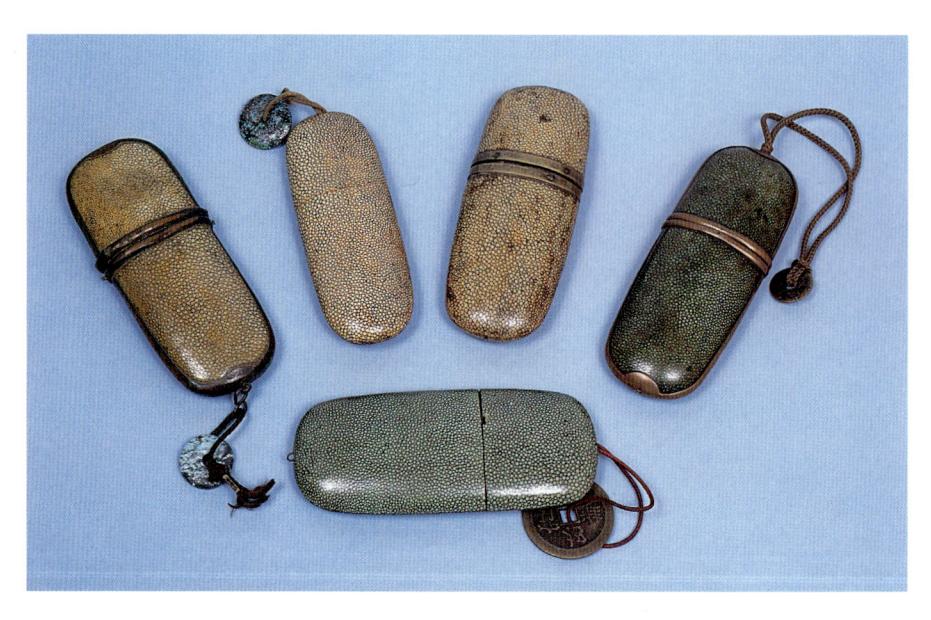

Figure 154. Shagreen spectacle cases circa 1800.

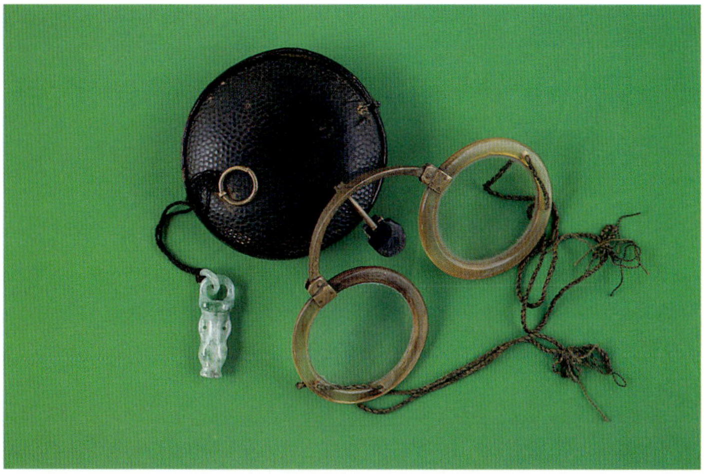

Figure 155. Cetorhinus skin-covered case and horn-rimmed folding spectacles with string temples.

Spectacle Cases in Author's Collection

Many in the author's collection are small (round and oblong) cases covered with the skin of a variety of smaller shark—the cetorhinus (Figure 155). The scales are smaller and resemble those of a lizard. The slip-top of the case was held on by a fancy loop, with crystal or jade beads holding it in place. A tassel hanging from the bottom was a finishing touch. In addition to collecting the types already mentioned, the author collected examples of spectacle cases covered with several types of lacquer:

1. Decorated (Figure 156)
2. Incised with allegorical sayings (Figure 157)
3. Carved (Figure 158)
4. Inlaid with mother-of-pearl, etc. (Figure 159)
5. Decorated with transfer (overlay or decal) (Figure 160)

The top of this last case almost completely covers the inside sleeve, which is retrieved by a handy finger cutout on the outer element. This case is additionally unusual in that the decoration gives a distinctive Persian impression.

Other cases are made of cloisonne, bamboo, and horn (Figures 161, 162, & 163). Several have the shape of a flat box with a pullout slide insert (Figures 164 & 165). These are cloth covered and decorated with embroidery. Even gold threads are used.

One old and rare case is made of ivory, circa 1700 (Figure 166).[4] It has the shape of a gourd, and the "tassel" is a piece of ruby glass (no longer made in China). This is a signed piece from the north of China. The calligraphy denotes eternal prosperity, like the pine tree. The carving shows a man sitting under a pine tree with a crane and deer as company. Its patina is marvelous.

Minute examination of the larger cases (Figure 167) reveals exquisite embroidery—some even with beads and faux jewels (Figure 168). The later examples do not carry fine embroidery, and some may be machine made (Figure 169). One of the larger cases (Figure 170), while flat, is embroidered with gold thread and clusters of gold grapes. (Figure 128 shows other embroidered cases.)

Tortoiseshell has not been ignored by the Chinese and Japanese in constructing their spectacle cases. The one illustrated here is lavishly encrusted with silver and gold scenes. It is the pullout-sleeve type of case and is shown front and back (Figures 171 & 172).

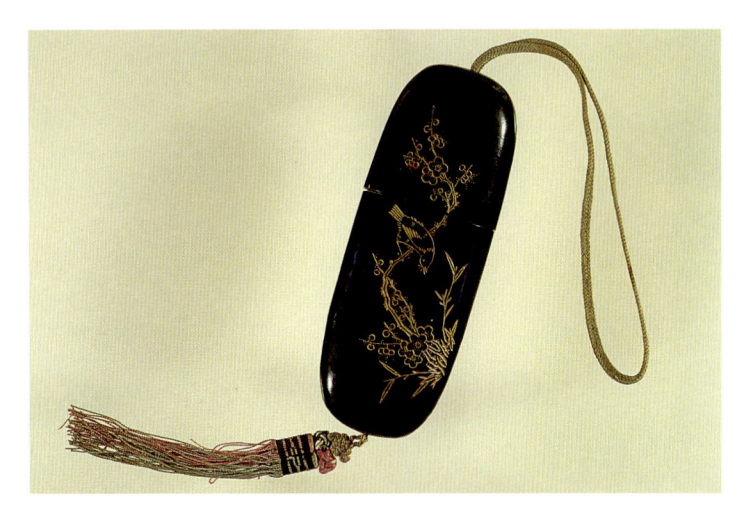

Figure 156. Decorated lacquer spectacle case.

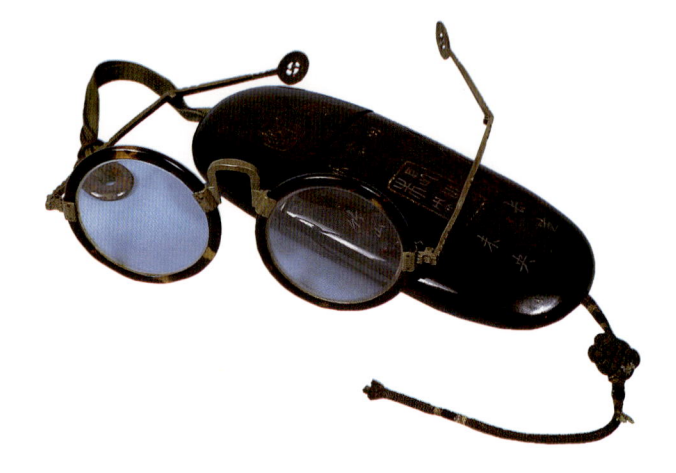

Figure 157. Incised lacquer spectacle case.

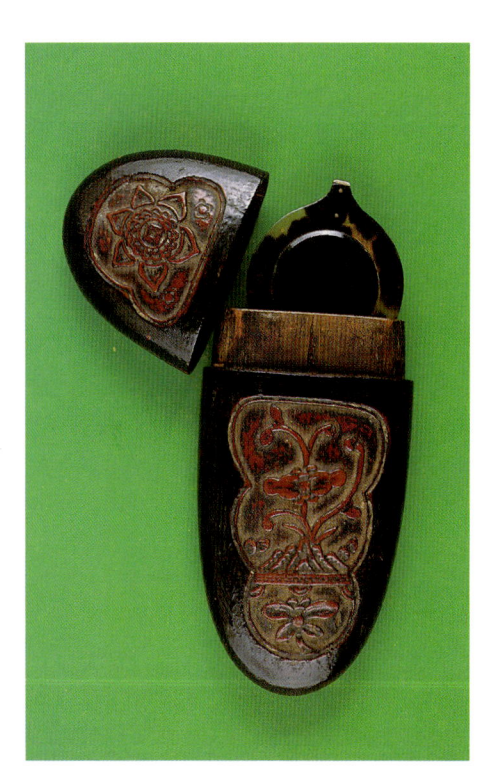

Figure 158. Carved lacquer spectacle case.

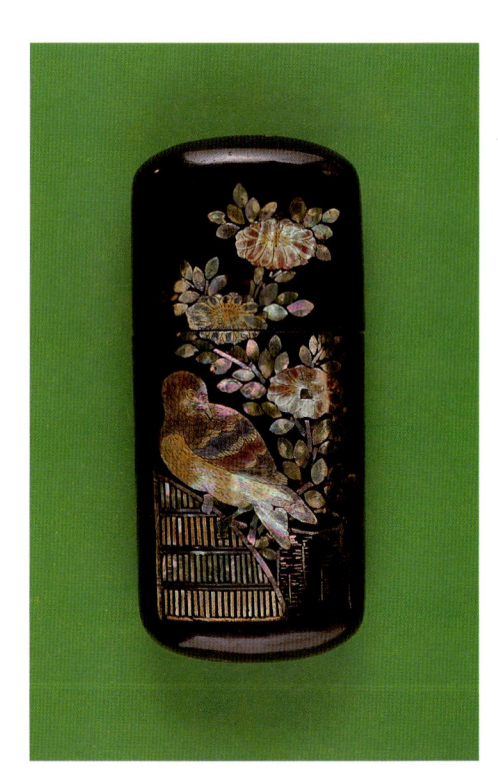

Figure 159. Inlaid lacquer spectacle case.

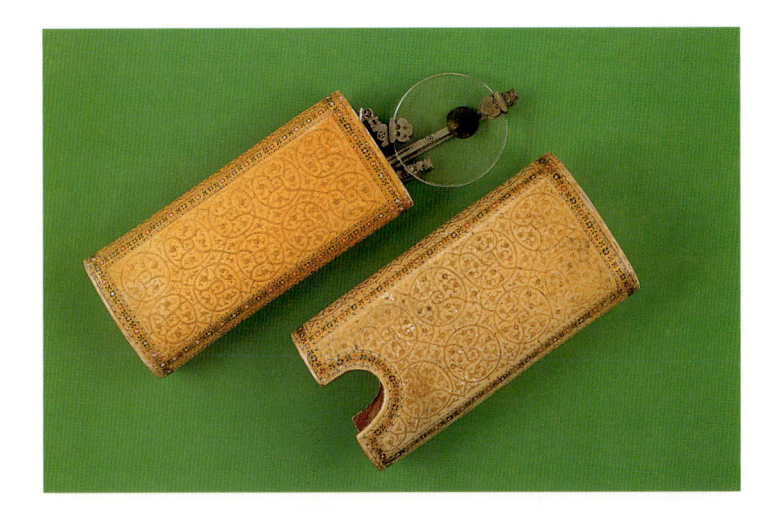

Figure 160. Transfer lacquer spectacle case.

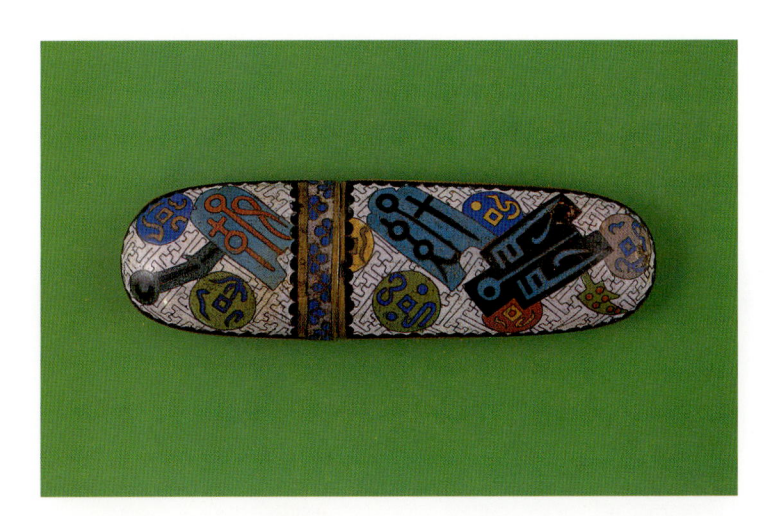

Figure 161. Cloissone spectacle case.

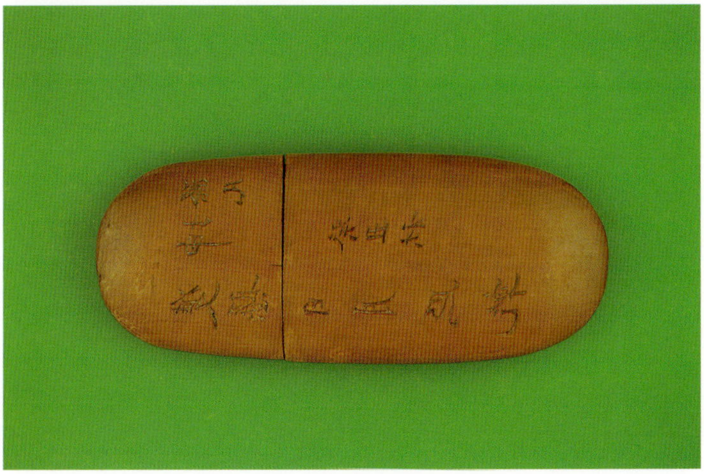

Figure 162. Bamboo spectacle case.

CHINESE EYEGLASS CASES

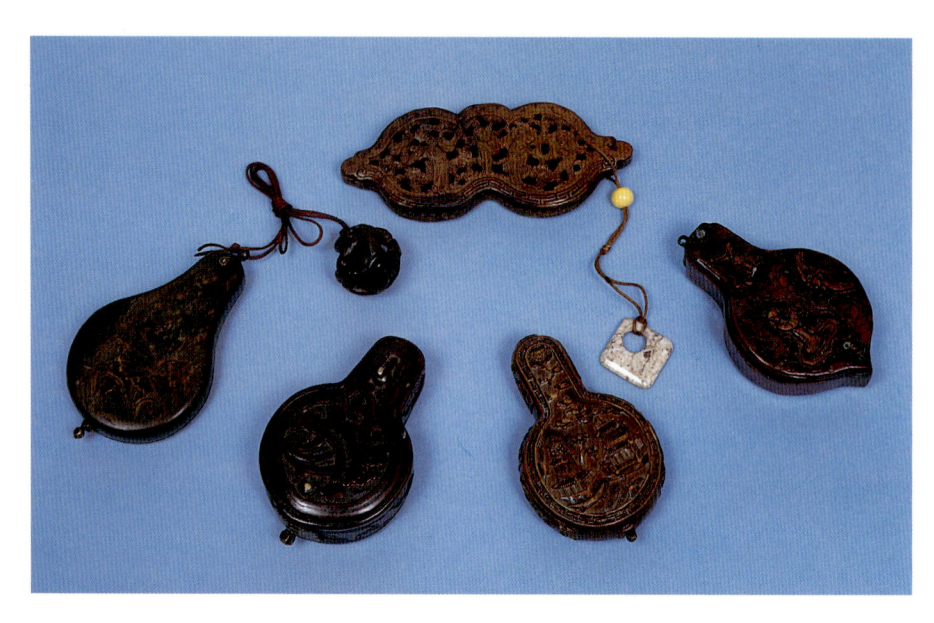

Figure 163. Horn spectacle case (first on left side).

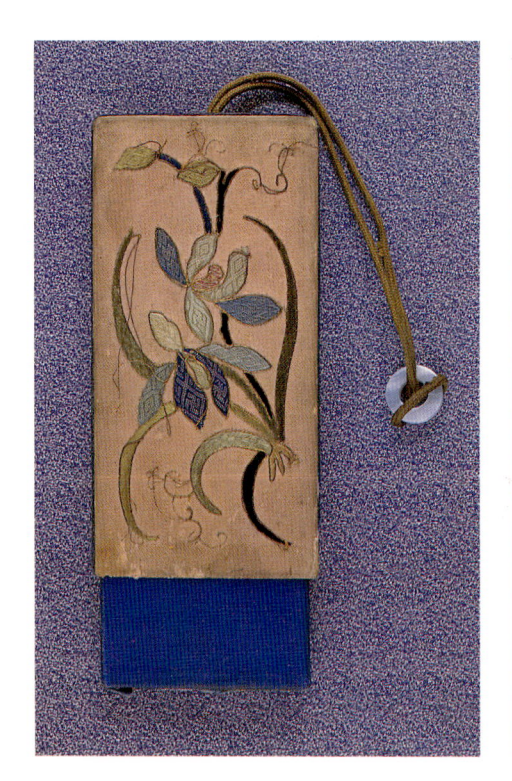

Figure 164. Flat Chinese spectacle case—embroidered.

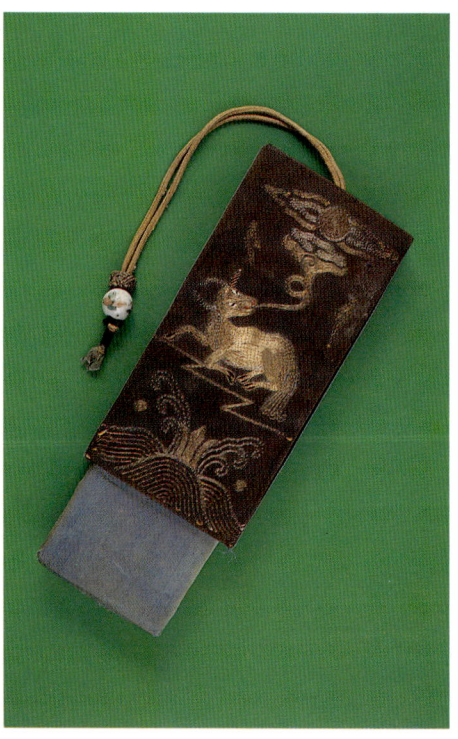

Figure 165. Flat Chinese spectacle case—embroidered using gold threads.

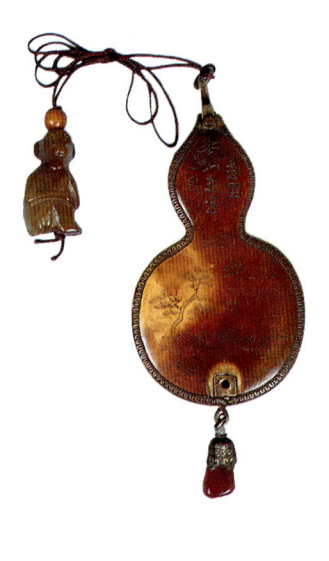

Figure 166. Ivory spectacle case in shape of a gourd.

92　CHAPTER 8

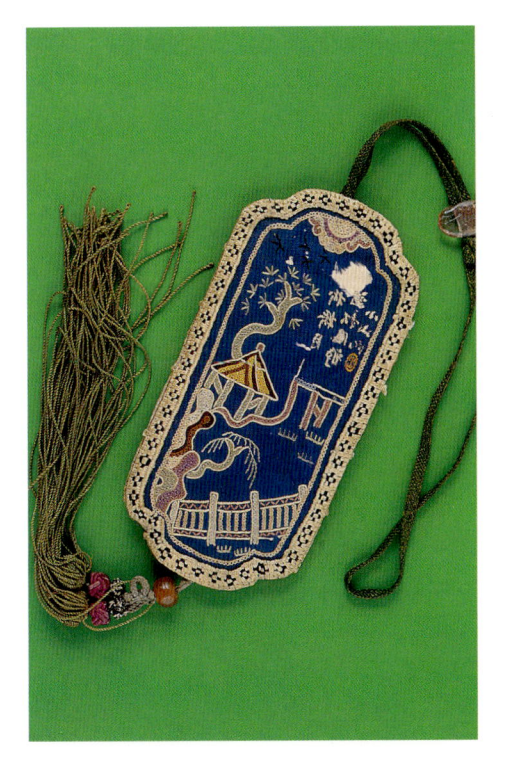

Figure 167. Embroidered spectacle case with fine handwork.

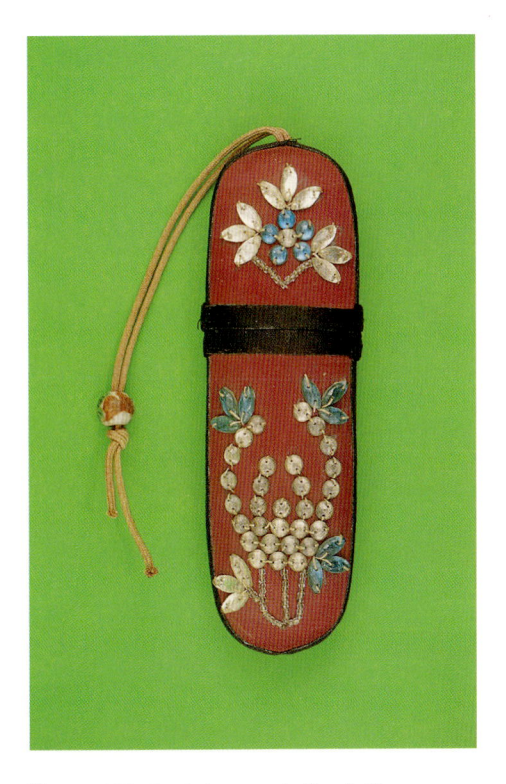

Figure 168. Spectacle case embroidered with beads and faux jewels.

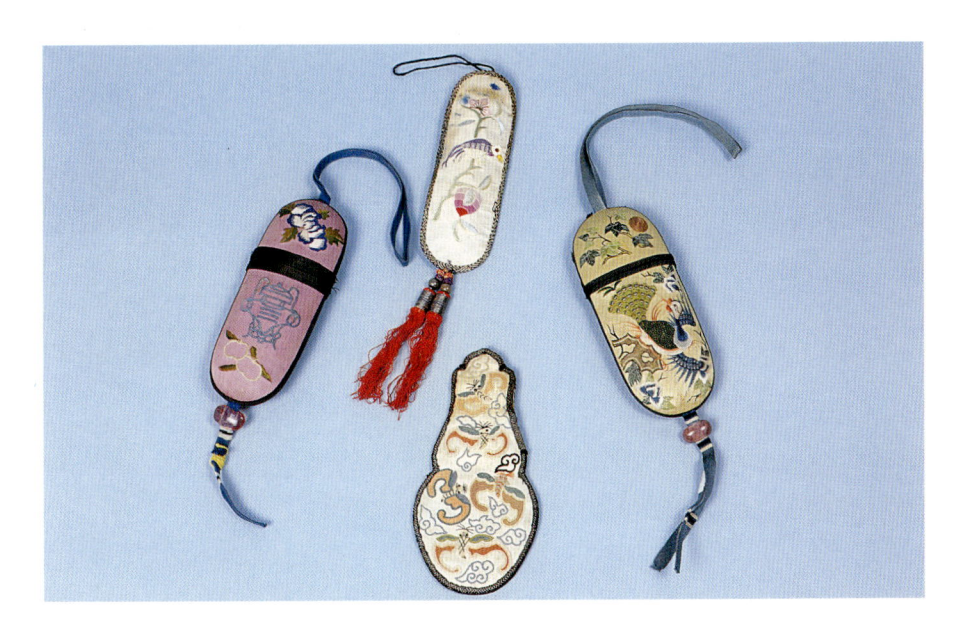

Figure 169. Embroidered spectacle cases—common varieties.

CHINESE EYEGLASS CASES 93

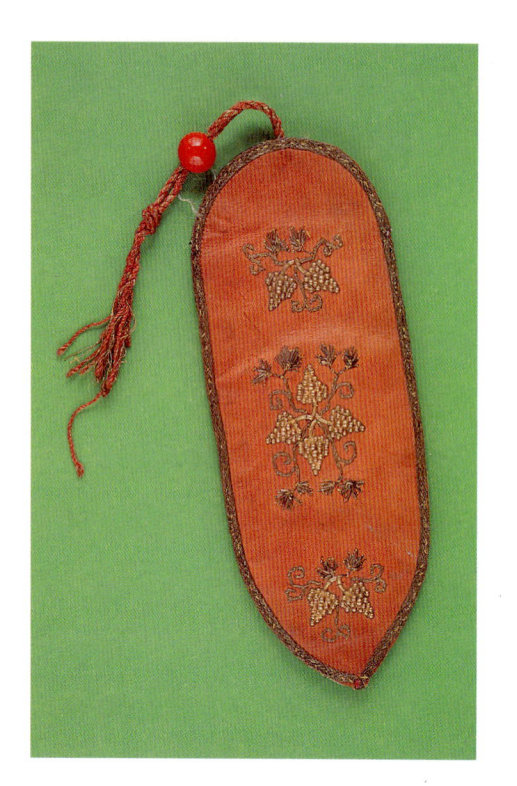

Figure 170. Spectacle case embroidered with gold.

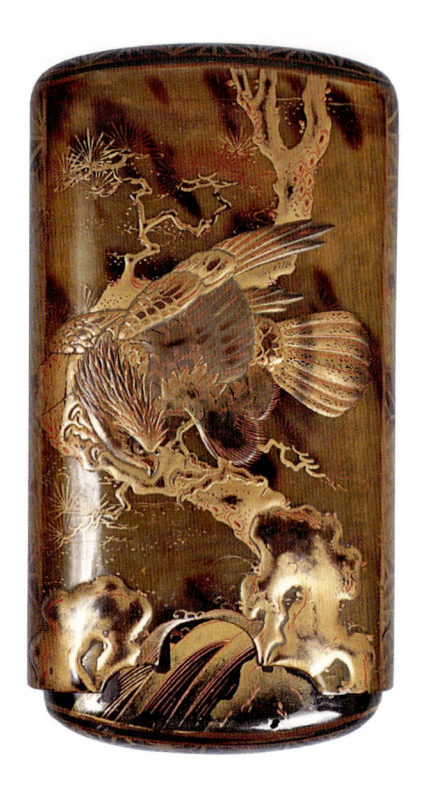

Figure 171. Front of tortoiseshell spectacle case.

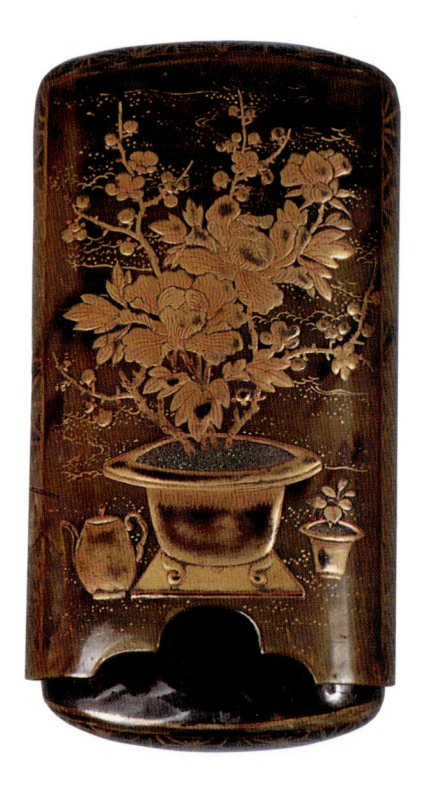

Figure 172. Back of tortoiseshell spectacle case.

94 CHAPTER 8

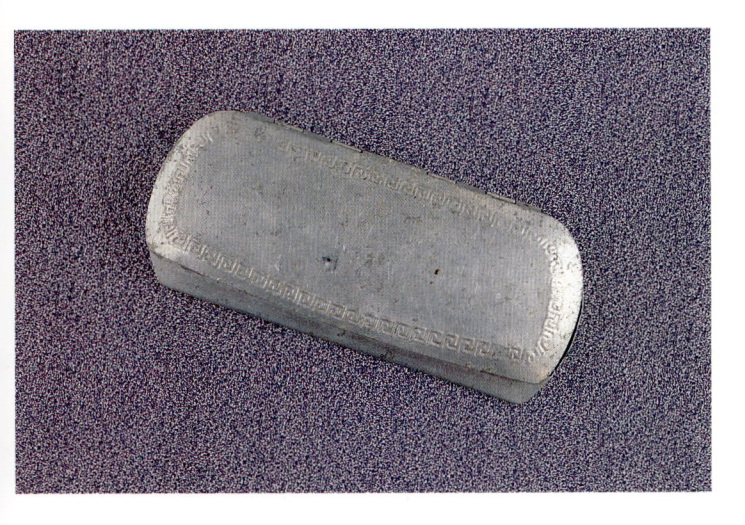

Figure 173. Pressed aluminum clamshell type of case.

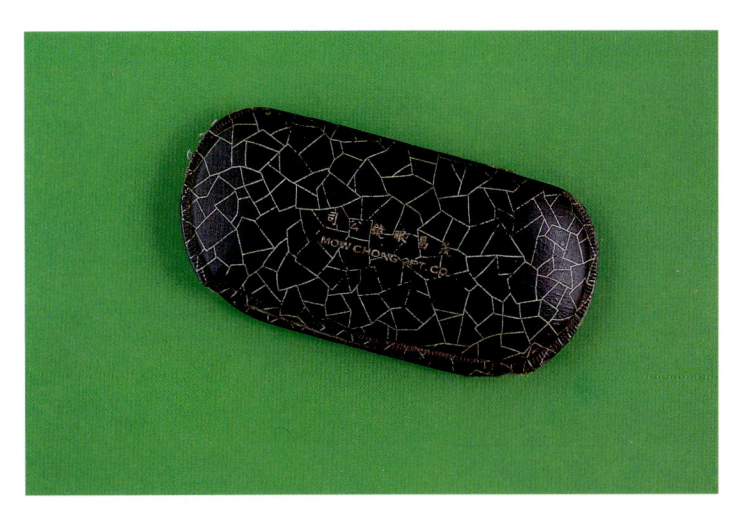

Figure 174. Plastic covered metal clamshell type of case.

Twentieth-Century Eyeglass Cases

Starting around 1900, the Chinese started making and using American- and European-style clamshell cases that snapped closed (Figure 173). Many were pressed aluminum—others covered with thin leather or plastic as we have seen in the United States until about 1960 (Figure 174). Since then, many types have become available: soft and hard, snap and flip, open-top and open-side, to name a few.

Conclusion

We see that a mundane article of everyday use—the spectacle case—was at the time an article of beauty or art, of endearing charm, of historical and religious distinction, and today a respected example of antiquity.

Notes

1. Raymond Li, *A Glossary of Chinese Snuff Bottles Rebus* (Kowloon, Hong Kong: Nine Dragons Publishers, 1976).
2. O. D. Rasmussen, *Chinese Eyesight and Spectacles* (Tonbridge, Kent, England, 1949).
3. Ibid.
4. C. Y. Tse, Personal communication, Hong Kong, 1992.

Other Sources Consulted for Chapter 8

1. Yui Kai Sze, Personal communication, Hong Kong, 1990.
2. Teng Tak, *Fine Arts* (Kowloon, Hong Kong: Nine Dragons Publishers, 1992).
3. C. A. S. Williams, *Outlines of Chinese Symbolism and Art Motives* (New York: Dover Pub., 1976).

9

Japanese Spectacles

Tracing the history of spectacles in Japan is somewhat like tracing the history of spectacles in general. There are different versions of their origin as well as the time frame in which they first appeared in Japan. Following is an article by Sekiya Shirayama, who has thoroughly researched this subject.

THE INTRODUCTION OF SPECTACLES INTO JAPAN
Spectacles are said to have been invented in Europe in the 13th century A.D. The question is how and when were they first introduced into Japan? We have two ways of knowing . . . firstly from the first appearance of the word meaning "vision aids" in literature, and secondly from examination of the oldest eyeglasses still in existence in Japan.

Starting with literature we find eyeglasses mentioned for the first time in the year 1551. Francisco St. Xavier (1506–1552) visited Japan in 1549 as a Christian missionary. He tried to see the most powerful Lord of Japan, at Metropolis, to get permission for missionary work. Unfortunately at that time, Kyoto the capital was in the midst of a civil war and therefore neither the Emperor nor the Shogun had real power. He had to leave Kyoto after eleven days without having had an audience with them. Francisco St. Xavier then visited Yoshitaka Ohuchi a secure and influential local feudal Lord in his domain (now Yamguchi). He was here granted an audience because he brought many gifts including eyeglasses. This story is found in many books in both Japan and Europe and is very reliable as historical fact. Here are the references:

JAPAN
1. *Honcho Tsukan*, compiled by the government during 1640–70.
2. *The Account of Yoshitaka Ohuchi*.

EUROPE
1. *Histoire de l'église de Japon 1689*, by Jean Crasset 1618–92.
2. *Histoire de Japon*, by Louis Frois 1532–97.

The oldest spectacles still in existence in Japan are to be found in the Daisenin Temple in Kyoto which is the temple of the Zen sect. They are of fairly high convex power and are pivoted eyeglasses. The frame and case are both made of ivory. The lenses are 25mm in diameter. According to legend the founder of this temple received these very glasses, which the tenth Shogun Yoshimasa Ashikaga 1436–90 had used, from the eleventh Shogun Yoshiharu Ashikaga 1511–50. If this story were true it would mean that they were in use more than sixty years before Francisco St. Xavier presented spectacles to Yoshitaka Ohuchi in 1551. Unfortunately the story is only temple tradition and there is no real evidence to corroborate it. There is also a view held in some quarters that these are in fact the spectacles which were brought to Japan by Francisco St. Xavier but that is impossible because

Shogun Yoshiharu Ashikaga died the year before Xavier visited Kyoto and there is no record of any meeting.

The spectacles are extremely decorative, beautiful and fine. They are not considered to be European because of their decoration and color, and it is hard to think of them as Chinese. (The Editor has seen a slide of the specs., and case. The case in particular is of a style also found in Ceylon.)

China was at that time in the era of the Ming Dynasty and in the literature of the years of the fifth Emperor Shuan Tsung 1399–1435 it is stated that they had no eyeglasses long ago but had them for the first time in the era of the Ming Dynasty 1368–1615 from the West. The literature also mentions that Shuan Tsung bought eyeglasses from foreign merchants and gave them to his father. The era of the twelfth Emperor of the Ming Dynasty Shih Tsung 1507–66 was contemporary with that of Yoshiharu Ashikaga 1511–66 in Japan. That eyeglasses were seldom then seen, and they were bought from foreign merchants who came from Malacca, Arabia or Samarkand, is mentioned elsewhere in the literature of this period. It is said that the manufacture of spectacles in China began in the 17th century in the Ching Dynasty which started in 1636.

In 1933 Dr. R. Greeff then a professor at Berlin University stated in his book "Aus Der Geshichte Der Brille" that spectacles were introduced into Japan by way of China around 1530, but the source of this information is not given and it cannot be proved.

Also in Japan there are two pairs of eyeglasses which belonged to the founder of the Tokugawa Shogunate Ieyasu Tokugawa 1542–1616. They are to be found in his Memorial Museum. They are of the rigid bridge type and are made of transparent yellowish spurious tortoiseshell. The lenses are glass and the eye sizes are 40mm diameter in one pair and 38mm diameter in the other pair. It is unknown how these eyeglasses came to be in the museum.

In conclusion we consider that the first spectacles to appear in Japan were the ones presented to Yoshitaka Ohuchi in 1551.[1]

Literature

We can thus see that the first spectacles were introduced to Japan in 1551 when Francisco St. Xavier (Portuguese, 1506–1552) presented a pair to Yoshitaka Ohuchi. Further information along this line came to the author from a book in Japanese by Dr. Hiroo Nagaoka of Kanazawa City, Japan.[2] The book was written in 1972 and is outlined in this chapter. Another Japanese book on the same subject is discussed here as well. Lacking language skills, the author apologizes for any errors here introduced.

On the dust jacket of his book, Dr. Nagaoka is described as "an expert oculist living in Kanazawa City, Ishikawa Prefecture. His family has been in the profession for nearly 200 years. He is well known for his study on ancient spectacles and the collection of them."

This well-illustrated book by Dr. Nagaoka contains about 150 pages. Ancient spectacles and cases are described in the first chapter. Photographs show rivet glasses (and case) owned by a shogun from Kyoto, slitbridge and Chinese-style glasses owned by a famous priest, and Dutch spectacles of the same period (1500–1600). Korean glasses pictured appear to be pure Chinese. Dr. Nagaoka shows a variety of old spectacles, some of which are unique in carving of ivory, folding technique, and bridge design. The European as well as the Chinese influence is easily seen on bridges, lenses, and temples.

One lorgnette is pictured, a Franklin type of bifocal, folding D clear and sun lenses, and protective glasses as made by American Optical Company. Spectacle cases appear to be handmade, and a few have *netsuke* type of objects to hang over the belt.

A line drawing of an Edo period spectacle shop (fifteenth to seventeenth century) is interesting in its simplicity and the fact that the optician is apparently grinding or edging a lens as a customer observes. Several pictures show various types of optical apparatus (transits, projectors, binoculars, etc.), as well as Chinese-style spectacles for women and those with strings to hold them behind the ears.

Dr. Nagaoka describes how the name "spectacles" came about (which the author could not translate). Other chapters included information on spectacles as the instrument of high culture, the artisans for spectacles and their dealers, superstitions, songs on spectacles, etc. Dr. Nagaoka's further illustrations show opticians' signs, a folding screen showing the Portuguese, city life in the Meiji Era, and the eyeglass-shaped bridges in Nagasaki and Tokyo. Many pages are filled with cartoons. Eskimo glasses are shown as well as Nuremberg type of pince-nez.

Another book on the history of spectacles in Japan was sent to this author by a friend, a Japanese ophthalmologist from Osaka, Dr. Okihiro Nishi.[3] The text in this book is totally in Japanese. By comparing the characters, the author noted that three of the five on each title page are identical. By combining that with the illustrations, the subject matter is identified. Unfortunately, this author was unable to translate the author's name. The book has 252 pages, the first half of which is devoted to early European spectacle development and its application to the Japanese. Several photographs, however, also show Chinese spectacles. Group photographs are shown before an imposing building. One is labeled in English: "Students of the Ophthalmological Course given at Osaka February 1926." Several other photographs show (apparently) typical opticians' shops, and others the inside of lens-grinding shops. A dozen pages picture spectacles from the rivet to the 1950s in typical Oriental and European styles. Fifteen cases are also pictured.

Conclusion

Both books are well illustrated and between the two of them show a selected collection of fine old spectacles and cases of Japanese, Chinese, Korean, and European styles. It is surmised that the Chinese had the most influence on the use of spectacles in Japan. Their development paralleled Chinese and European standards in technology and timeliness.

Notes

1. Sekiya Shirayama, "The Introduction of Spectacles into Japan," *Ophthalmic Antiques International Collectors' Club*, April 1991.
2. Dr. Hiroo Nagaoka, *History of Spectacles in Japan*, 1972.
3. Unidentified author, *History of Spectacles in Japan* (Osaka, 1989).

Other Sources Consulted for Chapter 9

1. Hukushima, M.D., "Giiti," *Amer. J. Ophthal.*, 1963.

10

Steel Spectacles and Cases

The use of steel for spectacle frames and cases started in the seventeenth century. (However, steel was not used in spectacle manufacture by the Chinese until the late nineteenth century.) After 1280, when riveted spectacles with wooden frames and beryl lenses were used, and after the fifteenth century, when a fixed bridge was used, steel cases and frames for "besicles"—with or without a "bonnet strap"—were employed. Additionally, a steel head band with steel spectacles was devised, but it was too uncomfortable to be popular. Although it is not uncommon to find steel cases and frames (including Martin's Margins) dating from about 1750 in the commercial antiques market today, examples of those just described are rarely seen.

Temples

Edward Scarlett, a London optician, perfected rigid temple pieces about 1727.[1] We find early hinges (see Thomin), screws with and without slots, and some recessed screws (Figure 175) Short temples, some with original padding, are available. (Figure 176). Double-hinged temples came later (1770), some with spatula-shaped ends. Then came extendable temples (first turn-pin [Figure 177], then sliding [Figure 178]), and following were those that hooked over the ear.[2]

Eighteenth-century steel spectacles had temples ending in small and large circles—some padded and others used for attaching ribbons to hang from the neck (Figure 179). Other endings were wheel-like, solid and fenestrated spatula-shaped, or spiral.

Bridges

The original bridge design was the C-shape (English bridge), followed by the X (Figure 180) and K (Figure 181) varieties, with simple and coil springs coming in later years, as well as the crank bridge (Figure 182).

Frames, Fronts, and Lens Rims

Documentation of the types of steel frames used is found in portraits, such as Anton Graff's oil of Daniel (Chodofeeki) Chodowiecki (1726–1801), Cherdin's self-portrait, and a portrait of Benjamin Franklin.[3] Rembrandt Peale, with two pairs of spectacles (1801), is a prime American example[4] (Figure 183).

Many examples of the spectacles used in the late eighteenth century are still available, as they were made of very durable steel. After the Industrial Revolution (1837), it was possible to draw wire for construction of frames and stamp out blanks for temples and frame fronts. This added a little finesse to the finished products.[5] These contained X- and K-bridges, double D lenses (Figure 184), and occasionally meniscus lenses. We find blued steel, nickel plating, chromium plating, and rhodium-coated steel frames.

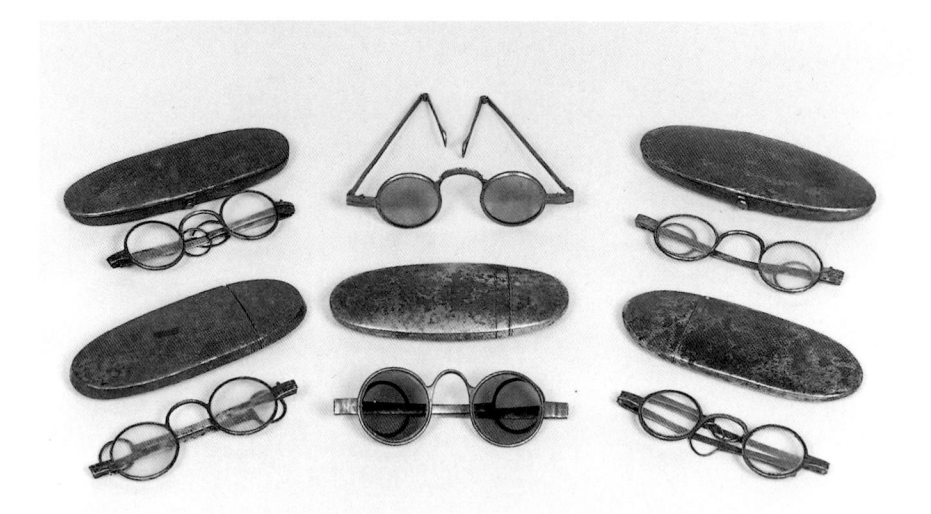

Figure 175. Early steel spectacles with C-bridge, raised and recessed screws, circular temple ends (except double hinge above) and steel cases.

Figure 176. Martin's Margins with original temple padding.

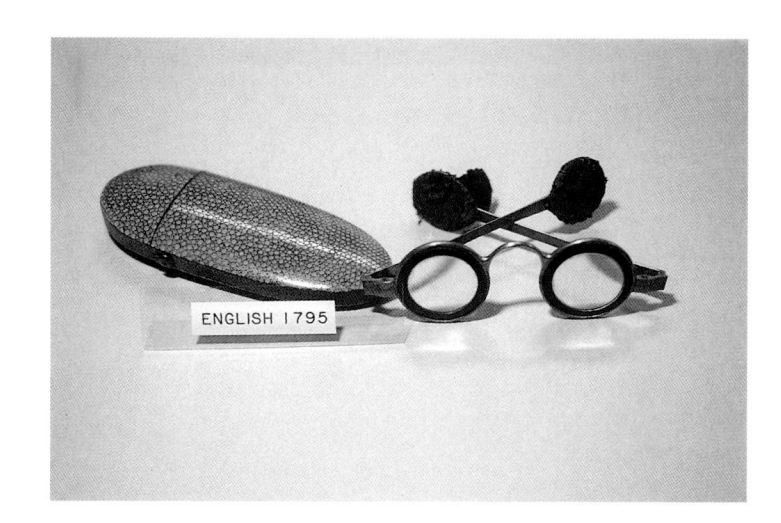

Figure 177. Turn-pin temples.

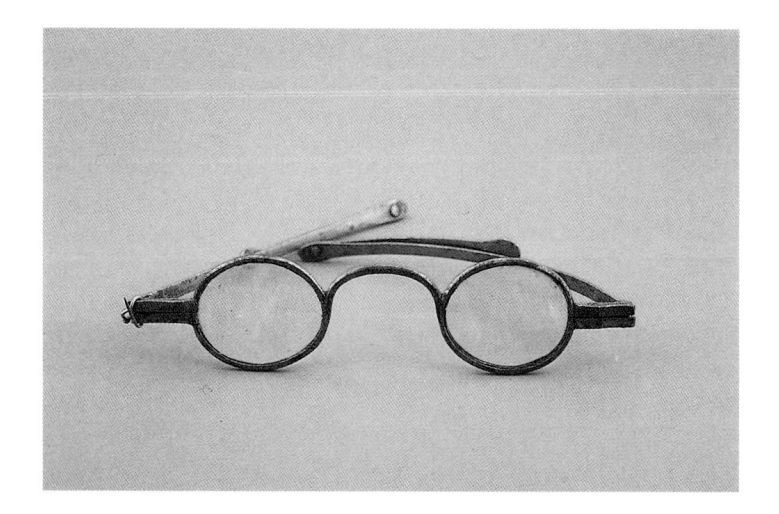

100 CHAPTER 10

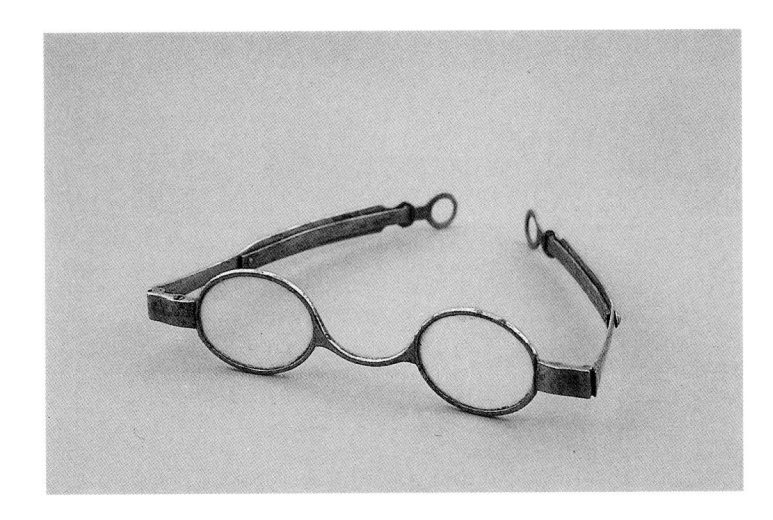

Figure 178. Sliding extension temples.

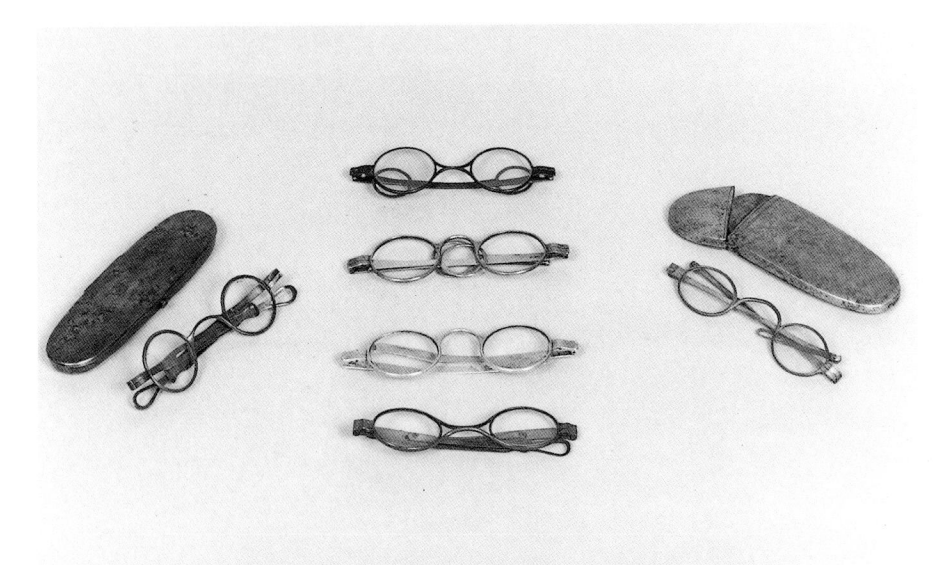

Figure 179. Various temples and bridge types used in the 1700s.

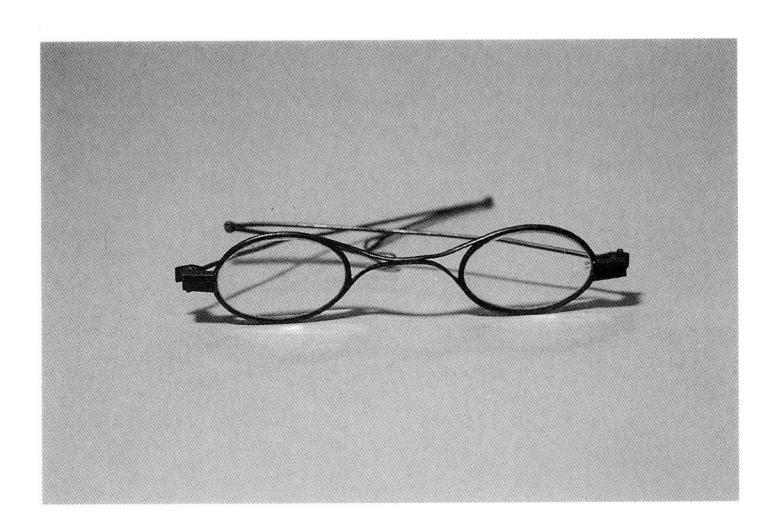

Figure 180. X-bridge.

STEEL SPECTACLES AND CASES 101

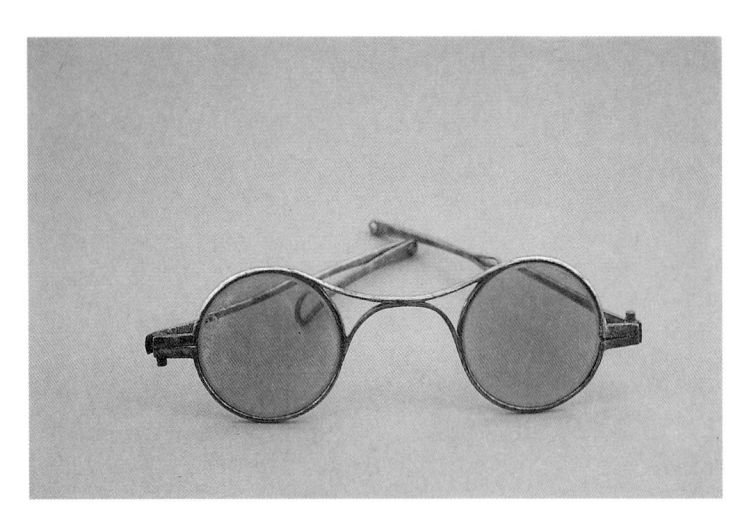

Figure 181. K-bridge.

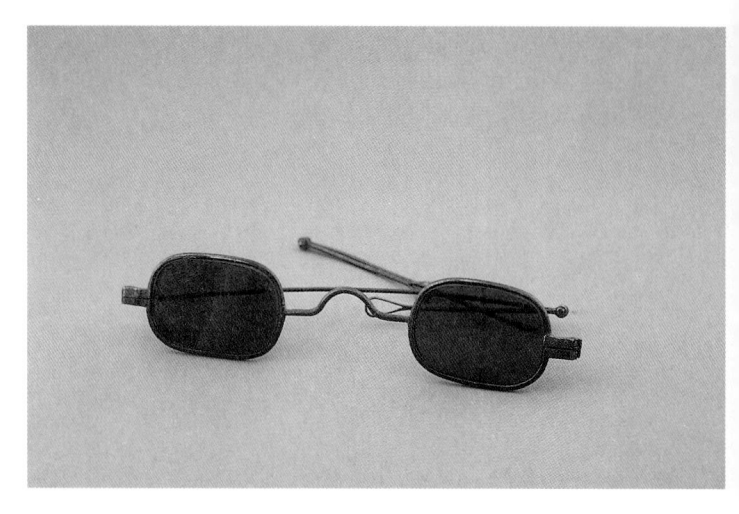

Figure 182. Crank bridge.

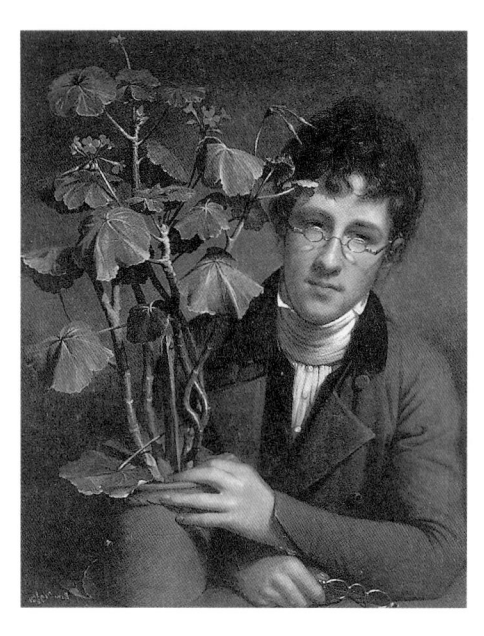

Figure 183. Rembrandt Peale.

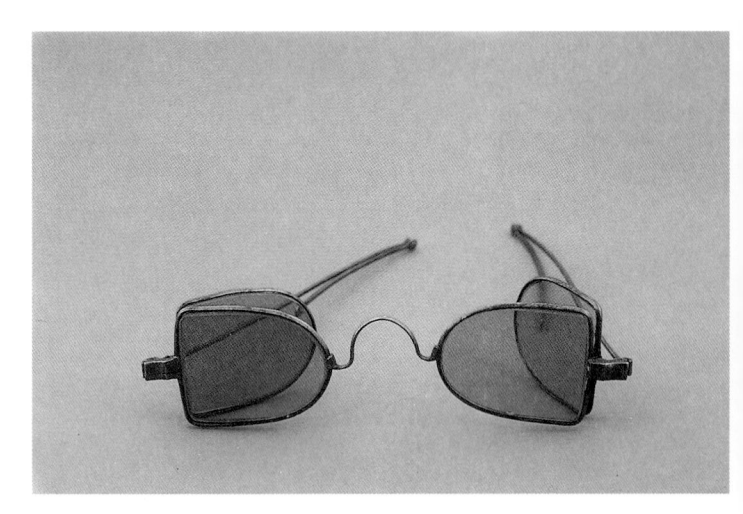

Figure 184. Double D lenses.

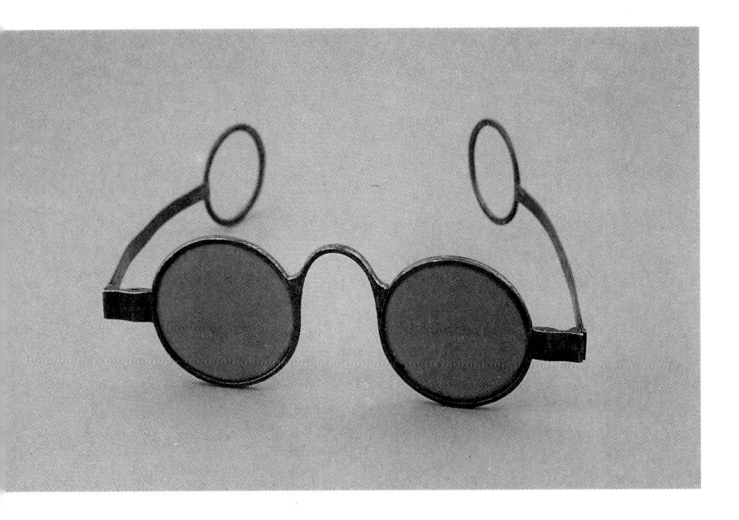

Figure 185. Round lenses.

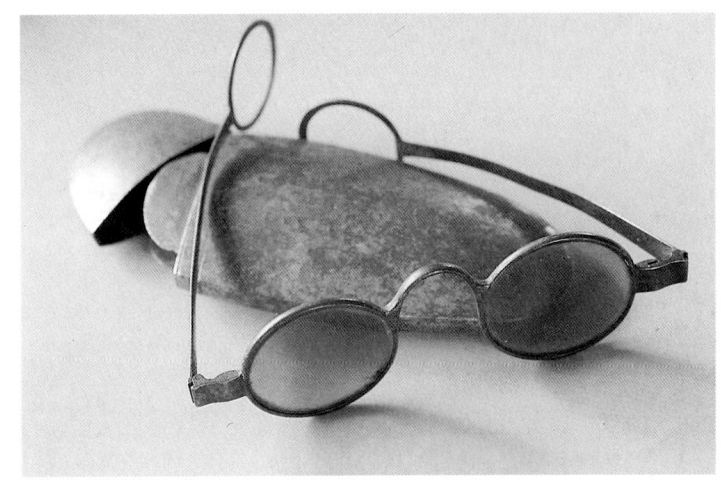

Figure 186. Oval lenses.

Tortoiseshell, celluloid, and, later, more sophisticated plastics also protected and augmented steel spectacle frames.

Some lens rims were lined with wood, but many contained tortoiseshell or horn inserts, such as Martin's Margins (as previously mentioned). These inserts held the lenses more securely than did steel. Lens shapes (i.e., spectacle rims) were originally circular and about 3 centimeters in diameter (Figure 185). About 1800, oval lenses (Figure 186) (2.5 × 3.5 cm.) were used to make it easier to glance over for distance viewing. Other shapes, such as the D lens and double lenses, came out around 1840. Even octagonal lenses are found.

Lens colors in steel frames were ordinarily absent. However, light and dark green and light blue were added for a therapeutic effect (noted in Dr. Samuel Johnson's journal). Smoked color was used for sun protection.

Although other metal alloys rapidly replaced steel as primary frame material, we still use steel in bridges, hinges, screws, and certainly in commercial protective goggles.

Spectacle Cases

Carved wooden cases protected early steel spectacles (Figure 187). Soon, however, steel cases of several varieties were available (Figures 175 & 179) and can still be purchased through antique dealers. Mostly found are clamshell designs, as well as hinged tops. Originally, the clamshell opening type was 12 centimeters long (Figure 188). It was then elongated to 15.5

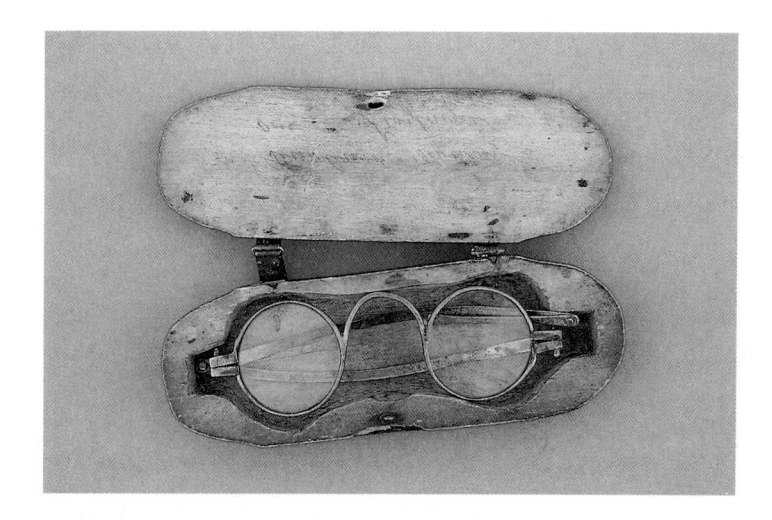

Figure 187. Carved wooden spectacle case.

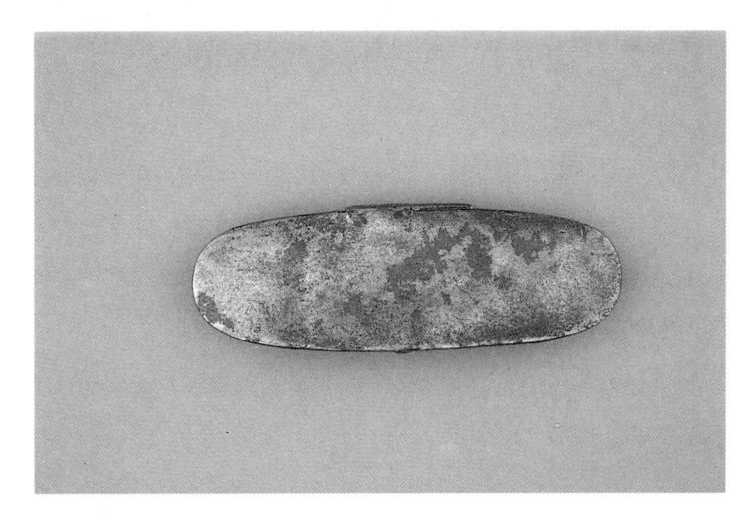

Figure 188. 12-centimeter clamshell pressed-steel spectacle case.

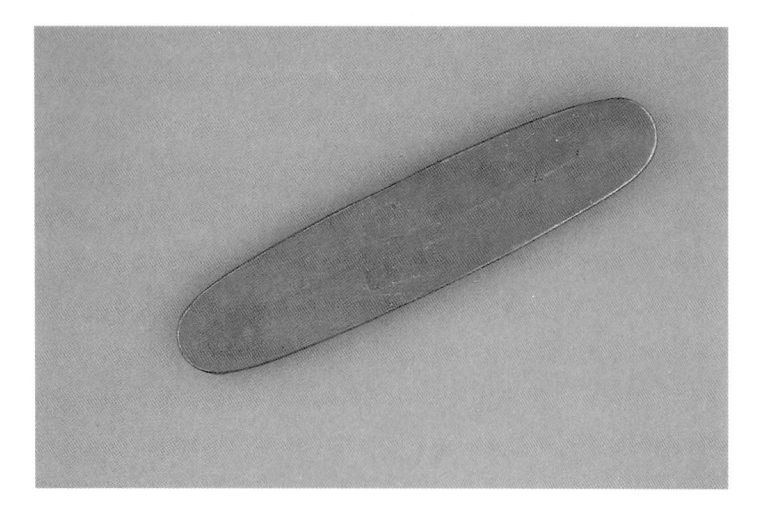

Figure 189. 15.5-centimeter clamshell pressed-steel spectacle case.

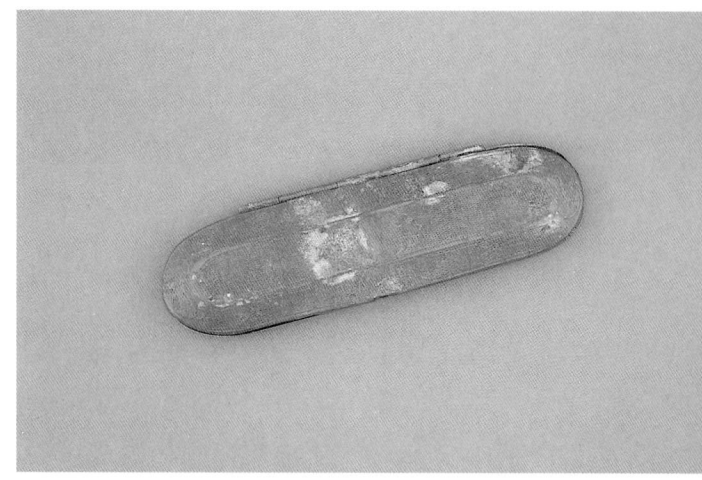

Figure 190. Coffin-shaped spectacle case.

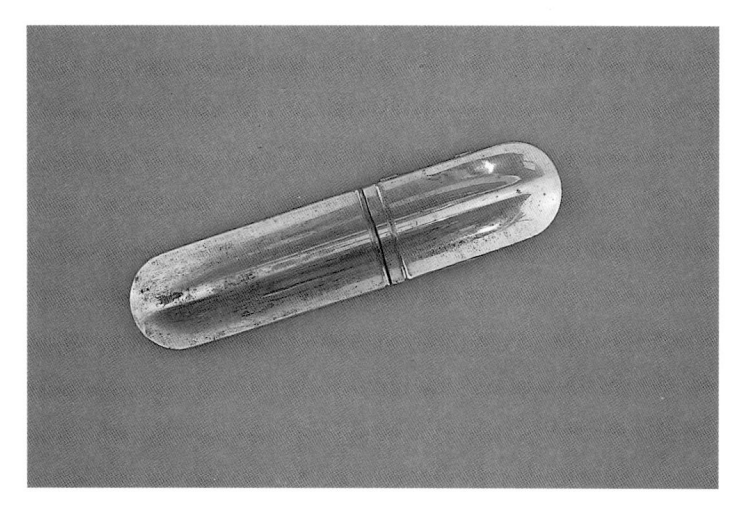

Figure 191. Coffin-lid opening.

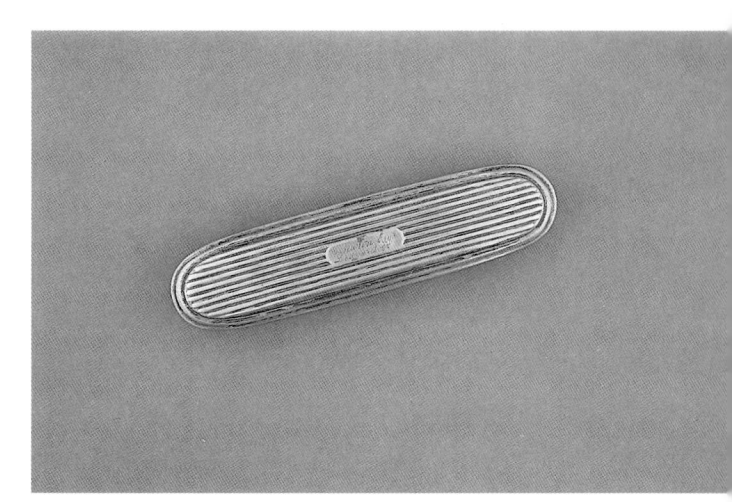

Figure 192. Decorative shaped pressed-steel case.

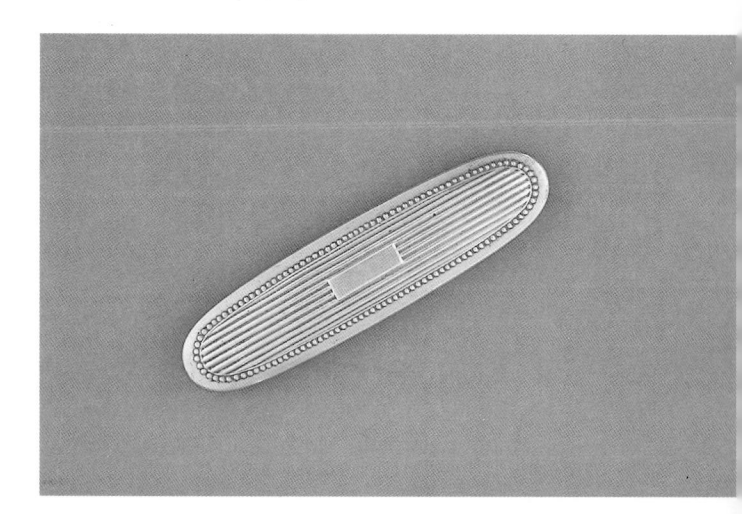

Figure 193. Decorative shaped pressed-steel case.

centimeters (Figure 189), and the coffin shape evolved (Figure 190). Coffin-lid openings followed (Figure 191), and fancy shapes thereafter. Pressed tin (tinplated steel) cases were patented in 1860 by C. Parker in the United States, and various designs of such have appeared since then (Figures 192 & 193).

From 1890 to 1960, use of steel cases with clamshell openings that snapped shut with a coil spring were almost universal. They were lined in a velvetlike material and covered with thin leather (later plastic).

Conclusion

It has been fascinating to trace the use of steel in the manufacture of spectacles and their cases—and to show that changes occurred predominantly in form and function from heavy durable steel to lightweight, tempered, wire alloy.

Notes

1. Richard Corson, *Fashions in Eyeglasses* (London: Peter Owen Ltd., 1980).
2. J. Wm. Rosenthal, personal collection.
3. Corson, op. cit.
4. Rosenthal, personal collection.
5. Rosenthal, personal collection.

11

Martin's Margins

In the early 1700s, a type of steel spectacle was made by several English manufacturers. The most prominent of these manufacturers was Benjamin Martin.

Personal History

Born March 1, 1704, the third son in a family of six children, Benjamin Martin, a self-educated scientist, was raised in rural Guilford, Surrey, England.[1] His father, John, was a farmer, and Benjamin helped till the land. Later Benjamin became a schoolmaster at Chichester, Sussex. This transformation was helped by a legacy that allowed him to purchase needed books. Later he became a writer of mathematical and scientific books, followed by a tour of lectures expounding on the new "experimental philosophy" or "natural philosophy."

In October 1729, Benjamin Martin married Mary Lover. They had at least one child, Joshua Lover Martin, who apprenticed to his father and later ran the business until Benjamin's death on February 9, 1782.

Martin was an instrument maker, author, and lecturer of prolific volume. To this end, he espoused advertisement, lectures, and publication of catalogs.

Ophthalmic Interest

To those of us interested in ophthalmic history, Martin's "visual glasses" are our only connection to this man, who made all sorts of microscopes, telescopes, celestial and terrestrial globes, parlor electrical apparatus, and the like. The glasses we associate with Benjamin Martin are, of course, Martin's Margins.

The title page of Martin's essay on visual glasses (vulgarly called spectacles), notes that ordinary glasses are prejudiced to the "rules of art," the "nature of things," and are prejudicial to the eyes. The essay was printed in 1756.[2] Martin stated that his glasses had partially obstructed apertures so that the eyes were not overloaded with light, and that the lenses were tilted inwards so that the axes of the eye converged on the object of regard. At first, the lens inserts reduced the apertures by one third, but this proved excessive, so that later models had less reduction. Martin considered a violet tint to be the most protective to the eyes, and he put this into his lenses.

Although these glasses were greeted with derision by other opticians, they became popular by their novelty. Martin eventually used them as a sign for his shop on Fleet Street in London.

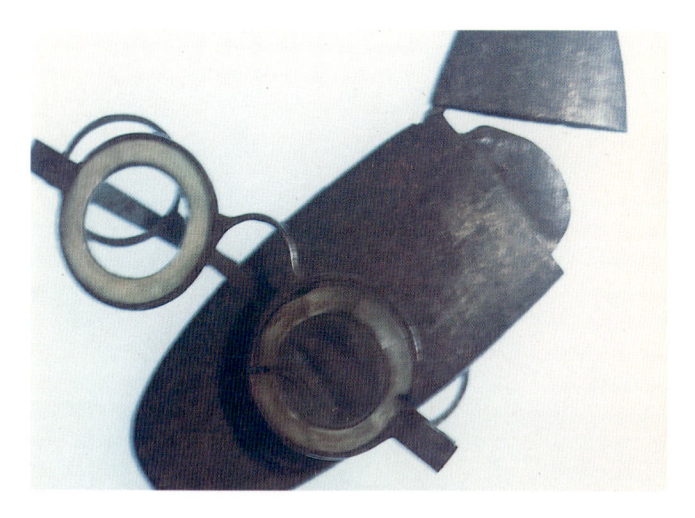

Figure 194. Martin's Margins, horn insert. Note the light-colored horn.

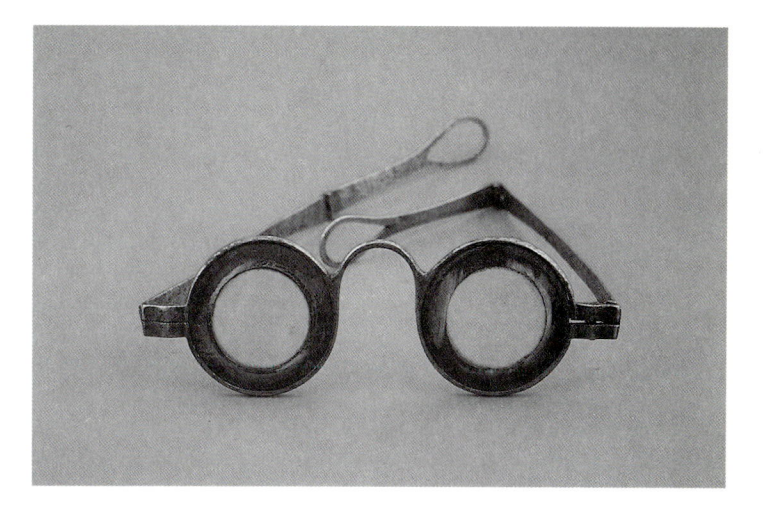

Figure 195. Silver Martin's Margins.

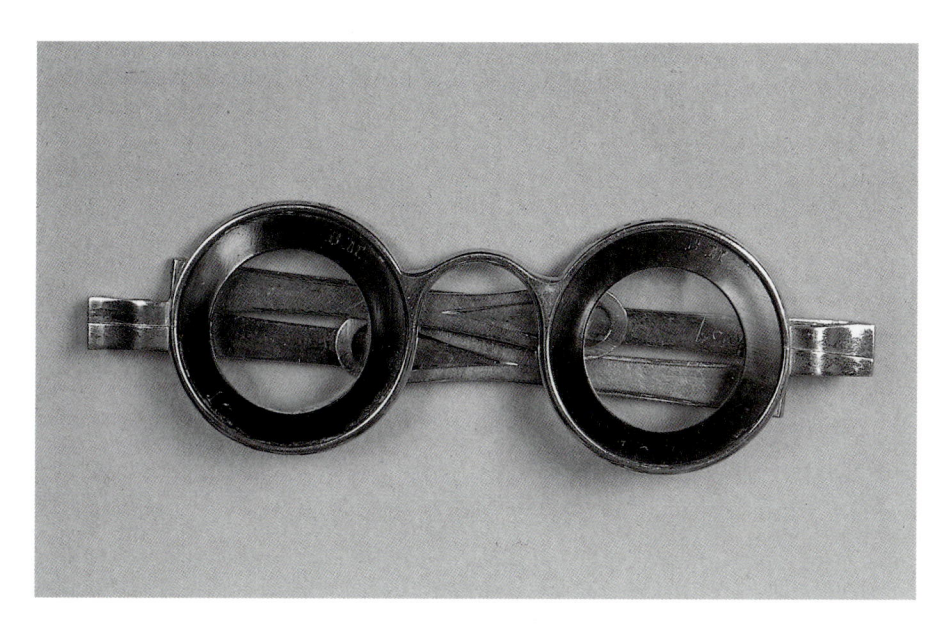

Figure 196. Martin's Margins, gold frame, horn inserts signed "B.M." on each side.

Description

Most examples of Martin's Margins spectacles offered for sale today are made of steel (Figure 194). The author, however, has a pair made of silver (Figure 195) and another that is also silver but plated with gold (Figure 196). There are invariably a C-bridge and round eye pieces (Figure 197, right). These measure 3.5 centimeters in diameter. Another pair in the author's collection is marked "C & W." The horn is very light colored, and the temples end in large (3 cm.) loops. The complementing flip-top case shows traces of gilding (Figure 198, above and right). Although the lens inserts are usually carved from cattle horn, luxury models sport tortoiseshell inserts. All lenses, whether of pebble or glass, were biconvex. Martin's Margins were also made in the form of a pince-nez type.

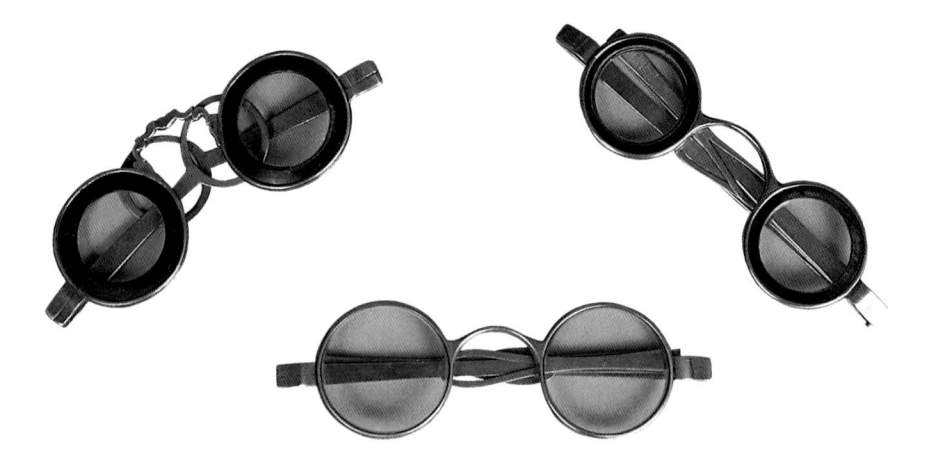

Figure 197. Center: silver Martin's Margins; left: inserts with fancy bridge; right: round eye inserts.

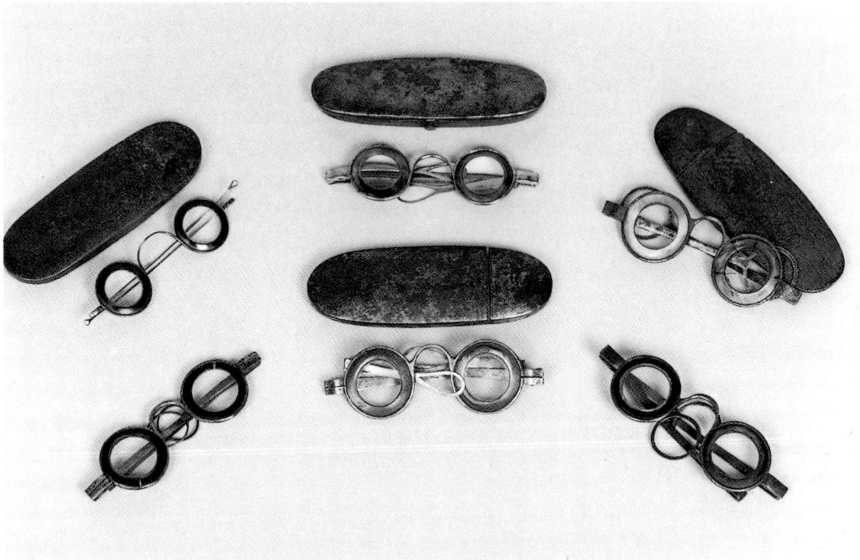

Figure 198. Various Martin's Margins and their cases. (Upper right case is gilded, top center case is clamshell, spectacles in top center and bottom row are double-hinged.)

Hinges

Temple hinges were solid and well-made, with two tines on the front and one fitted between them on the temple piece side.[3] Besides the screw to hold the hinge rotation, another was fitted to allow the lens to be properly placed (Figure 199). Some of the earlier models had raised screws without slots, while some are found with slots. Some later examples were even fitted with flush-headed screws. We must remember that Benjamin Martin was not the only one producing this type of spectacle.

Temples

Temples were usually straight, but some are found with double hinges for use of the glasses with or without a wig (Figure 198). Tips of the temple carried a steel circle at the end of the regular temple so that a cord or ribbon could be attached and the glasses hung around the neck. These circles are about 2.5 centimeters in diameter, some a little smaller. Occasionally, a circle was attached to the lower edge of the temple, at the end, of course. The ring ends of these temples were often padded with sewn-on dark material. Even today, some of these pads survive, which seems to indicate that the spectacles were used under wigs. Additionally, steel temples, although springlike, are less malleable than other metals and could have pressed on the wearer's skull. Therefore, perhaps some of them were ill-fitting from the date of purchase and were not worn much.

A Peculiar Type of Lens Insert

The author has purchased a peculiar type of lens insert not previously described. (Figures 200 & 201). In an ordinary steel frame of the 1750 period (more or less), lathed dowels are placed as shown in the figures. Each is drilled in the center so that a 1-centimeter tunnel is made. Lenses are secured in this aperture and act like spectacle lenses of positive power. The author unenthusiastically surmises that they were used for shooting, reading concentration, shielding from light, or whatever. (Can someone with superior information solve this mystery? This information is placed in the "Martin's Margins" area for lack of a more desirable location.)

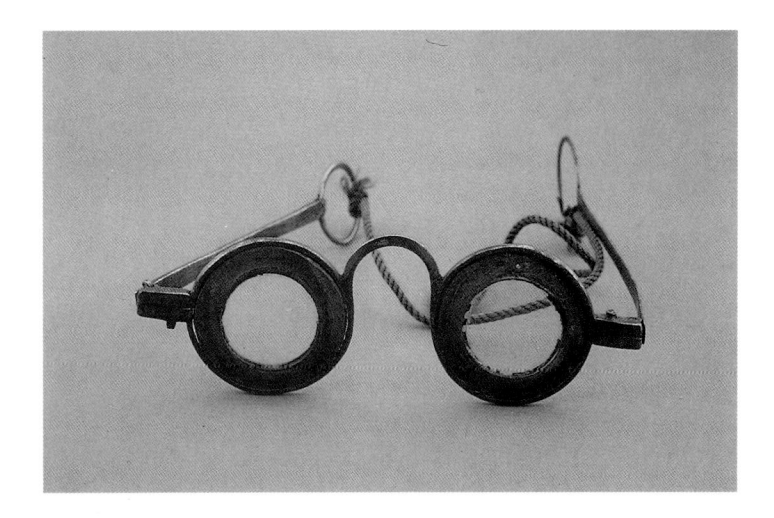

Figure 199. Martin's Margins with raised hinge screw.

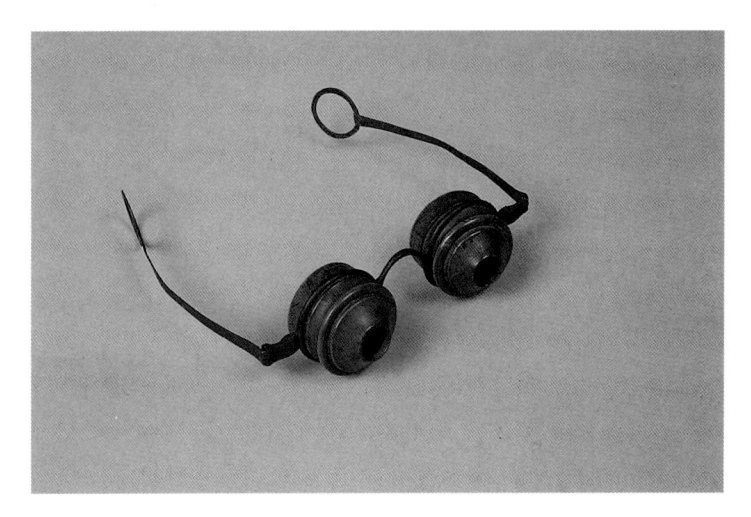

Figure 200. Martin's Margins type spectacles of the same period (1750).

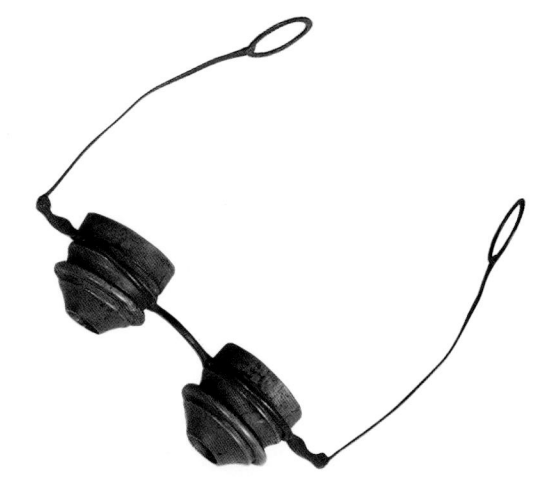

Figure 201. Top view of Figure 200.

Glasses Cases

Martin's Margins can be found in steel cases—usually of the flip-top variety, but also in the type called clamshell (Figure 198).[4] Individually carved wooden cases were also used.

End of an Era

When Martin's shop contents were auctioned following his death, 550 spectacles were offered for sale. A myriad of other scientific instruments—books, catalogs, and prints were disposed of at another sale.[5]

Notes

1. John R. Milburn, *Retailer of the Sciences* (London: Vade-Mecum Press, 1986), 13, 18, 56.
2. Ibid.
3. J. Wm. Rosenthal, personal collection.
4. Ibid.
5. Milburn, op. cit.

Other Sources Consulted for Chapter 11

1. Richard Corson, *Fashions in Eyeglasses* (London: Peter Owen Ltd., 1980), 93.
2. Stanley Newbold, *The Optician*, April 1961.
3. Fritz Rathschuler, *La Lente* (Genova, 1988), 146, 150.
4. Goetz Remus, personal communication. Frankfurt, Germany, 1993.

12

Wig Spectacles

When Edward Scarlett invented temple pieces in 1727, he was reaching for a logical design to keep spectacles on the face comfortably and practically.[1] One facet of the use of temples quickly became evident—their concurrent use with the wearing of a wig.

Wigs were in use by European and American men and women from the early 1700s. A wig must grasp the head to stay in place. Such pressure, when exerted against a temple piece, puts point pressure of the temple against the skin covering the skull, almost directly over bone. This skin, being squeezed between two hard objects, inevitably becomes sensitive. For comfort's sake, temples were shortened to rest on the user's temple or just in front of the ear (Figure 202). They were also made straight and relatively pointed to penetrate and rest in the wig itself. Thus, wig glasses.

Varieties

Most of the wig glasses seen are English or French, and later pieces are American. Most fronts are of tortoiseshell, with C-shaped bridges (Figure 203). Occasionally, spectacles made totally of silver are found. It is interesting to note the size of these bridges; some are rather small, but others are huge (1.5 to 2 cm.), indicating the wearer's obesity or rhinophyma. Occasionally, X-bridges are found, especially in French-made spectacles.

Lenses

Lenses were made of glass or pebble, many being oval, about 22 by 32 millimeters, but circular lenses abounded as well, measuring about 26 millimeters in diameter. Some of the glass lenses were tinted green or blue. The author has never found myopic lenses, though some convex lenses are rather weak (about +0.75D).

Temples

Many temple pieces are one piece, straight, tortoiseshell, about 12 centimeters long, with a squared-off tip, 2 × 3 millimeters. Some tips have been filed to a blunt point (Figure 204). The ends of others show a 1-centimeter circle that may be in line with the central axis of the temple or below this axis.

Pads are found on the inside of some straight temples and on the inside of circular tips on others (Figure 205). They seem to be made of a feltlike material.

In the later part of the eighteenth century, temples on wig glasses were made of metal, usually silver (Figure 205). This is fortunate, as it aids in dating the object as well as showing its manufacturer. For these relatively expensive spectacles to serve additional duty when wigs were off, extensions were placed on the temples so that they could hook behind the ears. At first, they were of the turn-pin type. In the early nineteenth century, sliding extensions were designed, and then the double-hinged temples performed the same task (Figure 206).

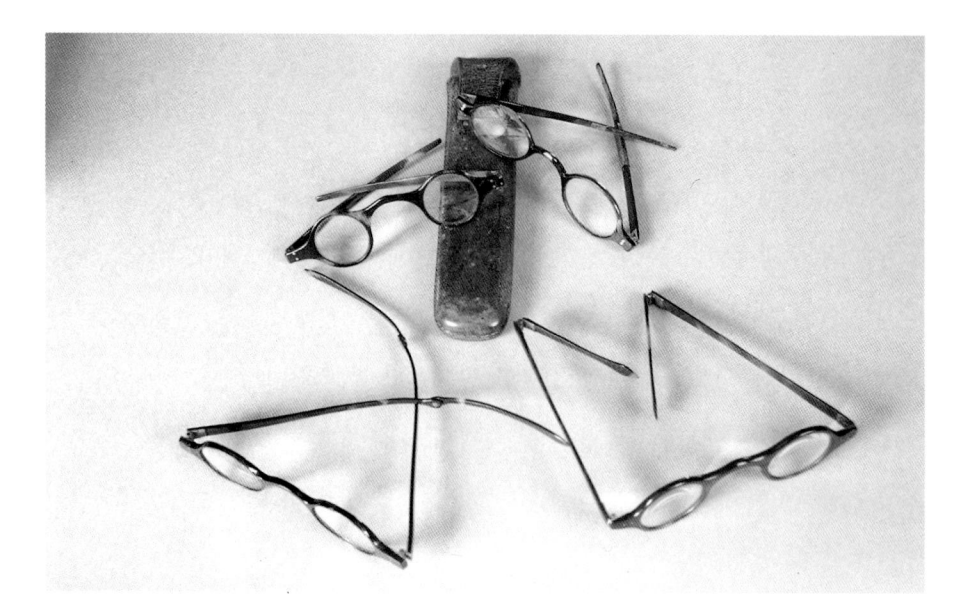

Figure 202. Tortoiseshell wig spectacles—above are short temples; below are extension temples.

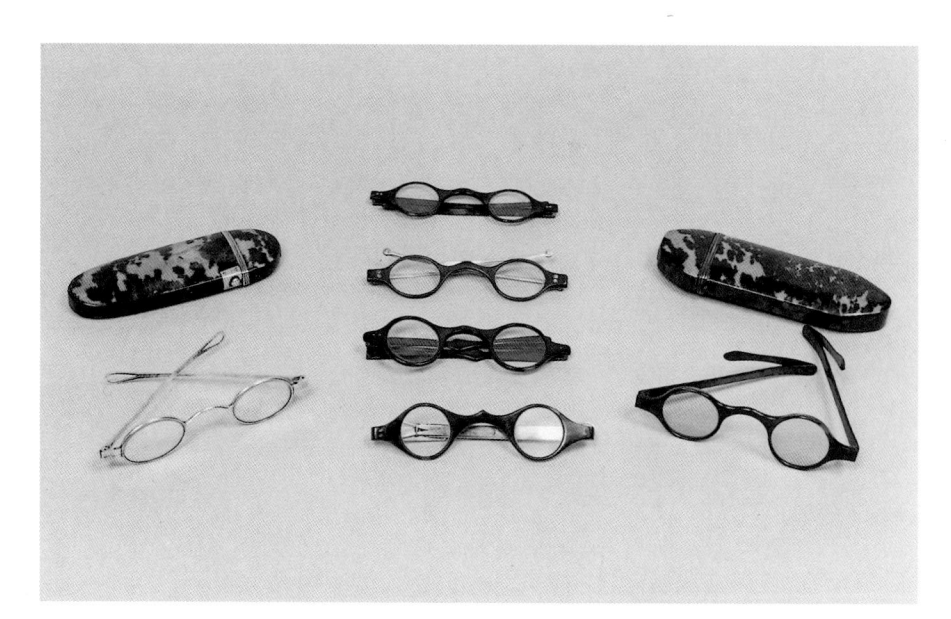

Figure 203. Varieties of wig spectacles.

112   CHAPTER 12

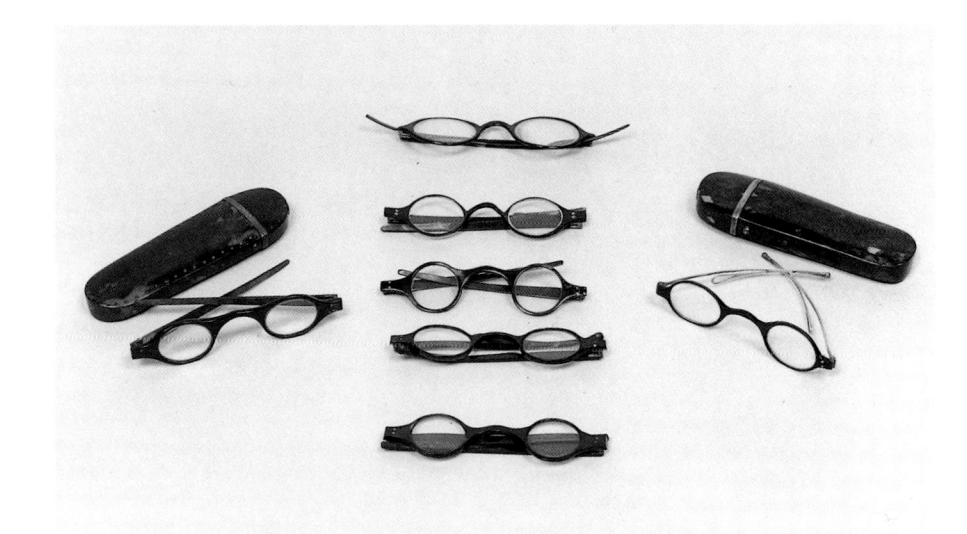

Figure 204. Temples changed according to need.

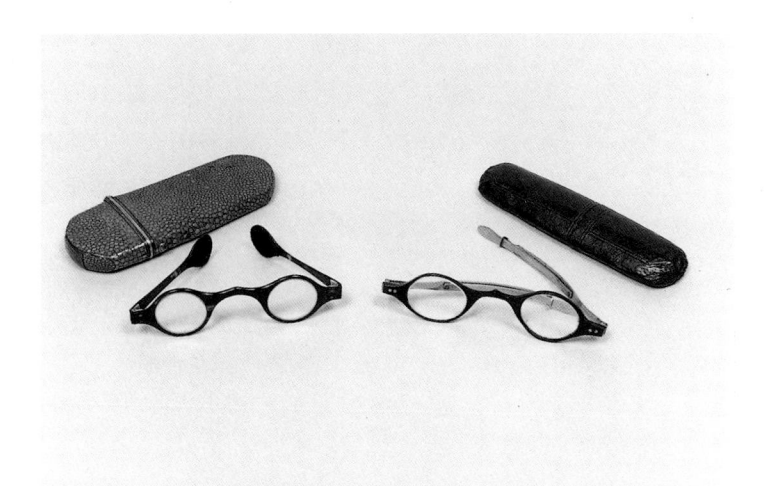

Figure 205. Padded temples.

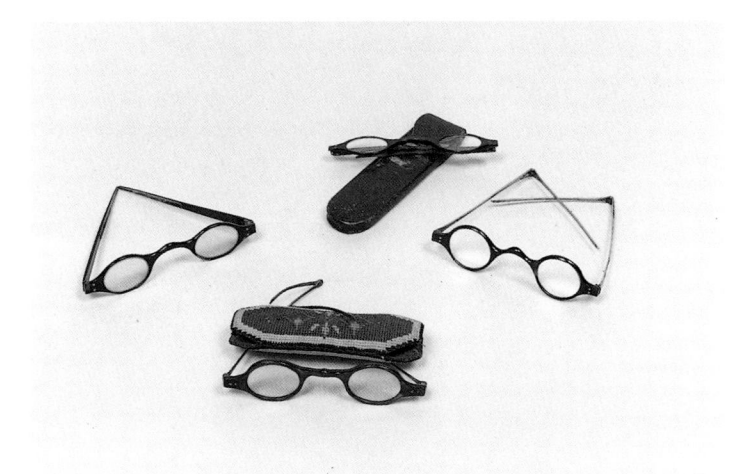

Figure 206. Extension temples (below and right).

WIG SPECTACLES **113**

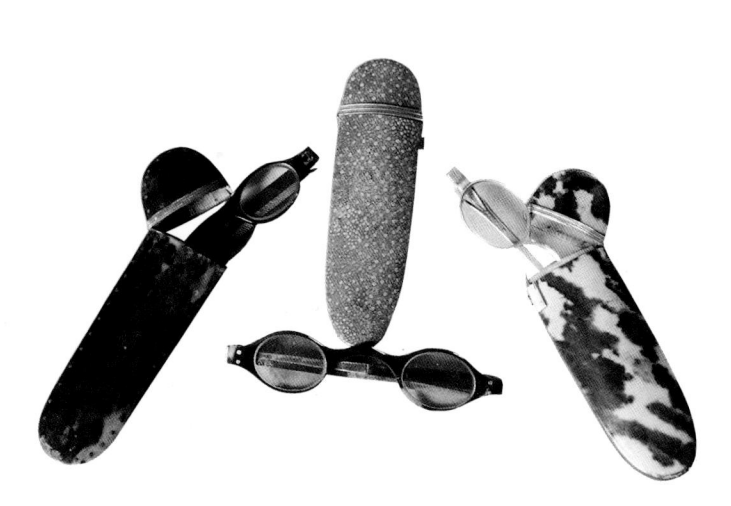

Figure 207. Types of cases used with wig spectacles.

Around the end of the nineteenth century, spectacles were produced with straight temples, but they were fairly long (about 14 cm.), with large round lenses about 4 centimeters in diameter. These glasses were plastic, tortoiseshell, or metal and were used until the 1930s.

Interesting to note is that many brass spectacles circa 1860 had the optician's name stamped on the front end of the outside of the temples. Such names as Habermeier and Schildknecht are found. The names are not in block letters, as are usually seen, but in script, all with similar lettering. Were these frames all made in Europe (possibly Germany) by the same manufacturer? Was the manufacturer of German descent, and did he make the frames and imprints in the United States? As the temples are not of a uniform style, perhaps the stamping machine was being used in the United States or abroad. Schnaitman was the first in United States to make his mark.

Spectacle Cases

Early wig spectacle cases were of beautiful tortoiseshell or shagreen, with silver banding and cartouche, silver hardware (hinges and catches), and occasionally silver pins as decoration. They had flip-tops (Figure 207). Other cases were made of soft material with petit point decoration. Still later, slip-top cases of pressed paper or leather were used to advantage but were not particularly decorative.

Conclusion

Although wigs are still used in some legal and ceremonial settings—also by some women—concurrent use of special wig glasses has not kept pace.

Notes

1. Richard Corson, *Fashions in Eyeglasses* (London: Peter Owen Ltd., 1967), 69.

13

Scissors Glasses

George Washington used a set of scissors glasses. This plays in juxtaposition with the usual connotation that scissors glasses were strictly European. It does additionally set a mental time frame for their use. The term *scissors glasses* comes from the French *binocles-ciseaux*, since the two stems from the handle come together under the nose and look as if they would cut it off[1] (Figure 208). Other notables who used scissors glasses were Goethe and Napoleon Bonaparte—both being myopic. Napoleon bought a pair in 1812 made of mother-of-pearl and gold.

According to Professor Albert von Pflugk, scissors glasses were invented in Germany in 1750. However, Karl von Greeff claims that George Adams of Fleet Street, London, first patented them in 1780[2] (Figure 209).

French models were usually more delicately made than others and only had a disc at the base where the two branches merged into a handle. There was also a ring to accommodate a ribbon to hang the glasses from the neck. Elegant gold and silver chains were also used (Figure 210).

Other models had handles made of tortoiseshell (Figure 209), mother-of-pearl (Figure 211), or horn (Figure 212). Two slabs of one of these materials were separated to allow the optical branches to fold inside for breakage protection when not in use. Sometimes, they were carried in a pocket.

The lenses were almost always round. Some arms holding the lenses were made of tortoise shell or horn, but most were made of steel, gold, silver, or an alloy. Odd varieties found reveal oval lenses and handles with a sliding or spring-loaded action.

During the directoire period (circa 1795–1799), scissors glasses were at their height in popularity, mostly in France, England, Germany, and Italy (Figure 213). They were used by the incroyables—mostly French dandies—with much affectation, posturing, and ostentatiousness. Originally, they were large but later were made smaller and otherwise refined. They were used by men and women alike.

Conclusion

Early in the 1800s, with the development of the lorgnette, use of this optical aberration—scissors glasses—came to an end (Figure 214).

Notes

1. Pierre Marley, *Spectacles and Spyglasses* (Paris: Hoebeke, 1988), 13, 94–95.
2. R. J. S. MacGregor, *Collecting Ophthalmic Antiques* (United Kingdom: Ophthalmic Antiques International Collectors' Club, 1992), 36.

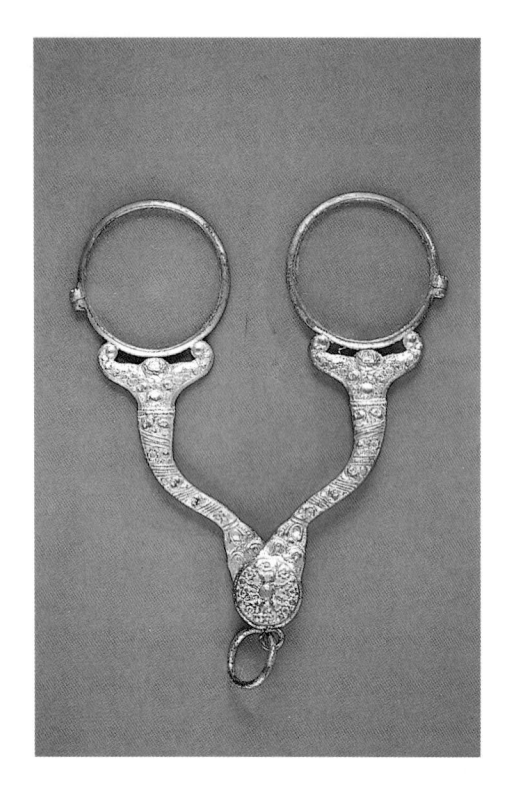

Figure 208. French gilt scissors glasses.

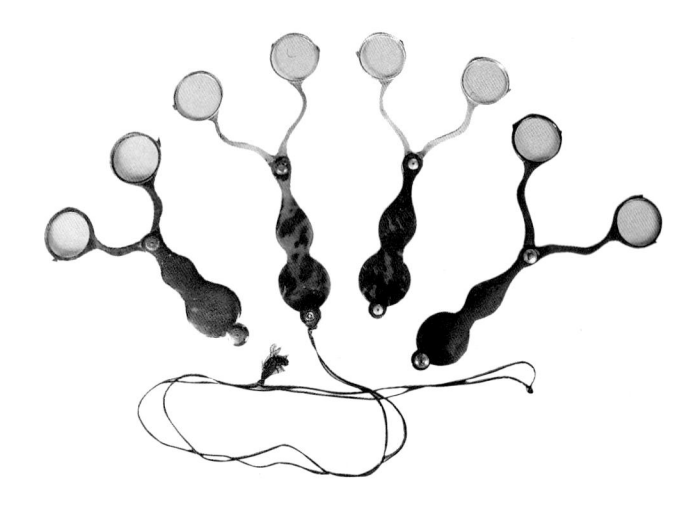

Figure 209. A variety of tortoiseshell scissors glasses.

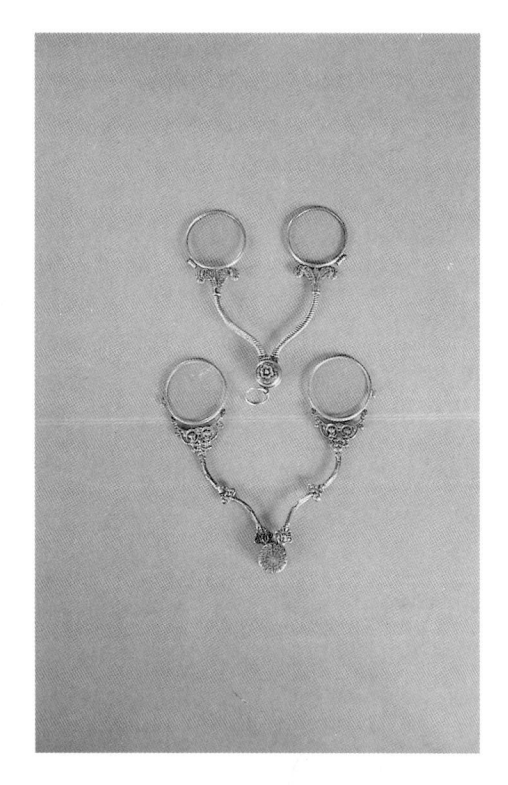

Figure 210. French scissors glasses.

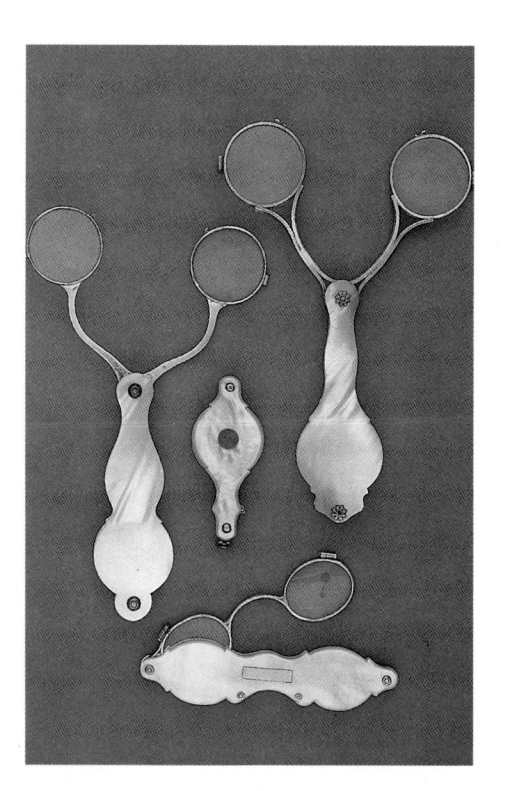

Figure 211. Mother-of-pearl and silver scissors glasses with lorgnette.

116   CHAPTER 13

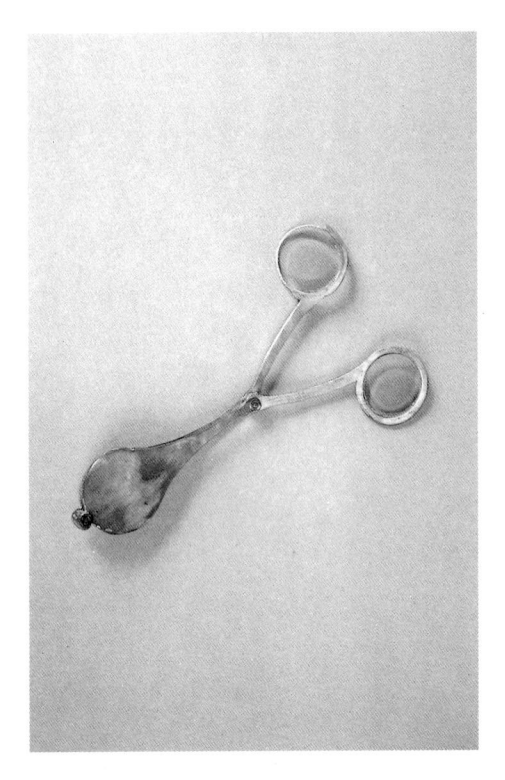

Figure 212. Scissors glasses made of horn.

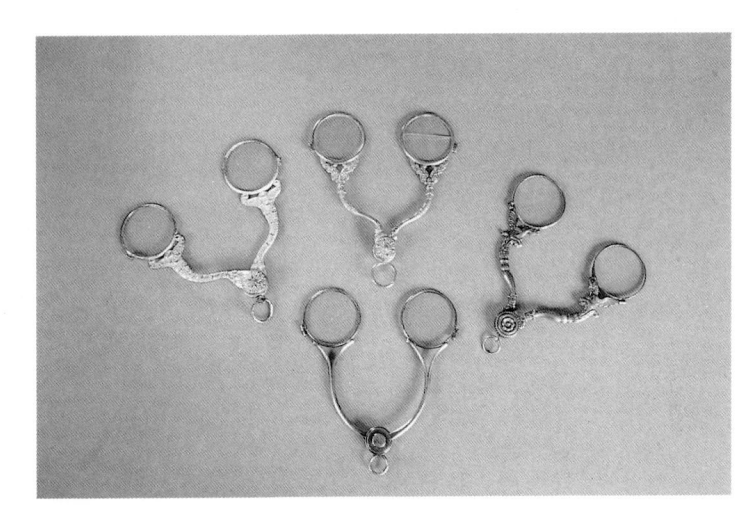

Figure 213. A variety of French scissors glasses.

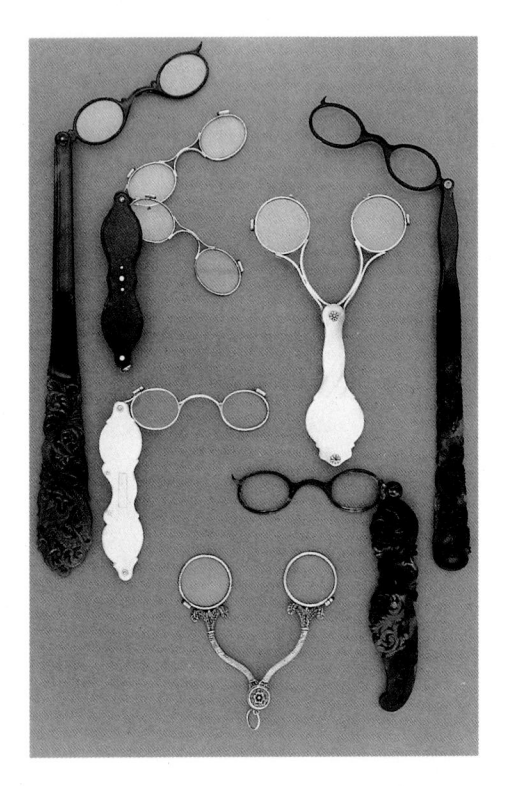

Figure 214. Scissors glasses and lorgnettes.

Other Sources Consulted for Chapter 13
1. *Il Museo dell'Occhiale*, Verona, pp. 73–83.
2. Hugh Orr, *Illustrated History of Early Antique Spectacles* (Kent, England, 1985), 84.

14

Lorgnettes

(From the French word *lorgner,* to leer or stare)

Origins

The forerunner of the lorgnette appeared in an illustration on the wall of the monastery of St. Marco of Florence in the fourteenth century. It was not until 1785 that the lorgnette's use became popularized, when the Englishman George Adams, the elder (an optician), designed a practical case.[1]

To be entirely clear, it should be stated that we are discussing here a pair of spectacles for women that can recess into a protective handle (Figure 215). We are not referring to the miniature telescope called prospect glasses by the English and also called lorgnette by the French during the seventeenth and eighteenth centuries and mentioned in Chapter 15 on monoculars.

George Adams

George Adams's early design was meant to be carried in the pocket. This form was so practical that it evolved into scissors glasses a decade later. (Scissors glasses are discussed in Chapter 13.) Small, oval lenses were fitted to (usually) silver or gold spectacle fronts. The latter were attached on one end between two parallel slabs of tortoiseshell, horn (Figure 216), metal, or mother-of-pearl (Figures 217, 218, & 219). These protective slabs were carved to fit the shape of the front and allowed the front to pivot to a nest in the manner of a pocketknife blade. Whereas some of the ends of the case had a bail, which did allow attachment of a chain or ribbon to go around the neck, such was not the primary design. Many of these were quite ornate, with carving and a cartouche suitable for engraving.

Robert Betell Bate

No further improvements were made until 1825, when Robert Betell Bate (an English optician) of London patented handled spectacles.[2] The handles were short and allowed the device to be hung around the neck (Figure 219). A hinge in the bridge permitted the two lenses to be folded on each other so that they could be used as a magnifying glass. At first there was no spring (Figure 220). Therefore, the lenses had to be manually opened and could be used as a spectacle (Figure 221). Later, a spring mechanism was added so that moving a small lever in the lorgnette handle would unlatch a catch and allow the lenses to spring apart (Figure 222). Ordinarily the lenses were round (Figure 223). An enlarged version of the latter style is known as the Louis spring lorgnette and may still be available new today.

It is interesting to note that although popular with women as a fashion accessory and as a necessity for clarity of vision, public use of the lorgnette was decried as poor decorum because it was often used for ogling neighbors or strangers.[3]

French Styles

In 1830, the French came out with a small, almost rectangular eyepiece that was hinged at the bridge with a spring and folded flat on its fellow lens (Figure 224). The whole device then rotated inside a decorated protective case with another spring on the end. Thus a touch of a fingernail on the catch in the handle would allow the two springs to activate, and voila—the spectacles were spread to a usable position.

Many of these French lorgnette cases were beautifully decorated. Materials used were gold, silver, copper (for the painting of miniatures), tortoiseshell, horn, bone, ivory, and mother-of-pearl (Figures 225 & 226). These cases often contained a silver cartouche. Some tortoiseshell examples were protected on the edges with a band of silver (Figure 225, center). Those made of metal were frequently fenestrated or decoratively reticulated. Further embellishment with enameling of decorative designs or pastoral scenes, encrusting with precious stones (Figure 227), including lockets (Figure 228), vinaigrettes, and timepieces, have all been seen in various collections (Figure 229).

In the following decade or two (circa 1840) lorgnettes of Continental, British, and American origin exhibited longer handles. They approximated 10 centimeters and were straight or curved, depending on the design. Foremost in construction was the use of many forms of embellishment to promote class, dignity, and opulence. Figures 230–234 exemplify those characteristics.

Long-Handled Lorgnettes

In the late nineteenth and early twentieth century, lorgnettes "grew" longer handles. Many were merely the French type of lorgnette with a longer handle (Figure 235). Some handles, however, were telescopic. A few years later, very long tortoiseshell (and imitation) or mother-of-pearl handles, called the dowager-duchess types, followed (Figure 236). They measured 20 to 30 centimeters in length. Some tortoiseshell types were carved, and some were plain, with set-in cartouche (Figure 237)—or even a watch. The imitation shell was frequently molded to a design or was reticulated. Some handles of silver were embossed (Figure 238), and others were richly engraved (Figure 239). Many came in their own "pin seal" leather slip cases, while others had a clamshell-opening type of case (Figure 240). Almost all sported a loop on the end of the handle (Figure 241). Any of these could have been made in America, in Britain, or on the Continent. One was even attached to an ear trumpet (Figure 242), while some were decorated with gold pins (Figure 243).

The 1890s

During the 1890s, a separate style of lorgnette appeared of American manufacture but closely copying the short-handled French styles. It was made entirely of metal, with handles about 6 centimeters long that flowed into the case that protected the lenses (Figure 244). The metal halves were embossed deeply and welded together in a seam finished so well that it could not be seen (Figure 245). The lenses were small, folded upon each other, and then placed into the case. A catch released them, and the two springs (French-style) flipped them open.

Many types of decoration and designs were embossed (Figure 246). One desirable type was the art nouveau style, originated by the artist Ungar. These styles are easily recognized currently, both by available examples and by viewing catalogs of that era. The author has examples decorated additionally with enamel (Figure 247) and diamonds (Figure 248). Many types are silver, gold, or gold-plated (Figure 249). All have loops on the end of the handle to hang from the woman's neck with ribbon or chain. The latter itself is a statement in gold, silver, and oftentimes, diamonds.

The 1920s

Lorgnettes became less fashionable in the 1920s and were less ornate (Figure 250). Most were of the spring variety but had smaller and plainer handles of around 10 centimeters (Figure 251). Certainly we find gold and silver examples (Figure 252), engraved and enameled (Figures 253–255), mother-of-pearl and the like, but these types were really utilitarian.

For the more sophisticated who desired to show off for formal affairs, lorgnettes were decorated with citrine, saphire, and diamond (Figures 256–259). Marcasite (Figures 260 & 261) and brilliants (rhinestones) (Figure 262) also appeared on the handle and the rim.

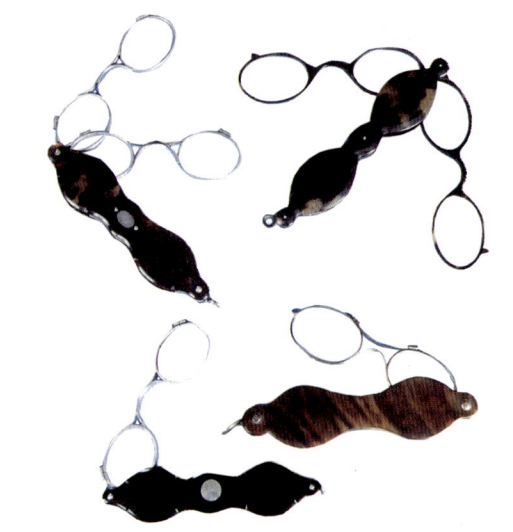

Figure 215. Varieties of tortoiseshell lorgnettes.

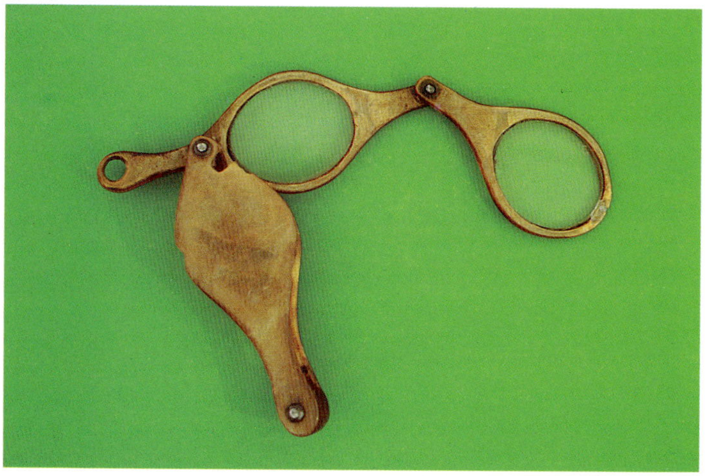

Figure 216. Lorgnette made of horn.

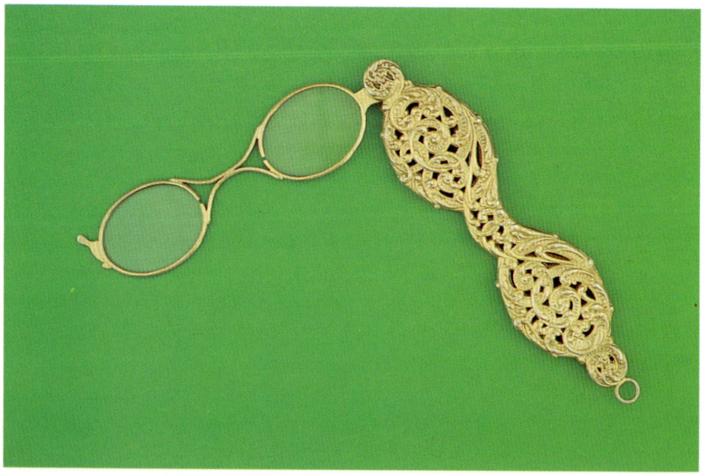

Figure 217. Gold lorgnette.

120   CHAPTER 14

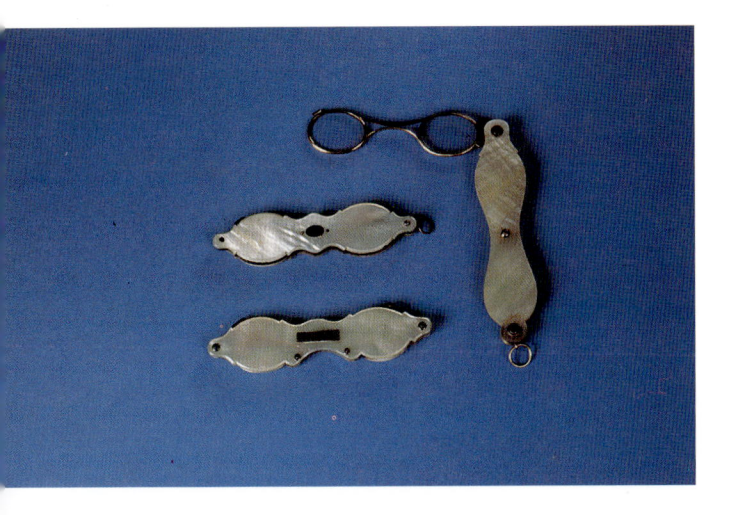

Figure 218. Mother-of-pearl and silver lorgnettes.

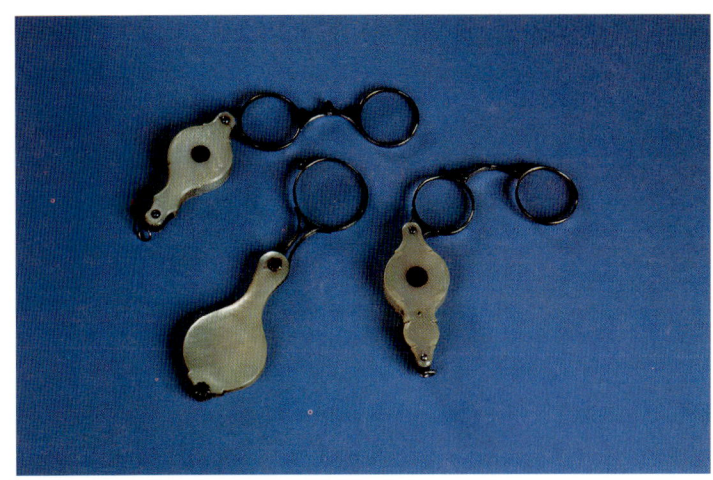

Figure 219. Mother-of-pearl and silver lorgnettes.

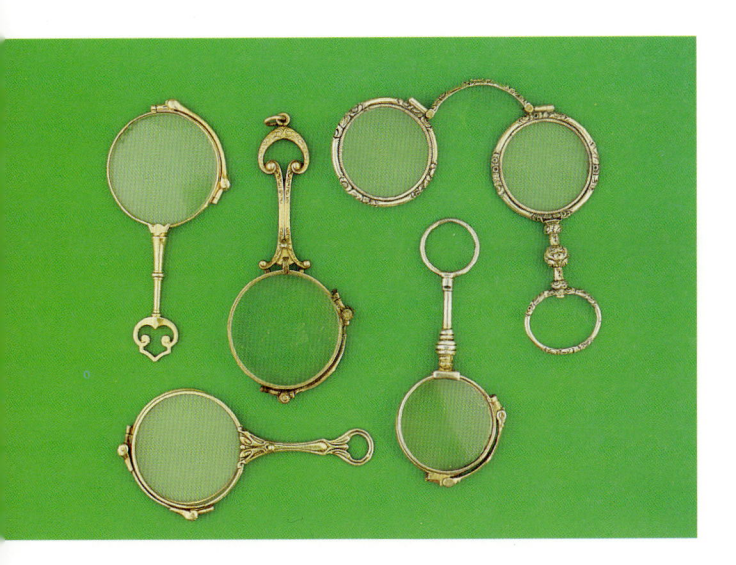

Figure 220. Gold lorgnettes manually opened.

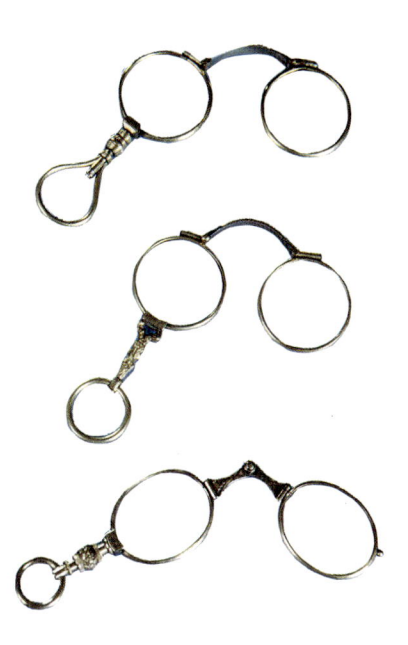

Figure 221. Gold lorgnettes manually opened.

LORGNETTES 121

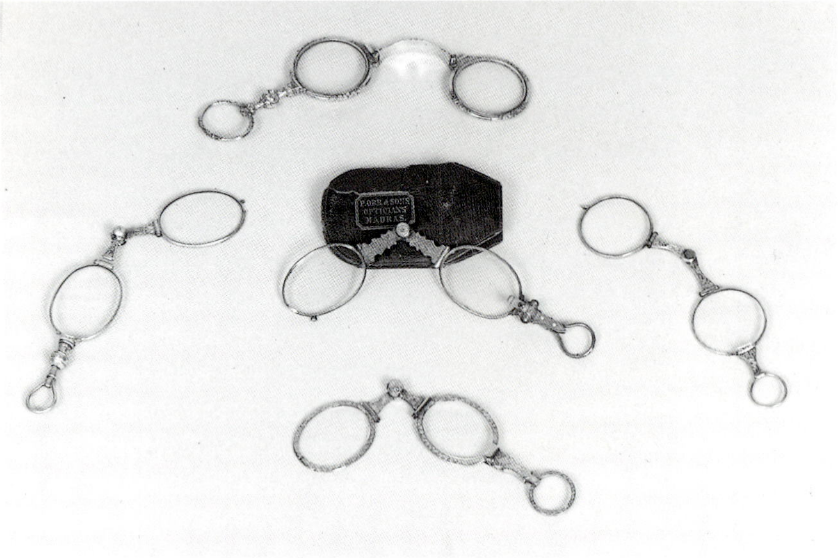

Figure 222. Gold lorgnettes with spring mechanisms.

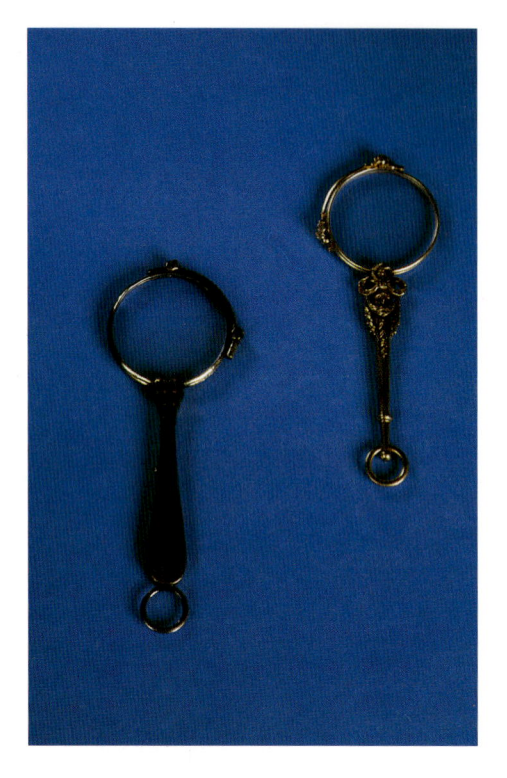

Figure 223. Spring lorgnettes.

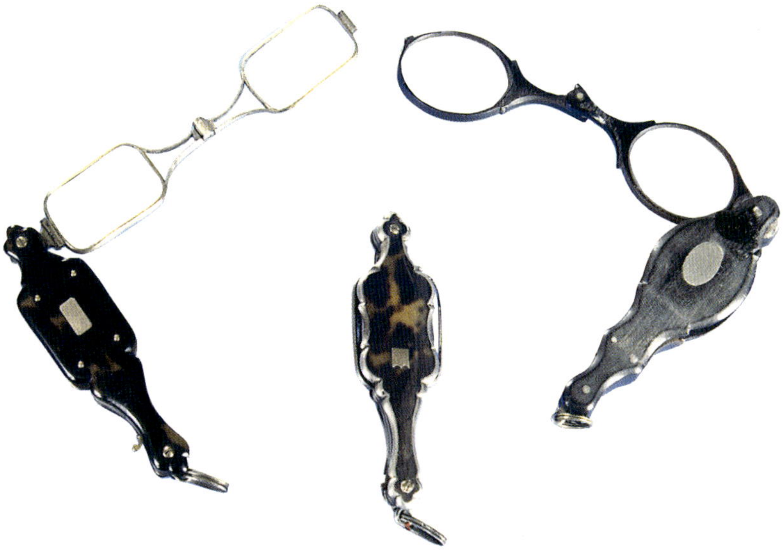

Figure 224. French lorgnettes circa 1830.

122   CHAPTER 14

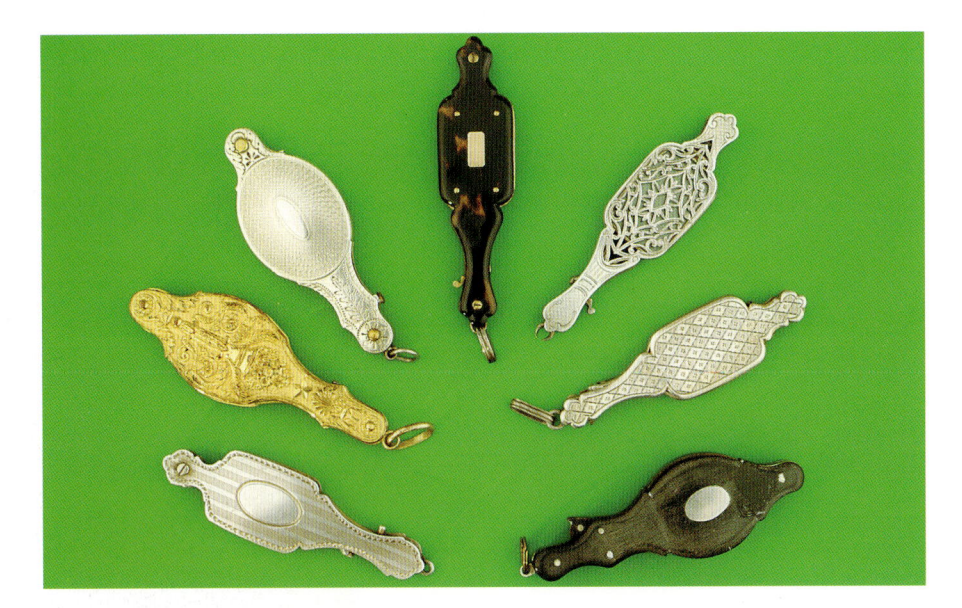

Figure 225. French lorgnettes' cases circa 1830.

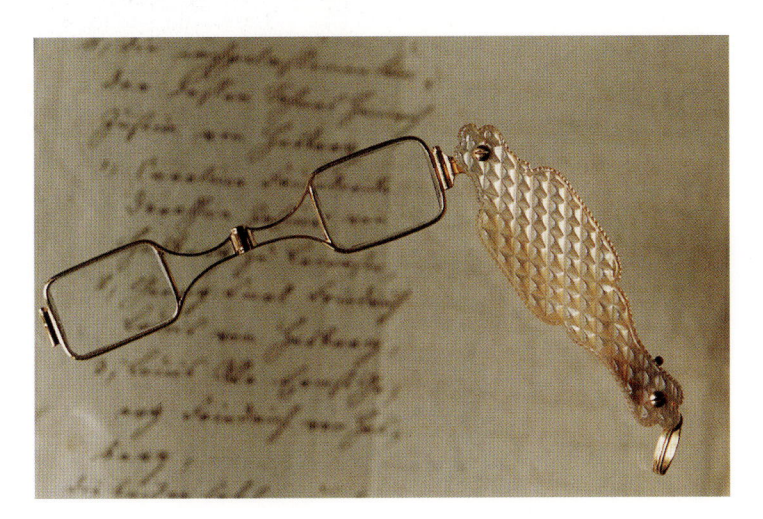

Figure 226. French lorgnette with mother-of-pearl case.

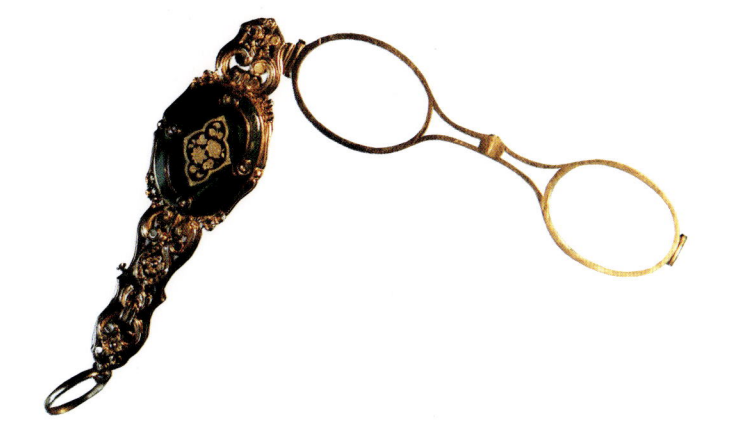

Figure 227. German gold, enameled, and jeweled lorgnette.

LORGNETTES **123**

Figure 228. Gold locket-style lorgnette.

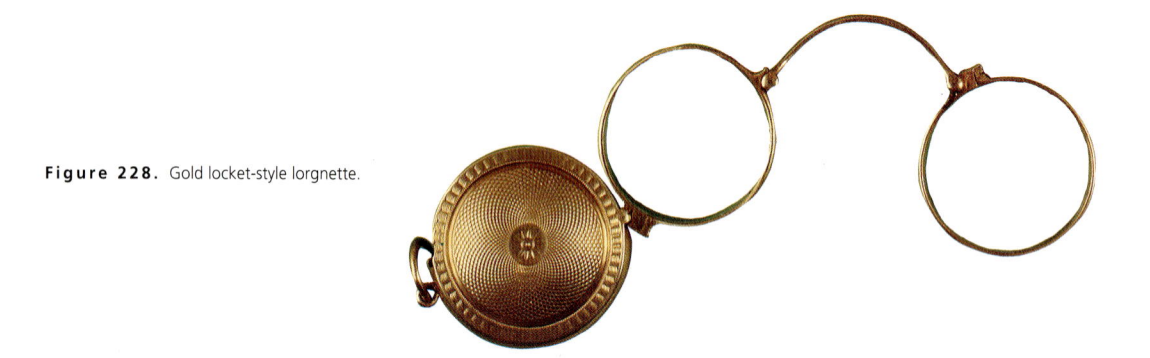

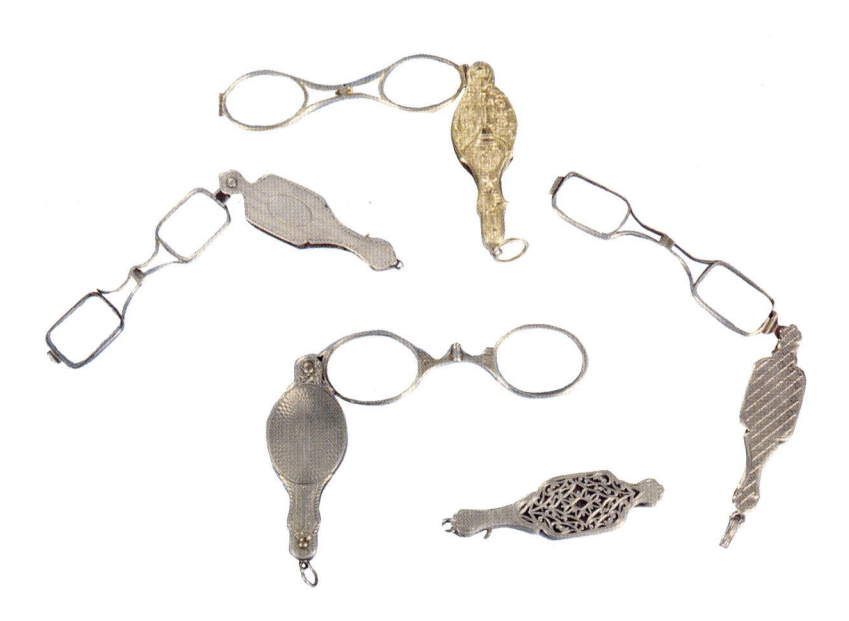

Figure 229. Various French lorgnettes.

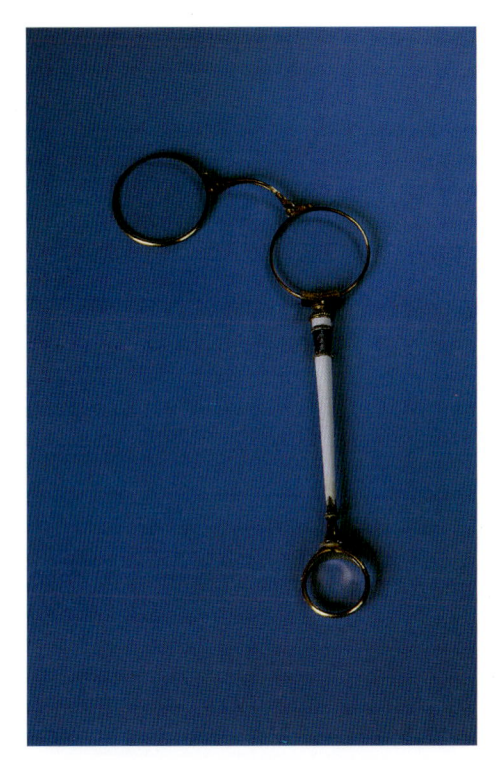

Figure 230. French enameled and jeweled lorgnette, Napoleonic period, with finger ring.

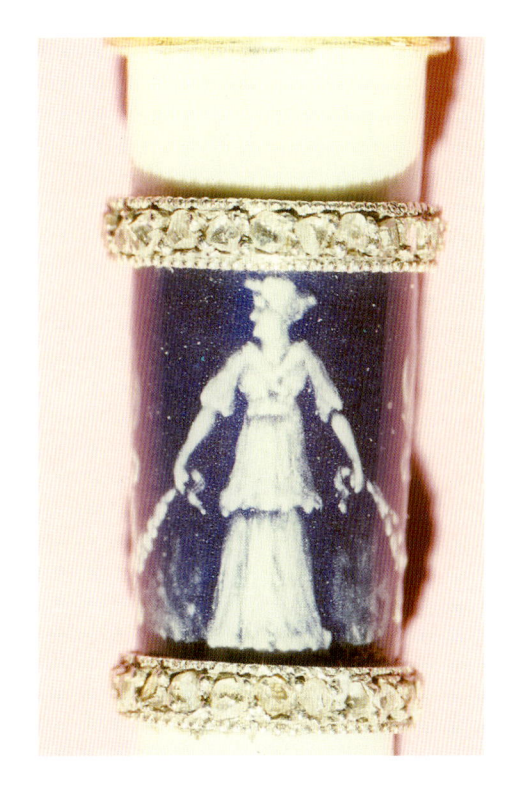

Figure 231. Same as Figure 230—close view of diamond-fringed frieze.

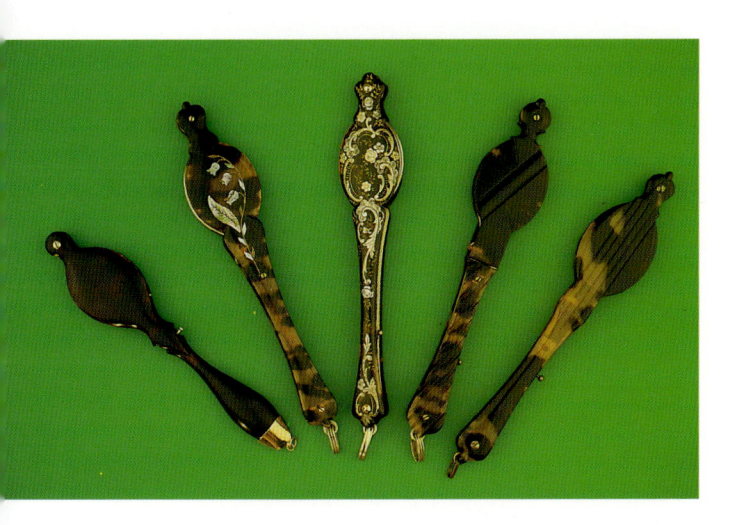

Figure 232. Tortoiseshell lorgnettes, carved, inlaid with gold and mother-of-pearl.

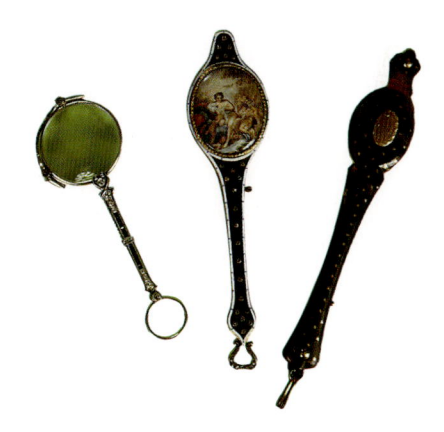

Figure 233. From left: White gold with sapphires, enameled with diamonds and central miniature, tortoiseshell with gold stars and cartouche.

LORGNETTES 125

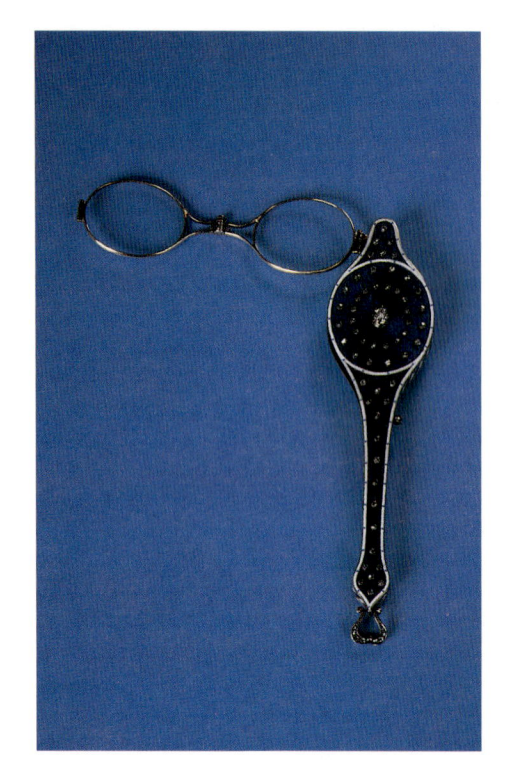

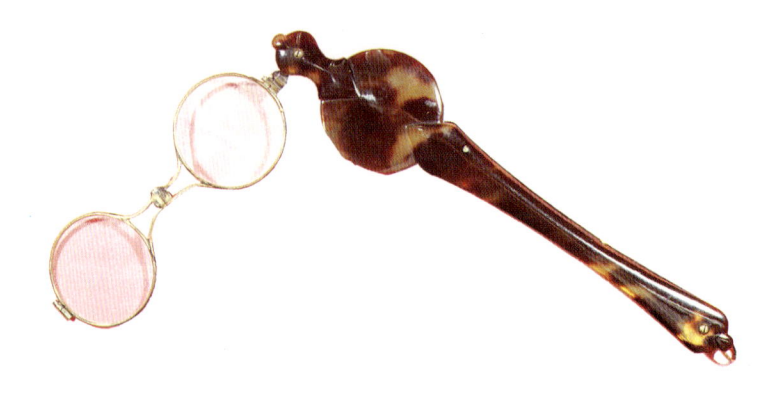

Figure 235. Carved tortoiseshell.

Figure 234. Reverse of Figure 233 (center).

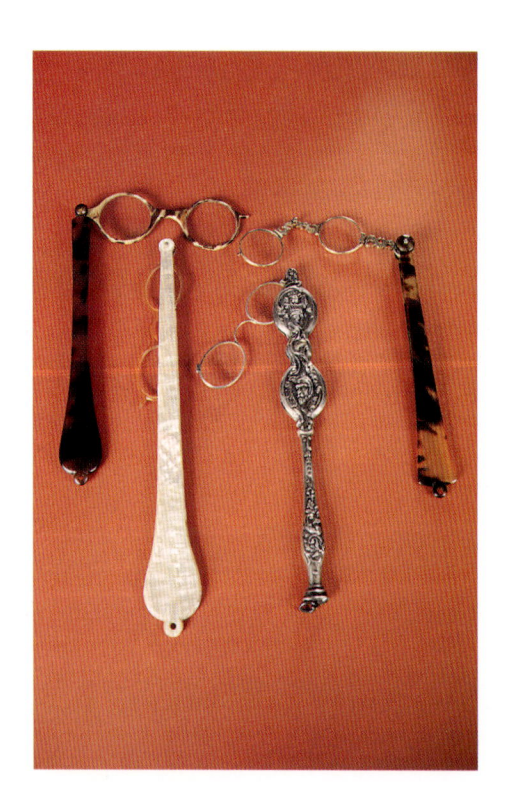

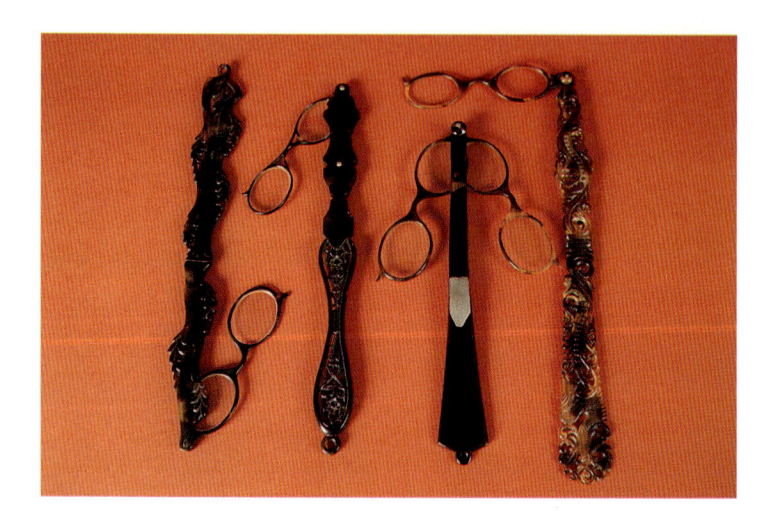

Figure 237. Tortoiseshell lorgnettes.

Figure 236. Mother-of-pearl, silver and tortoiseshell lorgnettes.

126   CHAPTER 14

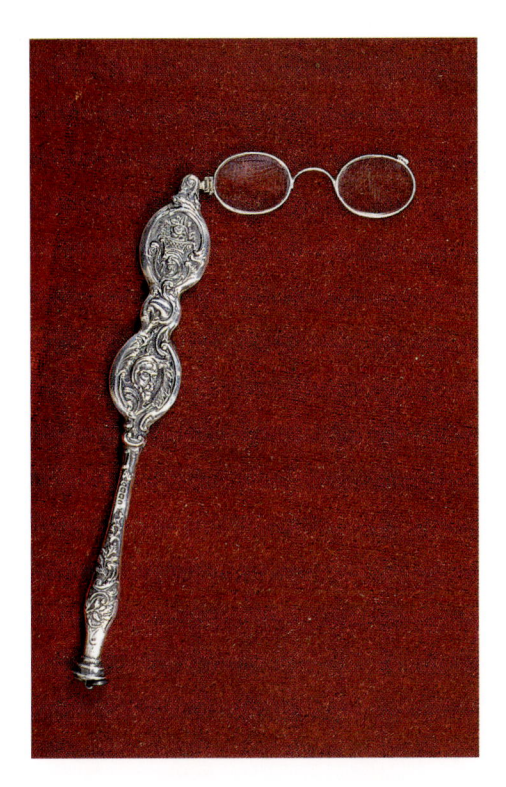

Figure 238. Embossed silver lorgnette (American).

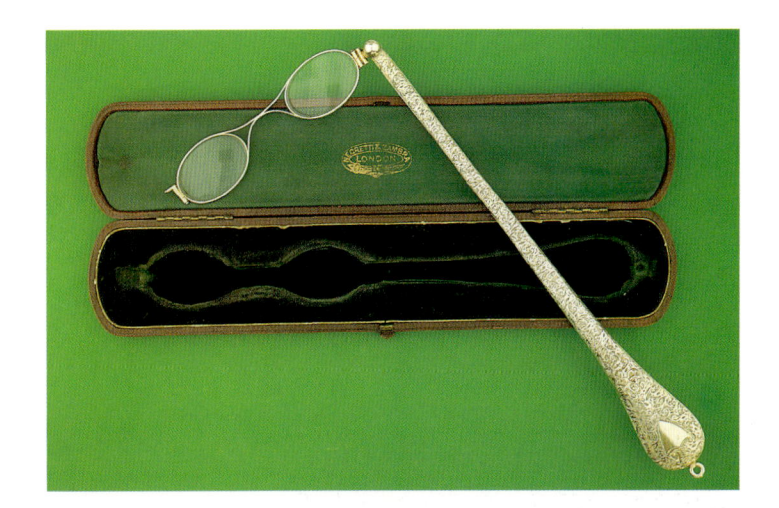

Figure 239. Engraved silver lorgnette (English).

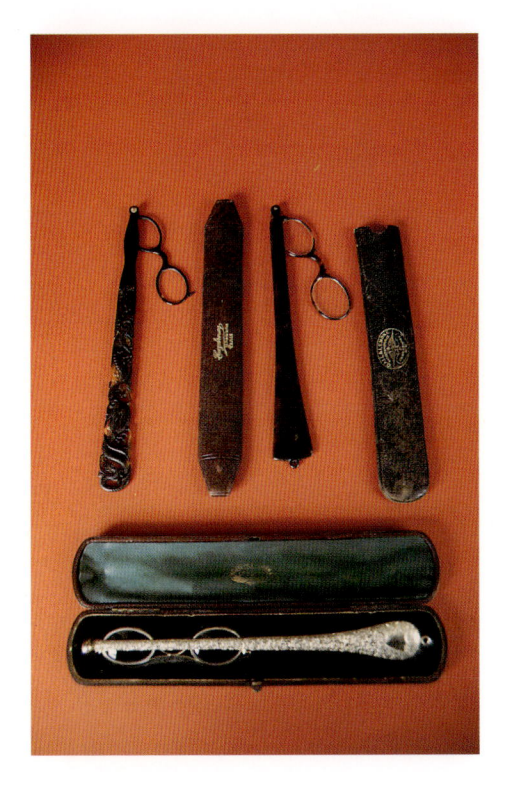

Figure 240. Types of cases.

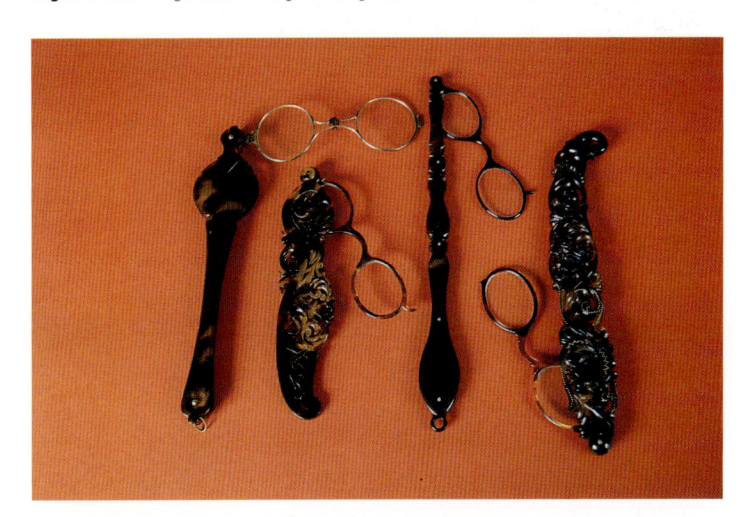

Figure 241. Tortoiseshell and plastic lorgnettes circa 1890.

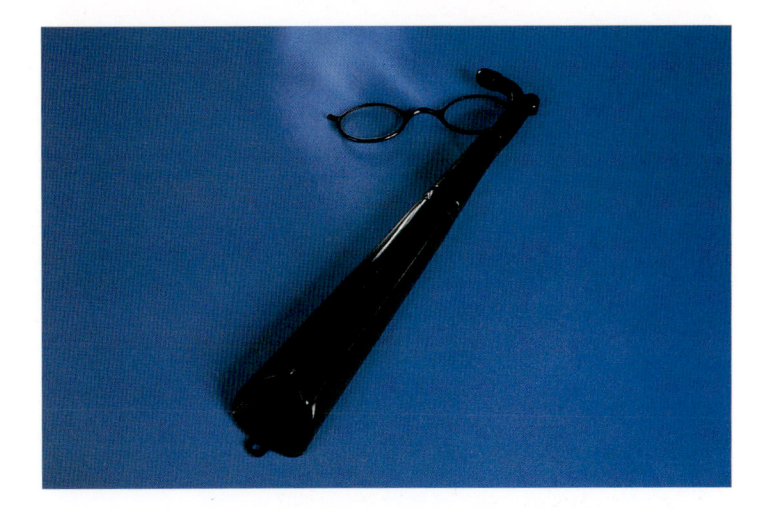

Figure 242. Combined ear trumpet and lorgnette.

LORGNETTES 127

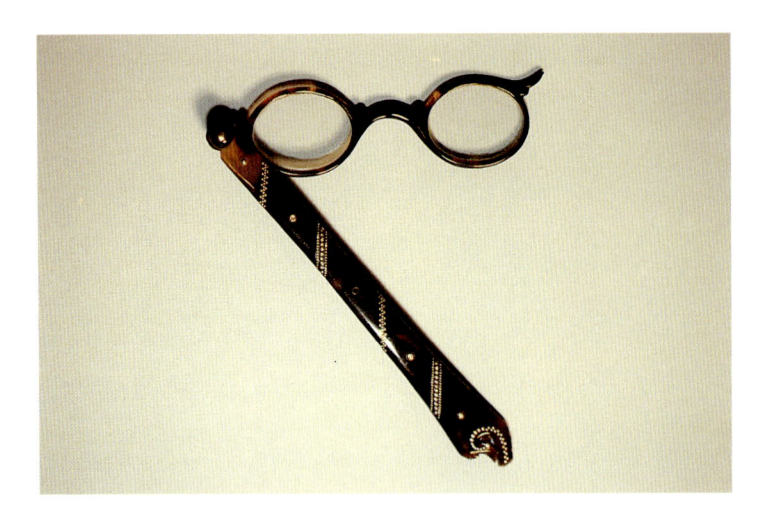

Figure 243. Tortoiseshell decorated with short gold pins.

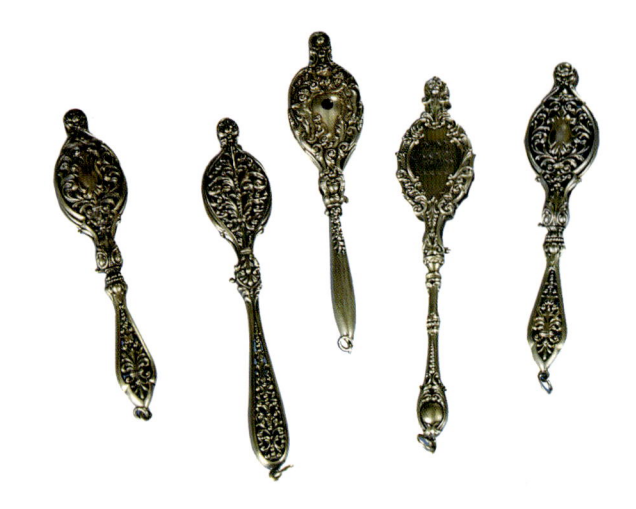

Figure 244. American gold lorgnettes circa 1895.

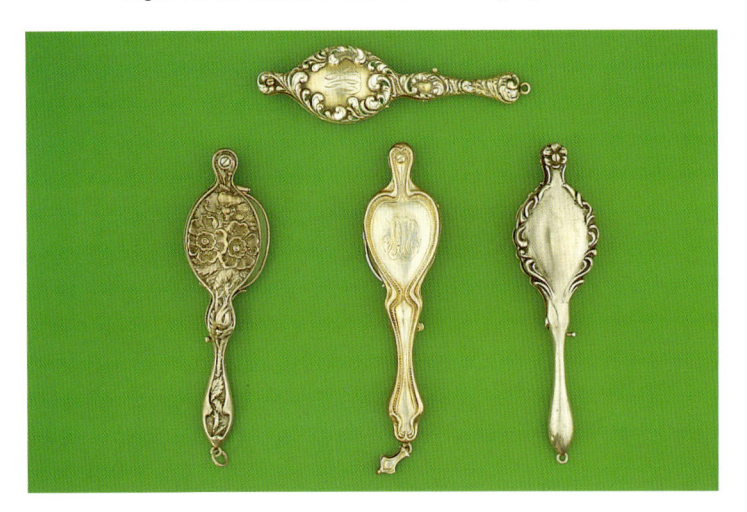

Figure 245. American silver lorgnettes.

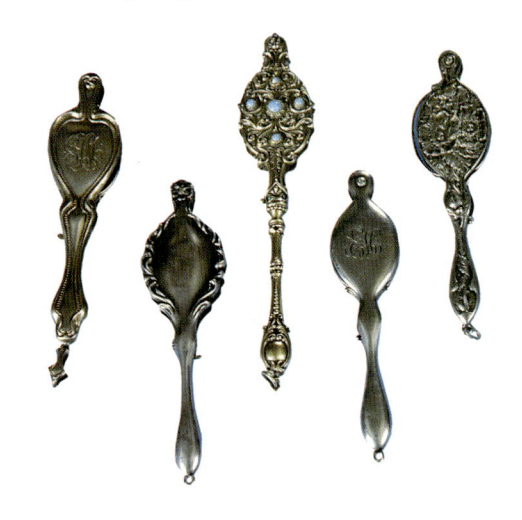

Figure 246. Embossed silver lorgnettes.

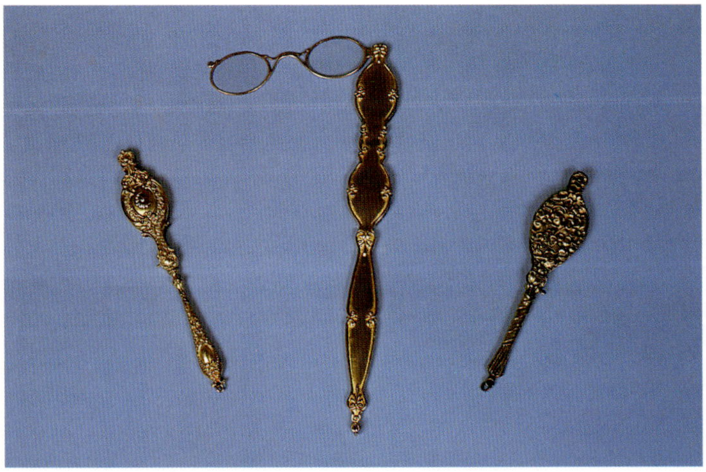

Figure 247. Enameled lorgnette (center).

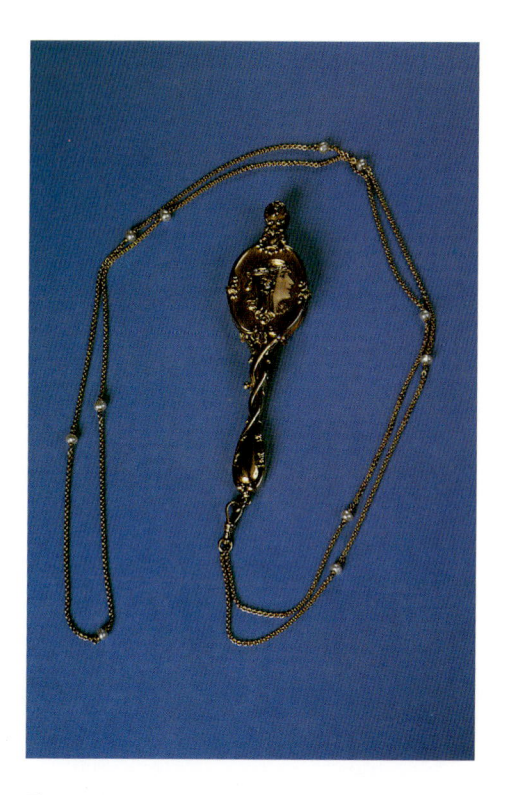

Figure 248. Enameled and diamond gold lorgnette.

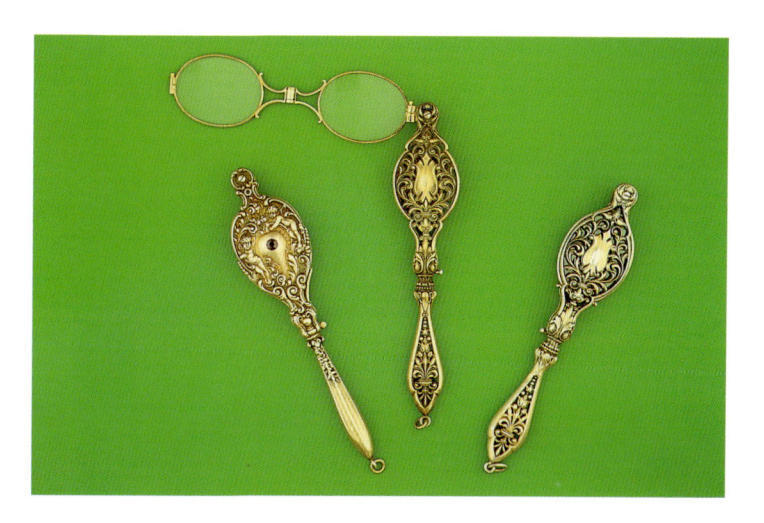

Figure 249. Reticulated gold American lorgnettes.

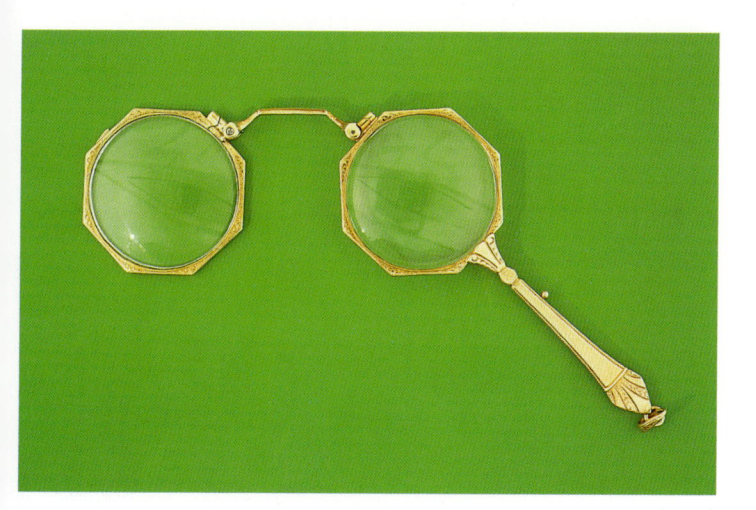

Figure 250. Belgian gold lorgnette circa 1920.

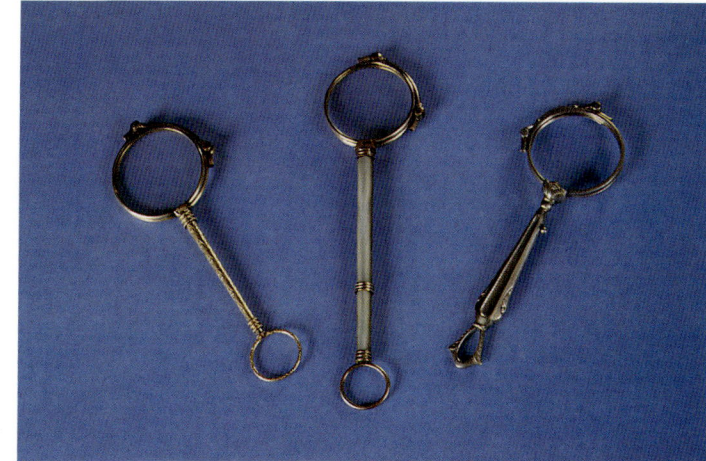

Figure 251. Ordinary 1920s lorgnettes.

LORGNETTES **129**

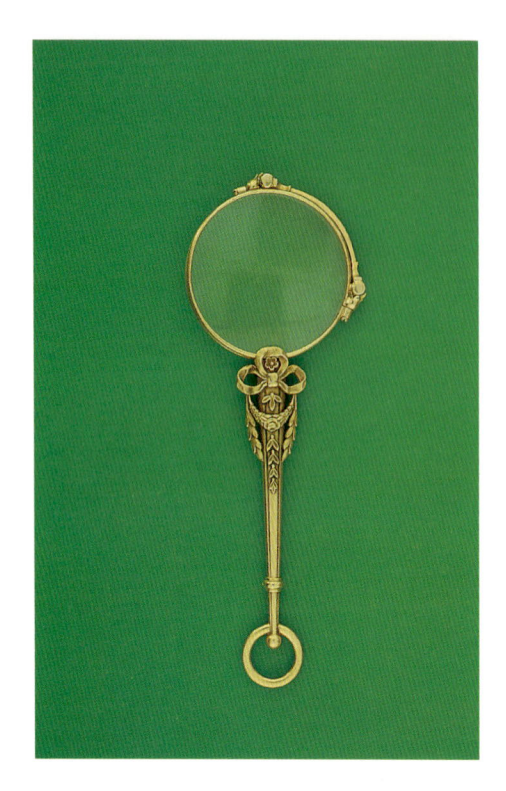

Figure 252. Classic gold lorgnette.

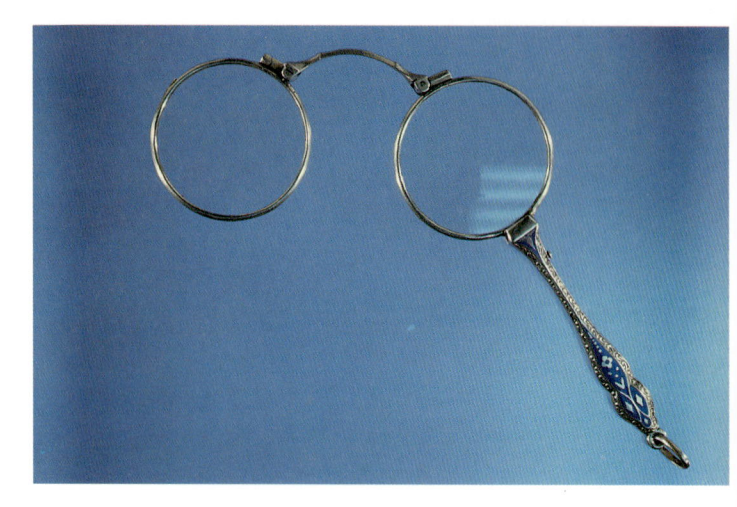

Figure 253. Enameled lorgnette.

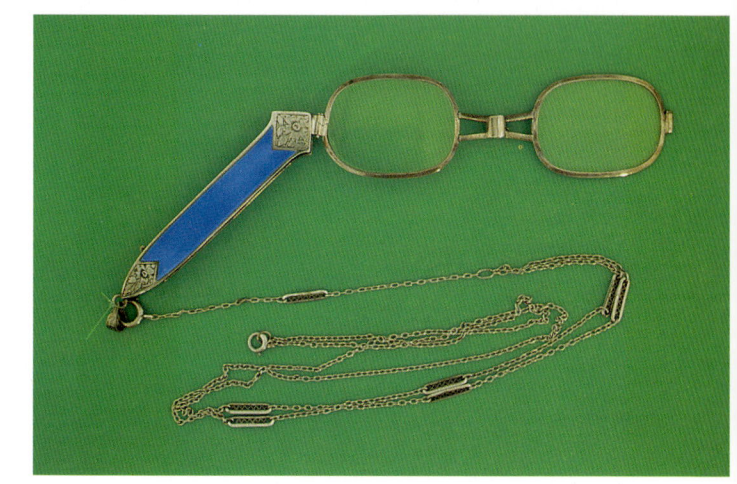

Figure 254. Enameled lorgnette.

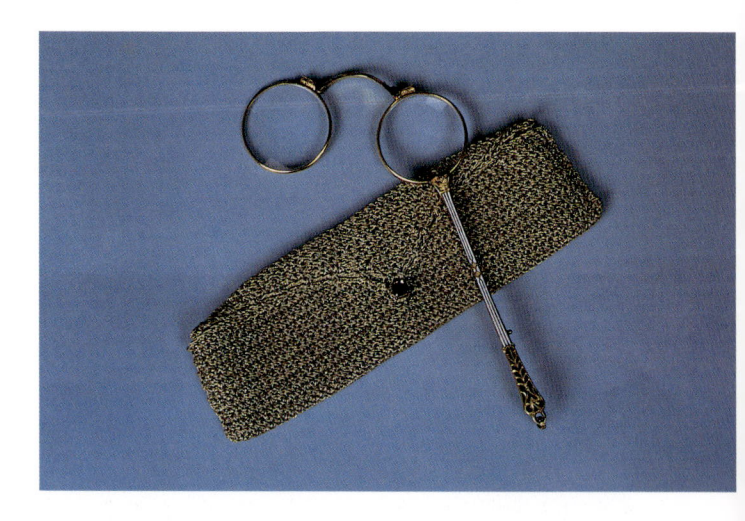

Figure 255. Enameled lorgnette.

130   CHAPTER 14

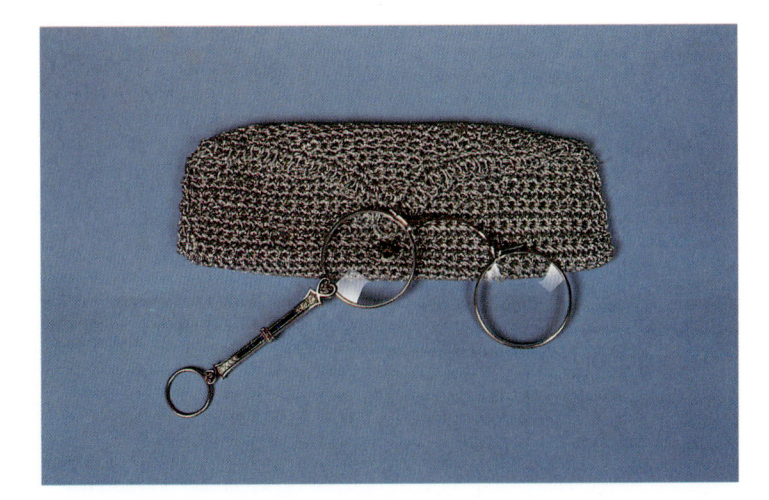

Figure 256. Sapphire and diamond lorgnette.

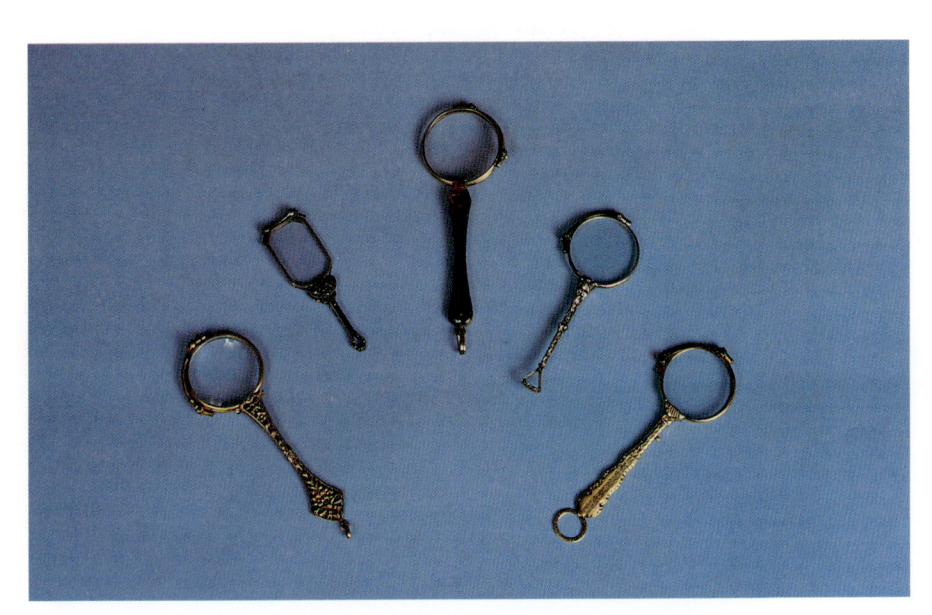

Figure 257. Gold, tortoiseshell, sapphire, and diamond lorgnettes.

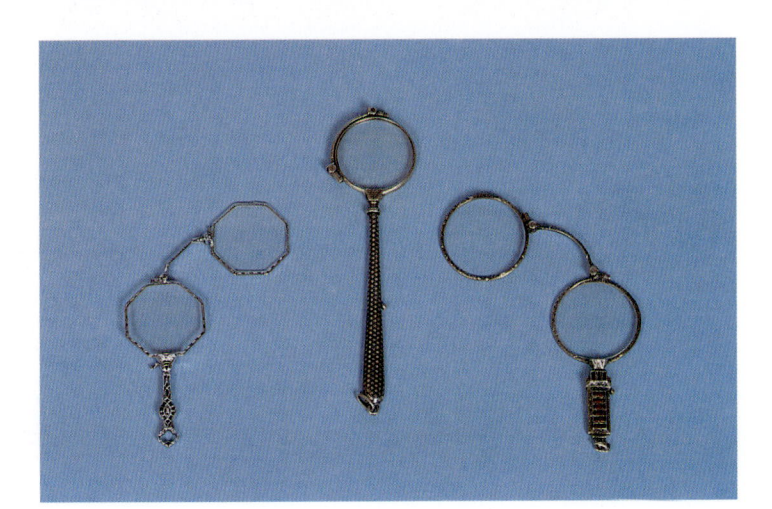

Figure 258. Diamond, niello (center), and ruby lorgnettes.

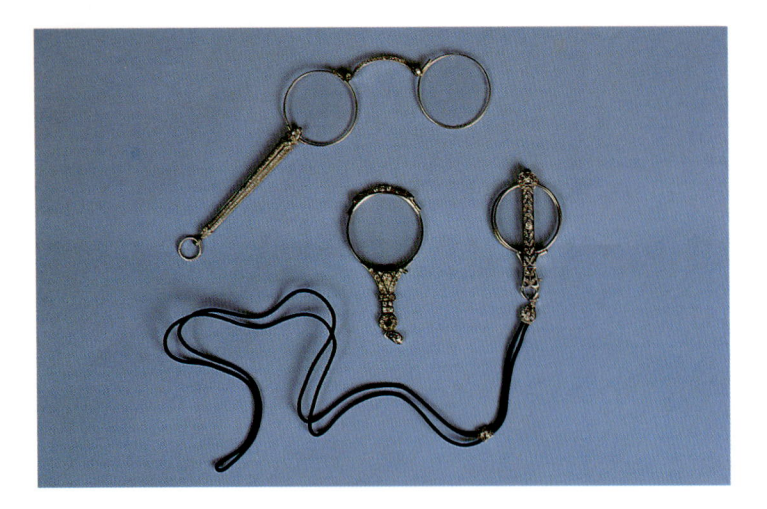

Figure 259. Diamond lorgnettes—above is French, below is American.

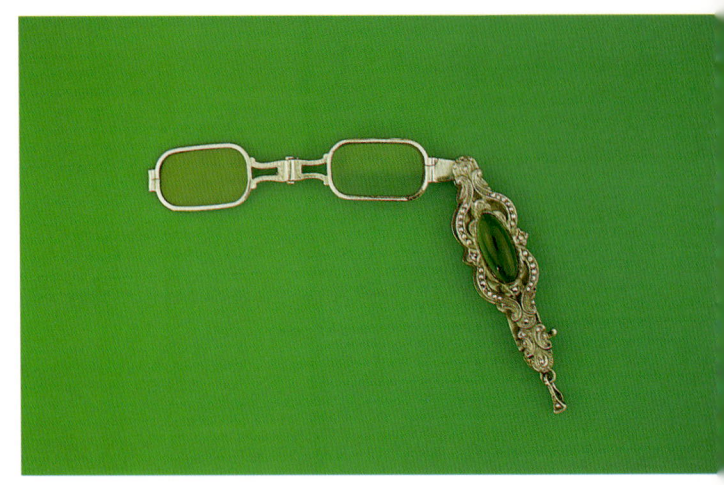

Figure 260. Marcasite and jade lorgnette.

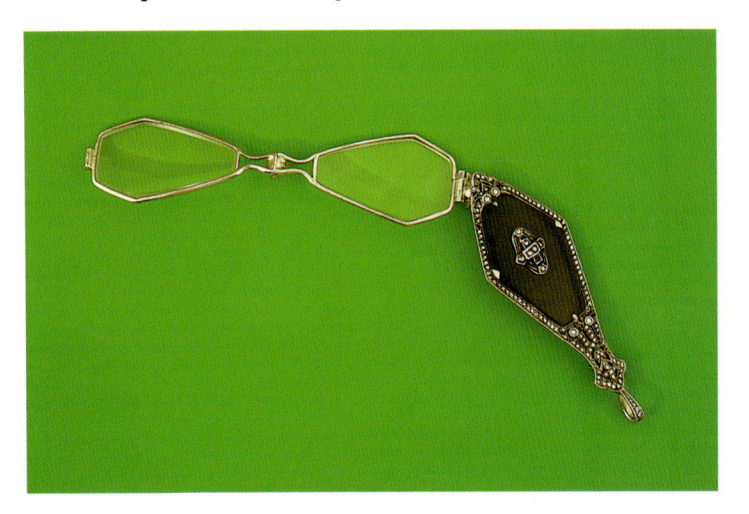

Figure 261. Marcasite and onyx lorgnette.

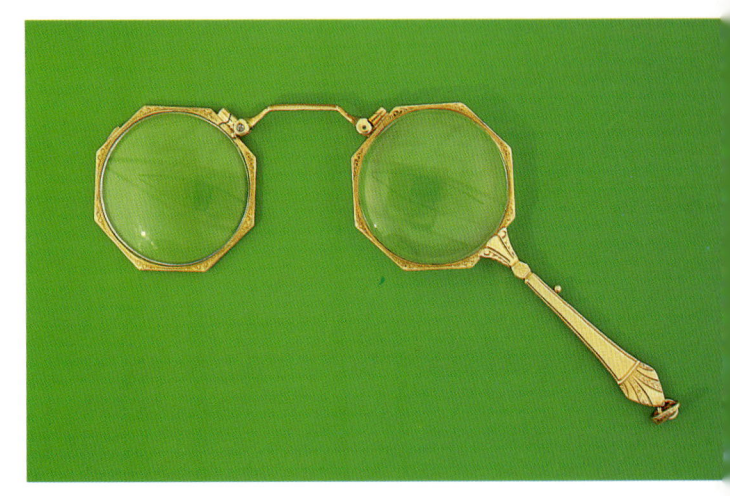

Figure 262. Lorgnette decorated with brilliants circa 1925.

1930s

Two distinct styles of lorgnettes were typical of the 1930 period. The classic (oxford) type (Figures 263 & 264), an American innovation, was produced. It is a type of pince-nez, with a spring for a bridge. It folded in one of two ways: (1) the spring was bent to a semicircle so that the lenses lay one over the other and were held by a catch (Figure 265), or (2) the Z-bridge was used, where the spring was hinged over each lens, allowing them to lie on each other (Figure 266). Handles were very short (about 3 cm.) and decorated with engraving or reticulation. They contained a loop for hanging with chain or ribbon. The lenses were held with metal frames of gold, silver, or plated metal.

A second type of lorgnette of this era was the clothes clip (Figure 267). Basically a side-to-side spring type of lorgnette, the handle was decorated to resemble a piece of jewelry (Figure 268). It clipped on to a woman's pocket or lapel. Some handles contained watches, marcasite, jewels, or enamel. Handles could be of any decorative shape. (Figures 269 & 270).

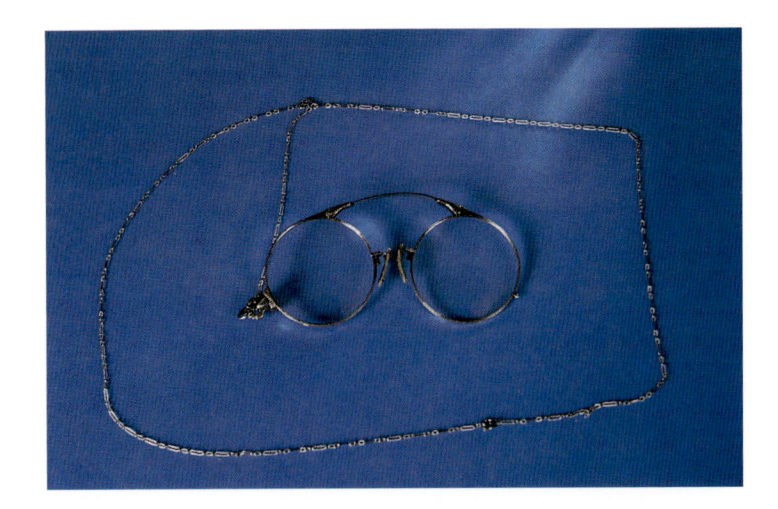

Figure 263. Silver oxford lorgnette.

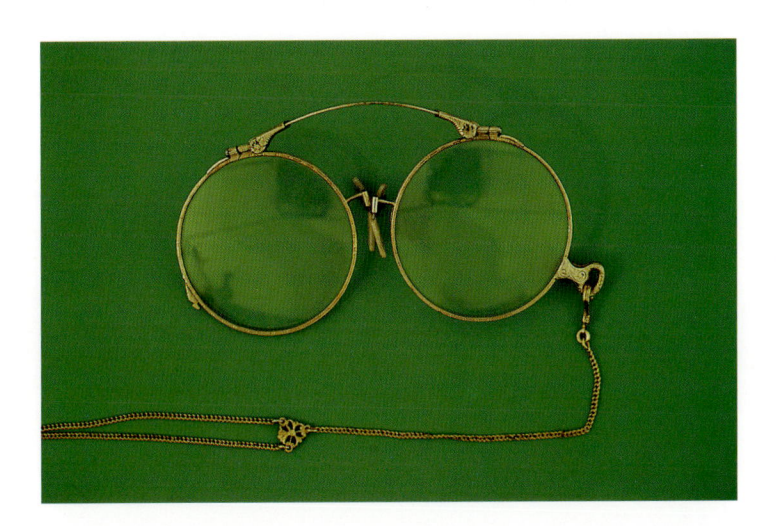

Figure 264. Gold oxford lorgnette.

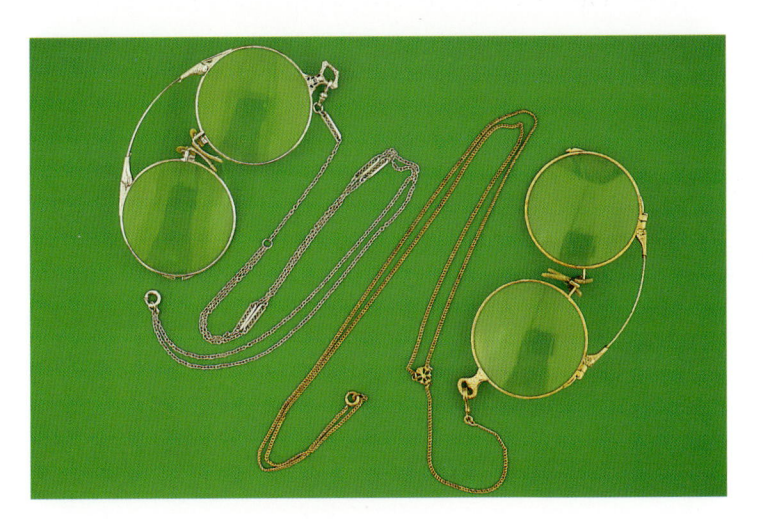

Figure 265. Pair of spring-loaded oxfords.

LORGNETTES 133

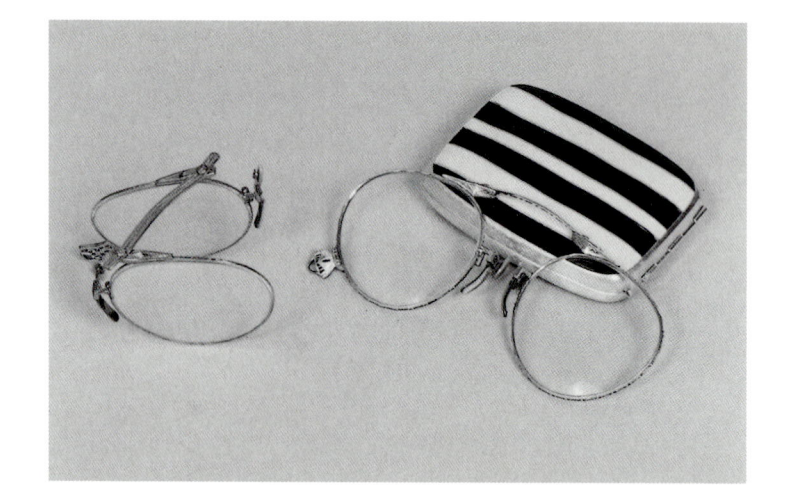

Figure 266. Z-bridge oxfords.

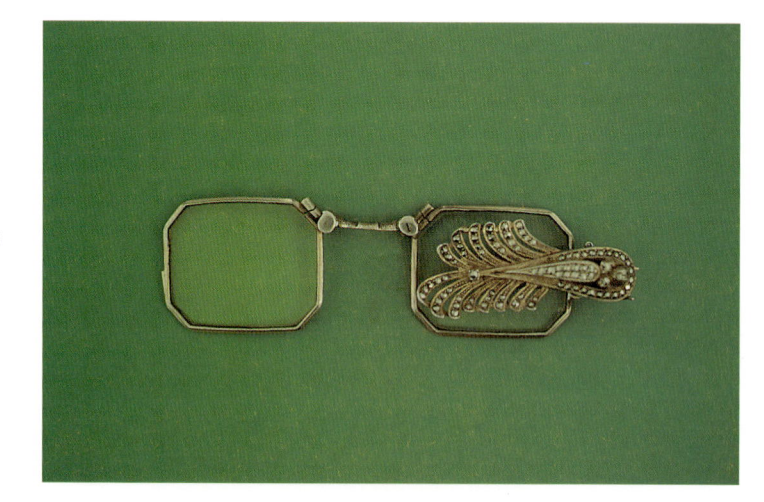

Figure 267. Rhinestone-decorated lapel lorgnette circa 1930, extended.

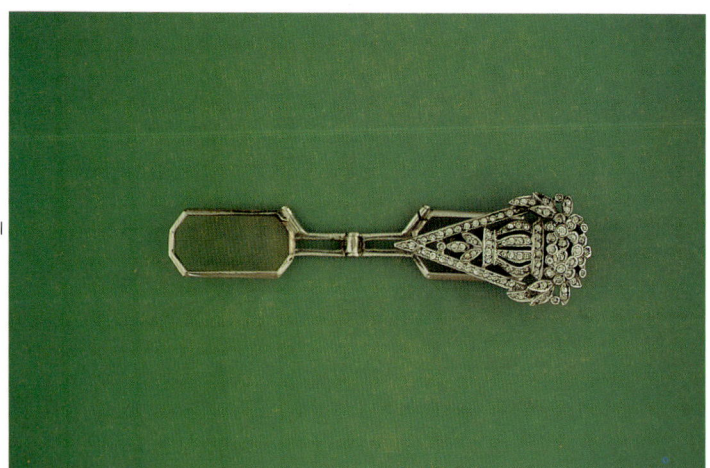

Figure 268. Rhinestone-decorated lapel lorgnette circa 1930, extended.

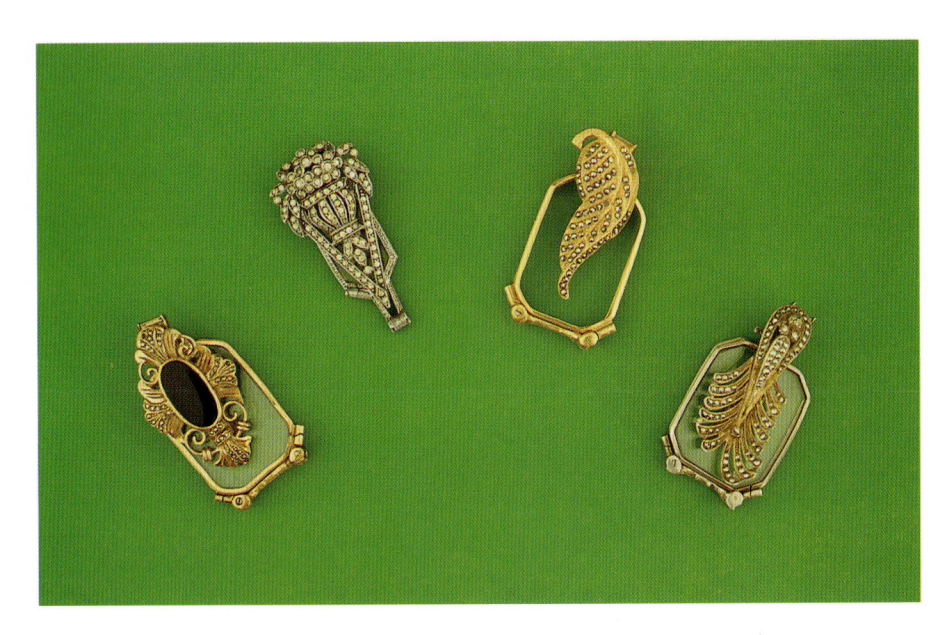

Figure 269. Various lapel clip lorgnettes, folded.

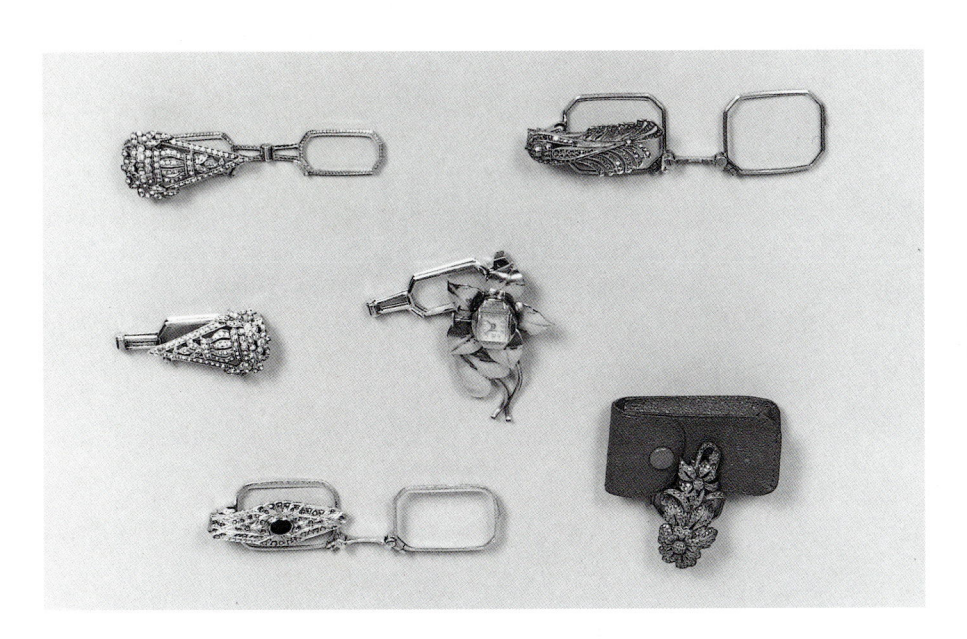

Figure 270. Various lapel clip lorgnettes, folded (note watch in center).

LORGNETTES 135

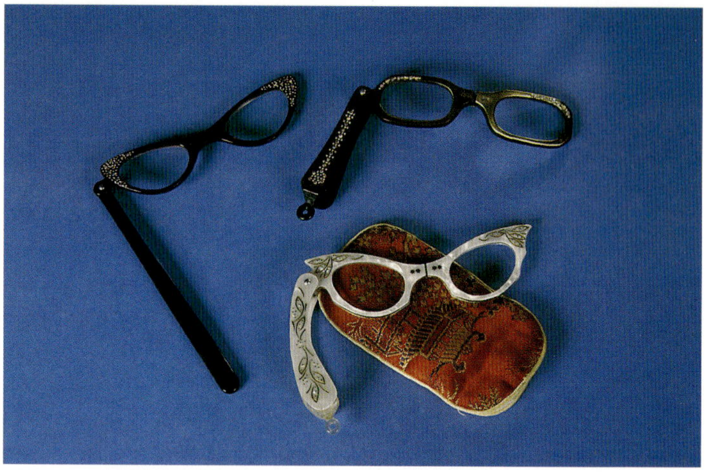

Figure 271. Various plastic lorgnettes circa 1960.

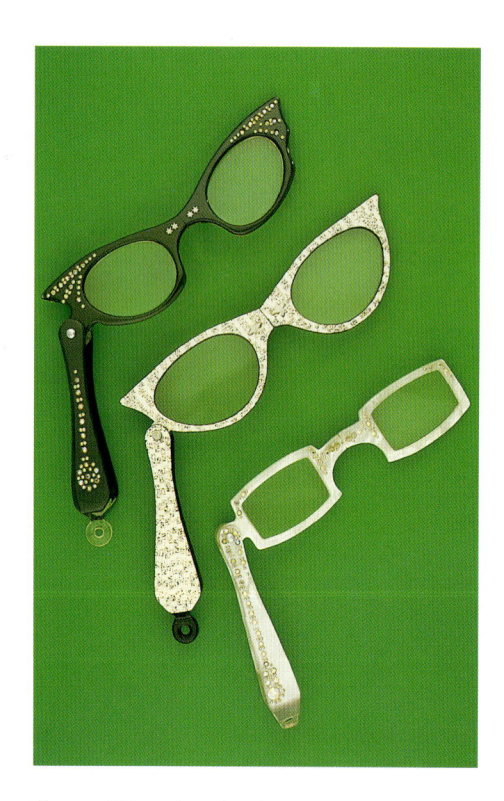

Figure 272. Various plastic lorgnettes.

Modern Lorgnettes

The lorgnette has been designed and used for several hundred years, and it has not been entirely abandoned as a practical vision aid or as decorative jewelry. Plastic lorgnettes in the 1980s and 1990s are made of many colors, many designs in the plastic and the shape, and many variations in the mechanics of the piece (Figure 271).

Being light in weight is an advantage of plastic, and the ease of inserting false jewels for "formal" wear enhances its use. The material is inexpensive, moldable, and adaptable to mass production. Commercial frame manufacturers find little trouble adapting their techniques to the making of these lorgnettes. Women find them handy to use during the daytime when hung around the neck and small enough to fit inside a purse for evening use. Many modern lorgnettes are furnished with complementing cases contained in the handles that enhance their decorative aspect (Figure 272).

Conclusion

At present, it is de rigueur to wear Grandma's lorgnette to the concert or opera for decorative and optical purposes. It incidentally establishes heirship to a long line of well-heeled ancestors. Nevertheless, lorgnettes are objects not only of beauty, workmanship, style, elan, and a little pomposity but but also of vision enhancement (Figures 273 & 274).

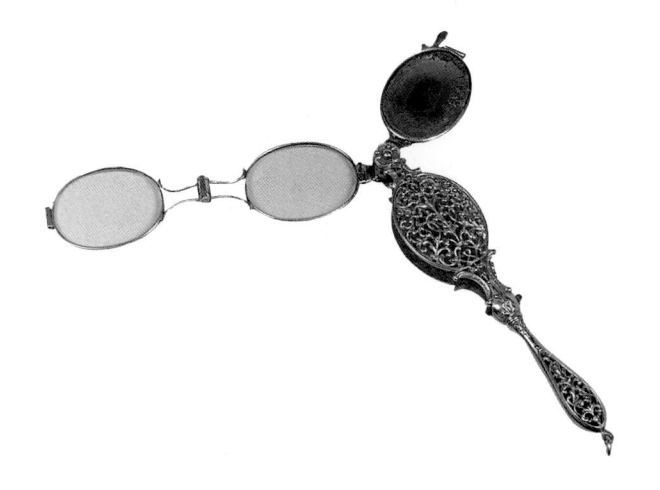

Figure 273. French gold lorgnette with side-polished steel convex mirror.

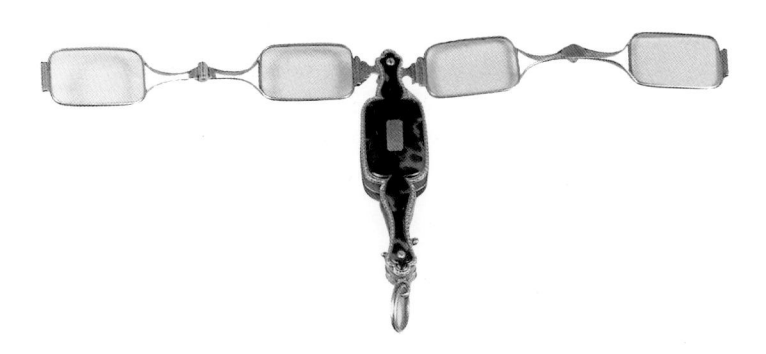

Figure 274. French double lorgnette—one set of lenses for reading and one set for distance.

Notes

1. Richard Corson, *Fashions in Eyeglasses* (London: Peter Owen, Ltd., 1980).
2. D. C. Davidson, *Spectacles, Lorgnettes and Monocles* (Aylesburg, Bucks, UK, 1989).
3. Corson, op. cit.

Other Sources Consulted for Chapter 14

1. Nils Jockel, *Vor Augen Formen, Geschichte und Wirkungen der Brille* (Hamburg: Museum für Kunst und Gewerbe, 1986).
2. Anita Kuisle, *Brillen* (Munich: Deutches Museum 1985).
3. R. J. S. MacGregor, *Collecting Ophthalmic Antiques.* (Ayrshire, UK: Ophthalmic Antique International Collectors' Club, 1992).
4. J. Wm. Rosenthal, *Lorgnettes*, Cecil O'Brien Lectureship. Tulane University, New Orleans, 1991.

15

Monoculars (Spyglasses) (1603–1830)

A monocular is a small, hand-held telescope (Figure 275). Various names such as prospect (by the English) or perspective glasses, lorgnettes (by the French), and spyglasses have all been used to describe what is basically the same thing—a monocular—a telescopic device with a single eyepiece. The evolution of the fashionable pieces used to inconspicuously spy on people at the theater and other places began with the discovery of the first telescope in the seventeenth century. According to Pierre Marley, the discovery was made by children of a Middleberg optician, Johannes Lippershey.[1] The children were playing with concave and convex lenses that their father had prepared, put them together, and accidentally discovered that they could see a distant belfry with the finest detail. Lippershey applied for a patent on his telescope in 1606.[2] Before reaching a decision, the committee asked Lippershey to build a "double" telescope with both tubes united. Two years later, Lippershey's claims were disputed by another inventor named Metius, who claimed priority because of his research on the single telescope. Concurrently, a third contender, Zach Janssen, entered the picture as well. The Janssens, father and son, also spectacle makers of Middleburg, are known to have made telescopes. In 1609, the government refused to patent Lippershey's telescope because he was not the only one to construct one. Despite the preceding facts, Galileo Galilei (1564–1642), who built his first telesope in 1609, is usually credited with its invention.

The invention of the telescope was the beginning of a new market, since the use of spectacles was frowned upon in the seventeenth and eighteenth centuries. As a result of improper fitting and grinding, spectacles did not provide good vision. Generally, ophthalmologists had little faith in the benefits of spectacles to their patients, and some ophthalmologists even denounced their use. This prompted patients to find alternate means of improving their vision, particularly at the theater.

By 1680, to accommodate the needs of society, smaller versions of the original telescope were being produced in England and on the Continent (Figure 276). Later, in the eighteenth century, theaters had grown in number and were frequented by polite society. Small English telescopes called prospect glasses (perspective glasses) and lorgnettes (in France) became enormously popular among men and women of fashion—not only because they magnified but also because they served to correct poor eyesight with a certain elegance (Figure 277). (The word *lorgnette* or the other currently used English version, *lorgnon*, probably comes from the French verb *lorgner*, to leer or stare.)

The first spyglasses (monoculars) were cylindrical, with one sliding tube inside another (Figure 278).[3] Until 1760, the

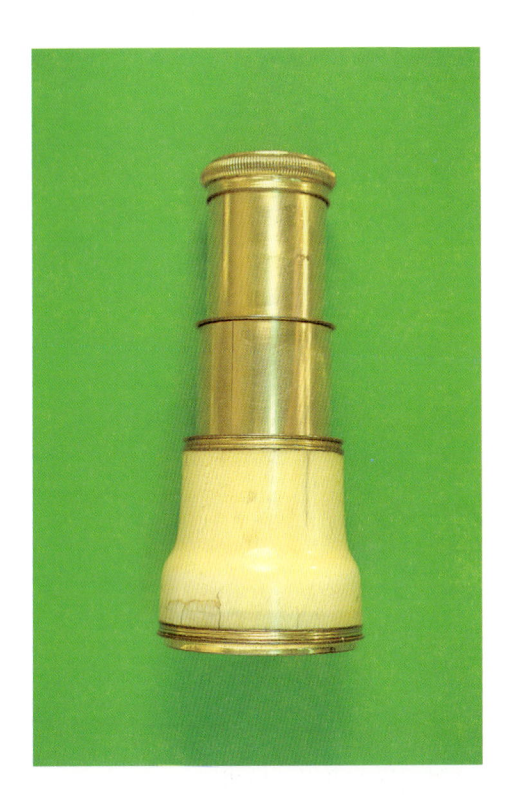

Figure 275. Pear-shaped French ivory monocular circa 1860.

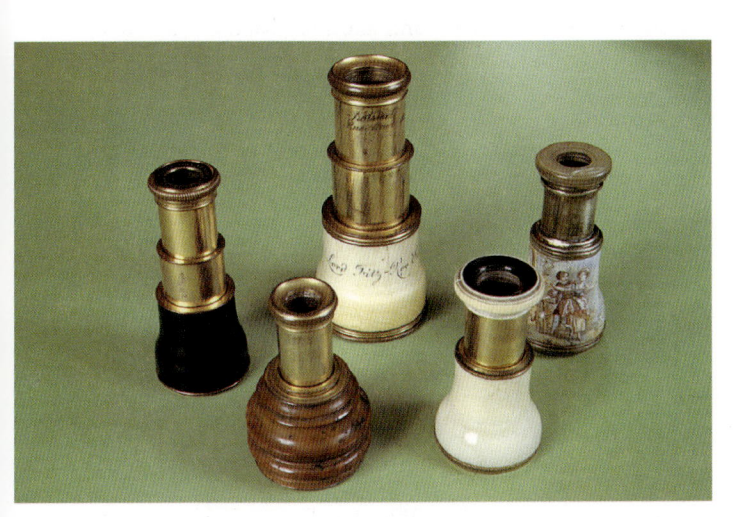

Figure 276. Group of metal, ivory, wood, and porcelain monoculars.

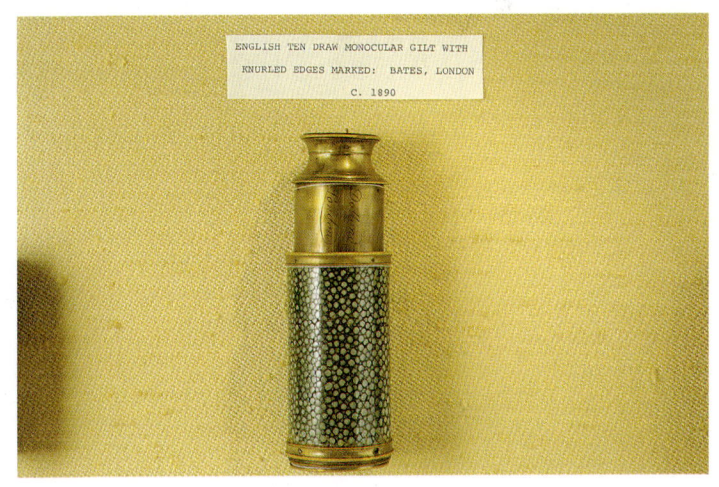

Figure 277. English one-draw monocular gilt with knurled edges, marked Bates, London circa 1890.

MONOCULARS

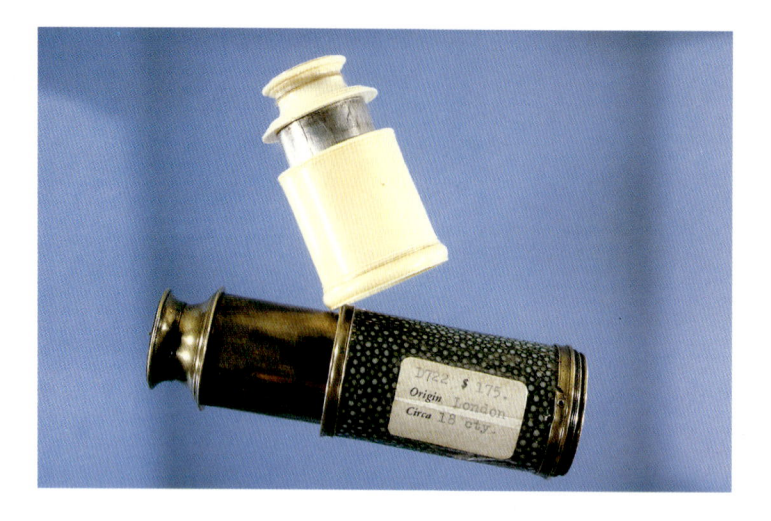

Figure 278. Single-tube sliding monoculars circa 1750.

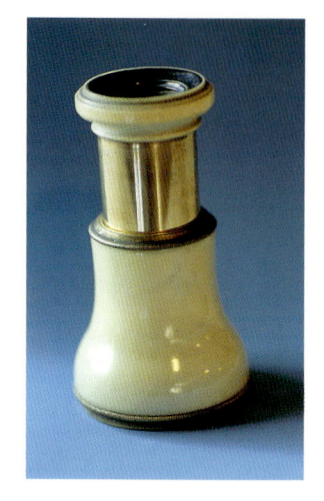

Figure 279. Lorgnette poire, French, circa 1840.

Figure 280. Group of multiple-draw monoculars.

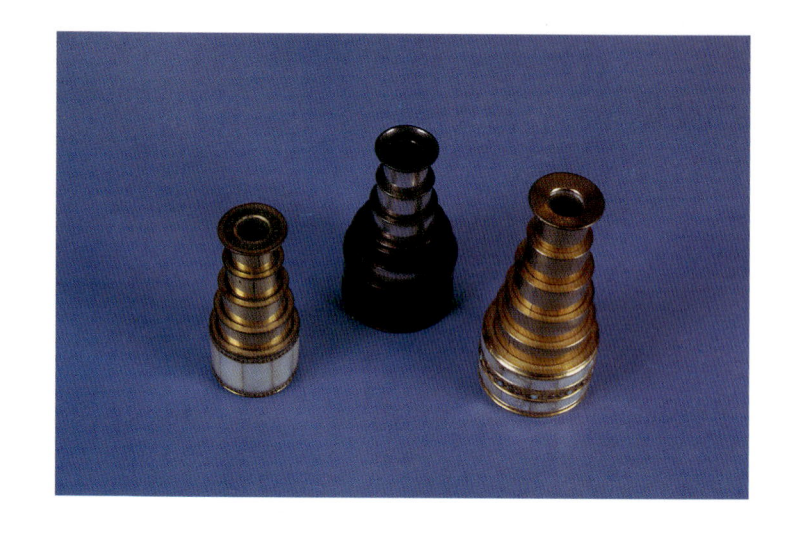

Figure 281. Jealousy glass and case circa 1750.

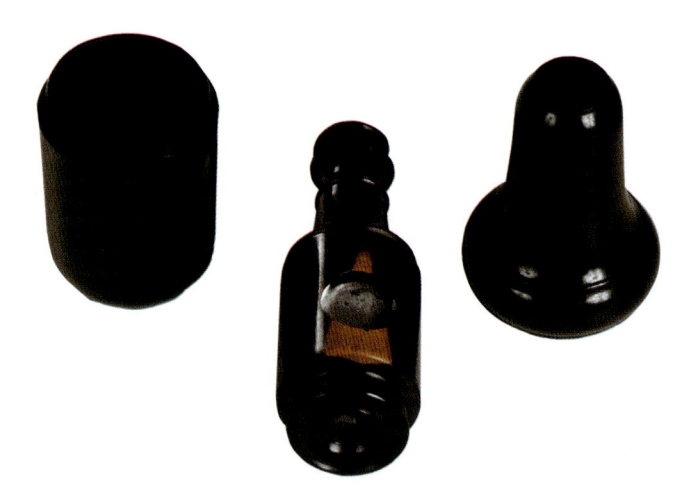

140 CHAPTER 15

lorgnette or prospect glass was usually found in the form of this single tube, with variations mainly in the covering and decoration. Later, the tube was made with one end larger than the other, and this was known in France as the pear-shaped glass (*lorgnette poire*) (Figure 279). This change from cylindrical to pear- or conical-shaped body tubes was due to the patenting of the achromatic lens by Dollond of London. Larger diameter objective lenses were possible, as no chromatic aberration was engendered. The next development was an inner sliding tube divided into a number of collapsible sections so that the glass could be closed into a more compact form for carrying (Figure 280). Some collapsed into the size and shape of a pocketwatch and were called *lorgnette pour la poche* by the French.

Other types of monoculars were available as well. One was described in 1749 by Thomin, optician to the Queen of France. Thomin stated:

> It is still another kind of opera glass [monocular] which is called "nounette du jalousie" (jealousy glass) which has the same proportions as the usual opera glass [monocular] but in which the difference consists of a plated mirror set in an angle in which the tube is pierced with an oval opening on one side [Figure 281]. It is sufficient to turn this opening in the direction of whatever one wishes to observe and the curiosity is immediately satisfied. Its usefulness is confined to letting us see surreptitiously a person we seem not to be observing. This lorgnette may have been called a decorum glass because there is nothing more rude than to use an ordinary opera glass for looking at some one face to face.[4]

The *nounette du jalousie* was used in a manner similar to the way a periscope is used today.

Another type of monocular was popular in the Empire period (1803–1814, Battle of Waterloo). It was cask shaped (like Napoleon's barrels of powder), and an *N* was frequently the pointed design.

Besides having different shapes, variations in the materials were used to make and decorate monoculars. They included cardboard or wood (Figure 282), covered with leather or parchment. Further decorations were of ivory (Figure 283), gold (Figure 284), silver, Wedgwood, pomponne, agate, enamel (Figure 285), studs (Figure 286), varnish, colored stones

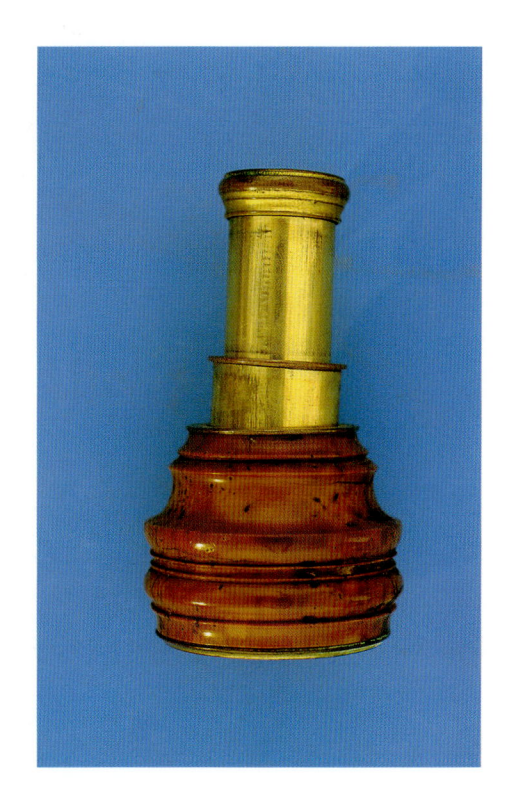

Figure 282. Burl wood and gilt, two-draw monocular, French circa 1810.

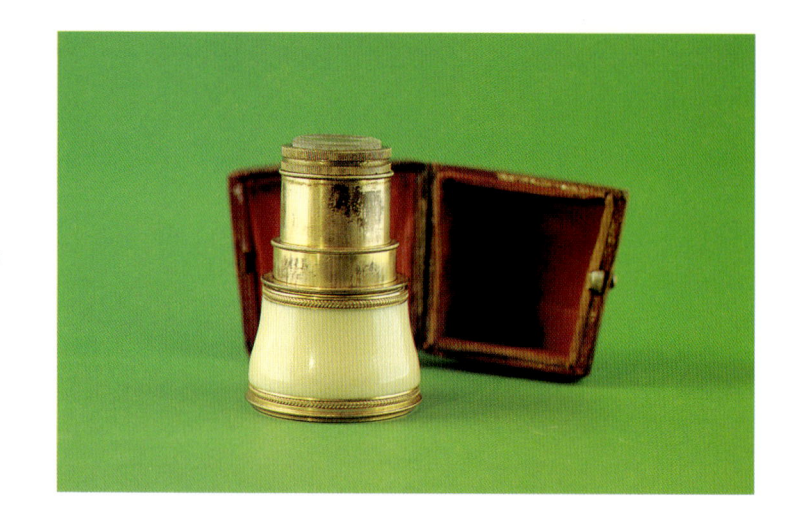

Figure 283. English ivory and gilt monocular.

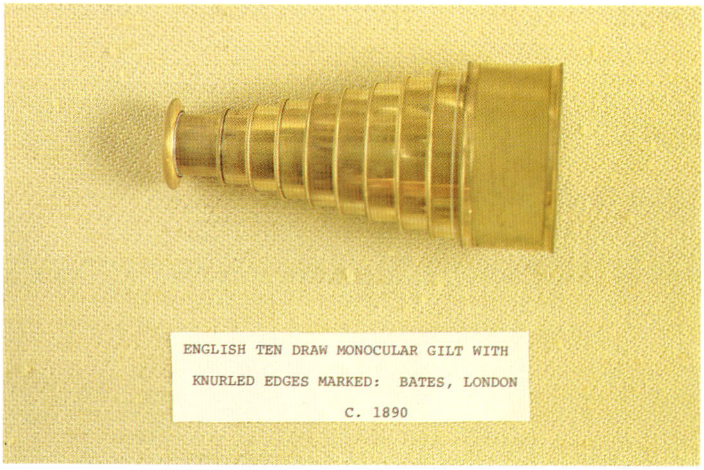

Figure 284. Ten-draw gilt monocular, Bates London.

Figure 285. Enameled monocular, replacement case.

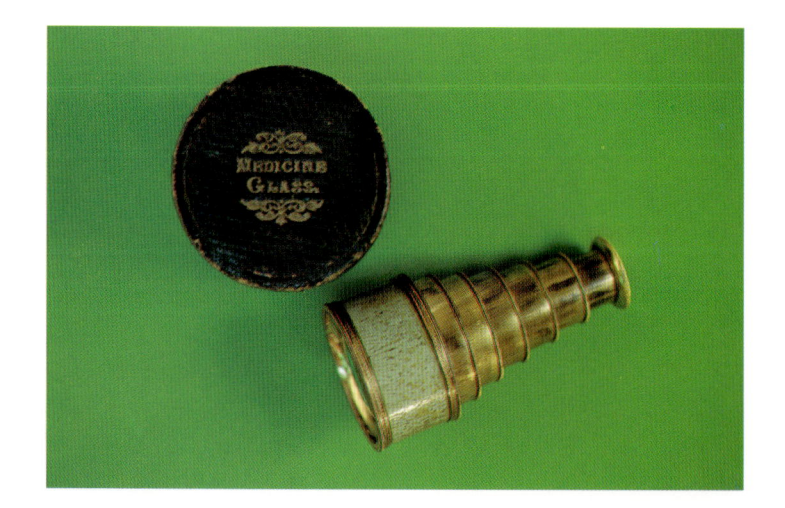

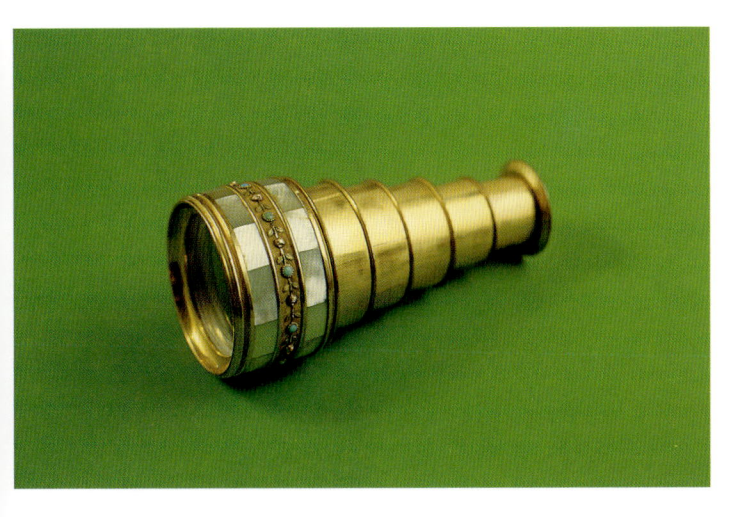

Figure 286. Mother-of-pearl and turquoise studs.

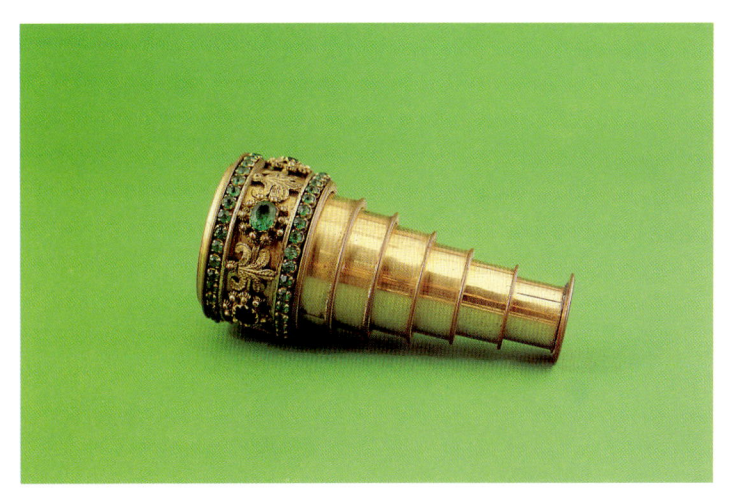

Figure 287. French gilt and green glass monocular.

(Figure 287), porcelain from Paris or Saxony, and marvelous miniatures (Figure 288). The fashionable pieces, crafted by artisans and artists, were treasured as works of art as well as for their practical use.

Apparently women's curiosity was not limited to the theater or other public places. The author has a boudoir hand mirror decorated lavishly with clear and green-faceted glass stones. The mirror's brass handle unscrews into three pieces, revealing a small telescope about 7 centimeters long, with one draw for focusing. This interesting piece, to be used about the home, was purchased in Frankfurt, Germany (Figures 289 & 290).

Although monoculars were beautifully decorated and considered works of art, their use began to cause controversy. They were, in fact, smaller versions of the original telescope but still were quite bulky and visible. One could not possibly inconspicuously spy at another, because of the large size of these glasses. Complaints of their use at the theater began to surface in 1745, when Anne Marie Lepage, a prominent socialite in Paris, stated, "I entered my box. Hardly was I seated when I noticed twenty glasses pointed toward me; I had sometimes seen at the Opera or Comédie the use of the lorgnette, but never with such effrontery."[5]

Similar protests continued throughout the eighteenth century. In *Tableaux de Paris*, published in Amsterdam in 1782, Mercier stated, "Paris is full of merciless oglers who place themselves in front of you and fix on you their bold staring

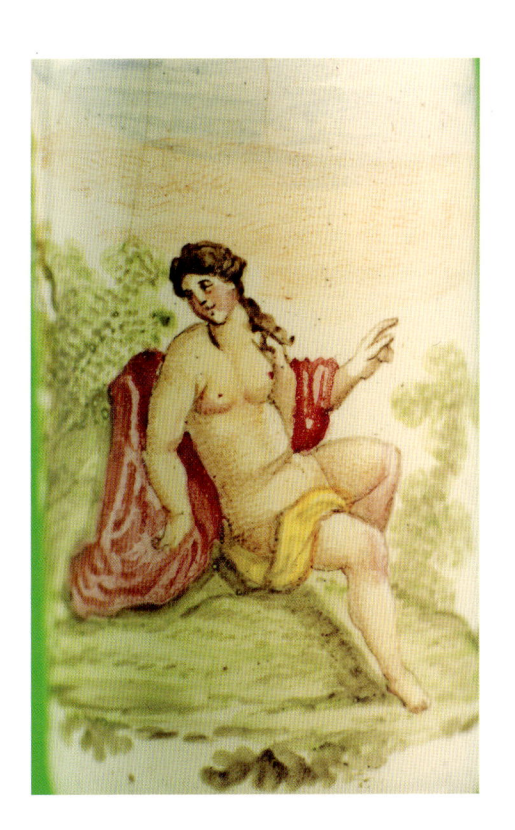

Figure 288. Enlargement of miniature on French etui.

MONOCULARS 143

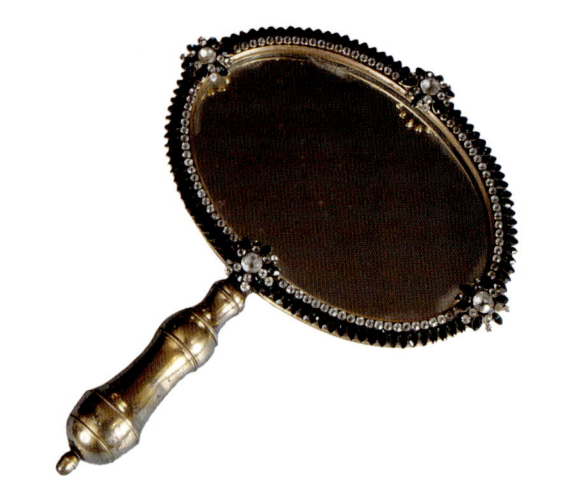

Figure 289. Woman's boudoir mirror with monocular in handle, assembled.

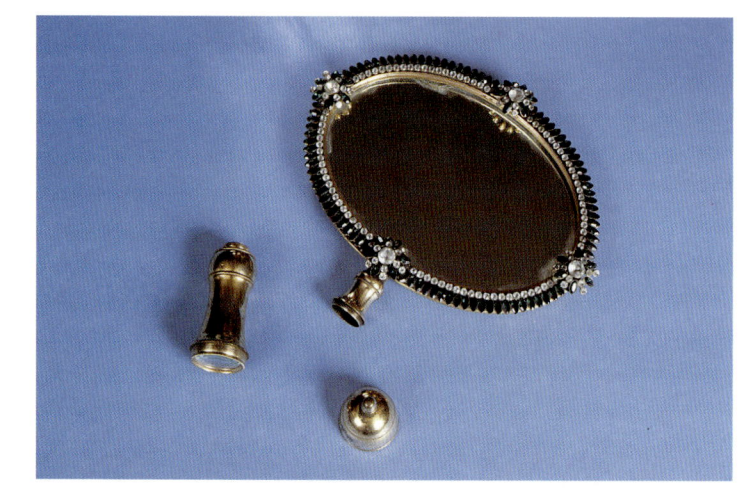

Figure 290. Woman's boudoir mirror with monocular in handle, unassembled.

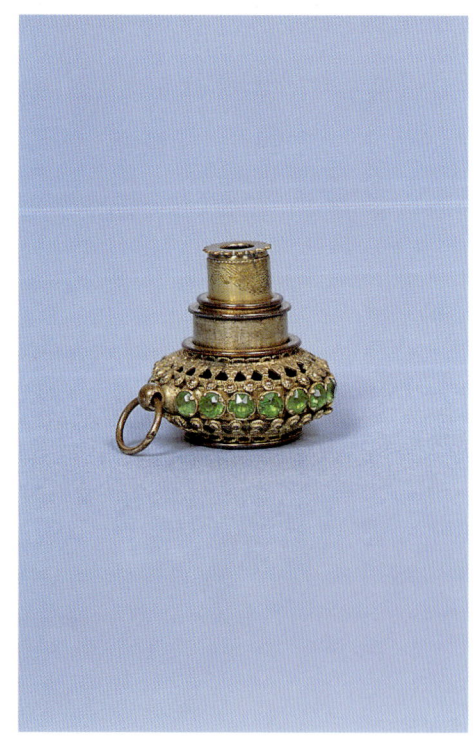

Figure 291. French locket two-draw monocular with green stones.

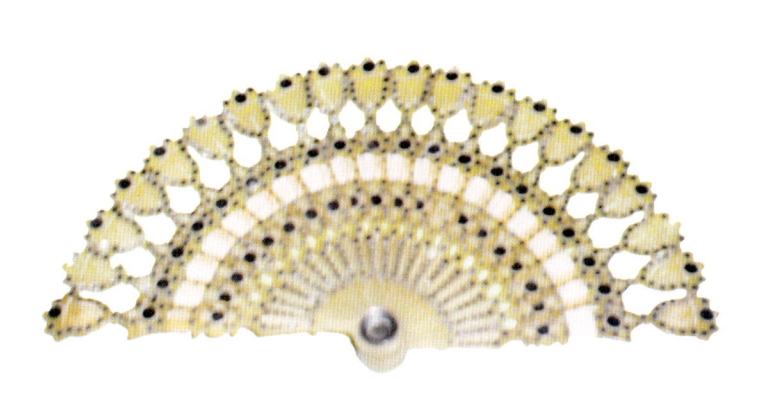

Figure 292. Telescope in fulcrum of fan circa 1790.

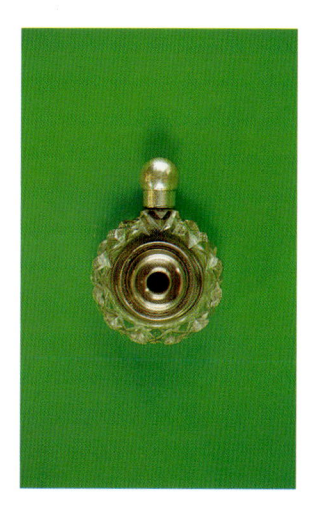

Figure 293. Small telescope in perfume flask circa 1780.

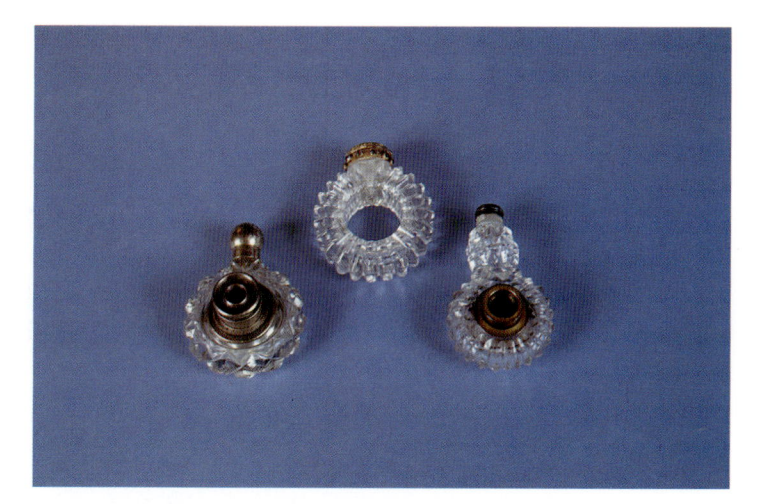

Figure 294. Small telescopes in perfume flasks.

eyes. This custom is no longer considered indecent because it is so commonplace."

As well as others, these complaints prompted craftsmen to further reduce the size of the spying mechanisms and conceal them in articles of everyday use (Figure 291). In the late 1700s, the more fashionable of these glasses were made so small that they could be fitted into fans (discussed in Chapter 18) (Figure 292) and parasol handles. Perfume flasks (Figures 293 & 294), smelling salts flasks, needle and toothpick cases, and sweet boxes were also used to conceal them. Ribright invented the highly fashionable etuis of the eighteenth century (Figure 295), and these were as well used as innovative camouflages (Figure 296). During the reign of Louis XVI, prospect glasses

MONOCULARS

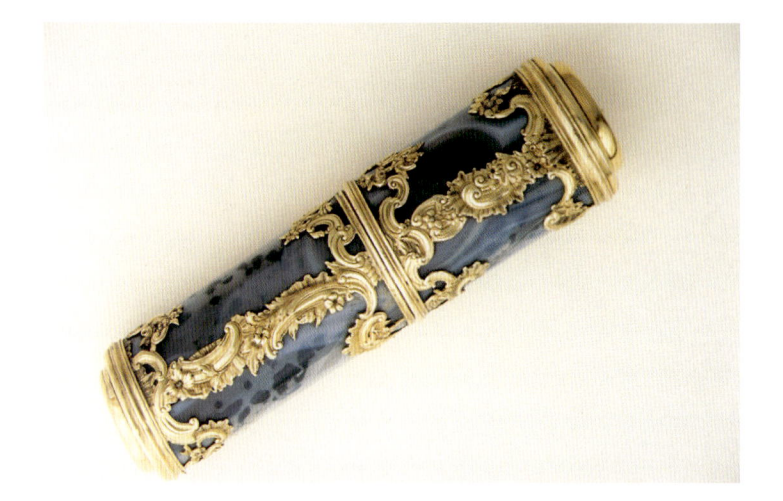

Figure 295. Agate and gold monocular and necessaire by Ribright Opticians, London. (Formerly property of King Farouk. Courtesy of Trevor Waterman, London.)

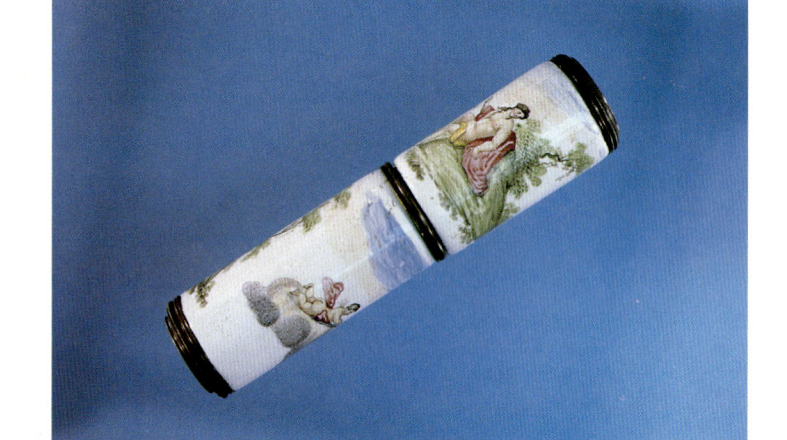

Figure 296. French porcelain etui circa 1830.

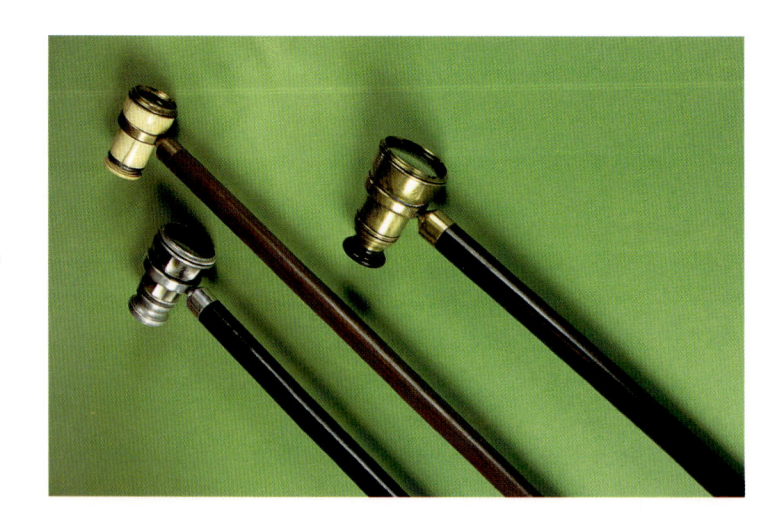

Figure 297. Group of men's canes using monoculars as handles.

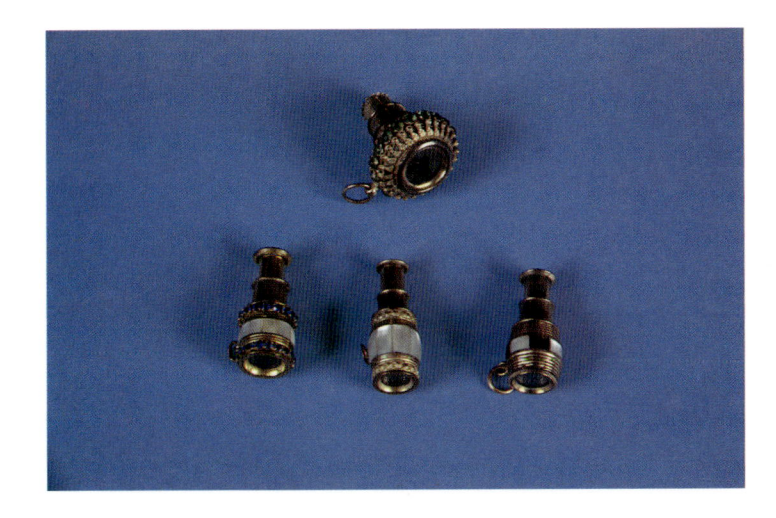

Figure 298. Group of charms with monoculars.

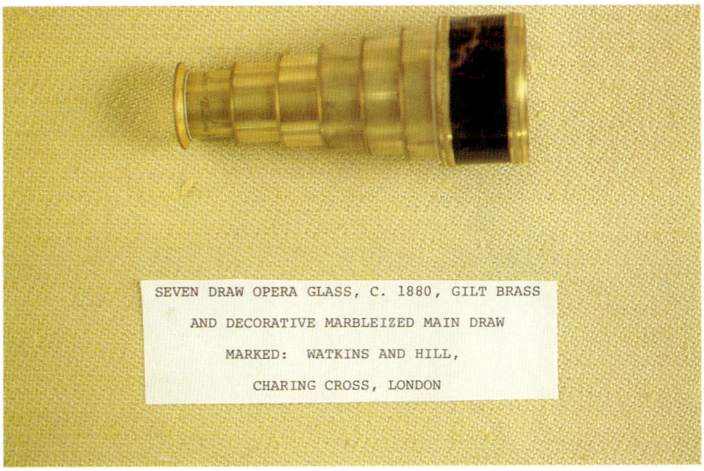

Figure 299. Seven-draw gilt and marbleized monocular by Watkins and Hill, London, 1804.

were mounted in the covers of elegantly decorated utility boxes used for holding such things as scissors, pencils, small rulers, knives, perfume, and sweets. In using the glasses, one appeared to be peering into the box. Additionally, the length of canes with glasses in the handle was so calculated that when the men were seated, the glass was exactly at eye level (Figure 297).

During the directoire period (1797–1803), lorgnettes were made so small that they were sometimes worn around the neck as charms (Figure 298). They also continued to be incorporated into various useful objects as previously stated, and their popularity carried into the nineteenth century. Many of these objects were signed by their makers—famous opticians of the times (Figure 299). They included Dollond of

MONOCULARS 147

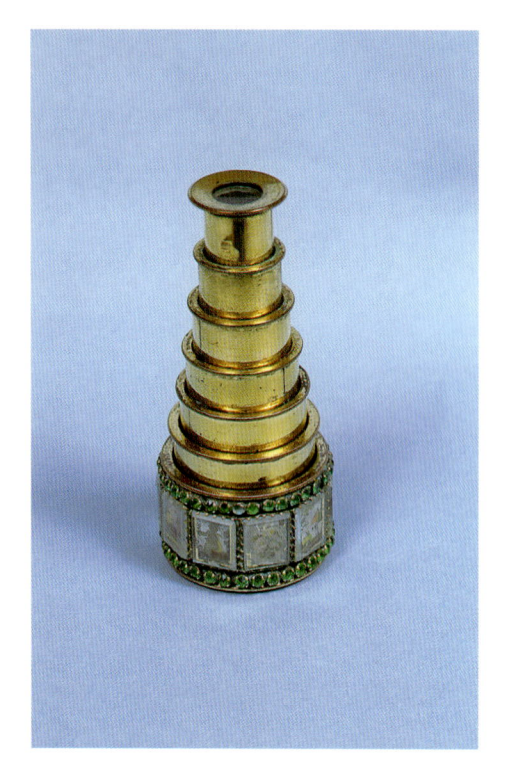

Figure 300. Gilt brass seven-draw French monocular circa 1790 with green jewels and miniature panels of paintings on glass.

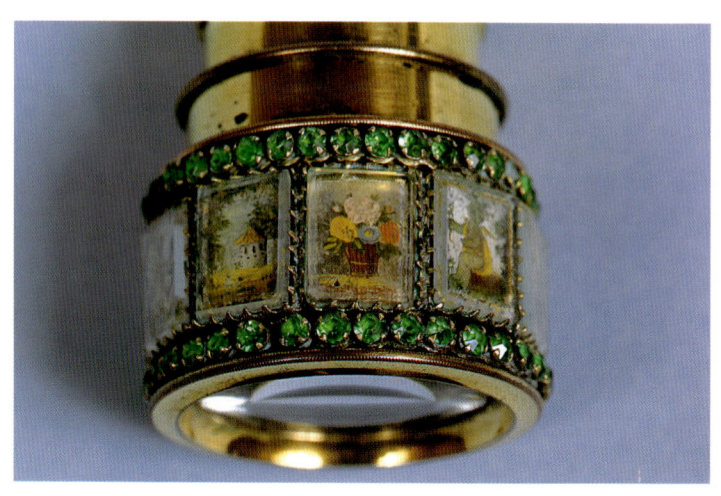

Figure 301. Details of reverse glass painting in Figure 300.

London; Dixey opticians (still in business today in London); Lumière of Paris, opera-glass maker; and others.

Although an enormous effort was made to conceal monoculars for inconspicuous use at the theater, their popularity began to die off. A new invention—the binocular or opera glass—by Lumière of Paris in 1825 began to lure people away from the use of the monocular. (Chapter 16 covers opera glasses in detail.) Since better visual acuity and depth perception are accomplished with the use of both eyes as opposed to only one eye, people soon found that this invention served them much better than the previously used monocular. The need to inconspicuously "spy" was superseded by a more practical need—good vision. Affording both good vision and good fashion, the popularity of the binocular soared. Therefore, the manufacture and sale of monoculars for all practical purposes ceased.

Notes

1. Pierre Marley, *Spectacles and Spyglasses* (Paris: Edition Hoebeke, 1988).
2. Richard Corson, *Fashions in Eyeglasses* (London: Peter Owen, Ltd., 1980), 55, 86, 88, 107.
3. R. J. S. MacGregor, 1992. *Collecting Ophthalmic Antiques* (Ayrshire, U.K.: Ophthalmic Antiques International Collectors' Club, 1992), 42.
4. Corson, op. cit.
5. Ibid.

Other Sources Consulted for Chapter 15

1. Hugh Orr, *Illustrated History of Early Antique Spectacles* (Kent, England, 1985), 98.

16

Opera Glasses

James H. Cohen, A.S.A.
J. Wm. Rosenthal, M.D.

History

Around 1800, attempts were made to coordinate two monoculars into a single instrument. (J. T. Hudson, an optician, stated in 1840 that opera glasses, formerly used singly, had been joined and used as double glasses since 1815 [Figure 302]). However, problems surfaced concerning the placement of two parallel lines of sight: focusing of individual eyes, simultaneous adjustment of both eyes, and interpupillary distances. In 1823, Voigtlander joined two monoculars with two bridging frames, allowing the user to adjust each draw tube to each eye separately. This, of course, was inconvenient for the user. In 1825, simultaneous adjustment of both eyes was accomplished by Lumière of Paris by using a patent of Monseret (1823) for an internal screw (Figure 303). By placing this screw centrally between the two barrels—and by also attaching the screw to a third frame that guided the focusing eyepieces in and out—the modern binocular (opera glass—for the theater [Figure 304], field glass—for horse races, etc. [Figure 305]) was produced.

Later, problems with interpupillary distances were addressed. One solution was offered when opera glasses and field glasses were made with folding bridges to more accurately conform to the interpupillary distance (Figure 306). Another solution involved oval-shaped lenses and body tubes to better fit these distances and increase the field of view (Figure 307). These solutions were partially successful but not very popular.

The third solution was the production of various-size instruments (small, medium, large) to conform to different facial configurations. This helped to make vision more comfortable and avoid diplopia. (The ability to focus each eye separately at the oculars was accomplished later.)

Another improvement in opera glasses came with the invention of the binocular roof prism by Ernst Abbe at Carl Zeiss Company, Jena, circa 1870–80 (Figure 305). Such a prism binocular enables the user to achieve greater enlargement of the image without having to deal with the increased length of the optical tube.

Demand

As stated in previous chapters, the theater was a large part of the social life in those times. Therefore, the demand for opera glasses was high. A great number of French opera glasses were brought into England, and almost every shop in London stocked them. All of these, however, were not of good optical quality. Hudson, the optician, preferred the best of the French glasses over the best of the English. The French were lighter and had great beauty and style and extraordinary lens power. The English, Hudson conceded, were, however, more durable. Interesting to note, Mr. Hudson was the first to offer opera glasses for sale or hire at her Majesty's Theater, the Theaters Royal Drury Lane, and Covent Garden.

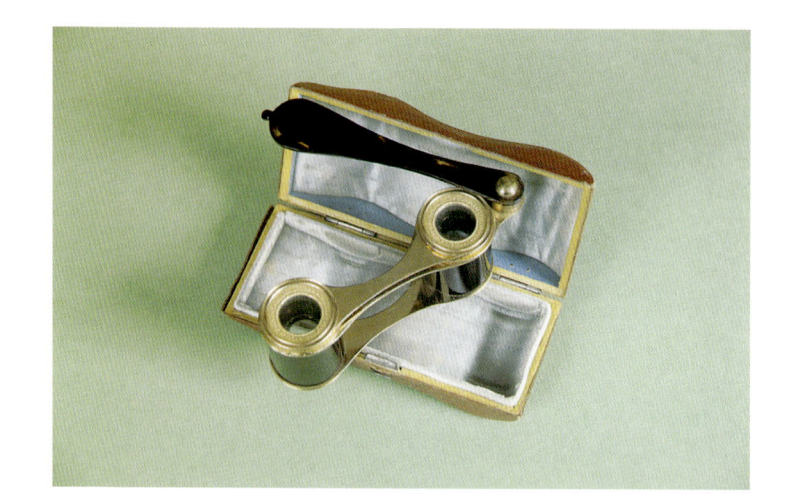

Figure 302. Tortoiseshell and gilt opera glass, Chevalier, circa 1825.

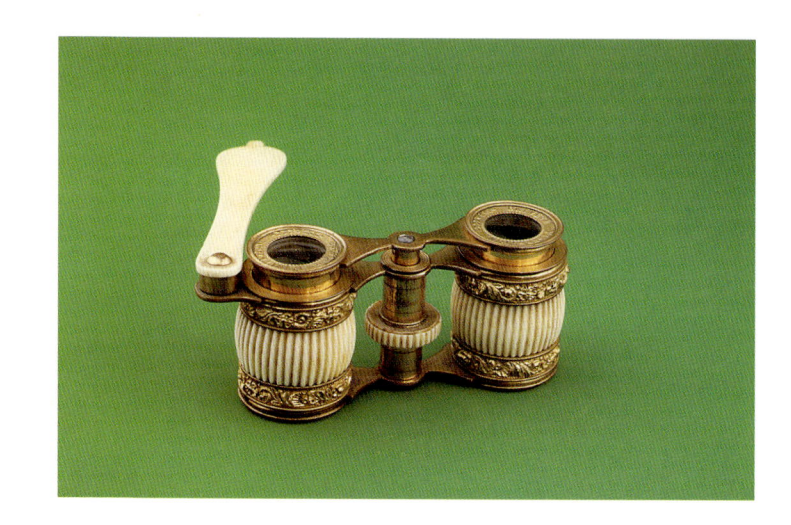

Figure 303. Utilization of a central internal screw.

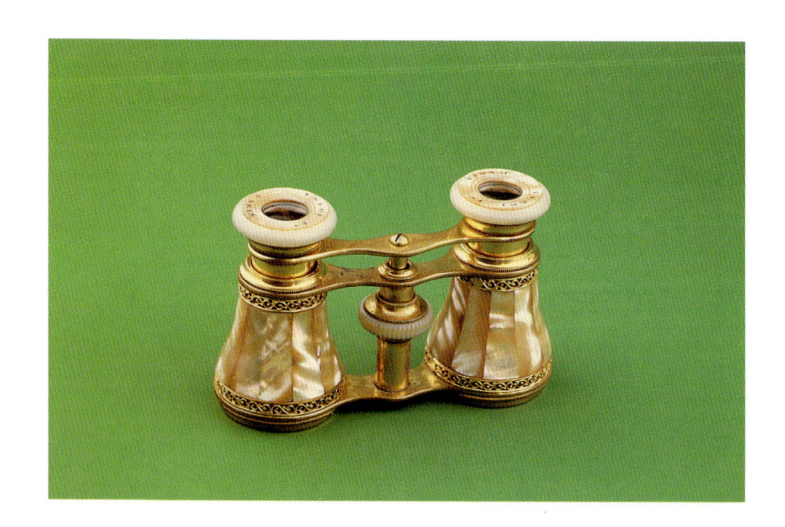

Figure 304. Sea snail and gilt opera glass, French, circa 1890.

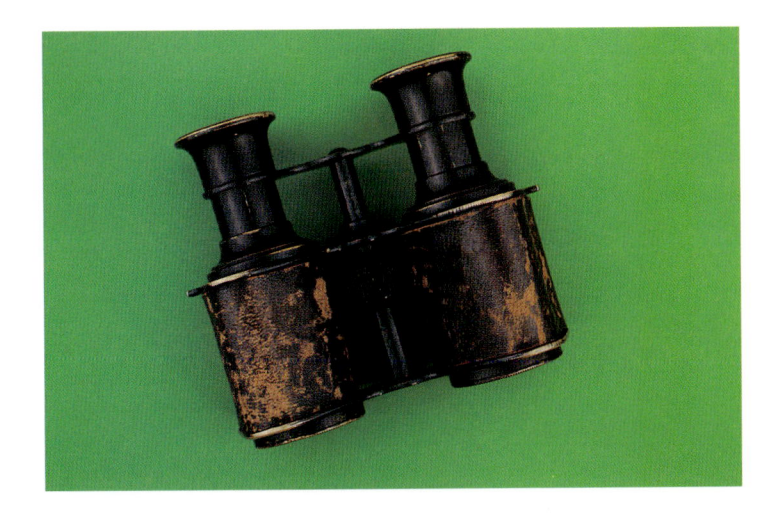

Figure 305. Leather-covered field glasses, prism type.

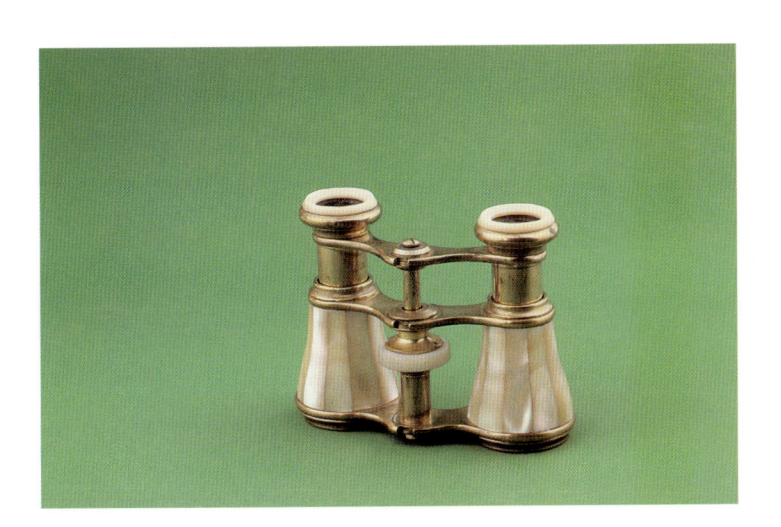

Figure 306. Opera glasses with folding bridge.

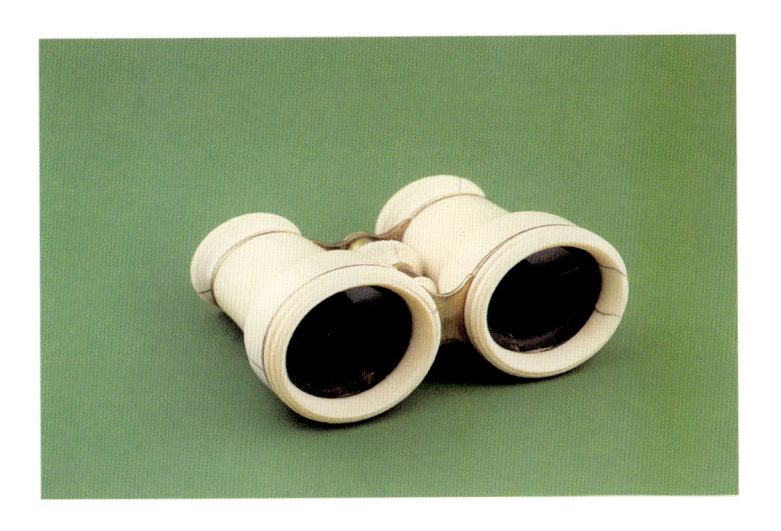

Figure 307. Ivory opera glasses with oval body tubes.

OPERA GLASSES 151

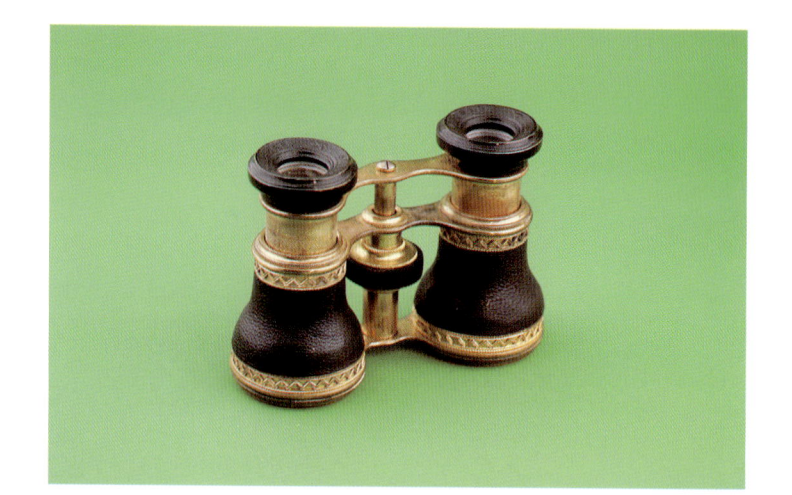

Figure 308. Brass and leather opera glasses.

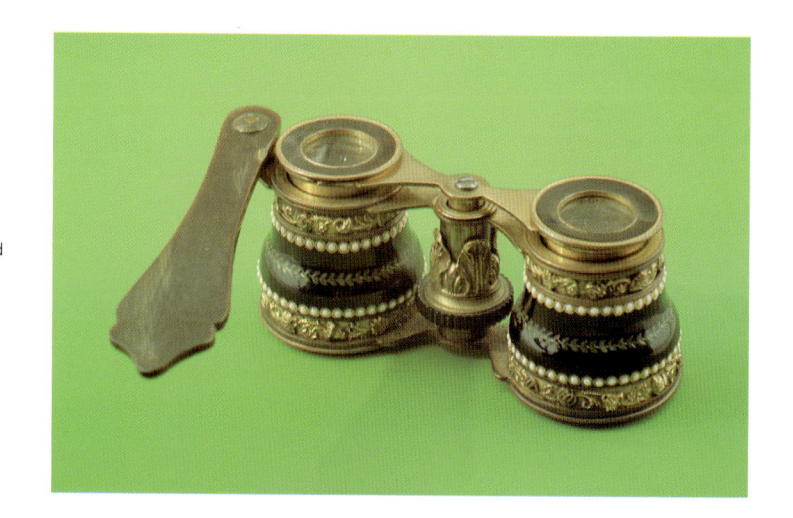

Figure 309. Embossed and decorated brasswork on opera glasses.

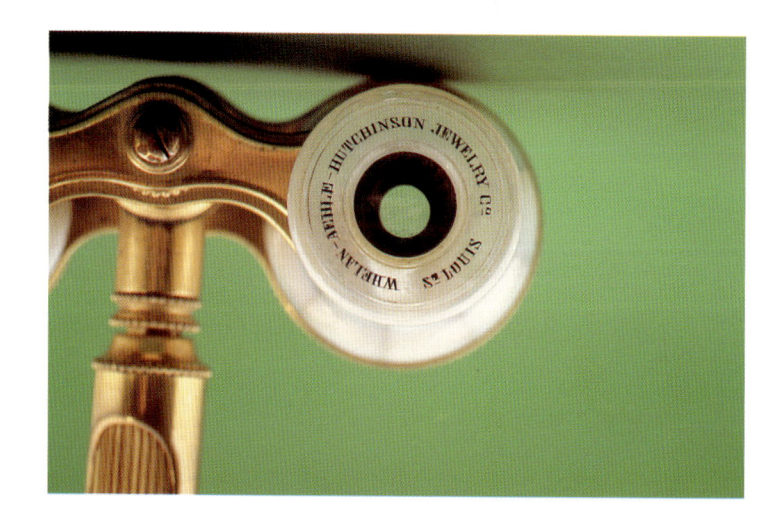

Figure 310. Opera glass lens cap showing retailer's information.

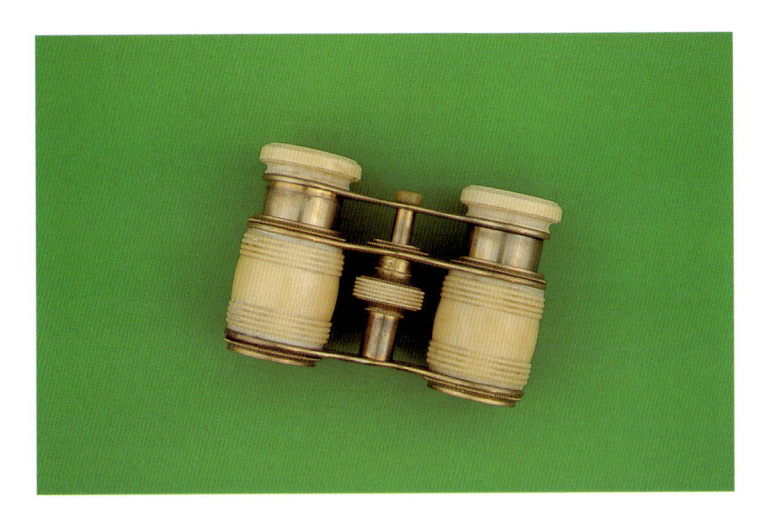

Figure 311. Bone-covered opera glasses.

Not only large cities but also smaller towns boasted of opera houses or theaters. These European, American, and Asian areas added to the need for opera glasses. Of course, since the richest woman of the smallest town had to have her own pair of opera glasses, the town jeweler or optician stocked a few.

The opera glass, which was not only utilitarian in nature but beautiful as well, created a new industry. Numerous manufacturers began production of this optical device, sparking a great deal of competition. Variation in form as well as decoration was used to attract buyers.

Embellishments

Opera glasses are "little jewels." Even early and common examples, made of brass and leather, can be most attractive (Figure 308). Other enhancements are offered by decorated, fenestrated, and embossed brass edgings (Figure 309). Some oculars have mother-of-pearl caps, engraved with the maker's name and city of origin, the name of the owner, or the company that sold the glasses (Figure 310).

Early barrels were made of cardboard, covered with shagreen in several colors. Ivory and bone were used later with wooden handles (Figure 311).

As manufacturing was perfected, the lenses were mounted in brass rings. The barrels supporting these rings were covered with tortoiseshell (Figure 312), mother-of-pearl (Figure 313), sea snail (Figure 314), abalone (Figure 315), and faux jewels (Figure 316). Combinations such as sea snail and black lip pearl (from the South Seas) abounded (Figure 317). The French embellished many with gorgeous enamels in a standard repetitious design (Figure 318) or with hand-painted floral designs (Figure 319). Repeated glazing of porcelains in several colors produces a three-dimensional and beautiful effect. As many as ten steps are used in some enameling processes. Dutch and Austrian products reveal hand-painted domestic, outdoor, and allegorical scenes (Figure 320).

Erika Speel states the following:

> The costliest examples were made by the firm of Fabergé, whose luxury glasses were of enamelled white gold and platinum or, occasionally, silver. The decoration for these was in the guilloche method with delightfully coloured translucent enamels fused over an engine turned surface, enhanced with gemstones. The name of Lemaire of Paris is the one most often found on elegant mother-of-pearl opera glasses [Figure 321] and this firm also produced quality

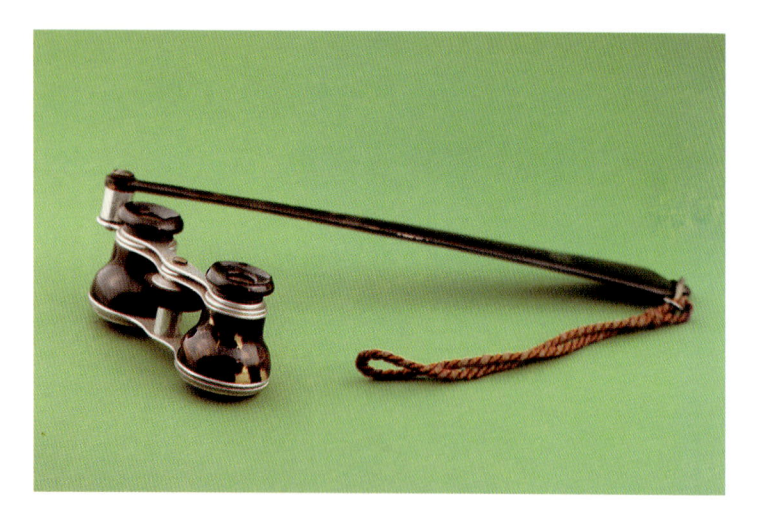

Figure 312. Tortoiseshell opera glasses.

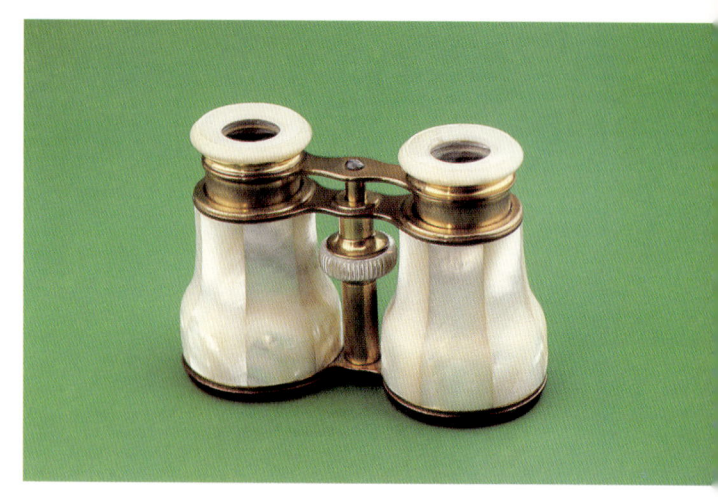

Figure 313. Mother-of-pearl opera glasses.

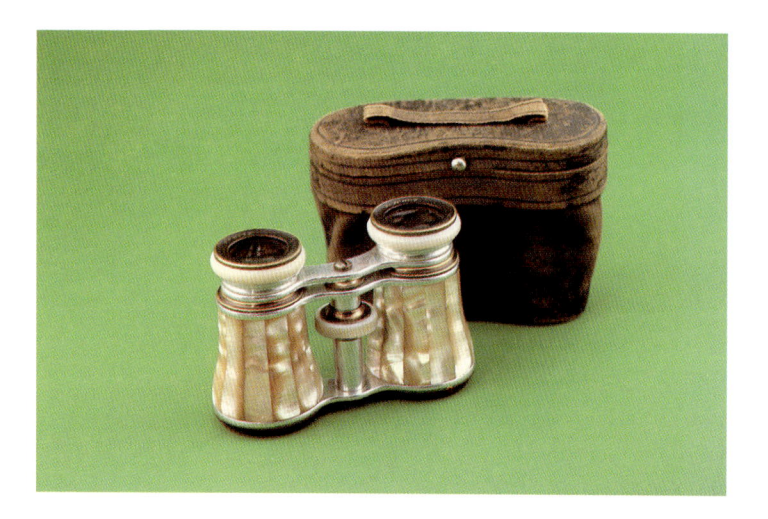

Figure 314. Sea snail opera glasses.

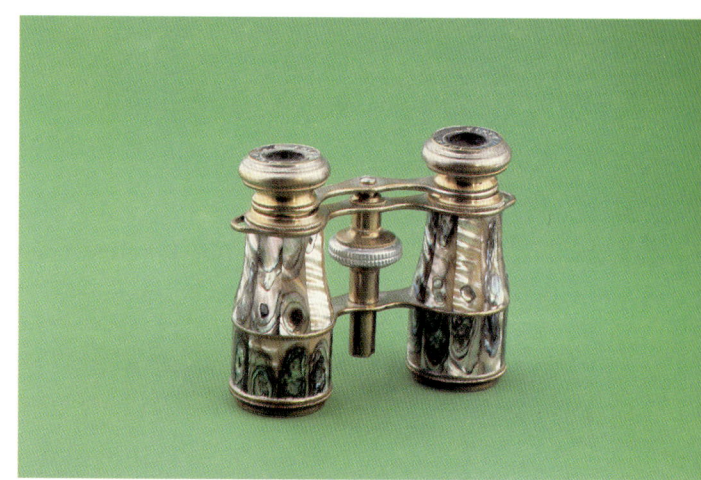

Figure 315. Abalone opera glasses.

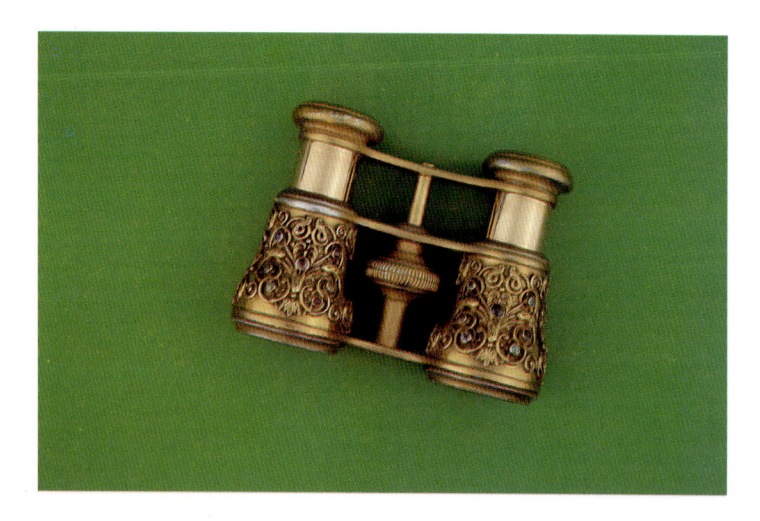

Figure 316. Opera glasses with faux jewels.

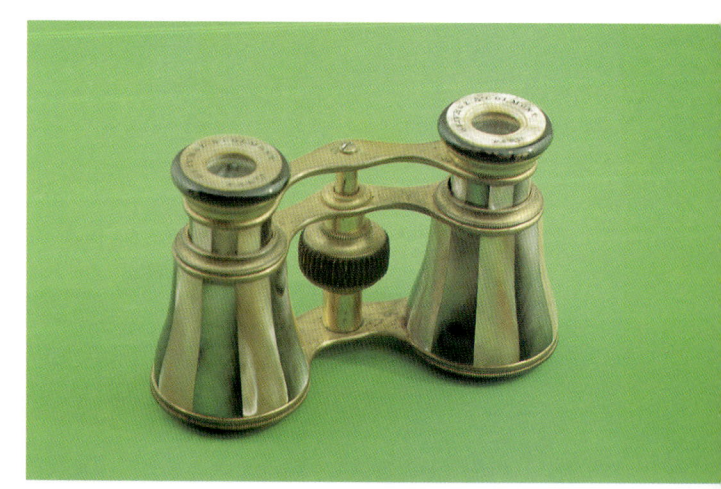

Figure 317. Sea snail and black lip pearl opera glasses.

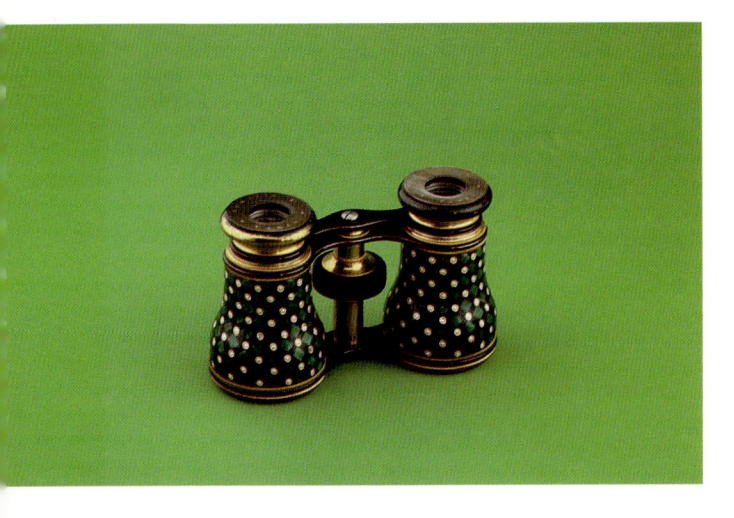

Figure 318. Emerald design opera glasses.

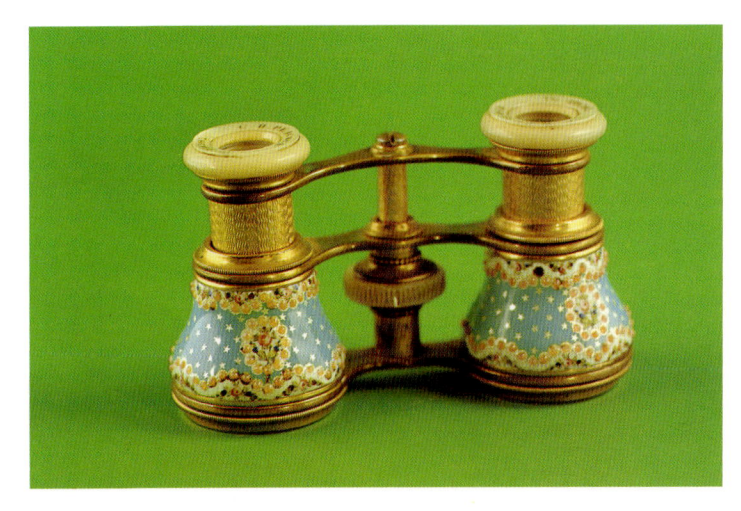

Figure 319. Floral designs on opera glasses (note engine-turned inner barrels).

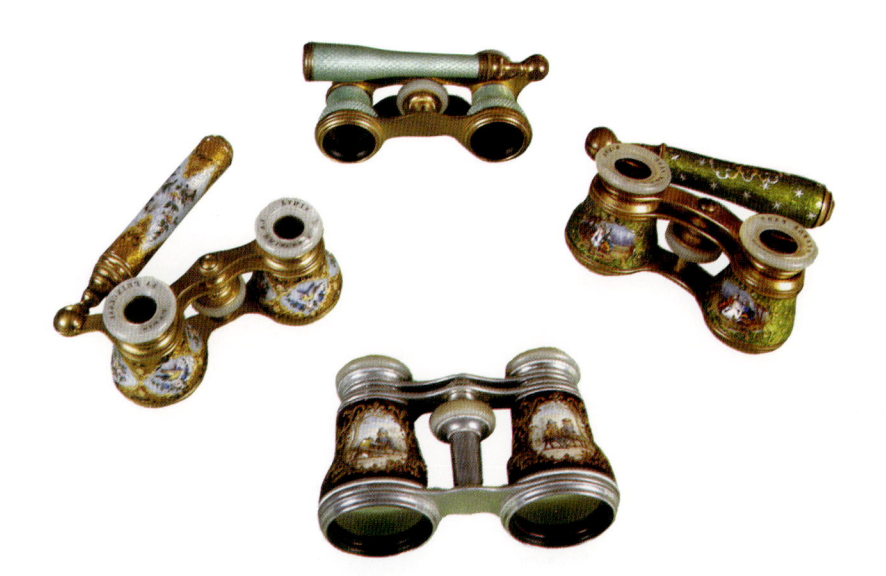

Figure 320. Opera glasses showing various scenes.

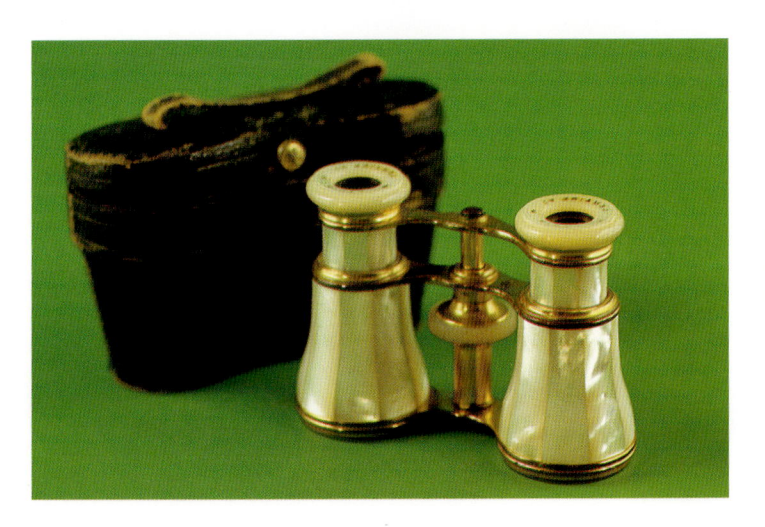

Figure 321. Lemaire mother-of-pearl opera glasses (note mother-of-pearl-clad inner barrels).

Figure 322. Limoges-style opera glasses.

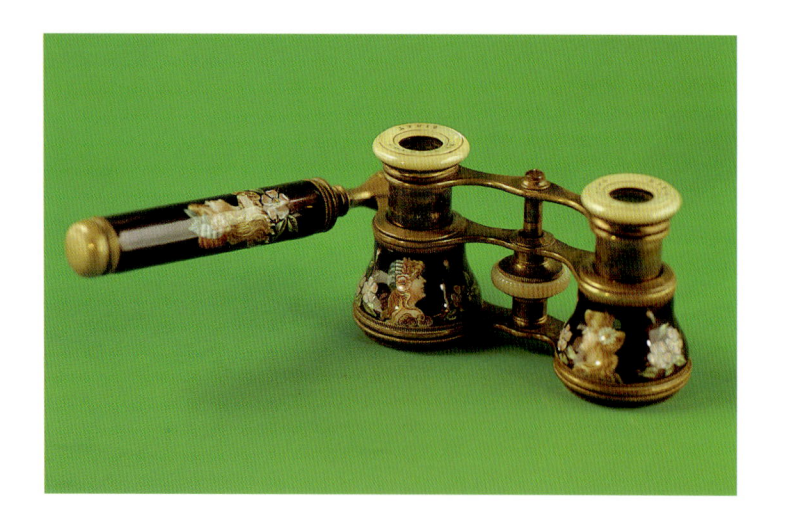

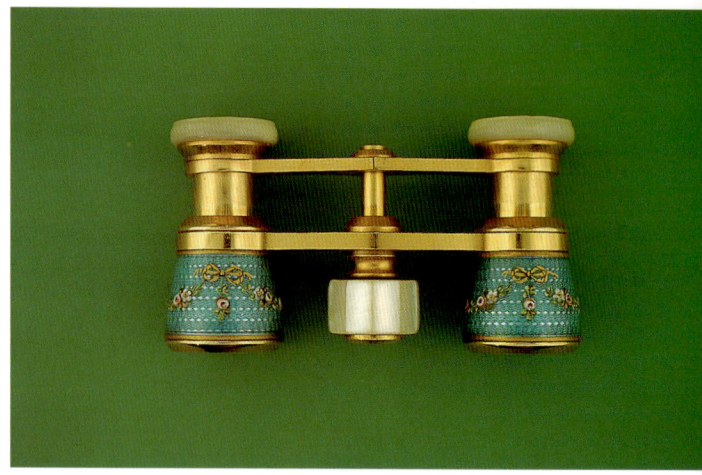

Figure 323. Blue enameled opera glasses with painted garlands.

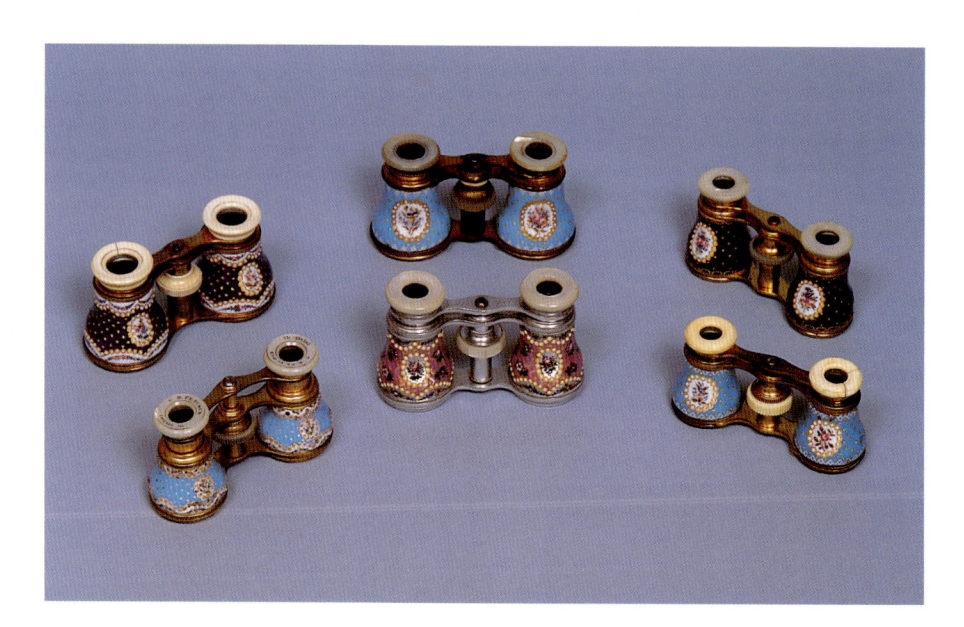

Figure 324. Various enameled French opera glasses.

156   CHAPTER 16

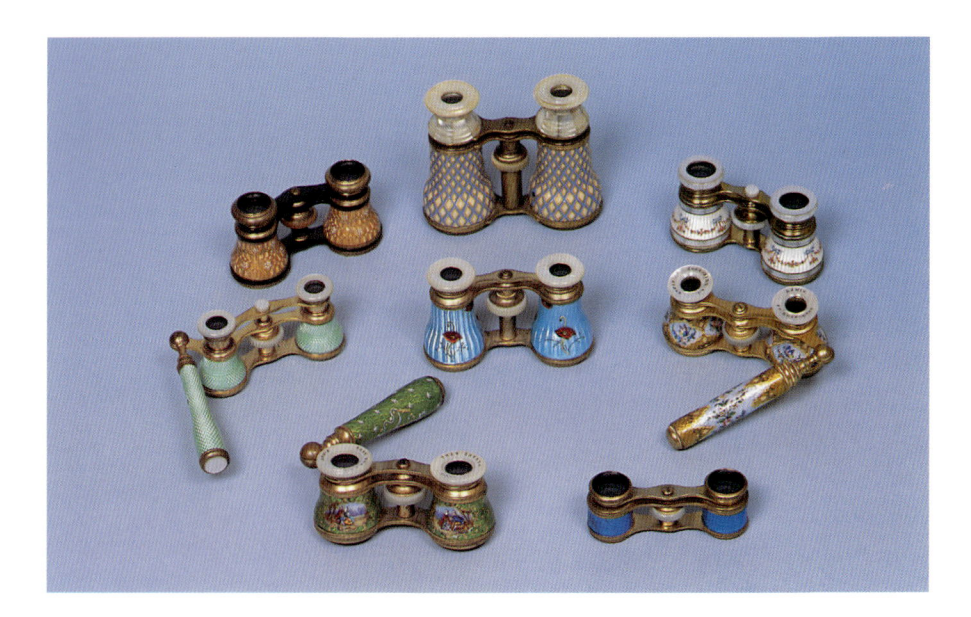

Figure 325. Engine-turned designs show through enamel (center).

enamelled ones. The Parisien makers who engraved their brand name "Hazebroucq Opticien" in the eye-pieces, offered finely painted "Limoges" style enamelled opera glasses [Figure 322].

A favourite enamelling style was an ornate design with the main body covered with a brilliant opaque glaze enlivened with tiny scattered gold stars or dots. This background contrasts with the borders and central oval reserves left with white enamel and painted with floral motifs. The painted centers and borders are framed with raised "beads" of white or opalescent enamel fused over circlets of gold, to simulate inset seed pearls [Figure 319]. This standard pattern was available in many permutations, and gave a symmetrical, rich looking finish, masking the rather squat, pear-shaped format of the barrels. Popular shades for these included rose pompadour, the many tones of blue, including turquoise, lapis, topaz fume, which simulated the semi-precious stones and pretty colors given such names as powder blue, lilac, violet, amethyst, duck egg green, or vert absinthe.

The most delicate enamelled styles were those with translucent colors, often with a small superimposed painted motif [Figure 323]. The translucent enamel surface was interspersed with very small stars or dots of pure gold or silver foil (paillons), sometimes with grains of red, blue or green enamel fused over, to sparkle like tiny rubies, sapphires or emeralds, within the surface of the glaze. With translucent glazes the color of the underlying metal shows through [Figure 324]. Applied over engine-turned silver, the finest high-key colors are produced with pale blue, green or mauve enamels [Figure 325]. The most admired glazes were of opalescent white or pink enamels [Figure 326]; they gave the very fashionable "changeant" effects with duality of color, these being at their best over white gold. Over yellow gold and brightened copper, ruby red and amber enamels are at their most brilliant.

Some of the enamelled opera glasses were painted in the method known as en plein, where a detailed scene in light, bright colors was superimposed and fused smoothly on a white enamel background. The enamel painters of Paris, Geneva, Vienna and London perfected the method to create delicate designs such as idealized landscapes and rustic couples. The French workshops excelled also in small scale painting with brilliant colors over translucent backgrounds, which called for great precision in the firing. A more complex style, known as Limoges School painting, was adapted for some of the most interesting opera glasses. These were paintings of tiny figural groups with a classical theme, or female profile heads, with slightly raised modeling [Figure 322]. For these, the painting was applied with opaque and translucent enamels, partly over foils to add depth and sparkle to the designs.

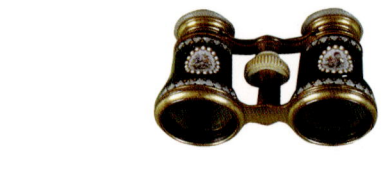

Figure 326. Pink enameled opera glasses (center).

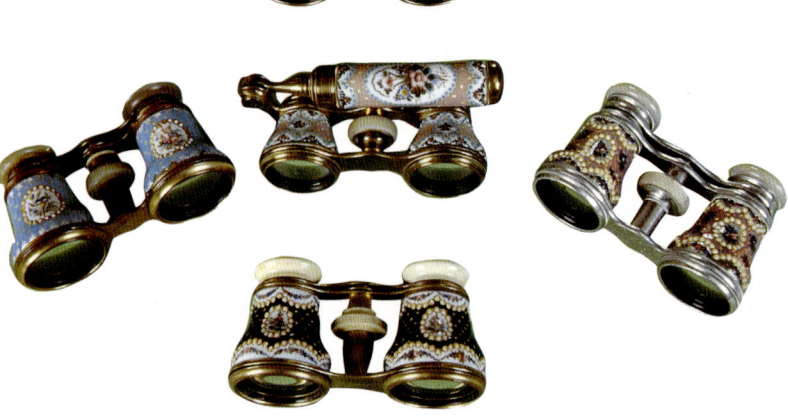

Figure 327. Aluminum opera glasses, circa 1890.

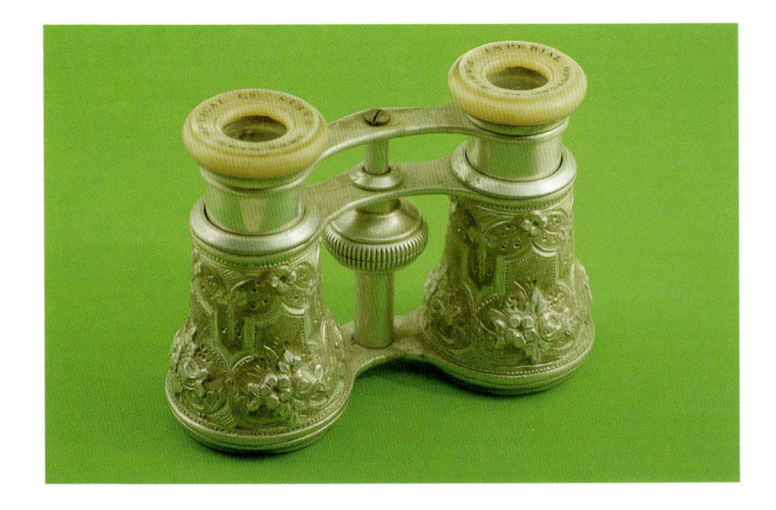

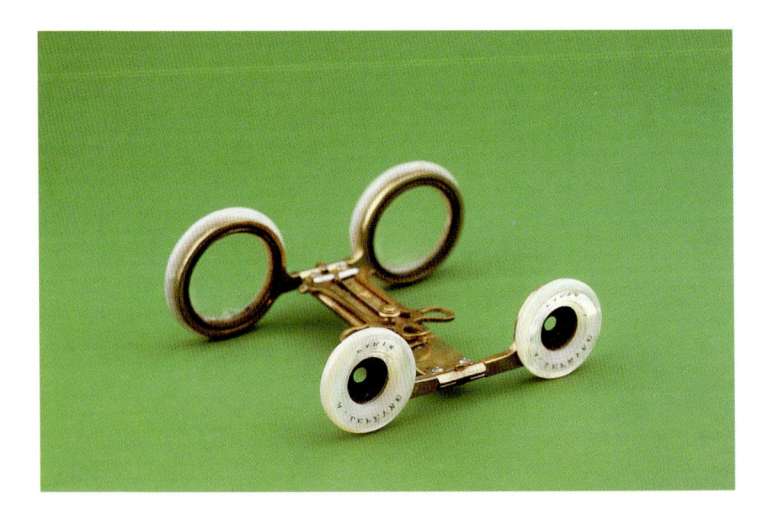

Figure 328. Folding British opera glasses.

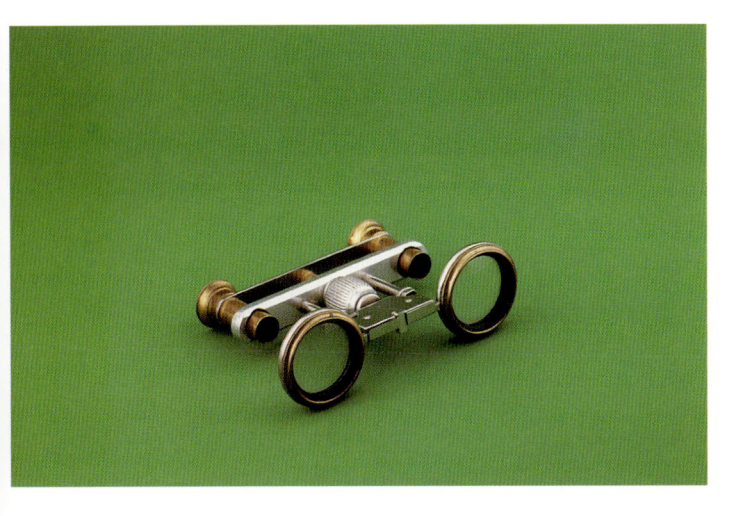

Figure 329. Folding British opera glasses.

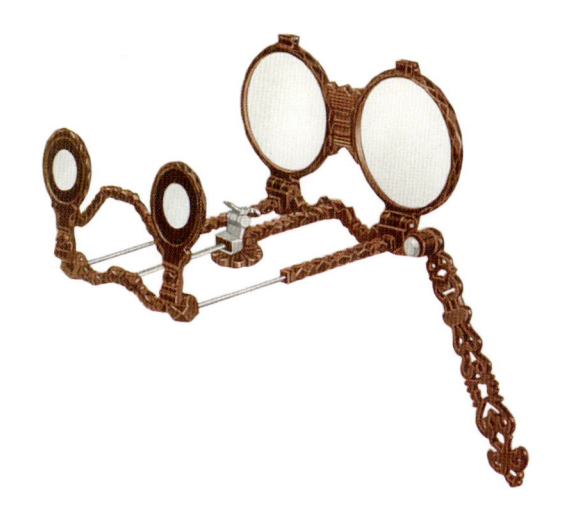

Figure 330. Folding French tortoiseshell opera glasses. (Courtesy British College of Optometrists.)

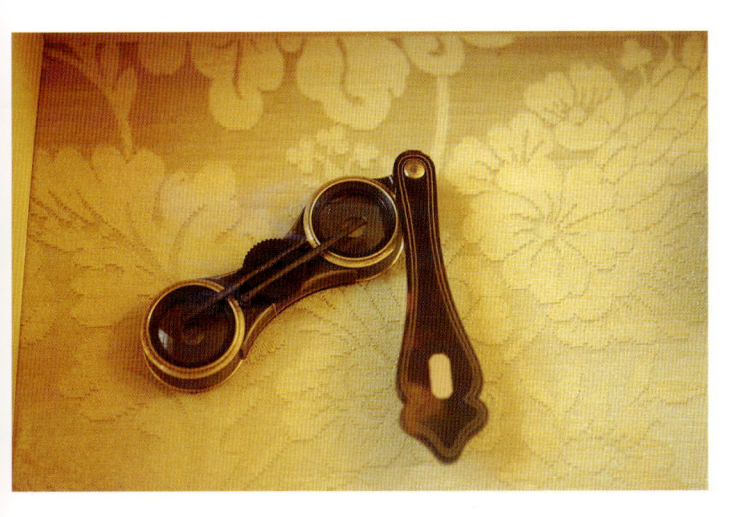

Figure 331. Folding French opera glasses, tortoiseshell and gold.

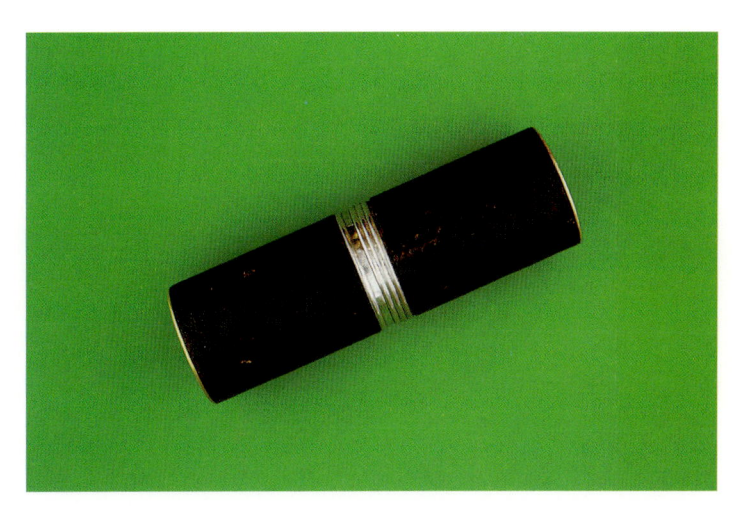

Figure 332. Cylindrical opera glasses, pull out for use.

We currently find opera glasses made of aluminum, with beautiful embossing and engraving (Figure 327). One may wonder why so much effort would be applied to this cheap metal. However, aluminum appeared on the market shortly before 1900—and was as expensive as silver. Therefore, it was considered very desirable and fashionable.

Oddities

Some early (skeletal) glasses (with brass or mother-of-pearl rings) folded flat into a flat case for easy transport (Figures 328 & 329). Others were made of tortoiseshell and were quite fragile (Figure 330). One French pair has a very intricate focusing system and a tortoiseshell handle (Figure 331). Another pair is cylindrical and pulls out to a useful binocular (Figure 332). In addition to these unusual varieties, many novelties have been made into the shape of opera glasses, such as salt and pepper shakers (Figure 333). Note the expanding British style in Figure 334.

OPERA GLASSES 159

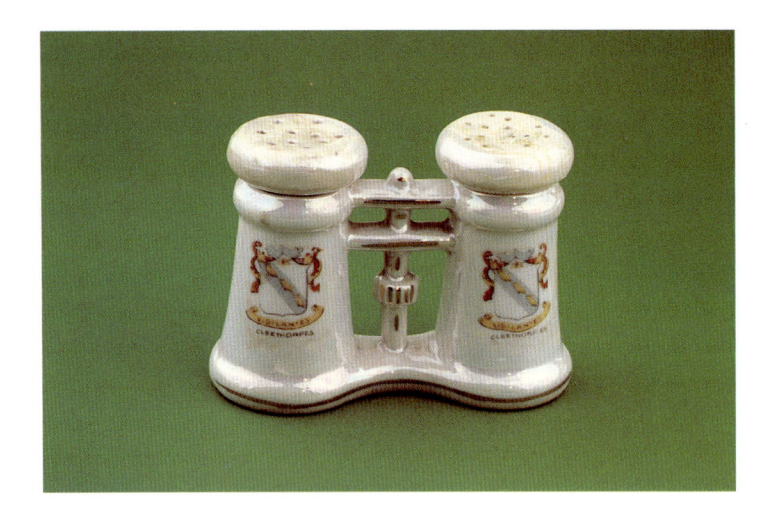

Figure 333. Salt and pepper shakers, modeled after opera glasses.

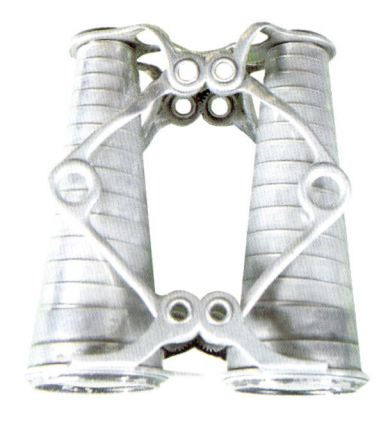

Figure 334. Aluminum British expanding opera glasses.

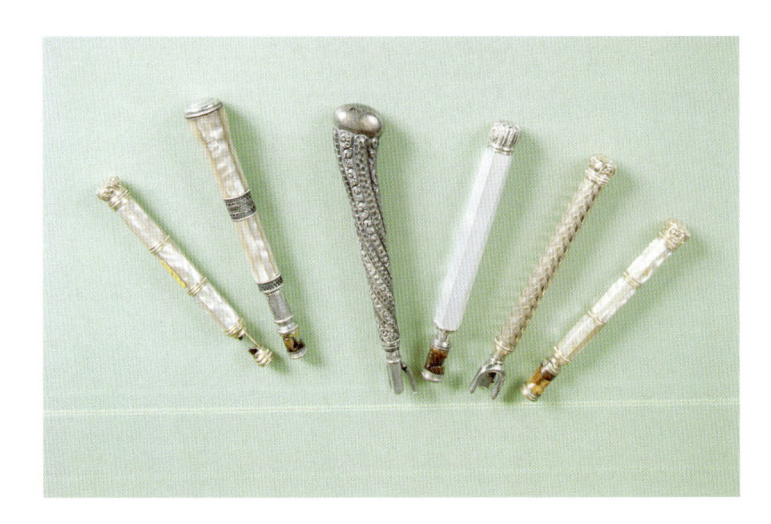

Figure 335. Group of opera glass handles separate from the glasses. (See also C391.)

160   CHAPTER 16

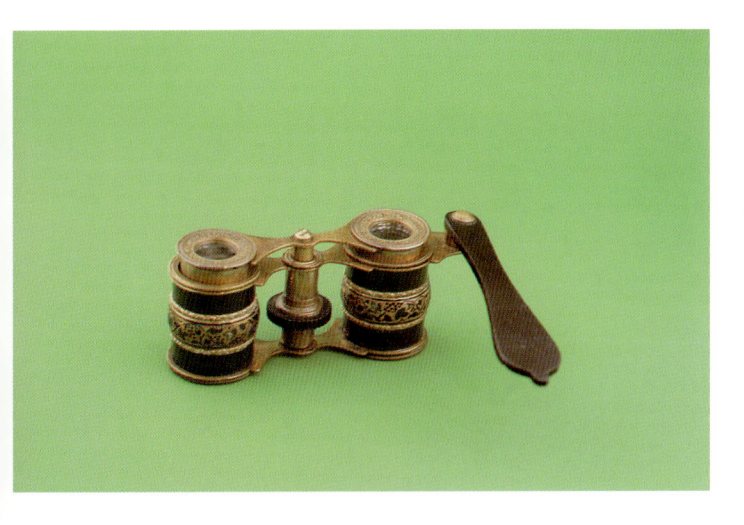

Figure 336. Short handle made of horn.

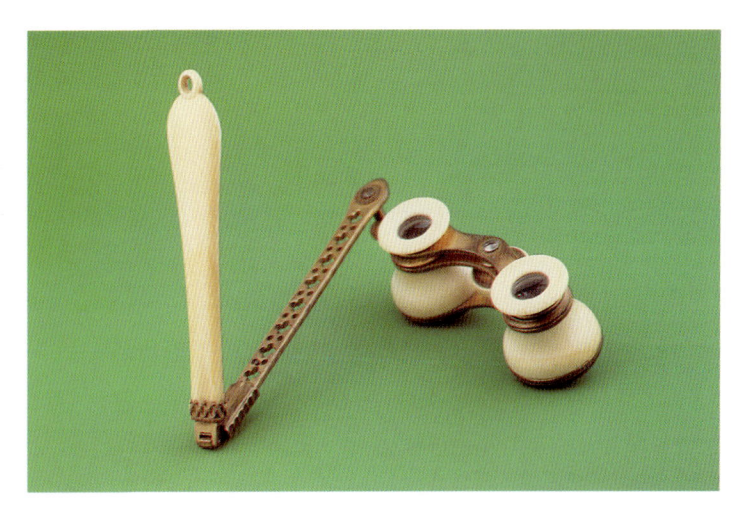

Figure 337. Ivory and gilt metal opera glass handle.

Handles

By the end of the nineteenth century, opera glass production was performed with such finesse that other attachments were needed to attract customers. Thus, handles were produced. At first, they were available separately for existing opera glasses (Figure 335). They may still be available but are usually found in flea markets—not in jewelry or optical stores.

Later, the handles were attached during manufacture to the central connecting frame. They pivoted across the width of the two barrels, and a stop lug held the glasses at the proper angle (Figure 336). The initial handles of the glasses were made of the same material as the barrels (ivory, mother-of-pearl, etc.). They were short and easily broken.

Another type of handle folded in the middle, making it longer (Figure 337). Although partially made of metal, it, too, was fragile. Then came a flat telescopic handle and a rounded metal handle, both with a three-draw telescopic length (Figure 338). Finally in 1895, Lumière advertised in the *Optical Journal* that his newly designed handle attached to the central screw. This enabled the focus of the opera glasses to be adjusted at the center pylon—as usual—or on the handle. This handle could be used in either hand (Figures 339–342).

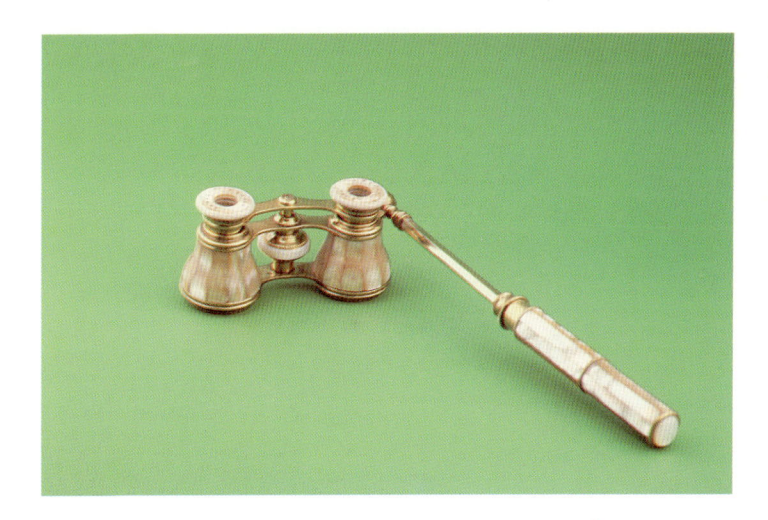

Figure 338. Telescopic opera glass handle.

OPERA GLASSES   161

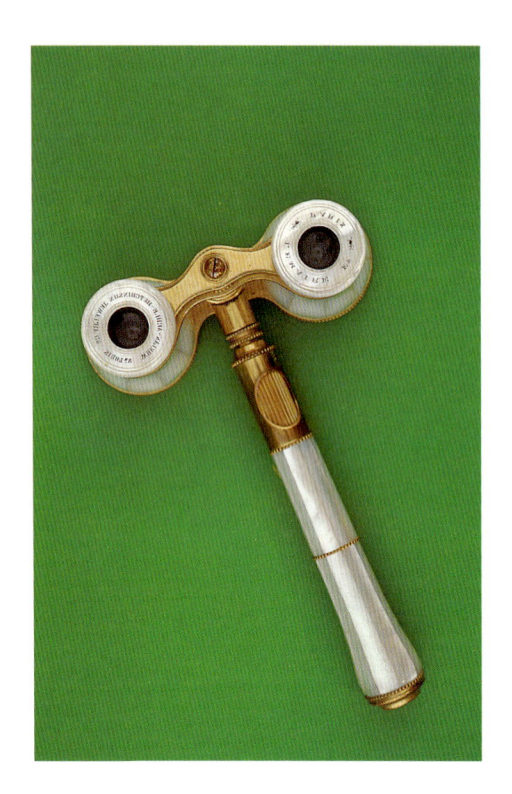

Figure 339. Opera glasses with handle at central screw.

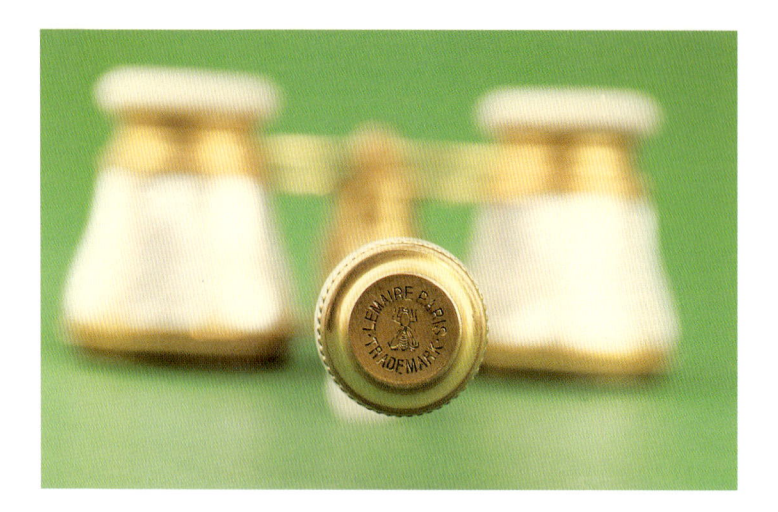

Figure 340. Lemaire marking on handle of Figure 339.

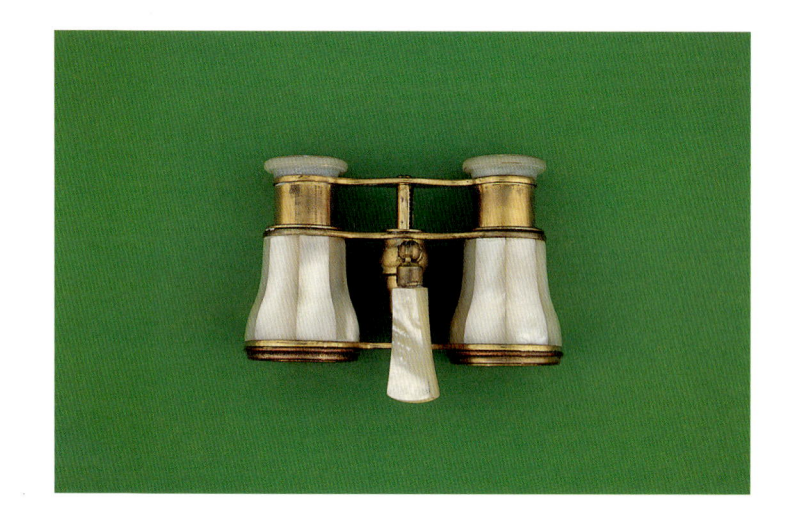

Figure 341. Another central handle type.

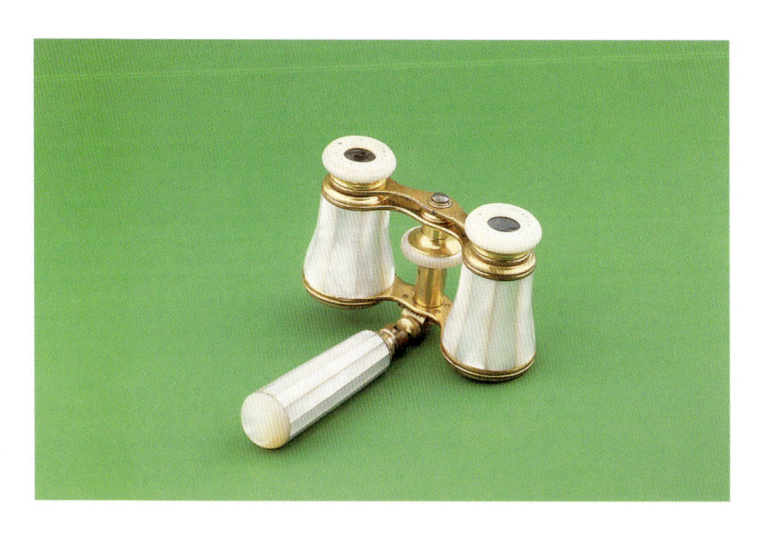

Figure 342. Another central handle type.

162   CHAPTER 16

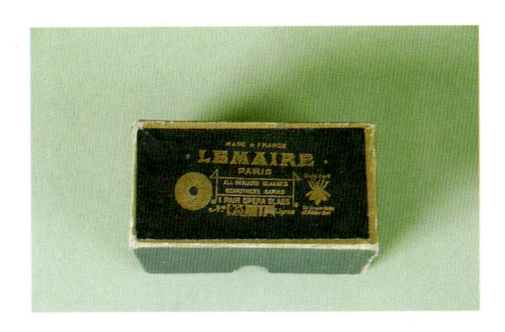

Figure 343. Outer cardboard box for opera glasses.

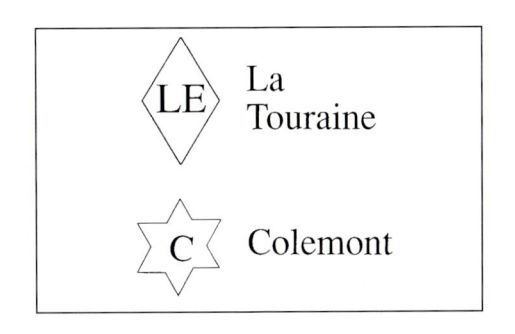

Figure 344. Identification names of makers found under the middle frames of opera glasses.

Cost

How much did opera glasses cost a century ago? We all recognize the effects of inflation and time on the price of any product. The same can be said of opera glasses. The prices presented here are found from sources dating from before and shortly after the turn of the century and should be viewed accordingly.

While it is obvious that not all opera glasses sold for the same amount a hundred years ago, none of the old bills of sale viewed by the authors actually list a specific price. Even if a figure was recorded, it would be impossible to tell whether the price represented a very plain or an elaborate pair. After extensive searching, the authors finally found a handwritten price on the bottom of a cardboard box (Figure 343), which originally housed a pair of opera glasses made by Lemaire of Paris. The sales figure was $12.00 for what is suspected to have been a pair of mother-of-pearl glasses with brass trim—and possibly carrying the Lemaire name on one or both lens caps. The reasoning for this is that the mother-of-pearl and brass trim are the more common of all the Lemaire opera glasses.

Another source of information on opera glass prices is sometimes found in catalog listings, as follows:

1. American Optical Company Catalog, circa 1890, page 11, Wellsworth Specialties, Opera Glasses, $5.00–$6.00.
2. Merry Optical Company Catalog, Kansas City, Missouri, circa 1910, pages 205–211, Opera Glasses, $9.00–$70.50.
3. Geneva Optical Company Catalog, Chicago, Illinois, circa 1922, pages 98–101, Field Glasses, $25.80–$76.80.
4. New Era Optical Company Catalog, Chicago, Illinois, circa 1940, pages 35–40, Opera and Field Glasses, $3.00–$27.80.
5. Benjamin Pike, Jr. Catalog #II, New York, circa 1850, pages 174–176, Opera Glasses, $8.00.
6. William McAllister Catalog, circa 1871, Philadelphia, pages 43–46, Opera Glasses, $4.75–$40.50.

While these listings unfortunately do not provide detailed information on specific specimens, they are helpful in determining general price ranges for opera glasses at that time.

Identification

Most opera glasses can be easily identified by looking under the supporting frames. Here you may find a bee stamped in the metal, indicating the manufacturers Lemaire; an LE within a diamond shaped outline—usually the manufacturer La Touraine; a six-pointed star containing a C—the manufacturer Colmont; etc. (Figure 344). Other designs/symbols are found as well and are outlined later in the chapter.

Another method of identifying opera glasses is by the ocular caps. The term *ocular caps* refers to the rings of metal, mother-of-pearl, etc., that hold the lenses in place—and are the part of the opera glass that rests against the eyes. Manufacturers and/or retailers often placed their names on one or both of the ocular caps. While some caps are interchangeable,

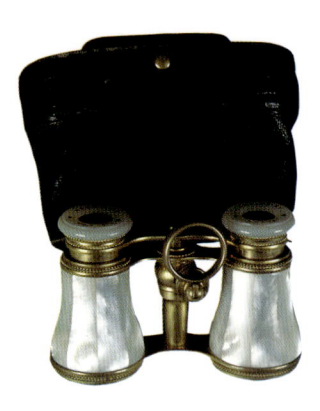

Figure 345. Mother-of-pearl opera glasses (note ring adjusting handle) and typical leather case.

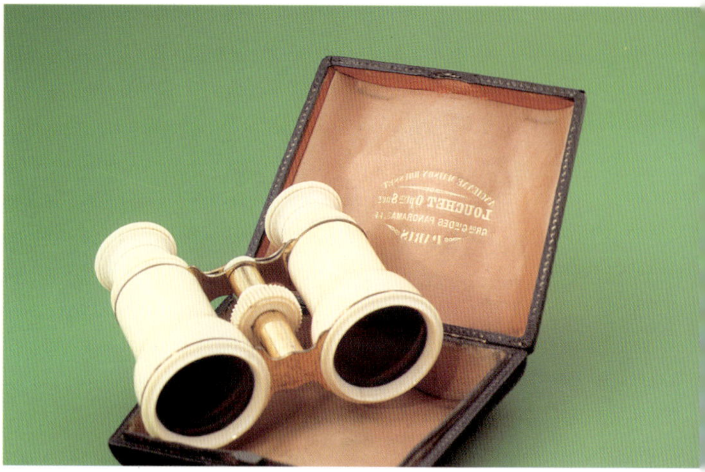

Figure 346. Hinged case conforming to shape of opera glasses.

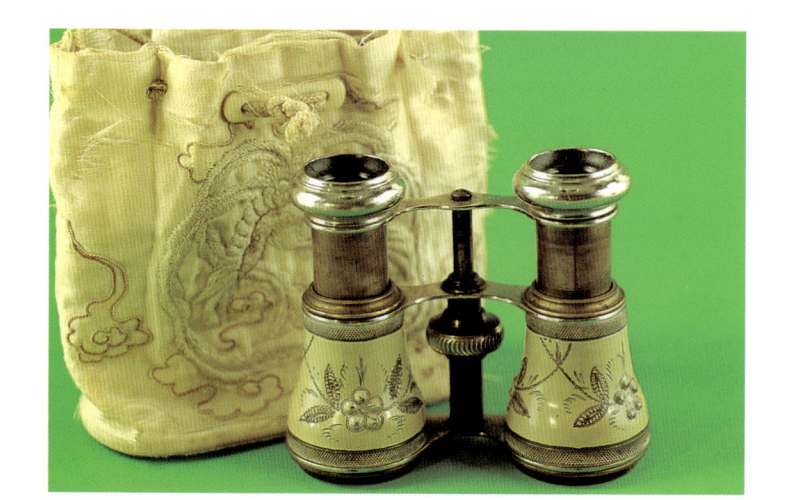

Figure 347. Silk drawstring pouch for opera glasses.

(e.g., one Colmont pair with another), many are not. Caps do not all have the same diameter and/or thread.

The type of decoration is sometimes so typical of a country that it is diagnostic in itself. Although it is not necessarily evident at first glance, each company offered several varieties of its product—much as automobile options are available now. Since Lemaire opera glasses were the most plentiful, more of this type are available today—making their many variations apparent.

Unfortunately, some opera glasses cannot be definitely attributed to any maker. During the course of commerce, some barrels were assembled by the manufacturer but were decorated elsewhere. Although the original manufacturer was identified on the lens caps, some retailers preferred to substitute their own caps, thereby surreptitiously taking credit for production of the opera glasses. Additionally, as known to happen today, skilled workers or partners left large firms and started their own businesses. In the process, patented names, brands, and designs may have been infringed upon. These things all play a part in the problems with identification of particular opera glasses. Later in this chapter is a detailed listing of the opera glasses in each author's collection as well as a list of the retailers who dealt with opera glasses.

Protective Cases

The great majority of opera glasses (especially those made in France) were offered in a case. Although these cases were not usually decorative, they did protect the article during transport from home to the theater. Some were made of soft leather (Figure 345), with tops and bottoms of wood or cardboard reinforcement. They were lined with red, purple, or blue silk—many with the company of origin or selling store embossed in gold. Early cases were covered with shagreen, and some (especially those for large glasses) came in a rigid case covered with embossed leather and hinged in half (Figure 346). The top and bottom of the rigid model were slightly hourglass shaped to conform to the shape of the glasses. The inside was covered with colored silk, like those previously mentioned. A small leather handle was connected to the center of the top, and the container was closed with a button-activated latch. The latch and hinges were of gold-colored metal.

Many of these cases are not found in pristine condition. Handles are detached, latches are lost, linings are worn or gone, etc. In fact, many of the opera glasses found in antique shops or flea markets today are not seen in their original cases. Collectors should be aware of this and note how the glasses fit into the case. The identifying marks of the glasses should be checked as well to see whether they coincide with those of the cases. Of the 230 examples in Dr. Rosenthal's collection, only 46 are housed in cases. This amounts to a 20 percent survival rate for cases.

The surviving cases do sometimes aid in identifying the origin of the glasses. Companies such as Lemaire and Colmont put their marks on the buttons of the latches. Additionally, the inside of the lids often are adorned with a print or label of the retailer or the manufacturer, as previously mentioned.

Since those opera glasses fitted with extension handles did not fit well in typical cases, some are found in drawstring bags or pouches (Figure 347). Some of these pouches were very fine and decorative, for a discriminating woman, no doubt. Others were rather ordinary and perhaps were a substitute for a lost or damaged original case.

Cases that are particularly delightful are those that serve additionally as a woman's purse (Figure 348). Each section of the case has its own function, but all are fitted together and decorated en suite. One such purse houses a scent bottle, folding fan, compact, pen and pad, as well as opera glasses!

Later in the chapter is a detailed list of cases in the authors' collections.

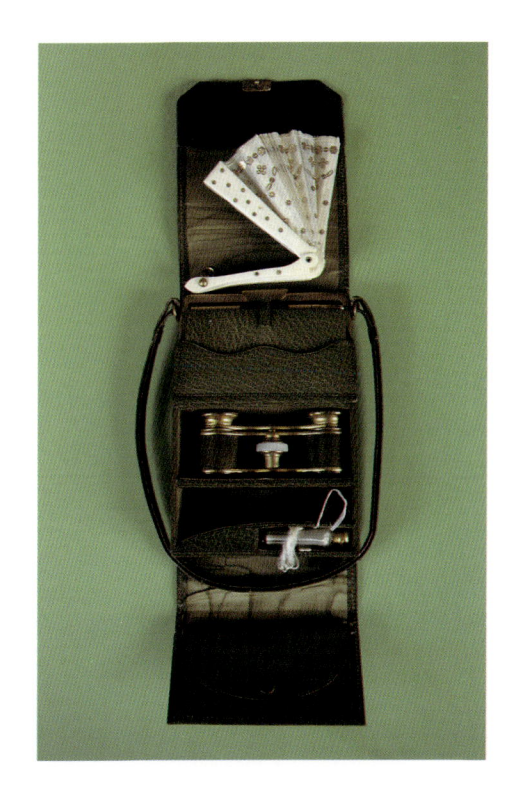

Figure 348. Woman's purse fitted with opera glasses and other accoutrements.

Cardboard Boxes for Initial Sales

The Lemaire Company of Paris, France, delivered its opera glasses in a cardboard box—covered with a dark green textured paper. The box measured approximately 4 ¾ inches by 3 inches by 2 ½ inches. The bottom half of the box was completely covered by the top half, which slipped over it. Identification was printed in gold letters stating the manufacturer (Lemaire), the bee, and other appropriate and advertising information. Other manufacturers doubtlessly employed similar outside protection for their products. Following is an example (Figure 343):

MADE IN FRANCE
LEMAIRE
PARIS

ALL GENUINE PARTS
BEAR THESE MARKS

1 PAIR OPERA GLASSES

NO 262–13 LIGNES

Because these cardboard boxes are rather frail, the number that have survived is woefully small when compared to the number of opera glasses with which they were originally paired. The collection of these two authors contains only two outside boxes, which in a collection of over 600 opera glasses is only a 0.3 percent survival rate.

What's in a Name?

While researching various publications for information regarding opera glasses, it becomes apparent that there is no name for a person who deals in, collects, or has an interest in opera glasses. Not even Webster's *Third New World Dictionary*, with its approximately 450,000 word listings, provides us with a term. Therefore, one of the authors—Mr. James H. Cohen—decided to invent such a word.

The French manufactured most of the early opera glasses, calling them *jumelles de théâtre*. Therefore, the base word *jumelle* was chosen. The suffix "ist" was chosen because two well-known fields of collecting have names ending as such: numismatist—a person in the coin field, and philatelist—one with an interest in stamps. Dropping the *e* from *jumelle* before adding the suffix—to conform to the usual American standards, the resulting term is *jumellist*—a person who deals with, collects, or has an interest in opera glasses.

Mr. Cohen submitted this word to Merriam Webster's dictionary for consideration. After doing their own research, the staff of Webster's notified Mr. Cohen that they would place this new coinage on their master file of new words—and if the word *jumellist* is found to be commonly used (i.e., printed in several different publications), it would then be used as an entry in the dictionary.

So, Mr. Cohen has created a new word with a pleasing sound, also making the authors the world's first *jumellists*!

Conclusion

Collecting opera glasses can be a delightful and perhaps an expensive pastime. Many types are available today, as exemplified by the combined collection of the authors—containing more than 600 examples. Amazingly, very few are exactly alike. James H. Cohen is a senior member of The American Society of Appraisers and a New Orleans antique dealer with a special interest in opera glasses—holding an extensive, varied collection of over 400 specimens.

Opera Glass Collection

Following are the descriptions of the opera glasses in the collection of both authors. The glasses are listed by manufacturer. Listings with numbers preceded by a *C* denote those in the collection of Mr. James H. Cohen. Those preceded by an *R* denote those in the collection of Dr. J. Wm. Rosenthal.

The name and location of the manufacturers are usually found on one or both of the lens caps. However, since some opera glasses did not carry the manufacturer's name, these companies ensured their due credit by stamping their marks (insignias) into the underside (usually) of the middle crossbar.

Sometimes, these insignias are so small that the use of a magnifying glass is necessary. Still, some opera glasses have no identifying marks whatsoever. Those glasses are listed at the end of this section under "Manufacturer Unknown." It should be noted that there are several variations in the spelling of certain manufacturers' names, as well as other names, words, etc.

The practice of subcontracting work has been going on since time immemorial, and in reference to opera glasses this practice has been no different.

Apparently one major firm manufactured opera glasses for at least seven other smaller businesses that in turn sold them to either jobbers, wholesalers, or perhaps even to individual businesses. In all cases, the same insignia was used:

⟨LE⟩

To date the following opera glasses all bear the same maker's mark placed under the center bar.

Since there is really no overwhelming number of marks indicating a specific firm as the prime manufacturer it will have to be assumed that no one company at present can be credited as the source.

The information listed below is the most current. Perhaps in time after seeing many more pairs of opera glasses with the mark on them a conclusion can be reached.

Different manufacturers using the insignia ⟨LE⟩:

Manufacturer	Location
M. Bertier Fab[1]	Paris
Hoffman	Columbus Ohio
La Corona	
The Elite (made in France)	
Wm. Kendricks' Sons	Louisville, Ky.
Merveille et Cie	Paris
I. A. Foye	Hot Springs, Arkansas
J. E. Milch	St. Petersburg
	Moscow
	Paris
Le Rogue	Memphis, Tennessee

The combined total of over 600 specimens was used to research this chapter.

Insignias

MANUFACTURER	LOCATION	INSIGNIA
Archimeder Deposse		
Audemaire	Paris	#1
Bartou 306	Paris	#2
M. Bertier	Paris	#3
Busch	Jena	(see La Princesse)
Emile Busch (A-G)	Rathenow / Brussels	#4
C. D.		
J. E. Caldwell & Co.	Paris / Philadelphia	
Carpentier	Paris	#5
Chavance & Co.	Paris	#6

Chevalier	Paris	#7 & #8	Dollond	London	
Guy Chevalier	Paris		V & H Dominelli, Frères	France	
			Duchesse		
Colmont	Paris	#2 & #9	Durand	Paris	
Crescent	Paris	#2	The Elite	Paris	#3
			Entrement	Paris	#3
Cresco	Paris	#10			
			Flammarion	Paris	#17
Cross	Paris	#11	Fleurigny	Paris	#18
			Fontaine	Paris	#19
Debutant	Paris				
Deraisme	Paris	#12, #13, #14, #15 & #16	Fowlers (Script)	Chicago (Block)	
			A. Fritsch	Graz	
Derepas Palais Royal			Geivroc & Colmont	Paris	#9
Dollard	London		Genroz & Colmont		#20

168   CHAPTER 16

IDA	Paris		La Favorite	Paris	
Iris	Paris	#21	La Fontaine	France	#26
Jelle Flammarion	Paris		Lamier		#19
Le Jockey Club	Paris	#22	Lafontine Optn	Paris 18 Palace Royal	
			La Gorona	Paris	
Jumelle	France		H. Lamay	Paris	
Krauss	St. Petersburg Leipzig Milan		Lamayre	Paris	
L & R			Lamier (La Mier)	Paris	#26 & #27
L B & Co	Paris	#23 & #24	La Mons	France	
La Belle	Paris		La Monte	Paris	
La Corona		#3	L'Amour	Paris	
			LAMY	Paris	
La Dauphine	Paris	#25	La Princesse	Jena (see Busch)	#28 & #29

OPERA GLASSES 169

La Princesse	Paris		Le Jeune	Paris	
La Reine	France	⟨LE⟩	Lemaire	Paris	🪰 #34
La Roque	Paris	#30 & #31	Le Maître Fab [1]	Paris	
Latour	France	#27	Lemière		
La Touraine	France	#3	Le Mieux	Paris	
La Touraine	Paris	⟨LE⟩	Le Miux	Paris	
Laval			Le Père	Paris	
Lavel	Paris	#32	Le Prince	France	
Lavière FI	Paris		Le Roi	Paris	
La Vil (Lavel)	Paris		Le Roque	Paris	#30 & #31
Le Clair	Paris	#33	Louchet	Paris	
Le Fils	France		Lumière	Paris	
Leglaire			Marchand	France	
			Marchand	Paris	

Marçon			
Marcon	Paris		
Mar Neil	Paris		
Meissonnier	Paris		
Merveille Et Cie	Paris		#3
J. E. Milch (Mielck)	St. Petersburg, Moscow		
Monroy F I	Paris		#35
Mourlon Fab¹	Paris		
Narcissus	Paris		
Noël	Paris		
Praecedo			#36
Precioptic Levallois			

Premier	Paris		#37
Rivera	France		#31
Rodenstock	Munich Charlottenburg		#38
Ross	London		#39 & #40
Paul Schaer	Brussels 94 Rue Neuve		#4
Semmons			
Société d'Optique	Paris		#41
Sportiere	Paris		#42
Sportreil	Paris		
Stenre Fabt	Paris		
Thézard			#27

OPERA GLASSES

Manufacturer	Location	Insignia
Unknown	Austria	
Unknown	England	
Unknown		#43
Unknown	Occupied Japan	
Unknown	Russia	
Verdi	Paris	
Waldstein	Vienna	
Wollensak	Rochester, New York	
Carl Zeiss	Jena	CARL ZEISS JENA #44

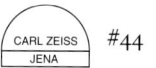

Opera Glass Collection by Manufacturer

Manufacturer	Location	Insignia

ARCHIMEDER DEPOSSE

C399 Collapsible, chrome over brass frame, no barrels: frame—Archimeder Depose.

AUDEMAIRE   Paris   #1

C058 Mother-of-pearl: caps—Audemaire Paris (deer heads separate the words): underside of center bar—Deer & France.

C074 Lorgnette handle: cap—Audemaire; other cap missing.

C171 Sea snail: caps—Audemaire Paris (words separated by deer heads on both sides).

C177 Mother-of-pearl: caps—Audemaire Paris (words separated by deer head): underside of top bar—#5.

C217 White mother-of-pearl, brass inner barrels, brass frame, trim and vertical stem, some reeded edges: caps—Audemaire Paris (deer heads on both sides); Chas. S. Frantz Lancaster: underside of center bar—Made in France.

C219 Sea snail, brass inner barrels, stem, trim, and frame: caps—Briely & Son Oshkosh, Wis: underside of center bar—Made in France and a deerhead.

C247 Mother of pearl: caps—Manufactured in Paris for *; Louis E. Shurtleff, New Bedford: underside of center bar—deerhead.

C264 Caps—Manufactured in Paris for E.W. Butlon & Co. Bridgeport: underside of center bar—deerhead and part of the word *France*; probably manufactured by Audemaire.

C311 Caps—Audemaire Paris (deerheads on both caps): underside of center bar—France and a deerhead. Sea snail.

C340 Black wood barrels, velvet ribbon: caps—Audemaire Paris (deerhead on either side of Paris).

C382 Aluminum, lightweight, outer barrels of highly chased flowers and leaves, single-pull lorgnette handle: caps—Audemaire Paris (two deerheads on each cap).

172   CHAPTER 16

R075 Leather outer barrels, brass inner barrels, brass trim: caps—Audemaire Paris (two deer heads on each).

R104 Mother-of-pearl, medium-size, handle with gears on bottom: "Audemaire Paris—Made in France": circa 1860.

R124 Embossed, gilt, in a case: Audemaire Paris.

BARTOU 306   Paris   #2

C224 Sea snail, brass trim, stem and inner barrels: caps—Bartou FI: underside of center bar—*CC* within six-pointed star.

C306 Mother-of-pearl, basket weave trim: caps—A. Bartou Paris.

M. BERTIER   Paris   #3

C274 Black finished silver outer barrels and single-pull lorgnette handle with carved design of birds in flight, flowers, plants, and leaves, aluminum frame, small pair, reeded aluminum turning knob: caps—M. Bertier Fab^T Paris: underside of center bar—Made in France and *LE* within a diamond shape: underside of bottom bar—Mollie from A-B-C-D July 25th, 1893 (after market).

C307 Dyed mother-of-pearl: caps—M. Bertier Paris.

R191 Embossed and engraved aluminum, mother-of-pearl caps: caps—M. Bertier Fab^T Paris: underside of center bar—Made in France and *LE* within diamond shape.

C130 Purple mother-of-pearl, split with a brass frame: bottom of turning knob—Busch Multinee D.R.C.M.

EMILE BUSCH (A-G)   Rathenow   #4
                     Bruxelles

C213 Mother of pearl, engraved brass trim, bell-shaped: caps—Emil Busch A-G Rathenow: underside of center bar—Fdr. M 4194/61, D.R.P. (mother-of-pearl turning knob in center).

J. E. CALDWELL & CO.   Paris/Philadelphia

C163 Sea snail: caps—J.E. Caldwell & Co. Paris; J.E. Caldwell & Co. Philad. Carpentier Paris #5

C204 Cobalt blue enamel glazed, ribbonlike surface, small bell-shaped, mother-of-pearl caps: caps—Carpentier FI 4 Paris; Bailey, Banks & Biddle Co.: top bar—6 lenses.

CHAVANCE & CO.   Paris   #6

C066 Green French enamel, paintings of women on barrels, double-pull lorgnette handle with cherub: caps—Chavance & Co., Paris; Jas. R. Reed & Co., Pittsburgh.

C116 Yellowed mother-of-pearl, lorgnette handle, single-pull: caps—Chavance & Co. Paris: underside of center bar—Made in France with *LE* within a diamond shape. (See M. Bertier)

C304 Mother-of-pearl, single-pull lorgnette handle of mother-of-pearl with cut work brass bands: caps—Chavance and Co. Paris: underside of center bar—*CE* within a diamond shape.

R047 Gold-dyed sea snail, gilt metal trim: Chavance & Co. Paris.

CHEVALIER   Paris   #7 & #8

C022 Mother-of-pearl, brass trim: caps—Chevalier Paris: bottom of top bar—indistinguishable marks.

C029 Mother-of-pearl, brass trim with some chrome plating: caps—Chevalier Opticiens Paris.

C054 White mother-of-pearl: caps—Chevalier Fab^T Paris: underside of top bar—Racehorse and rider.

C072 Mother-of-pearl, lorgnette handle: caps—Chevalier Paris.

C078 Blue enamel, many half-white beads: caps—Chevalier Opticians-Paris.

C084 White mother-of-pearl, bell-shaped, lorgnette handle: caps—Chevalier Paris.

OPERA GLASSES   173

C104 Leather outer barrels, chrome frame: caps—Chevalier, Paris (words separated by emblem).

C105 Mother-of-pearl, chrome over brass frame: caps—Chevalier Paris (words separated by emblem): underside of top bar— Made in France: underside of center bar—#67.

C110 Purple velvet barrel covering: caps—Chevalier, Opticien Paris.

C114 Sea snail, brass frame: caps—Chevalier Paris.

C118 Mother-of-pearl, chrome over brass frame: caps—Chevalier Paris (emblem separates words).

C122 Metal barrels with multicolored brown lacquer, chrome over brass frame: caps—Chevalier Paris: underside of center bar—Made in Paris (words separated by five-pointed star).

C131 Mother-of-pearl, brass frame and turning knob: caps—Chevalier Paris (words separated by emblem): underside of center bar—Made in France.

C183 Mother-of-pearl: caps—Chevalier Paris (words separated by a fine leaf flower): underside of top bar—Made in France: underside of bottom bar—*GL* (after market).

C215 Sea snail, aluminum frame, brass inner barrels: caps—Chevalier Paris (words separated by five petal flower): underside of center bar—Made in France.

C234 Gun metal with high relief figures of a deer being chased by hunting dogs in the woods: caps—Chevalier Paris (words separated by a five-pointed star): underside of top bar—Made in France.

C262 Mother-of-pearl outer barrels, brass inner barrels, frame, and turning knob: caps—Chevalier Paris: underside of center bar—Made in France.

C267 White metal outer barrels with raised design, chrome frame and inner barrels: caps—Chevalier Paris (in raised lettering): top of center bar—Made in France.

C272 Sea snail outer barrels, brass inner barrels and frame, double-pull lorgnette handle: caps—Chevalier Paris (far smaller caps than most).

C293 Sea snail outer barrels, brass inner barrels, stem, and frame: caps—Chevalier Paris: underside of top bar—Made in France.

C326 White-mother-of pearl: caps—Chas J. Noack Sacramento, Chevalier Opticien: underside of center bar—*CC* within six-pointed star.

C355 Mother-of-pearl, sky blue glazed barrels with half beads festooned in garland form with oval beading on each side of the barrel, pull-out lorgnette handle, brass trim: caps—Chevalier Opticien Paris.

C369 Sea snail, open work brass trim: caps—Chevalier Opticien Paris: underside of center bar—Made in France: underside of bottom bar—Joel H. Bates (after market).

C384 Grey gun metal in relief with birds, flowers, and grapes, brass inner barrels, chrome lens caps and frame: caps—Chevalier Paris (two five-pointed stars on each cap).

R021 Abalone, brass trim, double-pull lorgnette handle: Chevalier Opticien Paris.

R037 Fluted ivory, chrome over brass cap: caps—Chevalier Paris.

R147 Small, black-enameled metal and leather: metal caps—Chevalier Paris.

R195 Aluminum, turned, embossed, engraved, and octagonal: caps—Chevalier Paris (and five-dot symbol).

R210 Brass metal and cast pewter barrels: caps—Chevalier Paris: underside of top bar—Made in France.

R216 Chrome and brass (leather cover on barrels is missing), fancy brass decoration above and below: caps—Chevalier Paris (with five-dot design): underside of top bar—Made in France: underside of bottom bar—From John Miles.

R226 Gilt brass and tortoiseshell opera glass, no center pylon, in a case: Paris, Chevalier (see Corson, p. 157): circa 1825.

GUY CHEVALIER   Paris

R102 Bell-shaped tubes with incised and gold inlaid mother-of-pearl, garlands on mother-of-pearl caps, medium-size pair, aluminum body: inside tubes engraved—Maison de Guy Chevalier Opt., Made in France, Paris, France, 1 Rue Royale: c. 1850.

COLMONT   Paris   #2 & #9

C006 Sea Snail, very small size: caps—Colmont FI Paris; Henry C. Ahlers, San Jose, Cal.: MAI FROM ANNA (after market).

C008 Sea snail, small with handle: caps—Colmont FI Paris; S. Nordlinger & Son, Los Angeles: underside of top bar—Made in France.

C013 Mother-of-pearl, double-pull lorgnette handle, aluminum: caps—Colmont: underside of center bar— * with *C* within a six-pointed star: underside of top bar—France.

C033 Sea snail: caps—Colmont FI Paris; The Scribner and Loehr Co., Cleveland, OH: underside of center bar—France.

C038 Mother-of-pearl barrels and eyepieces: caps—Colmont: underside of center bar—*C* within six-pointed star.

C046 Black enamel with raised brass barrels-gold washed: caps—Colmont FI Paris; Kornblum Pittsburgh: top of center bar—*C* within six-pointed star.

C090 Sea snail, aluminum, in original case: caps—Colmont FI Paris; C.D. Peacock Chicago: underside of top bar—Omega symbol.

C097 Sea snail: caps—Colmont FI Paris: underside of center bar—*C* within six-pointed star: center guide located above center bar—Colmont Paris, *C* within six-pointed star.

C120 Sea snail, small size, lorgnette handle: underside of center bar—*C* within six-pointed star.

C153 Sea snail, single-pull lorgnette handle: caps—Colmont FI Paris: underside of center bar—*C* within six-pointed star: underside of top bar—Made in France.

C168 Sea snail: caps—Colmont FI Paris; Franklin & Co.—Washington D.C.: underside of top bar—Made in France: underside of center bar—*C* within six-pointed star.

C176 Sea snail: caps—Colmont FI Paris: bottom outside bar— PLL to ERH (in script) (after market).

C206 Brass inner barrels and stem: caps—Colmont FI Paris (words separated by *C* within five-pointed star): underside of center bar—*C* within five-pointed star: underside of top bar—France.

C207 Mother-of-pearl, aluminum frame, housed in leather pouch—dark blue satin lining with gold lettering: caps—Colmont FI Paris: 9/92 Beverly Ma (after market).

C242 Mother-of-pearl, brass barrels: caps—Meyrowitz Bros. New York (words separated by six-pointed stars); other cap is plain: underside of top bar—*C* within a six-pointed star.

C257 Mother-of-pearl, small pair, single-pull lorgnette handle divided by several beaded bands: underside of center bar—*C* within six-pointed star.

C260 Mother-of-pearl outer barrels, brass inner barrels and frame: caps—Simmons Bros. Columbus, O.; Colmont FI Paris: underside of center bar—J.S. & Co. and *C* within six-pointed star.

C312 Double-pull lorgnette handle: caps—Colmont Paris (words separated by *C* within six-pointed star): underside of bottom bar—*C* within six-pointed star: underside of center bar—*C* within six-pointed star.

C324 Green enamel with white mother-of-pearl trim: bottom and center bar—Taine Paris Colmont on eye "caps 2".

C329 Caps—E.B. Meyrowitz Paris; E.B. Meyrowitz New York: underside of center bar—*C* (for Colmont).

C334 Caps—Colmont Paris (six-pointed star on either side of Paris): underside of center bar—*C* within six-pointed star.

C364 Copper and brass outer barrels with raised figures of woman with long, flowing hair, floral design on rear of barrels, silver-plated trim: underside of center bar—*C* within six-pointed star.

C396 Bright, light blue glazed straight outer barrels and lorgnette handle, brass frame, white mother of pearl lens caps and trim, very small pair: caps—Colmont Paris:

OPERA GLASSES   175

underside of frame—*C* within six-pointed star: underside of center bar—*C* within six-pointed star.

R001 Mother-of-pearl and bronze: Colmont Paris.

R062 French brass and sea snail, extension handle, blue velvet case: Colmont Paris.

R071 Mother-of-pearl and sea snail, mother-of-pearl caps: caps—Colmont, Paris.

R079 Sea snail, double-pull lorgnette handle: caps—Colmont Fi Paris: underside of center bar—*C* within six-pointed star: underside of top bar—France: bottom bar—HHP 2 VMP souvenir Portland 1912.

R086 Sea snail, small size, lorgnette handle: bottom of outer barrel—Marguerite Colmont Fi Paris.

R098 White enamel over machine base with green and red garlands, double-glazed, mother-of-pearl borders, brass frame: underside of center bar—*C* within six-pointed star: underside of bottom bar—Colmont and *C* within six-pointed star, also *MES* (after market).

R105 Sea snail, medium-size, case: Colmont Paris: circa 1900: "Traub & Co., Detroit."

R110 Dark blue bell-shaped barrels with women's heads on porcelain, medium-size, brass body with side telescoping handle: "Colmont Bro. Paris": circa 1860.

R116 Gilded brass with mother-of-pearl caps, blue enamel bell-shaped barrels over machined brass with red poppies, medium size: Colmont: circa 1880.

R122 Nickeled brass with leather, in purse case, hard rubber caps: (Deposé), Colmont Paris: circa 1900.

R139 Small mother-of-pearl and black lip pearl stripes on brass: *C* within six-pointed star (Colmont): circa 1955.

R155 Brass and pink enamel with blue glass decorative spheres around floral enamel pictures, side-mounted three-draw telescopic handle, mother-of-pearl caps: caps—The McAllister Opt. Co.; 1116 Chestnut Street Philadelphia: crossbar—Made in France and *C* within six-pointed star.

R164 Brass and gilt with raised reticulated figures and enameled borders on brass base with mother-of-pearl caps:

caps—C. Ulrich Opticien; Paris, Vichy, Nice: crossbar—*C* within six-pointed star.

R215 Cast brass and chrome: underside of center bar—C.

CRESCENT   Paris   #2

C143 Mother-of-pearl: caps—Crescent Paris: underside of center bar—*CC* within six-pointed star.

CRESCO   Paris   #10

C220 White mother-of-pearl, brass inner barrels, trim, stem, and frame: caps—Cresco Co.: top of top bar—Made in France: underside of top bar—France.

CROSS   Paris   #11

C172 Black leather wrapped barrels: top bar—Cross (lion head over that): underside of center bar—HD Paris within symbol.

C279 Black leather outer barrels, brass inner barrels and frame, small pair: caps—CAOSS, PARIS (possibly Cross due to block lettering-separated by eight lines all pivoting in center on both sides): underside of center bar—#8 and Made in France.

DEBUTANT   Paris

C149 Sea snail: caps—Debutant Paris: underside of top, moveable bar—France.

DERAISME   Paris   #12, #13, #14 #15 & #16

C141 Sea snail, housed in original case with anchor symbol as button on case: caps—Made in France For: Andrew J. Lloyd Co. Boston: top of top bar—34X: underside of center bar—*D* and an anchor.

C185 Black enamel frame, leather wrapped, field glass type, adjustable swivel, 5 ¼ inches when extended: top of top bar—Deraisme Paris FAB[T]: underside of bottom bar—#580.

C302 White and brown mother-of-pearl in barber pole design on outer barrels and bottom of lens caps: bottom marked—Deraisme F^T Paris: underside of fixed bar—#81 and an anchor symbol with an inverted *D* and an *L*.

DEREPAS PALAIS ROYAL

DOLLARD London

C303 Green enamel over brass outer barrels, tops and bottoms convex and concave, decorated with flowers, gold crosses, and yellow dots, large pair: right barrel—LONDON (in script): left barrel—DOLLARD (in script).

DOLLOND London

R205 Brass and black pearl: caps—Dollond London.

V & H Dominelli, Frères, France

R069 French, aluminum, helmeted soldier atop center pylon: caps (brown enamel)—45 Avenue de Gare, Nice; V and H Dominelli, Frères: below—Isometrop.

DUCHESSE

C034 Mother of pearl: caps—Duchesse Fab I, Superior Glasses.

C047 Sea snail: caps—Superior Glasses Duchesse Fab I.

C162 Mother-of-pearl, brass frame: caps—Superior Glasses—Duchesse FAB^T.

R097 Triple glazed, light blue, four medallions with floral designs, brass frame, ivory lens caps and turning knob: top bar—Duchesse 12 verre: no markings.

R109 Navy blue barrels with flowers in circles, triple-glazed, medium-size brass with mother-of-pearl caps and twist central handle: "Duchesse 12 Verres" (12 lenses): circa 1880.

DURAND Paris

C281 Purple mother of pearl outer barrels, chrome inner barrels, black enamel eye caps, black crossbar: caps—Durand FaB Paris: underside of center bar—Deposé: underside of top bar—made in France (possibly added later due to double stamping of some of the letters).

THE ELITE Paris #3

C125 Caps—The Elite Paris: underside of top bar—*LE* within a diamond shape and Made in France: top of top bar—Extra Power. Dyed mother-of-pearl.

R094 Embossed and engraved aluminum, tortoiseshell lens caps, velvet bag: caps—The Elite Paris.

ENTREMENT Paris #3

FLAMMARION Paris #17

C087 Purple sea snail, aluminum: caps—J. Flammarion Paris: top of center bar—"Flammarion" and picture of flat open palm.

R032 Tortoise, brass, and black enamel, helmet design: bottom bar—Flammarion.

FLEURIGNY Paris #18

C003 Sea Snail, aluminum frame, small gold inset on one barrel: caps—Anderson & Randolph, San Francisco: underside of bottom bar—flower and #63.

C175 Mother-of-pearl: caps—Fleurigny Paris; Superior Quality (words separated by a flower): top of top bar—12 lenses (engraved): underside of top bar—France.

FONTAINE Paris #19

C270 Mother-of-pearl, brass frame: caps—Fontaine, Paris: underside of top bar—France and *N*.

A. FRITSCH　　　Graz

GEIVROC & COLMONT　　　Paris #9

C023 Caps—Geivroc & Colmont, Paris. Sea snail.

R013 Black lip pearl and sea snail alternating stripes inside and outside barrels: Geivroc & Colmont, Paris.

GENROZ & COLMONT　　　#20

IDA　　　Paris

C256 White mother-of-pearl, brass frame: caps—Ida Paris: underside of center bar—Made in France and #61.

IRIS　　　Paris　　　#21

C048 Mother-of-pearl, lorgnette handle in burgundy leather, housed in original black leather case: caps—IRIS Paris (words separated by six-pointed star).

C093 Caps—IRIS-Paris, raised letters and *I* within six-pointed star: underside of center bar—*I* within six-pointed star. Sea snail.

C136 Brown iridescent sea snail, dark brown eye cap trim and center turning knob: caps—IRIS Paris: underside of center bar—France Iris: underside of top bar—D.

C265 Sea snail, small pair: caps—Iris Paris (words separated by an *X*): underside of center bar—*I* within a six-pointed star.

C318 Mother-of-pearl inner barrels: caps—Iris Paris: underside of center bar—*I* within six-pointed star.

C338 Caps—Iris Paris (*I* within a-six pointed star on both side of Iris): top of top bar—Jumelle De Tir: underside of center bar—six-pointed star: bottom of center rod—a compass. Brass.

C376 Sea snail, brass trim: caps—Iris Paris: underside of center bar—Iris (in script).

R082 Sea snail outer barrels, brass inner barrels, single-pull lorgnette handle, three sections separated by brass trim: caps—Iris Paris (*I* within six-pointed star in two places on each cap): underside of center bar—*I* within six-pointed star.

R088 Mother-of-pearl, single-pull lorgnette handle: caps—Iris Paris (*I* within six-pointed star in two places on each cap): underside of center bar—*I* within six-pointed star.

R107 Sea shell tubes with brass, mother-of-pearl caps, small size, in a case: caps—Iris, Paris: circa 1930.

R134 Sea snail and brass: sea snail caps—IRIS France: marked France (IRIS): circa 1895.

R138 Gilt brass and abalone, mother-of-pearl caps, in leather case: caps—Iris Paris: crossbar—Iris France.

JELLE FLAMMARION Paris

C320 White mother-of-pearl with carved fleur-de-lis, lorgnette handle: caps—Jelle Flammarion Paris: underside of top bar—Made in France.

JUMELLE　　　France

KRAUSS　　　St. Petersburg, Leipaiz, Milan

C056 Mother-of-pearl, bottle-shaped: caps—Leipzig. Milan. St. Petersburg; E. Krauss & Cie, Paris. Londres.

L & R

L B & Co　　　Paris　　　#23 & #24

C081 Sea snail: caps—L.B. & Co.: bottom of bottom bar—"Aunt" from Katie (after market).

C103 Caps—L.B. & Co. Paris (raised letters) with a star on either side of Paris. Leather.

R022 Abalone and brass, abalone lens caps, mother-of-pearl trim, lido on bottom bar: L.B. & Co. Paris.

LA BELLE   Paris

C123 Sea snail, brass frame: caps—La Belle Paris.

C319 White mother-of-pearl, black enamel: caps—LaBelle Paris: underside of top bar—Made in France.

LA CORONA   #3

C082 Sea snail, lorgnette handle, one cap insert missing: caps—La Corona Paris: underside of center bar—*LE* inside of a diamond shape: underside of top bar—Made in France.

C101 Mother-of-pearl: caps—La Corona: underside of top bar—Made in France.

C277 White mother-of-pearl inner barrels and center turning knob: caps—La Corona: underside of top bar—*C* and Made in France: top of center bar—XTRA POWER (in script).

LA DAUPHINE   Paris   #25

C094 Mother-of-pearl: caps—La Dauphine (between two clovers), Paris (raised letters): underside of center bar—France.

LA FAVORITE   Paris

C024 Mother-of-pearl: caps—La Favorite, Paris.

C035 Mother-of-pearl, reeded center mother-of-pearl turning knob: caps—La Favorite Paris on eye caps.

LAFONTAINE OPTN   Paris   #26
18 Palace Royal

C221 Sea snail, brass inner barrels, white mother-of-pearl turning knob: caps—LaFontaine Opt, 18, Palais-Royal.

C252 Mother-of-pearl: caps—Lafontaine Opt N 18 Palais Royale 18.

LAMAIER   Paris

C253 Caps—Lamaier, Paris (five vertical lines depicting a bee between the words). White mother-of-pearl.

C395 Aluminum outer barrels with pink enamel pattern etched in afterwards, brass trim—partially chromed: caps—Lamaier FAB^T (two double leaves separating the words on each cap).

LAMAIRE   Paris

R197 Aluminum, turned, octagonal, two brass rings: underside of outer bar—Made in France: "Lamaire FAB Paris."

H. LAMAY   Paris

C229 Brass, octagon-shaped outer barrels, each panel has a bird in flight with branches above and below (in relief): caps—H. Lamay Paris.

C275 White mother-of-pearl: caps—Lamay Paris (symbol resembling a bee between words).

CAA1 Sea snail and dyed sea snail alternating strips—Brass inner barrels: caps—H. Lamay Paris.

LAMAYRE   Paris

C245 White mother-of-pearl, lorgnette handle frame without handle: caps—James Clegg, Buffalo; Lamayre, Paris: underside of bottom bar—M.E.A. (after market).

LA MERVEILLEUSE   Paris

R206 Brass and black pearl with fancy brass bands on barrels: caps—La Merveilleuse Paris *X*.

LAMIER (LA MIER)   Paris   #26 & #27

C070 Aluminum with red and gold-colored barrels: caps—Lamier FAB^T-Paris.

OPERA GLASSES   179

C088 Sea snail: caps—Lamier-Paris: underside of center bar— Made in France.

C089 Mother-of-pearl: caps—Lamier-Paris.

R198 Turned, embossed, and engraved aluminum with brass, in leather case: caps—Lamier FAB^T Paris.

LA MIGNONNE　　　Paris

C283 Folding pair in black-grained leather-covered case, inside label reads—U.S.A. Pat. Aug. 12-02, outside turning knob extends slightly out of case and reads—La Mignonne Paris: top of top bar—Gravière Paris.

R159 Flat pair simulating a purse, leather with brass floral garlands, in leather case, chain missing: "La. Mignonne, Patent B TE SGOG": "Cijuge Cissot Opticien 33 Ce Ole Opere, Paris" (engraved).

LA MONS　　　France

R015 Mother-of-pearl, chrome frame, black leather case: La Mons.

LA MONTE　　　Paris

L'AMOUR　　　Paris

R137 Mother-of-pearl and base metal, in leather case: caps—L'Amour, Paris.

LAMY, H.　　　Paris

R121 Mother-of-pearl: Lamy Paris: circa 1890.

LA PRINCESSE　　Jena (see Busch)　　#28 & #29

C201 White mother-of-pearl, bell-shaped, housed in alligator-grained leather case with "Busch" (in script) on closure button: caps—La Princesse Jena (within a design resembling a flower): underside of center bar—#61: underside of top bar—Busch: underside of bottom bar—Busch (in script).

LA PRINCESSE　　　Paris

R108 Gold tube outside barrel with birds and garlands on a blue background, medium-size brass tubes, telescopic handle on the side, mother-of-pearl caps: caps—La Princesse Paris: circa 1880.

C218 Purple-glazed enamel outer barrels with gold and silver trim, bell-shaped, brass inner barrels and stem, white mother-of-pearl turning knob, housed in Lemaire case: caps—La Princesse Paris: underside of top bar—Made in France.

LA REINE　　　France

C197 Mother-of-pearl, lorgnette handle: caps—La Reine Paris: underside of center bar—*LE* within diamond shape and Made in France.

C209 Sea snail, brass frame and inner barrels, single-pull lorgnette handle, vertical stem not connected: caps—La Reine Paris.

R019 Black leather barrels, black enamel frame, gold trim, black leather case with purple silk lining: La Reine.

R123 Aluminum and leather: La Reine France. (This specimen was donated to the Ellis Island Museum.)

R189 Embossed and engraved aluminum, tortoiseshell caps: caps—La Reine Paris.

R190 Aluminum with telescoping side-mounted handle: caps—La Reine Paris: underside of center bar—*LE* within diamond shape.

LA ROQUE　　　Paris　　　#30 & #31

LATOUR　　　France　　　#27

C031 Mother-of-pearl, brass trim, brass turning knob: caps—Latour: underside of top bar—Made in France.

C071 Sea snail: caps—Latour: underside of center bar—Made/ France.

C179 Caps—Latour Paris; L.J. Cooke Findlay Ohio: underside of center bar—#15: top bar—Made in France.

C328 Blue enamel with handle: caps—Latour Paris (five dots on the side): underside of top bar—Made in France.

R056 Brass and sea snail with extension handle: Latour Paris.

LA TOURAINE   France   #3
    Paris

C169 Sea snail, chrome over brass frame: caps—La Touraine Paris; H.Y. Loewenstein, St. Louis.

R085 Gold-dyed mother-of-pearl, brass inner barrels, single-pull lorgnette handle: caps—La Touraine Paris: underside of top bar—Made in France and *LE* within a diamond shape.

LAVAL

LAVEL   Paris   #32

LAVIÈRE FI   Paris

C290 Caps—Lavière F¹ Paris (lettering larger on one cap than the other): no other markings. White mother-of-pearl.

LA VIL (LAVEL)   Paris

C315 Enamel scenes on both barrels: caps—Lavil Paris (raised letters—symbol on each side).

LAVILLE   Paris

C086 Sea snail: caps—Laville Paris.

LE CLAIR   Paris   #33

C211 Black leather, gold trim, black metal inner barrels and vertical trim, copper bands above and below outer barrels, single-pull lorgnette handle: caps—Le Clair Paris.

LECLARE   Paris

C100 Caps—LeClare Paris. White MOP.

LE FILS   France

C036 Sea snail: caps—Lefils Paris (both caps, separated by symbol).

C064 Sea snail: caps—Le Fils, Paris: underside of center bar—Made/France.

C083 White mother-of-pearl, smaller than normal size: caps—LeFils Paris.

C235 Cobalt blue, brass trim, fleur-de-lis scattered on barrels and single-pull lorgnette handle: caps—LeFils Paris: underside of top bar—#8.

C251 White mother-of-pearl, brass frame: caps—Lefils, Paris.

C271 Mother-of-pearl, brass frame, reeded center turning knob: caps—Lefils Paris.

C313 Blue enamel: caps—Lefils Paris: underside of center bar—Made in France.

C374 Deep royal blue enamel background trim with fleur-de-lis, two similar 19th-century "ladies in waiting" portraits on barrels under glaze, matching double-pull lorgnette handle with portrait of cherub, brass frame, trim and inner barrels, white mother-of-pearl lens caps and turning knob: caps—Le Fils, Paris.

LEGLAIRE

LE JEUNE   Paris

C310 Colored mother-of-pearl: caps—LeJeune Paris.

LE JOCKEY CLUB   Paris   #22

C348 Brown leather: caps—Le Jockey Club Paris (clover on each side of Paris).

C368 Chased paisley pattern outer barrels with ovals for initials, indicating silver plate over brass, large brass inner barrels: caps—Le Jockey Club.

| LEMAIRE | Paris | #34 |

C001 Caps—Lemaire F¹ Paris; John A. Steinbach, San Francisco: bottom of center bar—flower and #63: bottom of bottom bar—Jane Reh 92 (for 1892—after market).

C004 Sea Snail: caps—Lemaire F¹ Paris; Henry Kahn & Co., San Francisco: underside of top bar—#31268A—Made in France: underside of center bar—Bee symbol.

C005 Mother-of-pearl: caps—Lemaire: bottom of bar just above adjustment set screw—J.W. Phila: other side of bar—Made in France.

C007 Mother-of-pearl, lorgnette handle: caps—Lemaire F¹ Paris; H.C. Warner, Fresno, Cal: underside of bottom bar—flower and #61: top bar—12 lenses.

C009 Purple sea snail: caps—Lemaire F¹ Paris; Max Meyer & Bro, Omaha: outside of bottom bar—1889: underside of center bar—symbol and #63.

C010 Mother-of-pearl: caps—Lemaire: underside of center bar— symbol and #21 Made in France.

C015 Mother-of-pearl, straight lorgnette handle affixed from bottom center: caps—Lemaire: symbol in center of pat. 95: *K* in center of 268112 pat. Nov. 28th '82.

C018 Purple sea snail, aluminum trim, black enamel caps—Lemaire: underside of center bar—#G3B–33.

C021 Caps—Lemaire: outside of bottom bar—J. Curley & Bro. New York: underside of center bar—#632–See symbol.

C025 Sea snail: caps—Lemaire F¹-Paris; Archie Ligtmeyer—Milwaukee, WI.: underside of center bar—symbol and #6 Made in France.

C028 Sea snail: caps—Lemaire Paris: underside of top bar—28213: bottom of center bar—symbol and France.

C037 Mother-of-pearl, chrome finish, straight handle from base: caps—Lemaire F¹ Paris: underside of center bar—symbol and 539006 Pat May 7–95: underside of top bar—D-16449 Made in France: *K* surrounded by 139 Pat 82–Nov. 28 266112.

C039 Mother-of-pearl: caps—Lemaire FAB¹ Paris; F.W. McAllister Co., Baltimore MD: underside of top bar—#35880B-France: underside of center bar—#61–B38.

C045 Sea snail: caps—H.J. Blair Bristol: center bar—a bee and #63.

C049 Aluminum/mother-of-pearl: caps—Lemaire FAB¹ Paris; E.B. Meyrowitz Paris New York: underside of center bar—#2838 Made in France.

C050 Gilt raised metal barrels, black enamel frames: caps—Lemaire FAB¹ : underside of center bar—Paris #63B.

C051 Sea snail: caps—Lemaire F¹ Paris; J.W. Webb Dallas, Texas: bottom bar—Dec 6, 1890 (after market): underside of center bar— #63 and a bee.

C052 Iridescent sea snail, chrome finish, black, grey color: caps—Lemaire F¹ Paris; Jobe Rose Jewelry Co. Birmingham: under center bar—a bee.

C053 Caps—Lemaire F¹ Paris; F.W. Badger Beaumont Texas: underside of center bar—bee and Made/France #5: button on end of lorgnette handle reads "Pat. Dec. 8, 1896."

C062 White mother-of-pearl, brass: caps—C.D. Peacock, Chicago, Lemaire: underside of center bar—a bee and Made/France.

C063 Sea snail: caps—A. Webster, Brooklyn, N.Y., Lemaire F¹ Paris; A.A. Webster & Co., Brooklyn: bottom of center bar—a bee and #63.

C065 Purple mother-of-pearl: caps—Lemaire F¹ Paris: underside of center bar—a bee and #63.

C068 Mother-of-pearl: caps—Lemaire-Paris; W.S. Taylor & Son, Utica, N.Y.: underside of center bar—a bee and #63.

C069 Black leather/black enamel, in case: caps—Lemaire Paris: underside of center bar—a bee and Made/France: underside of top bar—#27437.

C075 Black enamel, black leather: caps—Lemaire-FAB¹ Paris.

C079 Light blue enamel barrels, garland half pearls, fitted for straight lorgnette handle: caps—Lemaire FI Paris: underside of top bar—Made in France: underside of center bar—Pat. Nov 28–82 #268112: Pat 539006: A bee surrounded by May 7, 95.

C098 Chrome tricolor basket weave: caps—J.E. Caldwell & Co., Philad.; J.E. Caldwell & Co., Paris: underside of center bar—#63, a bee and #5.

C107 Purple mother-of-pearl: caps—Lemaire F^I Paris (words separated by a bee): underside of center bar—#63 and a bee.

C108 Purple sea snail, brass frame: caps—Lemaire F^I Paris (words separated by a bee): underside of center bar—#63 and a bee.

C109 Caps—Lemaire FAB^I Paris (bee on each side of name, raised lettering): underside of center bar—#63.

C111 Caps—Derepas Palais Royal (star separates the words): underside of center bar—a bee (Lemaire). Black pearl.

C112 Caps—Lemaire Fabricant Paris (words separated by bee): underside of center bar—a bee. White mother-of-pearl.

C117 Sea snail, brass frame: caps—Lemaire FAB^I Paris (words separated by a bee): underside of center bar—#61 and a bee: underside of top bar—G26053.

C119 Black enamel over chrome, flat-folding leather-covered four-piece flip covers, adjustable knob on magnifying lenses, turning knob inside center stem (a bee on the underside of the stem): caps—Lemaire F^I Paris (words separated by a bee).

C124 In original case: caps—Lemaire FAB^I Paris; George P. Tuthill, Saint Paul Minn.: underside of bottom bar—Ruth E. Wilson (after market): underside of center bar—#61 and a bee: underside of top bar—Made in France and #17092B.

C128 Mother-of-pearl, chrome frame, double-pull lorgnette handle: caps—Lemaire F^I Paris; Chas F. Artes Evansville: underside of top bar—#21926A: underside of center bar—a bee and Made in France: outside of bottom bar—NMG after market.

C134 Mother-of-pearl: caps—Lemaire F^I Paris; B. Olbricht, Brooklyn, N.Y. (words separated by a bee): underside of center bar—#16, a bee, and Made in France: bottom of bottom frame—AMR (after market).

C137 Iridescent sea snail: caps—Lemaire Paris (block letters): bottom of bottom bar—"Bee France".

C138 Mother-of-pearl: caps—Geo. C. Shreve & Co. San Francisco: underside of center bar—#63 and a bee: bottom outside bar—Mar 7, 1888.

C140 Mother-of-pearl, brass frame: caps—Lemaire Paris (words separated by a bee): underside of center bar—*C* within a six-pointed star (unusual for Lemaire glasses to have a Colmont marking. Repaired?).

C142 Sea snail, small pair, single-pull lorgnette handle: caps—Lemaire FAB^I Paris (words separated by a bee); W.T. Hixson Co. El Paso Texas: underside of center bar—#61 and a bee: underside of top bar—Made in France G1730.

C145 Sea snail, in original case: caps—Lemaire F^I Paris (words separated by bees); A. Stowell & Co. Boston: underside of center bar—a bee: top bar—12 Glasses.

C146 Sea snail: caps—Lemaire F^I Paris; E. Bausch & Son, Rochester NY: underside of top bar—Made in France, Serial #25208A: underside of center bar—a bee and #61: top of top bar—12 lenses.

C151 Mother-of-pearl, in original case: caps—Lemaire F^I Paris, (with bee symbol): Dachtera Bros, N.Y.

C152 Bright-colored gold outer barrels, bell-shaped; mother-of-pearl inner barrels, floral design: caps—Lemaire F^I Paris (bee separates the words): underside of center bar— #12.

C154 Sea snail, frame is part black enamel and part brass: caps—Lemaire FAB^I Paris (in raised letters, words separated by a bee): underside of center bar—#68 and a bee.

C156 Mother-of-pearl: caps—Lemaire F^I Paris (words separated by a bee): underside of center bar—Made in France, and a bee: bottom of bottom frame—Collins (after market).

C161 Sea snail, aluminum frame: caps—Lemaire F^I Paris; Bailey Banks & Biddle Co.—Phila: underside of center bar—a bee and Made in France #27: top of top bar—12 glasses.

C164 Mother-of-pearl: caps—Lemaire F^I Paris; Kings Achromatic: underside of center bar—a bee and #63.

C173 Purple mother-of-pearl: caps—Lemaire of Paris; J. Robinson, Optician, Broadway New York: underside of center bar—a bee.

C174 Mother-of-pearl: caps—Lemaire FAB^I Paris (words separated by a bee): underside of center bar—a bee and #61 J.W. Phila: top bar—G.26551 Made in France.

C182 Black enamel with leather barrel covering: caps—Lemaire FAB[I] Paris (raised lettering, words separated with two bees): underside of center bar—#63 and a bee.

C184 Black enamel over brass, leather-covered outer barrels, large field glass type-8 inches overall when fully extended, including pullouts: caps—Lemaire FAB[I] Paris (words separated by two bees).

C187 Mother-of-pearl, 3 ½ inches when extended: underside of center bar—a bee (Lemaire): barrel near cap—Montreal.

C194 Sea snail, brass trim: caps—Ferd Wagner Cincinnati, Oh; Lemaire F[I] Paris: underside of center bar—#63 and a bee.

C196 Black enamel frame with leather outer covering resembling two flasks, pair folds flat into case, which is also used as a base or handle, center turning knob to raise and lower eye caps, fitted with frame to hold a strap on each side: caps—Lemaire FAB[I] Paris: inside of center bar—a bee.

C200 Sea snail, brass leaf design and bead trim on inner and outer barrels: caps—S.C. Mac Keown Lawrence; Lemaire F[I] Paris: underside of center bar—a bee and #13, Made in France.

C205 Mother-of-pearl: caps—Lemaire Paris; Joslin & Park, Salt Lake City, Utah.

C208 Original case, cobalt blue satin lining with gold lettering—E. Borhek & Son, Opticians, 623 Chestnut St., Philad (printed like a ribbon type banner), center knob turns when barrels are removed first: caps—Lemaire F[I] Paris; E. Borhek, Philadelphia: underside of center bar—#23, #63, and a bee.

C210 Deep red lacquer with gold fleur-de-lis trim outer barrels, brass frame, inner barrels, and vertical stem, mother-of-pearl eye caps, double-pull lorgnette handle: caps—Lemaire Paris: underside of center bar—a large bee and Made in France: underside of bottom bar—Kittie F (engraved after purchase).

C212 Pebbly grained black leather, bell-shaped, glossy black metal frame, stem, and inner barrels, small case lined in purple satin with bee clasp: caps—Lemaire FAB[I] Paris (words separated by five-pointed stars): underside of center bar—bee, R, and #63/13 (L).

C216 Kelly green enamel outer barrels bordered by flowers, brass frame and inner barrels, beaded trim: caps—Lemaire F[I] Paris (words separated by stylized bee designs): underside of center bar—a bee and #63.

C222 Dark mother-of-pearl, brass trim, stem, inner barrels and frame, housed in original case: caps—Andrew J. Lloyd Co. Boston; Lemaire FAB[I] Paris: underside of center bar—Made in France and a bee: underside of top bar—G04843 and C4899.

C223 Purple mother-of-pearl, brass braid type, black enamel top center and bottom bars, brass inner barrels, stem and trim: caps—Lemaire F[I] Paris (words separated by a bee): underside of center bar—#63 and a bee.

C232 Leather, black enamel over brass, black leather case with a bee on the snap—gold stamp lettering on chestnut silk—White & Mac Naught: caps—Lemaire FAB[I] Paris (words separated by a bee); White & Mac Naught, Minneapolis: underside of top bar—17992A: underside of bottom bar—a bee, #61 and Made in France.

C237 White mother-of-pearl, housed in original black leather case with dealer's address: caps—R. Harris & Co., Washington, D.C.; Lemaire F[I] Paris: underside of center bar—Made in France, #16, and a bee: underside of bottom bar—E. Harper (in script—after market).

C246 Caps—C.D. Peacock, Chicago; Lemaire, Paris: underside of center bar—Made in France and a bee: top bar—#14 Tensis. White mother-of-pearl.

C249 Caps—Andrew J. Lloyd & Co.: underside of center bar—#9, a bee, and Made in France: top of top bar—#12 lenses (in script) (probably Lemaire). Sea Snail.

C254 Sea snail, brass barrels with beadwork trim: caps—Jas. R. Armiger, Baltimore; Lemaire, Paris (words separated by a bee): underside of center bar—#28 and a bee: underside of bottom bar—ECN 1895 within a square (after market).

C258 Caps—Lemaire F[I] Paris: underside of center bar—a bee, #27, and Made in France. Sea Snail.

C259 Purple sea snail, black enamel frame: caps—Lemaire Paris (words separated by bees): underside of center bar—#63, #10, and a bee.

C261 Mother-of-pearl, brass inner barrels and stem, large pair: caps—Lemaire F^I Paris: underside of center bar—#23, a bee, and #63: underside of bottom bar—R.E. (after market).

C266 Caps—Williams, Brown & Earle, Philadelphia, Pa.; Lemaire F^I Paris: underside of center bar—bee and Made in France. Sea snail.

C269 Mother-of-pearl outer barrels, brass inner barrels and frame: caps—Bacon Bros, Lowell: underside of center bar—#63 and a bee.

C284 Mother-of-pearl outer barrels, brass rings of leaf design trim at top, brass inner barrels and frame: caps—Lemaire F^I Paris and a bee: underside of center bar—Made in France, #2, and a bee.

C291 Mother-of-pearl outer barrels, brass inner barrels and frame: caps—Lemaire F^I Paris: underside of center bar—Made in France, #23, and a bee.

C305 Gold-colored mother-of-pearl: caps—Lemaire F^I Paris (words separated by bees).

C332 Detached handle: caps—Lemaire F^I Paris (Bee on both sides of Paris): underside of center bar—a bee surrounded by May 7 95 Pat 539006: top of center bar—*K* surrounded by 268112 Nov. 28 82 Pat.

C335 Black enamel: caps—Lemaire F^I Paris; J. Winreurgh and Son Utica: underside of center bar—a bee.

C341 Caps-Lemaire Paris; Jos Linz and Bros. Dallas Tex.

C342 Adjustable: caps—Spaulding and Co. Paris: underside of center bar—a bee. White mother-of-pearl.

C343 Caps—Mermod and Jaccard Jewelry Co. St. Louis; Mermod and Jaccard Jewelry Co. Paris: underside of center bar—a bee: top of center bar—#3076. White mother-of-pearl.

C356 Sea snail, double-pull lorgnette handle: caps—Lemaire: underside of top bar—#30652: underside of center bar—Made in France and a bee.

C357 White mother-of-pearl, fixture for lorgnette handle but none attached: caps—Lemaire: underside of center bar—a bee, C4, and Made in France: top of center bar—EXTRA.

C358 Purple mother-of-pearl, brass trim: caps—Lemaire F^I Paris: underside of center bar—#63 and a bee: Lemaire bee on four spots of dark lens caps.

C360 Black enamel inner barrels, silver outer barrels, chased with bee, flowers and leaves on each barrel: caps—Lemaire, Paris (two Lemaire bees on each cap): underside of center bar—#63 and 3C with a bee.

C362 Chrome and mother-of-pearl trim, double-pull mother-of-pearl lorgnette handle, cupped lenses: caps—Lemaire FAB^I Paris: flat top of glasses—3X Prism Opera.

C363 Purple mother-of-pearl, beaded brass trim, beet-color lens caps: caps—Lemaire F^I Paris (two Lemaire bees on each cap): underside of center bar—Made in France, a bee, and #12.

C385 Purple mother-of-pearl outer barrels with leaf design chased in brass on top and bottom, brass inner barrels and trim: caps—Lemaire F^I Paris (two bees on each cap): underside of center bar—Made in Paris and a bee: J.M. Dec. 25/97 (after market).

C387 Purple mother-of-pearl, chrome over brass frame and crossbars: caps—Lemaire F^I Paris (two bees on each cap): underside of center bar—#61 and a bee.

C389 White mother-of-pearl, brass trim: caps—Lemaire F^I Paris (two bees on each cap): underside of center bar—Made in France and a bee, also AD EL (engraved after market).

C391 Sea snail outer barrels and double-pull lorgnette handle, reverse-bell mother-of-pearl trim between top bar and lens cap bottom, all brass trim: caps—Lemaire F^I Paris (two bees separating the words): underside of center bar—#63 and a bee.

CAA2 Snail outer barrels, gold-washed frame and inner barrels: caps—James Prentice & Son: underside of center bar—#10, #63, and Lemaire bee: in original black leather case.

CAA3 Mother-of-pearl outer barrels and lorgnette handle, handle fits into base of glasses and has turning knob at front end: back end of handle—539006, bee, May 7, Pat 95: caps—The Rushmer Jewelry Co. Pueblo; Lemaire F^I Paris (bee separates words).

CAA6 Caps—M Arnold Ann Arbor; Lemaire F^l Paris (without bee symbol): underside of center bar—Made in France, bee, and #27.

R009 Mother-of-pearl, center pylon screw adjustment, black leather case with blue silk lining: Lemaire.

R011 Mother-of-pearl, gilt, black leather case marked Ross & Co. New Bond St. London: Lemaire Paris.

R020 Black enamel, black leather, black leather case: Le Maire FAB^T/Bee.

R033 Tortoise and aluminum, single-pull lorgnette handle that attaches to a set lug: caps—Le Maire Fabricant—Paris.

R039 Mother-of-pearl and brass, large size: underside of center bar—Le Maire bee.

R043 Sea snail: Le Maire Paris F^l.

R048 Aluminum and mother-of-pearl, double-pull lorgnette handle: Le Maire FAB^T Paris; J.E. Caldwell & Co. Philadelphia.

R059 Aluminum and sea snail: Le Maire Paris; made for John Wanamaker N.Y.: # K 94546.

R068 Brass, black enamel, and sea snail: Le Maire Fab. Paris (with a bee).

R073 Sea snail: caps—Le Maire, Paris; A.A. Webster & Co. Brooklyn, N.Y.: center bar—a bee and Made in France: bottom bar—owner's monogram.

R074 Mother-of-pearl, straight adjustable Loumiere handle coming out of the center of the side of the glasses: caps—The B.H. Stief Jewelry Co., Nashville, Tenn.; LeMaire Fi Paris.

R077 Sea snail outer barrels and double-pull lorgnette handle: caps—Le Maire Fabi Paris: top bar—12 lenses: underside of top bar—No. 23719: outer side of bottom frame—MRD. After market?

R078 Mother-of-pearl, turning handle affixed to bottom of glasses: caps—Le Maire Fi Paris (bees on both): underside of center bar—No. 5, a bee, and Made in France.

R081 Mother-of-pearl, brass inner barrels, Loumiere handle: caps—Le Maire Fi Paris; Whelan-Aehle-Hutchinson Jewelry Co. St. Louis (two bees on each cap): center bar—No. 5 and *K* surrounded by Pat. Nov. 28, 82 and Sn. 266112, a bee surrounded by Pat. May 7–95 Sn 539006.

R092 Pink enamel with four floral medallions, aluminum frame and inner barrels: top bar—April 16, 1894: underside of center bar—#63 and a bee: underside of bottom bar—JMC from JCB (after market).

R096 Turquoise, teal blue, triple-glazed, four medallions with floral insets: caps—Le Maire Paris; Theo Eagle St. Louis.

R100 Triple-glazed enamel, dark blue, four medallions, brass frame and inner barrels, mother-of-pearl lens caps: underside of center bar—#63, a bee, and #12.

R117 Brass and black enamel skeleton with black lip pearl caps, green enamel over machined metal bell-shaped barrels with black cross hatching and silver overlay baked into intersections, medium-size: caps—Le Maire Paris, #63, and a bee: circa 1880.

R126 Gold-dyed mother-of-pearl and brass, solid handle in center: Lemaire, Paris (bee): "K" pat. (268112) Nov. 28, 1882: owner's initials M.B.L.: 539006 pat. May 7, 1895: caps—Geo Bausch, Syracuse, N.Y.

R127 White mother-of-pearl and brass, solid adjustable handle: Lemaire, Paris (bee).

R133 Mother-of-pearl and brass, mother-of-pearl caps: caps—Exposition Universelle 1867; Lemaire Fabricant Paris: top bar—Duchesse 12 Verres (engraved).

R135 Mother-of-pearl and brass, telescoping mounted handle, mother-of-pearl layered inner barrels, center adjusting pylon: Lemaire, Paris.

R136 Mother-of-pearl and brass, mother-of-pearl caps, in leather case: caps—Lemaire Fab. Paris (bee in center): center bar—a bee and #61: top bar—Made in France.

R143 Sea snail and brass: sea snail caps—Lemaire, Paris: left crossbar—#63: right crossbar—#24 & Bee?

R156 Brass, dark green French enamel with gold stars and floral bouquets, hourglass-shaped ivory caps, large-size, triple-glazed: crossbar—#6 and a bee (Lemaire): circa 1875.

R161 Gilt brass and reticulated gilt over sharkskin, mother-of-pearl caps: crossbar—a bee (Lemaire): no other markings.

R162 Gold-dyed mother-of-pearl and brass with fancy brass borders: caps—Lemaire Paris: crossbar—a bee and #63.

R168 Sea snail, gilt, brass, no case but in original cardboard box: caps—Lemaire Fab, Paris; The Harvey Lewis Co. USA: left crossbar—#61: right crossbar—a bee (Lemaire).

R187 Brass and mother-of-pearl lined inner barrel, in leather case: caps—Lemaire Paris (two bees): underside of top bar—Made in France (twice): underside of center bar—Made in France and a bee.

R200 Aluminum and black pearl, fitted for separate telescoping handle, which is black pearl and locks in place: caps—Lemaire Paris (with two bees on each cap): underside of crossbar—a bee and #61.

R202 Black enamel and black pearl: caps—Chavonnoz Ingenileer Opticien; Bordeaux 37 Cours de L'Intendance: underside of crossbar—a bee (Lemaire): top bar—Lumelle Duchesse: underside of bottom bar—owner's initials *BC*.

R203 Chromed metal with beaded rings and black pearl: caps—Lemaire F¹? (two bees on each cap): underside of center bar—#61, a bee, and Made in France.

R218 Brass with black enameled caps, extension separate handle on the side: caps—Lemaire Paris; Platt and Goodthein, Cincinnati, O.: underside of center bar—Made in France and a bee.

LE MAITRE FAB I   Paris

C133 White mother-of-pearl caps, outer barrels and reeded turning knob, brass frame and inner barrels: one lens cap—Lemaitre FAB¹ Paris; other cap—T.H. Lynch, 1 & 3 Union Square.

LAMARYE   Paris

C295 Caps—LaMarye, Paris: no other markings. Sea Snail.

LEMIERE

C159 Mother-of-pearl, single-pull handle: caps—Lemiere: Optician Fabricant; #5 Av. De L'Opera, Paris.

LE MIEUX   Paris

C148 Mother-of-pearl: caps—LeMieux Paris: underside of bottom bar—LENA (in script).

C255 White mother-of-pearl: caps—Lemieux, Paris.

LE MIUX   Paris

LE PÈRE   Paris

C292 Mother-of-pearl outer barrels and lens caps, brass inner barrels, center bar and frame: caps—LePere Paris.

LE PRINCE   France

C061 Sea snail: caps—Le Prince Paris: underside of top bar—Made in France: bottom of bottom bar—12-25, 1902 (after market).

LE ROI   Paris

C135 Sea snail, brass frame: caps—Le Roi.

C359 Sea snail, corrugated vinelike brass trim, single-pull lorgnette handle: caps—Le Roi Paris: underside of center bar—Made in France and *LE* within diamond shape.

LE ROQUE   Paris   #30 & #31

C085 Chip on barrel: caps—LeRoque-Paris: underside of center bar—Made in France. Sea Snail.

C147 Brass barrels, chrome over brass trim: caps—LeRoque-Paris: underside of center bar—Made in France.

LOUCHET   Paris

R057 Ivory and brass, circa 1845: Louchet Paris.

LUMIÈRE   Paris

MARCHAND   France
             Paris

C043 Sea snail: caps—Marchand-Paris: underside of top bar—Made/France.

C044 Sea snail: caps—Marchand-Paris: underside of top bar—Made/France.

C132 Mother-of-pearl: caps—Marchand Paris: underside of top bar—Made in France.

C016 Sea snail, three-pull turn knob: caps—Marchand-Paris: underside of top bar—Made in France.

C199 Sea snail, brass frame: caps—Marchand Paris: underside of top bar—Made in France.

C289 Mother-of-pearl, brass frame and center step: caps—Marchand, Paris: underside of top bar—Made in France.

MARCON   Paris

C102 Mother-of-pearl, lorgnette handle of engraved brass: caps—Marcon-Paris.

MAR NEIL   Paris

C127 Mother-of-pearl, brass frame: caps—Mar Neil Paris: underside of center bar—France: outer side bottom bar—*AEM* (after market).

MARQUISETTE   Paris

C091 Miniature-size: caps—Shreve & Co. San Francisco: underside of middle bar—*C* within six-pointed star: bottom bar—Marquisette Paris. Sea snail.

MEISSONNIER   Paris

C020 Mother-of-pearl, thin barrels, bottle shaped: caps—Meissonnier-Paris.

MERVEILLE ET CIE   Paris   #3

C012 Sea snail, lorgnette handle, with cardboard box—Balcony April 23: caps—Merveille et Cie Paris; I.A. Foye—Hot Springs, Ark.: underside of center bar—*LE* within diamond shape.

J. E. MILCH (MIELCK) St. Petersburg,
             Moscow

C055 Mother-of-pearl: caps—J.E. Mielck, St. Petersburg Moscow.

MONROY F I   Paris   #35

C331 Caps—Monroy FI Paris (symbol between words): underside of center bar—fleur-de-lis. Mother-of-pearl.

MOURLON FAB I   Paris

C096 Mother-of-pearl, single-pull lorgnette handle: caps—Mourlon FAB¹ Paris; Mourlon FAB¹ France.

NARCISSUS   Paris

C126 Iridescent sea snail, single-pull lorgnette handle: caps—Narcissus Paris: underside of bottom bar—B.C.M. (after market).

C349 Abalone: caps—Narcissus Paris. Nerdi Paris

C059 Sea snail, mother-of-pearl eye caps: top bar— Nerdi-Paris.

NOËL   Paris

R125 Filigree and sea snail: Noël, Paris: circa 1886.

PRAECEDO #36

C230 Black leather, black enamel inner barrels and frame, outer barrels—The Praecedo within a diamond shape: caps—Queen & Co. Phil.

PRECIOPTIC LEVALLOIS

C225 Mother-of-pearl, brass trim and frame, very small unique design—folding single central bar closes pair to less than 3" length, 1 ½" height: caps—Precioptic Levallois: bottom of eyepieces—slight adjustment markings.

PREMIER   Paris   #37

C321 Grey, lorgnette handle: caps—Premier Paris.

C336 Sea snail with chased brass trim: caps—Premier Paris: underside of center bar—Made in France and a rose.

RIVERA   France   #31

C027 Black enamel/leather: caps—Rivera Rivera; France: underside of center bar—Made in France.

RODENSTOCK   Munich   #38
Charlottenburg

C322 Caps—Berlin-Munchen * Charlottenburg; Josef Rodenstock * Optiker: underside of top bar—V.Z.G. 2832: bottom bar—Busch (after market).

R186 Aluminum and sea snail, in leather case: caps—Josef Rodenstock, Berlin; Josef Rodenstock Munchen: underside of cross bar—*LE* within diamond shape.

ROSS   London   #39 & #40

C144 Mother-of-pearl, double-pull lorgnette handle: caps—Bruxelles #94 Rue Neuve; Paul Schaer, Optician.

SOCIÉTÉ D'OPTIQUE Paris   #41

C202 Alternating mother-of-pearl and sea snail outer barrels, chrome over brass trim and inner barrels: caps—Société D'Optique.

SPORTIÈRE   Paris   #42

C080 Gun metal, raised hunting scene: caps—Sportier-Paris: underside of center barrel—Made in France.

C113 Gun metal with raised hunting scene, chrome over brass frame: caps—Sportière Paris (words separated by a star): underside of top bar—Made in France.

C180 Gun metal finish, raised design of birds and fruit: caps—Sportière Paris (words separated by five-pointed star): underside of top bar—Made in France.

C280 Mother-of-pearl: caps—Sportier, Paris (raised block letters, words separated by solid five-pointed stars): underside of top bar—Made in France.

C288 White mother-of-pearl, chrome over brass lens caps: caps—Sportier, Paris: underside of top bar—Made in France.

C294 Dark grey gun metal outer barrels with raised design of birds, flowers, and berries, brass inner barrels, chrome eye caps: caps—Sportier, Paris (words separated by raised five-pointed star).

C392 Gun metal outer barrels with hunting scene of dogs and stag in high relief, parts of brass frame are chrome-plated: caps—Sportier, Paris (two five-pointed stars one on each cap separating words): underside of top bar—Made in France.

R166 Black enamel and black leather: caps—Sportière Paris: cross bar—Made in France.

R209 Chrome and case pewter barrels: caps—Sportière Paris: underside of cross bar—Made in France.

SPORTREIL   Paris

STENRE FABT   Paris

R091 Iridescent green enamel outer barrels and single-pull lorgnette handle, medallion on each barrel with male and female figures, medallion on lorgnette with female figure: caps—Stenre Fabt Paris: underside of center bar—*LE* within a diamond shape.

THÉZARD   #27

C347 Ivory, large pair: caps—Thezard 141 Palais-Royal (raised lettering—five dots on either side of Thezard).

TUMELLE DUCHESSE

C158 Mother-of-pearl stripes, alternating colors: top of top bar—Tumelle Duchesse (handwritten) after market.

R084 Mother-of-pearl, brass inner barrels, twist-type focus: atop center bar—Tumelle Duchesse: underside of bottom bar—Isadora F. McIntyre: no maker's marks.

VENDÔME   Paris

C278 White mother-of-pearl outer barrels, chrome inner barrels, center turning knob and frame: caps—Vendôme, Paris (raised lettering).

R192 Aluminum, turned and anodized red and pink barrels: caps—Vendôme, Paris.

R193 Aluminum, turned and octagonal barrels, red anodized: caps—Vendôme, Paris.

VERDI   Paris

C095 Sea snail: caps—Verdi F^l Paris; H.C. Graffe-Fort Wayne, Ind.

C155 Iridescent purple and white sea snail, inner and outer barrels are of multiple alternating stripes: caps—Verdi F^l Paris.

C178 Mother-of-pearl, brass frame: caps—Verdi F^l Paris.

C233 Brass, silver-plated, designs on outer barrels of an ear of corn and leaves on a stalk: caps—Verdi F^l Paris (words separated by circular design within a diamond shape).

C244 White mother-of-pearl, brass frame, small pair: caps—Ball, Black & Co., New York (words separated by stars): top of top bar—Marquise #12 Verdi (in script).

R066 Sea snail and gilt, circa 1895: Verdi (F^l Paris).

VERNE   Paris

C195 Sea snail, brass trim: caps—Verne Paris.

VERTIER   Paris

R064 Fluted black leather and gilt (?): Vertier Paris.

WALDSTEIN   Vienna

C014 Mother-of-pearl, green enamel, lorgnette handle, Napoleonic feeling, gold wreaths festooned: caps—Wein I Kohlmarkt 20; J. Waldstein, Optikea: Vienna.

WOLLENSAK   Rochester, New York

R012 Black enamel, texturized metal, black leather case: Biascope, Rochester USA, Wollensak.

R171 Black enamel and black leather, in black leather case: B.L. Wollensak, Rochester U.S.A. Bioscope.

MANUFACTURER UNKNOWN   Austria

R101 Porcelain, bell-shaped tubes with signed outdoor scene of man and woman, brass body, mother-of-pearl caps, medium-size pair: Austrian circa 1850: no markings.

R112 Porcelain bell-shaped barrels with silver background and man and woman in forest, small-size, brass with mother-of-pearl caps: no markings—Austrian?: circa 1880.

R103 Manufacturer unknown: Occupied Japan

R018 Chrome frame, embossed copper: occupied Japan.

R211 Chrome and pewter barrels: marked Made in Occupied Japan, underside of bottom bar (1945–51).

R003 Russian yellow plastic, black leather case: marked USSR, manufacturer unknown.

R229 Maroon enamel: on case—Made in USSR: marked "cccp" etc.: circa 1970.

MANUFACTURER UNKNOWN

C002 Mother-of-pearl, aluminum: caps—Hammersmith & Field, San Francisco.

C011 Sea snail, decorated center stem: caps—American Optician Paris; E.B. Meyrowitz, New York.

C017 Sea snail, odd shape, taller than most: no name.

C019 Sea snail: caps—Hirsch & Kaiser, San Francisco: top bar—Made in France (in script).

C026 Purple sea snail: caps—no name: top bar—G.E. Pryor-Ingopt (#1–B Rue Huber Paris).

C030 Mother-of-pearl, lorgnette handle: caps—Wm Kendricks Sons, Louisville KY: underside of middle bar—*LE* within diamond shape: bottom of bottom bar—Karrier Gardener (after market). (The symbol *LE* within a diamond shape was used by the following manufacturers: Bertier, Elite, La Corona, La Touraine, Le Roque and Le Roi.)

C032 Mother-of-pearl, lorgnette handle: caps—The G.W. Jewelry Co., Peoria, IL.

C040 Mother-of-pearl, chrome and brass trim: caps—Thompson Jeweler; G.R. Thompson Optician.

C041 White mother-of-pearl barrels/caps: caps—Made in France for; Andrew J. Lloyd & Co. Boston.

C042 White mother-of-pearl: caps—Made in France for James Mc Creery & Co, New York: underside of top bar—Made in France.

C057 Short glasses, brass gilded rings on each barrel, lorgnette handle: caps—Mermod Jaccard & King, N.Y.; Mermod Jaccard & King Co., St. Louis: bottom of bottom bar — Tris Paris.

C060 Caps—Estberg & Sons, Waukesha. Wis: No other marks.

C067 White enamel, gold festoons: caps—L. Ulrich, Opticien; #4 Jardin Public-Nice-"Foreign".

C073 Blue enamel, paintings of French women, enamel lorgnette handle: caps—Schumacher & Toreman; Baltimore MD.

C076 White mother-of-pearl miniature, chrome metal, small case: no name.

C077 Sea snail: caps—Fowlers (in script), Chicago (block letters): underside of center bar—France.

C092 Sea snail: caps—Made in France for Wm. Senter & Co. Portland ME: underside of top bar—Made in France.

C099 Sea snail: caps—C.C.: underside of center bar—#63: bottom bar—E. Schmutz (after market) (possibly Lemaire).

C106 Brass frame, odd shape, two-tiered barrels separated by a bell-shaped brass fitting: No markings.

C115 Bakelite-type outer barrels: base of turning knob—Broy's Special Patent (arrow under Broy and #2 above).

C121 Cloisoine barrels, very short pair: caps—La Haye Heijnen; La Heijnen, Opticien.

C129 Abalone barrels, aluminum frame: caps—F.W. Richter, Dresden-Foreign: underside of center bar—*Z*.

C139 Mother-of-pearl, chrome over brass frame: caps—Optical Institute-Paris (in script).

C150 Sea snail, brass frame: caps—Goldsmith & Son-Washington.

C157 Mother-of-pearl, single-pull lorgnette handle: caps—Mulford-Memphis Tenn: top of side bar—Made in France:

bottom of outside bar—October 15, 1902 and EHC: underside of center bar—*LE* within diamond shape: underside of top bar—Made in France.

C160 Mother-of-pearl, single-pull lorgnette handle, small pair: only marking is *RT* within diamond shape.

C165 Mother-of-pearl: caps—C. Muller-San Francisco: front of round vertical knob—*M* over winged horse (Pegasus)—gives the effect of a unicorn.

C166 Black leather, brass trim: caps—(Vienna) Semmons Wien.

C167 Mother-of-pearl: caps—Made in France Specially For; Andrew J. Lloyd & Co., Boston: underside of top bar—Made in France.

C170 Purple sea snail, double-pull lorgnette handle, aluminum frame: underside of bottom bar—Asprey: underside of center bar—RT within symbol.

C181 Bone, brass inner barrels, taller than most.

C186 Ivory single-lens monocular, brass inner barrel, brass rings at top, center and bottom: barrel—Sleulen (in script) and London (in print).

C188 Black enamel leather-covered outer barrels, black enamel inner barrels: caps—Dinard Paris; A. Perain Optician.

C189 White mother-of-pearl, aluminum frame, housed in brown leather faux alligator-design case (stamped in gold inside lid—Diplom-Optiker Cravel Bremerhaven): caps—Cravel with sunburst; Bremerhaven with sunburst: underside of bottom bar—Bond.

C190 Chrome, black enamel trim: caps—Meyrowitz Bros. Albany.

C191 Purple mother-of-pearl, frame fitted for lorgnette handle (not attached): caps—J.H. Johnston and Co. New York: underside of center bar—*LE* within diamond shape.

C192 Sea snail, brass frame: caps—J.W. Batchelder, Buffalo, N.Y.

C193 Dark blue enamel with raised turquoise stones set in leaf designs, brass trim, single-pull lorgnette handle: underside of top bar—Made in France and #8.

C198 Mother-of-pearl, single-pull lorgnette handle: caps—no name.

C203 Sea snail: caps—Hardy & Hayes Pittsburgh, PA: underside of top bar—reverse bracket symbols.

C214 Mother-of-pearl, brass frame: caps—William Nagel Paducah KY: top of top bar—Made in France.

C226 Purple grosgrain effect under lacquer, brass bars, stem and inner barrels, 1 ½" high when closed, 2" high when opened, housed in blue leatherette case: caps—E. Gome Opticien; 2 Rue Duphot Paris.

C227 Reptile leather, taupe-colored, chrome inner barrels, eyepieces, stem and support, housed in matching taupe-colored reptile leather case: underside of top bar—Made in France.

C228 Glazed dark red enamel with gold stars in field, floral designs, bell-shaped, large size—5 ¼" when extended, double ivory tops and turning knob: no markings.

C231 Caps—Heinrich Rath, Hof-Optiker; Residenz Str. 21 Munchen.

C236 Purple mother-of-pearl, lorgnette handle affixed to bottom of frame: caps—J. Wiss & Sons, Newark, N.J.: underside of center bar—horsehead: top of center bar—Made in France.

C238 Brass, ivory and horn lens caps, housed in original case with markings: caps—Negretti & Zambra; Opticians to the Queen, London: corner underside of top bar—#12. (possibly Lemaire)

C239 Mother-of-pearl, chrome, in original case: caps—G. Santi Opticien; G. Santi Marseille: underside of top bar—#20, 57, T.N. (scratched on—after market).

C240 Brass, in original case: caps—Negretti & Zambra Opticians (in script); Holborn.

C241 White mother-of-pearl: caps—Optical House of M.H. Harris: underside of top bar—Made in France: underside of center bar—A.S. inside of a star within a triangle.

C243 Mother-of-pearl, brass frame, very small pair: underside of center bar—*RT* within diamond shape.

C248 Sea snail outer barrels, brass inner barrels, black enamel frames: caps—J.J. Freeman, Toledo, O.

C250 Ivory outer barrels, brass inner barrels and frame: no other markings.

C263 Mother-of-pearl, brass frame: caps—Hauserman's, Patterson, N.J.: underside of center bar—Made in France and #8.

C268 White sea snail, fitted for lorgnette handle but none attached: caps—Challoner & Mitchell Victoria, B.C.: Inscription reads "Presented by C & M Devel Teague to Madge Robinson Watt for Literary Work".

C273 Aluminum outer barrels, alternating silver color and fuchsia, brass inner barrels, aluminum frame with raised lettering, design on barrels is incused.

C276 White mother-of-pearl outer barrels, alternating brass/copper inner barrels and frames, two-tier barrels, one larger than the other.

C282 Black enamel outer barrels, brass inner barrels and frame, attached swivel lorgnette handle made of horn: caps—Par Brevet D'Invention Et De Pref nt; other cap is blank.

C285 Brown-grained leather outer barrels (diamond pattern), brass frame, black enamel eye caps, larger size-4" extended length.

C286 All brass, black enamel bars: no markings.

C287 Brass inner and outer barrels and frame, black enamel eye caps extended, Wall of Troy type circular trim on top and bottom: no markings.

C296 Horn outer barrels, brass inner barrels and frame, fitted for lorgnette handle, center stem embossed with leaf design brass overlay: caps—Conichon, Place, Des Victoires A. Paris (followed by a cluster of six dots).

C297 Tan leather-wrapped outer barrels, brass inner barrels and frame, leather-wrapped single-pull lorgnette handle, housed in matching leather case that reads—Made in France for Besthoff (in script) New York: underside of center bar—#6: top of top bar—Besthoff (in script) New York and made in France.

C298 Sea snail outer barrels, brass inner barrels, center stem and base caps, chrome eye caps, top, center and middle bars: no markings.

C299 Ivory outer barrels and center turning knob, brass inner barrels, frame, and center rod: no markings.

C300 Ivory outer barrels, eye caps, and center turning knob, center of eye caps enameled with black over ivory, brass inner barrels, top, center, and bottom bars: no markings.

C301 Mother-of-pearl, metal frame, inner barrels read: Joseph Godchaux Optician; 9 Bard Des Italiens Paris (black enameled square letters).

C308 Mother-of-pearl, lorgnette handle: caps—Chas. Noack Sacramento.

C309 Non-USA: underside of center bar—J. Hoen Optn Lyon Brotteaux.

C314 Pink enamel: caps—Lance L Paris.

C316 Red enamel: caps—Arnhold Opticien; 13 Rue Auber Paris.

C317 White mother-of-pearl: caps—Kornblum Pittsburgh PA; Kornblum Pittsburgh, PA.

C323 Mother-of-pearl inner barrels: caps—Lange and Lange Debuque.

C325 Tortoiseshell: caps—Dixon and Hampenstall Dublin.

C327 Ridges on barrels, lorgnette handle: caps—Made in France For; A. J. Stark and Co. Denver: underside of top bar—Made in France.

C333 Handle: caps—Steward Dawson and Co. Ltd; Regent St. W.

C337 Caps—F. Gscheidel Koenigsberg.

C339 Ridge wood black lens caps: caps—Theodore B. Starr New York.

C344 Caps—A. Meulemans Opticien; Rue de La Madeleine 70 Bruxelles (four "bugs" separate words).

C345 White mother-of-pearl: caps—A. Stowell and Co. Boston.

C346 Caps—Prosper Bunoust Ingr Opticien; Palais-Royal #3 Paris.

C350 Abalone, handle: caps—Hofman's Columbus O.: top bar—Made in France: underside of center bar—*LE* within diamond shape.

C351 Brass, large pair: caps—Hayes Brothers; Barry Dock and Cardiff.

C352 Grained leather: top of top bar—Derress and #8.

C353 Leather: right barrel—Ross London: left barrel—I 1905.

C354 Green enamel barrels with glaze finish, brass trim, black eye caps, half beads forming oval frames: no markings.

C361 Greenish abalone, brass-bronze combination eye caps and frame, copper trim, highly chased brass floral design at top and bottom of barrels, more square than most.

C365 Horn outer barrels with high lacquer finish (due to small chip near bottom), brass inner barrels and frame, black center, top and bottom bars, very light weight.

C366 Sky blue enamel, half beads festooned into oval and garlands—flowers in the ovals.

C367 High relief of flower garlands at top of outer barrels, violin over a bagpipe on both sides, brass inner barrels, chrome eye caps, top, bottom, and center bars.

C370 White mother-of-pearl straight barrels, brass frame, very small pair: top of center bar—Made in France.

C371 Pink enamel with high gloss, many pearllike half beads including brass oval frames as trim: underside of center bar—Made in France: unmarked caps.

C372 Ivory, highly polished, brass inner barrels and trim: no markings.

C373 White mother-of-pearl and darker sea snail in alternating vertical stripes on outer barrels, brass inner barrels and trim, bars show some chrome plating: underside of top bar—J (possibly after market).

C375 White mother-of-pearl, matching single-pull lorgnette handle, brass trim: no markings.

C377 Snakeskin-covered outer barrels, brass inner barrels, brass trim with chrome top, center, and bottom bars, ivory eye caps: underside of top bar—Made in France.

C378 Fine black leather-covered outer barrels, brass inner barrels, frames, eye caps, and bars: no markings.

C379 Highly designed brocade gold and cream fabric outer barrels, highly lacquered, polished brass (pink in color) trim, inner barrels, and frame, small pair: underside of center bar—#61 and France.

C380 Tan and brown snakeskin-covered outer barrels, brass inner barrels and trim, ivory lens caps: underside of top bar—Made in France.

C381 Ivory, barrel-shaped outer barrels, brass inner barrels and trim, ivory turning knob: no markings.

C383 Brass inner barrels, frame and center bar, chrome lens caps and crossbars (3): underside of center bar—c2: (French).

C386 White mother-of-pearl outer barrels and eye caps, matching top-folding lorgnette, brass inner barrels, frame, center pole, and bars, rather small pair: no markings.

C388 White mother-of-pearl outer barrels and eye caps separated by copper trim, all other trim is brass with chrome plating: no markings.

C390 Ivory and brass outer barrels, brass inner barrels and trim (quite elaborate), eye cap has extra ivory base between top of top bar and bottom of cap: no markings.

C393 Deep red, reeded outer barrel, brass inner barrel, black trim, single-lens spyglass type: no markings.

C394 Ivory single-lens spyglass type, brass inner barrel: no markings.

C397 Fabric-looking pale yellow underglaze material on outer barrels, brass inner barrels, frame, and trim, very small size, single-pull lorgnette handle: no markings.

C398 Ivory outer barrels with many carved designs—circles, half moons, and half dots, brass inner barrels and trim, folk artlike : no markings.

CAA4 White mother-of-pearl outer barrels, brass frame and inner barrels: caps—H. Rosenberg-Canon City COLO: top and bottom of top bar—Made in France: no other markings, housed in what is probably the original case, case has a bee on the lock button.

CAA5 White mother-of-pearl inner and outer barrels: caps—Hight & Fairfield Butte-Mont; Butte-Mont: latter cap is half mother-of-pearl and half replacement wood: underside of center bar—France.

R002 French enamel, adjustable P.D. gold lamé case, circa 1930: on base—France.

R004 Black lip pearl, aluminum frame.

R005 French enamel and gilt: Brevet d'Invention.

R006 French enamel and gilt, folding horn swinging handle: "Jumelle Par Brevet d'Invention."

R007 Abalone, sea snail caps and turning knob, brass frame.

R008 French vermeil and enamel, swinging horn handle.

R010 Black enamel frames, leather outer barrels, black leather case.

R014 Green leather woman's evening set, perfume bottle, folding fan, opera glasses, brass and green leather: underside of bar—R.T.

R016 English field glasses, black leather and black enameled metal leather purse, compass between lenses.

R017 Mother-of-pearl, aluminum frame: Bailey Banks & Biddle Philadelphia.

R022 Pink brushed aluminum: French, circa 1895.

R023 Same as #22, no markings, larger size.

R024 Abalone and brass, single-pull lorgnette handle: French.

R025 Abalone and brass, abalone single-pull lorgnette handle, mother-of-pearl tip.

R026 Abalone and chrome, single-pull lorgnette handle, mother-of-pearl tip, velvet bag.

R027 Abalone and brass, long barrels: caps—Paris.

R028 Tortoise and aluminum with long swinging tortoiseshell handle, silver open-book design near tip of handle (cartouche).

R029 Small red enamel with pink roses: French, circa 1890.

R030 Tortoise and aluminum.

R031 Tortoise and machined aluminum.

R034 Ivory and brass Greek key trim.

R035 Ivory and brass, ivory caps.

R036 Ivory and chrome, cloth purse.

R038 Embossed, engraved, and enameled aluminum, brass inner barrels.

R040 Ivory and brass, ridged tips and bottoms of outer barrels.

R041 Engraved mother-of-pearl, brass and gilt trim, handle swings over top of glasses, leaf design on center stem: Fab Brevet d'Invention.

R042 Engraved and embossed long-length barrels, ivory lens caps and turning knob.

R044 Engraved mother-of-pearl and copper: Par Brevet d'Invention et de Perf NT.

R045 Striped ivory barrels and gilt, swinging lorgnette handle: Brevete d'Invention.

R046 Drilled bone barrels (fenestrated).

R049 Black lacquer elliptical eyepieces: Jumelle Elliptique Brevetée S.G.D.G.

R050 Sea snail and brass, adjustable frames.

R051 Elliptical-shaped ivory glasses, large size, elliptical eyepieces, brass trim.

R052 Edwardian embossed brass.

R053 Brass and embossed silver, small, French, circa 1890, with extension handle.

R054 Embossed, small-size, (?) U.S. circa 1930.

R055 French, small-size, chrome, circa 1935.

R058 Aluminum and sea snail, French, inner and outer barrels covered.

R060 Fluted brass and black enamel: unmarked.

R061 Mother-of-pearl and brass, large-size: caps—OB & T 529 Broadway N.Y.: crossbar—opera glasses 8 verres.

R063 French mother-of-pearl, large-size: unmarked.

R065 Brass and sea snail, French manufactured circa 1910: cap—Knight and Son, North Hampton.

R067 Black enamel and brass, orange French enamel.

R070 Aluminum and brass, French: unmarked.

R072 Aluminum and leather over aluminum barrels, circa 1890, 4X, adjustable P.D.: caps—Paul A. Meyrowitz, 287 Fifth Ave.; Made in France for Prism Optics.

R076 Sea snail outer barrels, brass inner barrels: caps—Made in France expressly for; Jaeger Bros. Portland, Oregon: underside of center bar—*LE* within a diamond shape.

R080 Mother-of-pearl, chrome trim, swivel ring at rear end, lorgnette handle.

R083 Sea snail outer barrels and double-pull lorgnette handle, aluminum frame and inner barrels: underside of center bar—#61.

R087 Mother-of-pearl: caps—M. Burt and Co. Jewelers; Cleveland, Ohio: no maker's marks.

R089 Brass inner barrels and center rod, light blue enamel gold trim, four floral arrangements, triple-glazed: no markings.

R090 Brass frame and inner barrels, ivory lens caps and center turning rod, triple-glazed navy blue with four floral medallions.

R093 Reticulated brass overlay on bell-shaped aluminum barrels, aluminum top, bottom and center bars, anodized inner barrels and center stem, pierced work.

R095 Triple-glazed enamel, primarily red with gold and silver overlays, brass frame, mother-of-pearl eye cap trim: no markings.

R099 Leather-wrapped outer barrels, brass frame, aluminum eye caps and bars, housed in cloth snap-lock pouch: underside of center bar—No. 30: no markings.

R103 Cylindrical tubes of pieces of pink-dyed mother-of-pearl, small-size, chromed brass, case: "Made in France."

R106 Japanese black metal with plastic mother-of-pearl, CHEAP, medium size.

R111 Red porcelain bell-shaped barrels with picture of two men sitting, gold overlay, large-size, aluminum with mother-of-pearl caps: no markings: circa 1875.

R113 Aluminum, bell-shaped barrels of navy blue porcelain with angels, large-size: no markings—French?: circa 1895.

R114 Brass with cylindrical barrels, turquoise enamel over machined brass, small-size: no markings—French?: circa 1900.

R115 Brass with hourglass-shaped mother-of-pearl caps, bell-shaped barrels with pink diamonds on blue enamel background, large-size: "Tiffany & Co. N.Y.": circa 1880.

R118 Folding ivory with mirror and compass: circa 1920.

R119 Dark blue French enamel with handle: circa 1880.

R120 Monocular, French enamel, four-draw.

R128 White mother-of-pearl with mother-of-pearl telescoping handle on side, aluminum base: French, *LE* within a diamond shape (manufacturer, France): Made for H. Murr's Sons, Phila.

R129 Mother-of-pearl and brass, medium-size: marked *X* with a line above it on the crossbar.

R130 Mother-of-pearl and aluminum: made for Tiffany & Co., New York (by unknown maker): no markings.

R131 Typical French mother-of-pearl and brass with mother-of-pearl caps, barrels inlaid with gold in oriental motif: no markings.

R132 Large (4_" high) mother-of-pearl and brass with hourglass-shaped caps, continental type make: no markings.

R140 Dyed dark gold mother-of-pearl and brass, medium-size: crossbar—#7.

R141 Brass and snakeskin with mother-of-pearl caps: no markings.

R142 Mother-of-pearl and brass, medium-size: English?: no markings.

R144 Brass and brass filigree on barrels, bordering black leather chrome crossbars, hard rubber caps: one cap—leaf bouquet: no other markings.

R145 Ivory and brass barrels and lens caps, folding out handle: English: marked "Patent Ste SGBO" around G.P.

R146 Aluminum and leather, large-size, in leather French case: crossbar—#59 and C3: circa 1910.

R148 Folding cylindrical, chrome and leather: pylon cap—B TE SGOG: crossbar—":" : French: circa 1980.

R149 Black enamel metal, folding: English: "James Sinclair Co. Ltd, 54 Haymarket, London S.W.": Busch "Winett" Binocular Patent": circa 1925.

R150 Long, thin, cylindrical French-type barrels of black enamel metal, hard rubber and black leather, adjustable P.D. with unique screw top.

R151 Collapsible flat English nickel and brass: circa 1910.

R152 Collapsible flat French brass and mother-of-pearl with numbered focus marked "A. Lefevre Paris" on mother-of-pearl caps, in flat leather case: left cap arm—a symbol: right cap arm—France: center pylon—Jumelle Mars. BT EES France Etranger.

R153 Flat collapsible black metal, heavy and rather crude: Eastern European make?: no markings.

R154 Small brass and turquoise enamel over machine turnings with side-mount telescopic handle: French: no markings: circa 1895.

R157 Small brass and red enamel with mother-of-pearl caps, pink rose design on barrels: French: top of crossbar—#8: no other markings.

R158 Flat pair simulating a purse, gilt brass and mother-of-pearl, gold-tooled tan leather trim, perhaps worn as a chatelain: one cap—POCOSCOPE Patent 13411; other cap missing: English?: circa 1890.

R160 Gilt brass and filigree with faux jewels, brass caps: caps—Theodore B. Starr, New York: crossbar—Made in France and *LE* within a diamond shape.

R163 Light blue enamel and brass, triple-glazed floral garlands with mother-of-pearl caps: caps—C.D. Peacock, Chicago, Ill: cross bar—Made in France.

R165 Aluminum and tortoiseshell, in leather case: underside of crossbar—S: top of crossbar—Selfridge, London.

R167 English expanding, all aluminum with spinal barrels: "Aitchison's Patent 1016."

R169 Aluminum and black enamel with black leather panel: caps—Wall and Ochs, Philadelphia; Wall and Ochs Opticians 1716 Chestnut St., Philadelphia: top of crossbar—Jena Special Glass: underside of crossbar—Perimegashop.

R170 Black enamel, blue pseudo mother-of-pearl barrel, in brown leather case: Japanese: marked Pat. 237915: circa 1950.

R172 Black enamel brass and prism type: top of top bar—Prisma Paris: underside of top bar—Made in France.

R173 Brass and black leather, compass under lower bar, in black leather case: caps—Sporting Glass (three stars on each cap): underside of top bar—Made in France.

R174 Liquor bottle in shape of binoculars, glass with plastic top in brown leather case: bottle marked "Federal law forbids sale or reuse of this bottle": Label—"Personal Binocular bottle."

R175 Simulated opera glass in glass and plastic: labeled on left—"Juliette," and on right—"Romeo."

R176 Ceramic salt and pepper shakers simulating opera glasses: Souvenier of Sandown IW England: marked foreign on bottom.

R177 Ceramic salt and pepper shakers simulating opera glasses: from Cleethorpes, England with amorial on both sides: marked foreign on bottom.

R178 Ceramic salt and pepper shakers simulating opera glasses with salt container integral from Blackpool, England: marked foreign on bottom: England.

R179 Duplicate of #175.

R180 Ceramic salt and pepper shakers simulating opera glasses from "Niagara Falls, N.Y. Prospect Point": Label on bottom—"M S product — Made in Japan."

R181 Ceramic salt and pepper shakers simulating opera glasses: "Florida" on barrels: "Japan" on bottom.

R182 Orange salt and pepper shakers simulating opera glasses: "Rough Sea of Blackpool" and picture on left barrel: "Rough Sea Princess Parade Blackpool" and "Made in Japan" on bottom.

R183 Large black enamel and leather binoculars with extendable barrels: top bar—Made in France.

R184 Black enamel and leather, barrel extenders and loops for leather strap: caps—F. Bernhard Carlsbad: Triple ocular focus "Marine," "Field" and "Theater."

R185 Ivory and brass, in leather case: caps—W. Hooper Point Portsmouth: top bar—12 glasses: triple ocular focus—"Campagne," "théâtre" and "marine."

R188 Embossed and engraved aluminum, mother-of-pearl caps: caps—Imperial Optical Co. Paris: underside of crossbar (left)—*LE* within diamond shape, (right)—Made in France.

R194 Polished aluminum with twisted fluting on barrels and caps: "Jumelle Fin de Siecle."

R199 Aluminum, embossed, engraved, and grey enameled, in silk drawstring embroidered case: underside of top bar—Modern France: no other markings.

R201 Brass and black pearl: no markings.

R204 Brass and black pearl with brass garlands around barrels: underside of crossbar—*LE* within a diamond shape.

R207 Brass and black pearl (South Sea pearl), in velveteen pouch: no markings.

R208 Chrome metal and black cast barrels with black enamel: underside of crossbar—Foreign: Japanese?

R212 Aluminum and engraved brass barrels: English: circa 1900.

R213 Brass and engraved barrels: caps—Sporting Club Paris: underside of top bar—B H A in a design: top box—6 Verres: underside of center bar—#55.

R214 Black enamel and cast bronze barrels, chinoiserie decor: top of top bar—Superior glasses.

R217 Black enamel and leather (missing) on barrels, in leather case: caps—L. Bach Munchen: ocular focal lenses—"Campagne, Marine and Théâtre."

R219 Sea snail and gilt brass handle for opera glasses: no markings.

R220 Same as #219.

R221 Sea snail and base metal opera glass holder, marked "Julius King Opt. Co.," Patented Nov. 28, 1892, and Patented March 12, 1889.

R222 Gold-filled opera glass holder, machined and embossed: no markings: circa 1890.

R223 Mother-of-pearl and chrome opera glass holder, marked as #221.

R224 Silver embossed opera glass holder: no markings.

R225 Gilt brass and tortoiseshell opera glass, triple-draw: marked "12 Verres": French: circa 1860.

R227 Brass, black enamel, and black pearl, engraved and silver inlaid: caps—Klein Dezso: Budapest: circa 1880.

R228 Gilt, brass, mother-of-pearl, inner barrels covered with material: Prague bought: Made in Paris by H.D.: circa 1875.

R230 Black enamel, in chamois case: marked "Schmura, Budapest" and "Busch, Multinett": circa 1950.

New Orleans Opera Glasses

Mr. James H. Cohen, A.S.A.

C400 Sea snail, double-pull lorgnette handle: caps—Lemaire F^I Paris; Coleman E. Adler New Orleans (Lemaire bee separates the words): underside of center bar—a bee and #67: underside of top bar—Made in France and #7373.

C401 Sea snail, brass frame, single-pull lorgnette handle with brass trim: caps—read A. Bauman New Orleans, La.: underside of center bar—Made in France and *LE* within a diamond shape.

C402 Sea snail outer barrels with alternating stripes of two different kinds of vertical grain, chrome inner barrels, center rod, top, middle, side, and bottom bars, mother-of-pearl eye caps with black incised letters: caps—E & L Claudel New Orleans.

C403 Black enamel with very dark brown leather outer barrels: caps—E & L Claudel New Orleans: no other markings.

C404 Iridescent sea snail outer barrels and lens caps, brass frame with cut work in brass trim at bottom and top of outer barrels: caps—E & L Claudel New Orleans; Lemarie Paris (bee between words): Rumor says that these glasses belonged to "Miss Lottie", a minor French Quarter personage.

C405 Purple mother-of-pearl (dyed) outer barrels with beaded trim, brass frame, housed in typical Lemaire black leather case with a bee on the pushbutton: caps—Frigerio New Orleans; Frigerio 161 Canal St.

C406 White mother-of-pearl outer barrels, caps, and stem knob, rest is brass with many rings of brass beads on the barrels, turning knob and under the eye caps: caps—Frantz & Opitz New Orleans: Made in France (attempts to remove this after manufacture by gouging into the metal).

C407 Sea snail outer barrels and eye caps, rest is brass: caps—Frantz & Opitz N.O.; Lemaire F¹ Paris: underside of center bar—a bee and #63.

C408 Sea snail outer barrels and eye caps, brass frame, reeded top part of middle turning rod: caps—Frantz & Opitz New Orleans: underside of center bar—France: underside of the bottom crossbar—JLM (after market).

C409 Sea snail, double-pull lorgnette handle with a brass ring in the center, reeded mother-of-pearl turning rod, mother-of-pearl button that covers center screw at top of center bar: caps—A.B. Griswold & Co. New Orleans; Lemaire FAB¹ Paris (bee on each side of Paris): underside of top bar—Made in France and #15725: underside of center bar—#61 and a bee.

C410 Pink enamel with figures of two winged cherubs centered around an easel, reverses depict an outdoor urn, brass frame, black enamel crossbars, turning knob, and outside portion of eye caps—inside rings are sea snail: caps—A.B. Griswold & Co. New Orleans: underside of center bar—a bee and #63.

C411 Aluminum with raised design; flowers have 3D effect, white mother-of-pearl reeded center turning knob and caps: caps—A.B. Griswold & Co. New Orleans; Lemaire F¹ Paris (Paris separated by a bee design on both sides): underside of center bar—Made in France, #20, bee, and #33: top of the top bar—Nov 16, 1900 (after market): bottom bar—Chaille' Jamison ([a New Orleans physician]etched in after market).

C412 White mother-of-pearl, single pull lorgnette handle: caps—Le Fils Paris; A.B. Griswold & Co. New Orleans, La.

C413 Sea snail, 5/8" bell leading to eye caps, reeded white mother-of-pearl turning knob, brass trim: caps—Colmont FI Paris; A.B. Griswold & Co. New Orleans, La.: underside center bar—*C* within six pointed star: underside of top bar—France: underside of top bar—#30 (after market).

C414 Sea snail, chrome frame and inner barrels, handle near bottom of glasses that sticks straight, outfitted with a reeded turning knob to extend eye caps from the handle, also has turning knob at center rod for use when lorgnette handle is not in place: caps—Lemaire F¹ Paris (a bee on each side of Paris); A.B. Griswold & Co. New Orleans: underside of center bar—*K* surrounded by 268112 Pat. Nov 28, 82 (for 1882), also a bee surrounded by #539006 Pat May 7, 95: base of handle—a bee and "Trade Mark—Lemaire Paris".

C415 Sea snail outer barrels and eye caps, brass inner barrels and frame, straight removable lorgnette handle: caps—Lemaire F¹ Paris (a bee on each side of Paris); A.B. Griswold & Co. New Orleans, La.: underside of top bar—Made in France: underside of center bar—a bee surrounded by #539006 Pat May 7, 95, also *K* 268112 Pat Nov 18, 82: end of handle—a bee and "Trade mark—Lemaire Paris."

C416 Sea snail, black enamel frame, brass-beaded rings around base and top of outer barrel with two others below eye cap and three around center turning rod: caps—A.M. Hill New Orleans.

C417 Light blue enamel outer barrels festooned around top and bottom with gold fleur-de-lis, white oval background highlighted by many ½-pearl type of white enamel with floral design, small pair, brass frame, stem and inner barrels, reeded center turning knob of mother-of-pearl as are both eye caps and stem guide on top part of center bar: caps—Hyde & Goodrich: top bar—Duchesse 12 verres (in script).

C418 White mother-of-pearl, brass frame: caps—Lemaire F¹ Paris (a bee on each side of Paris); L. Jansen New Orleans: underside of center bar—Made in France and a bee: the initial *L* is for the name Leopold.

C419 Mother-of-pearl outer barrels, eye caps, and reeded center turning knob, brass frame and center rod: caps—Lemaire F¹ Paris; M. Scooler New Orleans: underside of center bar—#12, a bee, and #29.

C420 Sea snail outer barrels and eye caps: caps—Lemaire F¹ Paris (a bee on each side of Paris); M. Scooler New Orleans La.: underside of top bar—Made in France and #18506: underside of center bar—a bee and #61.

C421 White mother-of-pearl outer barrels and single-pull lorgnette handle (with brass tip and ring in center), brass and copper frame: caps—By Marchand Paris; and Weinfurter New Orleans—La: underside of center bar—Made in France and a rooster with *O* and *C* on either side of its feet.

C422 Brass barrels (formerly leather-wrapped), black enamel center bar: caps—Lemaire F¹ Paris (and a bee); Weinfurter, New Orleans, La.: underside of top bar—#775A: underside of center bar—Made in France, #61, and a bee.

C423 Sea snail outer barrels, eye caps, center turning knob screw cover, brass frame, inner barrels, and center turning knob, small pair: caps—Colmont F¹ Paris (six-pointed star and *C* separating words): underside of center bar—six-pointed star and *C*: underside of bottom bar—Comus 1926 (after market).

Retailers

The names of the following retailers below are usually found on one or both of the lens caps, as stated previously.

RETAILER	LOCATION
Coleman E. Adler	New Orleans LA
Henry C. Ahlers	San Jose CA
Anderson & Randolph	San Francisco CA
Jas. R. Armiger	Baltimore MD
Arnhold	Paris
Chas F. Artes	Evansville IL
Asprey	London
Bacon Bros.	Lowell MA
F. W. Badger	Beaumont TX
Bailey Banks & Biddle	Philadelphia PA
Ball, Black & Co.	New York NY
A. Bardou	Paris
J. W. Batchelder	Buffalo NY
A. Baumann	New Orleans LA
E. Bausch & Son	Rochester NY
Geo Bausch	Syracuse NY
Besthoff	New York NY
H.J. Blair	Bristol
Borhek & Son Opticians	Philadelphia PA
Briely & Son	Oshkosh WI
M. Burt and Co. Jewelers	Cleveland OH
Emile Busch A.G.	Rathenow
E. W. Butlon & Co.	Bridgeport CT
J. E. Caldwell & Co.	Philadelphia PA
J. E. Caldwell & Co.	Paris
Challoner & Mitchell	Victoria

Chavonnoz Ingenileer Opticien	
E & L Claudel	New Orleans LA
James Clegg	Buffalo NY
Cornichon	Paris
L. J. Cooke	Findlay OH
Cravel, Diplom-Optiker	Bremerhaven
Cresco Co.	France
Curley & Bro.	New York NY
Dachtera Bros.	New York NY
Steward Dawson and Co.	Regent St. [London]
Derepas Palais Royal	
Dixon and Hampenstall	Dublin
Barry Dock	Cardiff
Dollard	London
Dollond	London
Theo Eagle	St. Louis MO
Estberg & Sons	Waukesha WI
J. Flammarion	Paris
Fleurigny	Paris
Fowlers	Chicago IL
I.A. Foye	Hot Springs AR
Franklin & Co.	Washington, D.C.
Chas. S. Frantz	Lancaster MO
Frantz & Opitz	New Orleans LA
J. J. Freeman	Toledo OH
Frigerio	New Orleans LA
The G.W. Jewelry Co.	Peoria IL
Joseph Godchaux	Paris

Goldsmith & Son	Washington, D.C.
E. Gome Optician	Paris
H. C. Graffe	Fort Wayne IN
Grey	Paris
A. B. Griswold & Co.	New Orleans LA
F. Gscheidel	Koenigsberg
Hammersmith & Field	San Francisco CA
Hardy & Hayes	Pittsburgh PA
H. M. Harris	France
R. Harris & Co.	Washington, D.C.
Hauserman's	Patterson NJ
A. M. Hill	New Orleans LA
Hirsch & Kaiser	San Francisco CA
W. T. Hixson Co.	El Paso TX
Hofman's	Columbus OH
Hyde & Goodrich	New Orleans LA
Imperial Optical Co.	Paris
J. W.	Philadelphia PA
Jaeger Bros.	Portland OR
Jansen	New Orleans LA
J. H. Johnston and Co.	New York NY
Joslin & Park	Salt Lake City UT
Henry Kahn & Co.	San Francisco CA
Wm. Kendrick & Sons	Louisville KY
Kornblum	Pittsburgh PA
E. Krauss & Cie.	Paris, London
E. Krauss & Cie.	Leipzig, Milan
E. Krauss & Cie.	St. Petersburg

L. B. & Co.	Paris
La Heynen	
La Mignonne Gravière	Paris
Laine	Paris
L. Lance	Paris
Lange and Lange	Dubuque IA
Lavil	Paris
The Harvey Lewis Co.	USA
Archie Ligtmeyer	WI
Jos Linz and Bros.	Dallas TX
Andrew J. Lloyd & Co.	Boston MA
H. Y. Lowenstein	St. Louis MO
S. C. Mac Keown	Lawrence KS
Mar Neil	Paris
Marcon	Paris
McAllister Opt. Co.	Philadelphia PA
F.W. McAllister Co.	Baltimore MD
McCreery & Co.	New York NY
Max Meyer & Bro	Omaha NE
Mermod Jaccard & King Co.	St. Louis MO
Mermod and Jaccard Jewelry Co.	St. Louis MO
Meulemans	Brussels
Meyrowitz Bros	Albany NY
Meyrowitz Bros	New York NY
E. B. Meyrowitz	New York NY
J. E. Mielck	Moscow, St. Petersburg
Monroy	Paris
Mulford	Memphis TN

C. Muller	San Francisco CA
Busch Multinee D.R.C.M.	
H Murr's & Sons	Philadelphia PA
William Nagel	Paducah KY
Negretti & Zambra	London
Negretti & Zambra	Holborn
Nerdi	Paris
Chas. J. Noack	Sacramento CA
S. Nordlinger & Son	Los Angeles CA
OB & T	NY
B. Olbricht	Brooklyn NY
Optical Institute	Paris
C.D. Peacock	Chicago IL
A. Perain Optician	Paris
Platt and Goodthein	Cincinnati OH
Prosper Bunoust Ingr	Paris
Pryor-Ingopt	Paris
Queen & Co.	Philadelphia PA
Heinrich Rath	Munich
Jas. R. Reed & Co.	Pittsburgh PA
F. W. Richter	Dresden
J. Robinson Optician	Broadway New York
Josef Rodenstock	Berlin
Josef Rodenstock	Munich-Charlottenburg
Jobe Rose Jewelry Co.	Birmingham AL
Ross & Co.	London
G. Santi	Marseilles
Paul Schaer	Brussels
Scribner and Loehr Co.	Cleveland OH
E. Schmutz	

M. Scooler	New Orleans LA	J. W. Webb	Dallas TX
Schumacher & Toreman	Baltimore MD	A. A. Webster & Co.	Brooklyn NY
Semmons-Wein	Vienna	Weinfurter	New Orleans LA
Wm. Senter & Co.	Portland ME	Whelan-Aehle-Hutchinson Jewelry Co.	St. Louis MO
George C. Shreve & Co.	San Francisco CA	White & Mac Naught	Minneapolis MN
Shreve & Co.	San Francisco CA	Williams Brown & Earle	Philadelphia PA
Louis E. Shurtleff	New Bedford MA	J. Winreurgh and Son	Utica NY
Simmons Bros.	Columbus OH	J. Wiss & Son	Newark NJ
Simon Bros.	Columbus OH	Wollensak	Rochester MD
James Sinclair Co. Ltd.	London	Jacob Young	New Orleans LA
Sleulen	London		
A. J. Stark	Denver CO		
Theodore B. Starr	New York NY		
John A. Steinbach	San Francisco CA		
B. H. Stief Jewelry Co.	Nashville TN		
A. Stowell & Co.	Boston MA		
W. S. Taylor & Son	Utica NY		
Thezard	Paris		
G. R. Thompson	USA		
Tiffany	New York NY		
Traub & Co.	Detroit MI		
George P. Tuthill	St. Paul MN		
C. Ulrich, Opticien	Paris		
L. Ulrich Opticien	#4 Jardin Public Nice		
Vendome	Paris		
Ferd Wagner	Cincinnati OH		
Waldstein	Vienna		
Wall and Ochs	Philadelphia PA		
John Wanamaker	New York NY		
H. C. Warner	Fresno CA		

Description of Cases in J. Wm. Rosenthal's Collection

Art.#

R002 Gold lamé purse lined in gold velvet, rectangular, snap closure. French circa 1910.

R003 Black leather slip in case with snap closure. Russian circa 1989.

R009 Typical black leather French case, lining missing on top. No identifying marks.

R010 Typical French type. No identifying marks. Small.

R011 Typical French type, red interior, marked Rose & Co. 111 New Bond St. London.

R012 Black leather slip-in case, French circa 1930. Two snaps. No marks.

R014 Green leather case in the shape of woman's small purse holding small opera glasses, change purse, fan, scent bottle, pencil and pad, all en suite, circa 1925. Lined in green moiré. Probably U.S.

R016 Small glasses in grey suede purse lined in blue velvet. English circa 1910. Snap top.

R019 Typical black leather French case, lining missing on top. No identifying marks. Silk lining is purple. Snap has a bee.

R020 Typical black leather French case, lining missing on top. No identifying marks.

R026 Lorgnette-type glasses in tan velvet pouch case, closed by pullstring, lined in blue silk.

R029 Small typical French black leather case. Bee on latch button.

R034 Same as R029.

R036 Blue cloth pouch with snap top, lined in material.

R037 Hard wooden case covered with black leather outside and red silk inside. Marked "Louchet Opt. Sone-Paris, etc."

R062 Soft blue velvet pouch with drawstring. No marks.

R064 Typical French black leather case. No marks.

R093 Typical French black leather case. No marks.

R093 Typical French black leather case. Bee on button.

R094 Burgundy-colored velvet pouch. Drawstring.

R105 Typical French black leather case. "Traub Bros. & Co. Detroit" on inside.

R107 Gold lamé box lined in tan velvet, Irish circa. 1930.

R122 Brown velvet purse with snap top above and space for small glasses separately below. No mark on case.

R124 Typical French black leather case. No marks.

R136 Typical French black leather case. Bee on button.

R137 Typical French-style case. No marks.

R138 Typical French-style case. Blue silk lining. Fleur-de-lis on latch button.

R146 Typical French black leather case. Bee on button.

R152 Flat English folding glasses in slip-in case.

R159 Special green leather over hardboard-shaped case for flat purse type of glasses. Marked "DÉPASÉ."

Appendix

Many opera glasses are found devoid of identification except for certain numbers found on the crossbars. Probably, these are model numbers restricted to a particular manufacturer. This is not certain, however, and the numbers and frequency of findings with their associated manufacturers (if known) are presented as an introduction to their use and identification by collectors.

Numbers on Crossbars by Manufacturers

Manufacturer	Number	No. of Instances
Lemaire	2	1
	3C–63	1
	4	1
	5	1
	5/63	1
	6	1
	8	1
	9	1
	10/63	1
	10/21926	1
	12	2
	12/29	1
	13	3
	13/63	1
	16	2
	20/33	1
	21	1
	23	2
	23/63	2
	27	1
	28	1
	61	8
	61/775	1
	61/17092	1

	61/17992	1
	61/18506	1
	61/25208	1
	61/B38	1
	61/G1730	1
	61/G26053	1
	61/G26551	1
	63	31
	67	1
	67/7373	1
	68	1
	632	1
	2838	1
	3076	1
	17992A	1
	23719	1
	266112	1
	268112	5
	268112/539006	1
	27437	1
	28213	1
	30652	1
	31268A	1
	539006	3
	C4899	1
	D16449	1
	G04843	1
	G3B–33	1
Rodenstock	UZG 2832	1
Deraisme	81	1

IDA	61	1
Sporting Club-Paris	55	1
No name	7	1
	8	1
	30	1
	59	1
	63	2

Figures from the Authors' Collections Not Referenced in the Text

The following figures are additional samples of opera glasses and cases from the authors' collections that are not mentioned in the text. An R before the figure number indicates that the item is from Dr. Rosenthal's collection; a C before the figure number indicates that the item is from Mr. Cohen's collection.

Figure R349. Aluminum opera glasses.

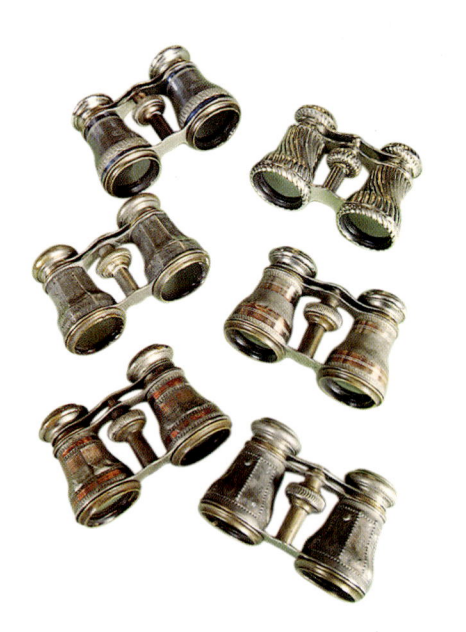

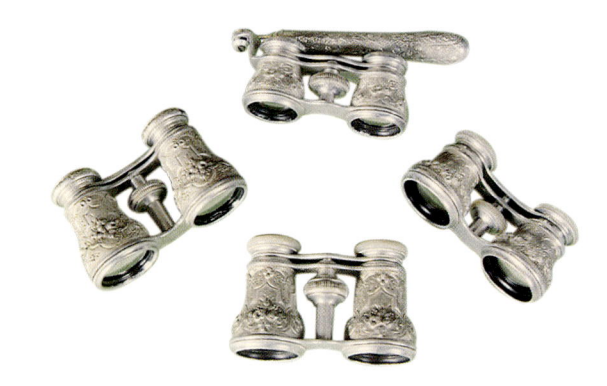

Figure R350. Aluminum opera glasses.

Figure R351. Aluminum and brass opera glasses.

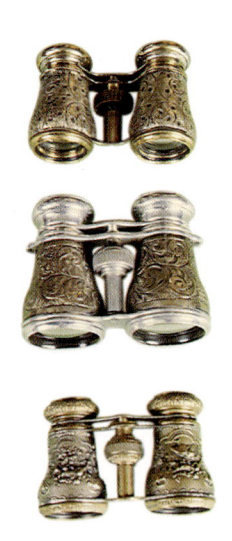

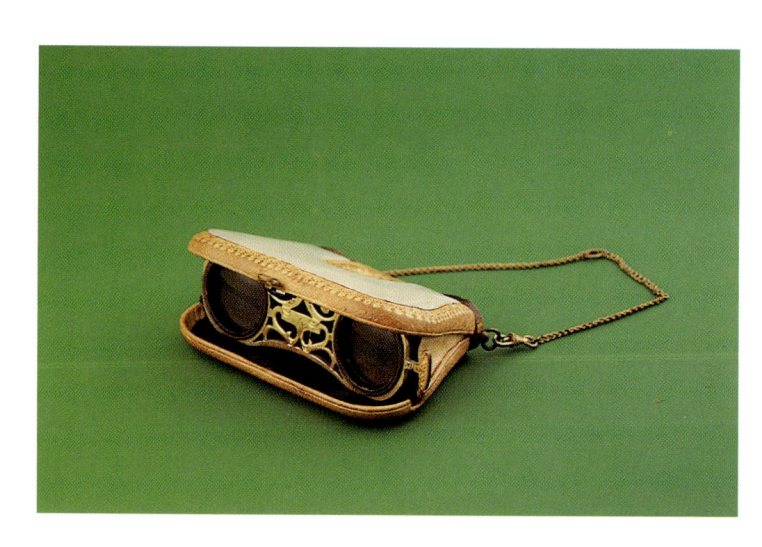

Figure R352. Mother-of-pearl case with folding opera glasses.

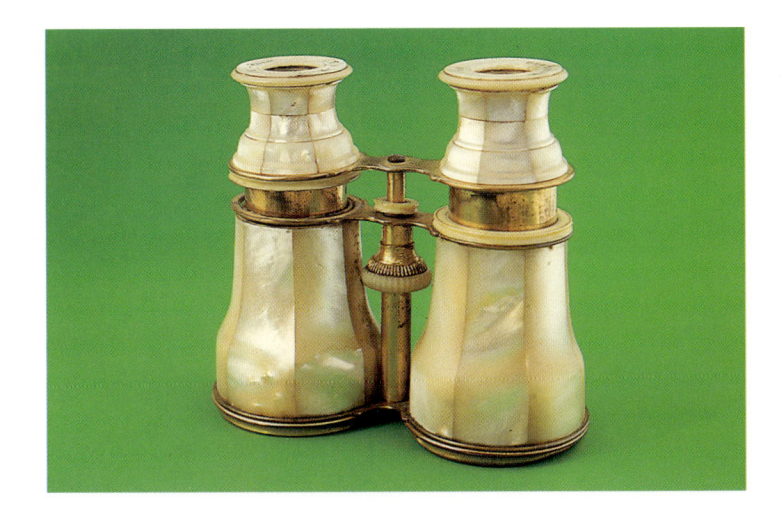

Figure R353. Mother-of-pearl opera glasses, produced in Brussels.

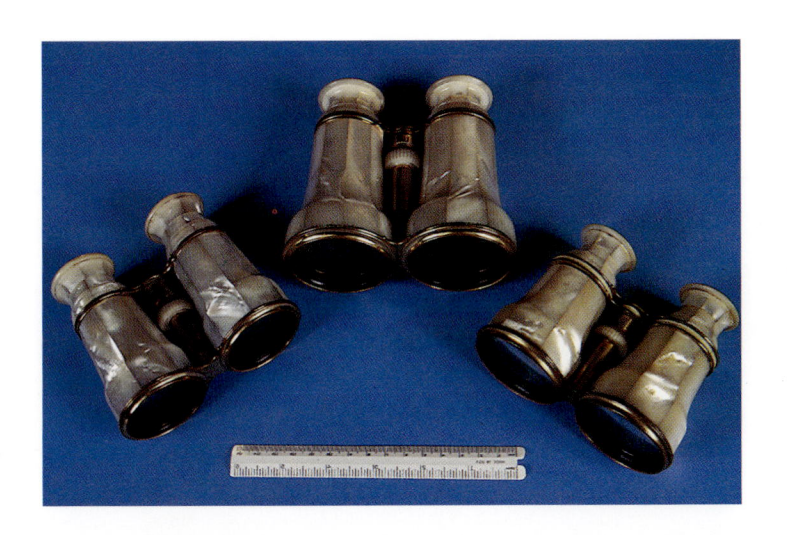

Figure R354. Group of large mother-of-pearl opera glasses.

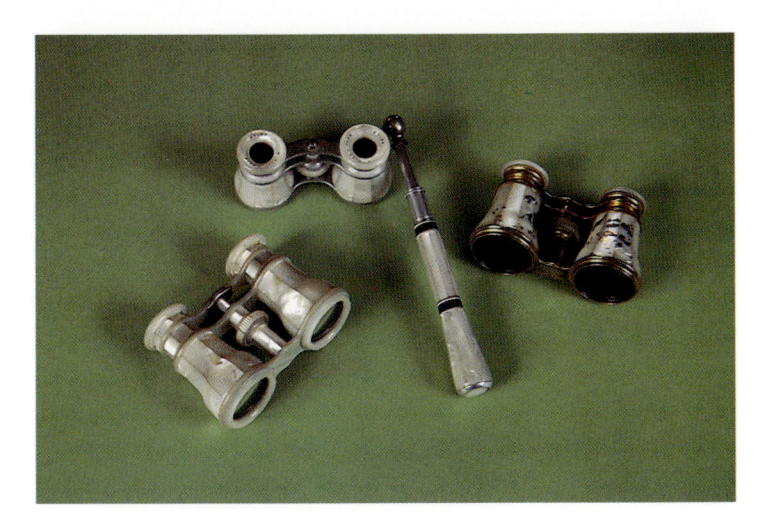

Figure R355. Types of mother-of-pearl opera glasses, including gold inlay.

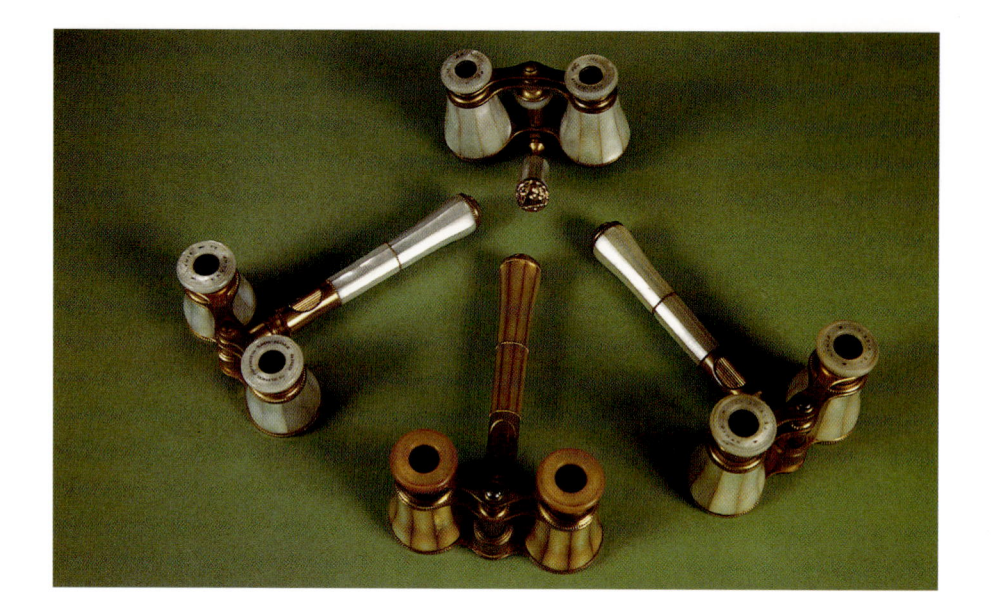

Figure R356. Types of mother-of-pearl opera glasses, including gold-dyed.

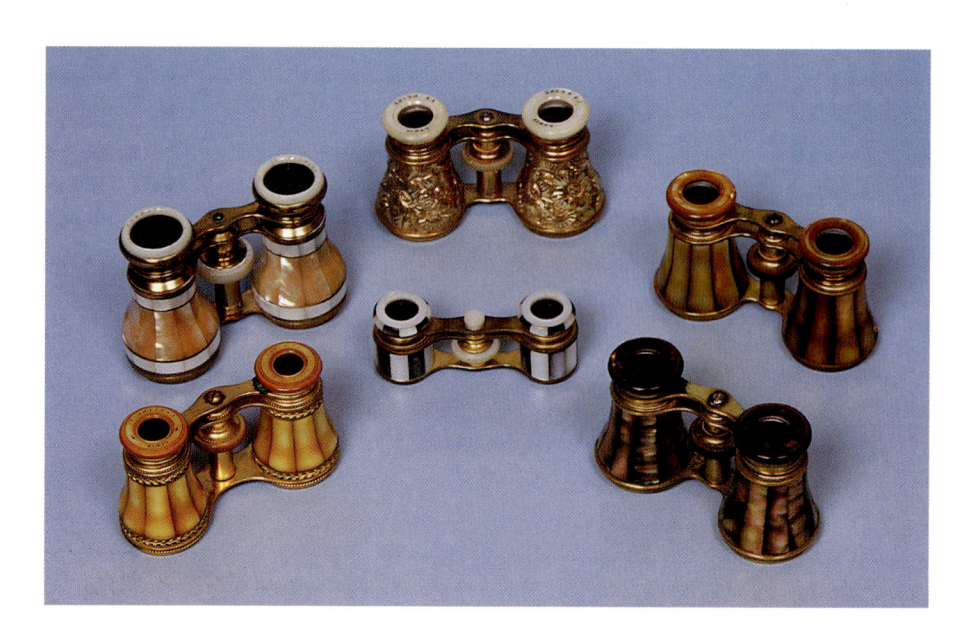

Figure R357. Mother-of-pearl combinations in opera glasses.

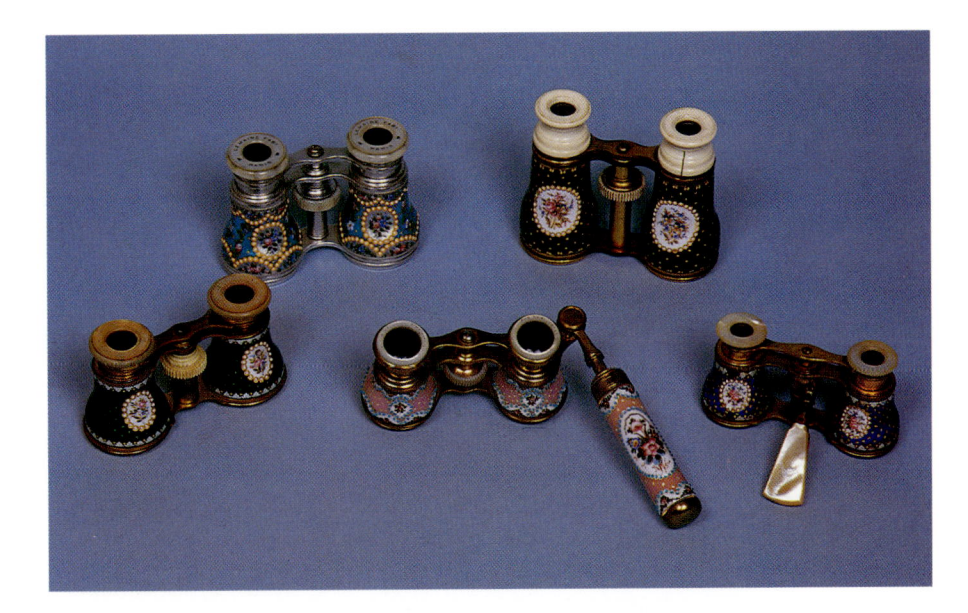

Figure R358. French porcelain opera glasses. Pink pair marked "McAllister".

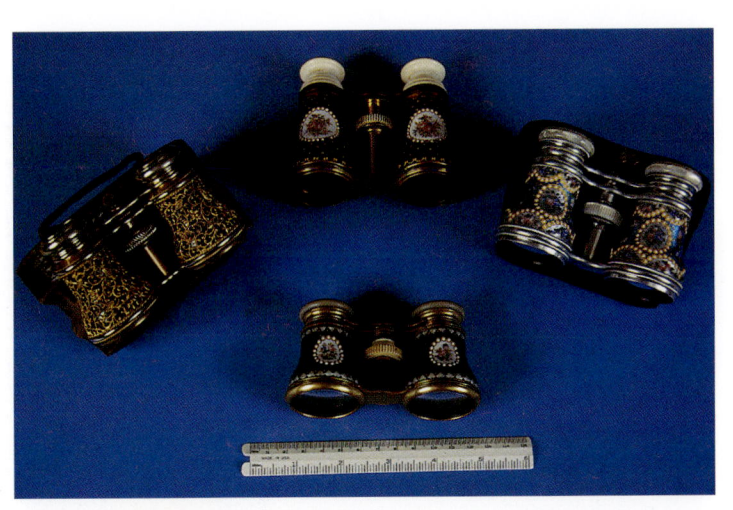

Figure R359. French porcelain and jeweled opera glasses.

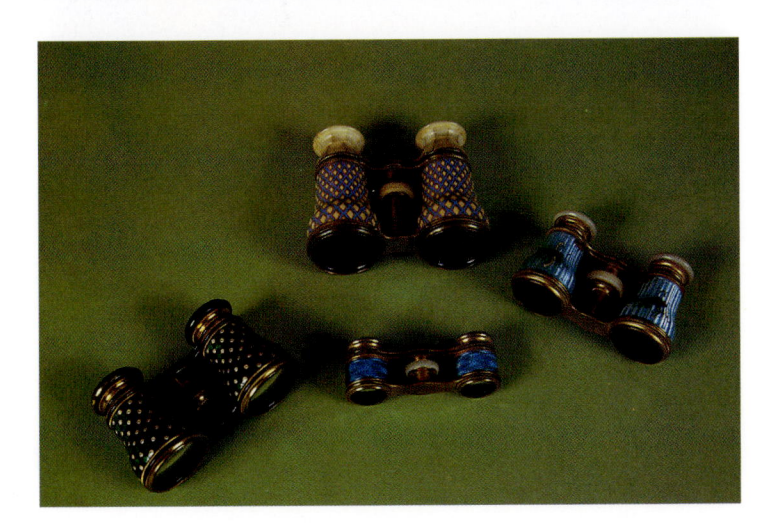

Figure R360. French enameled opera glasses.

OPERA GLASSES **209**

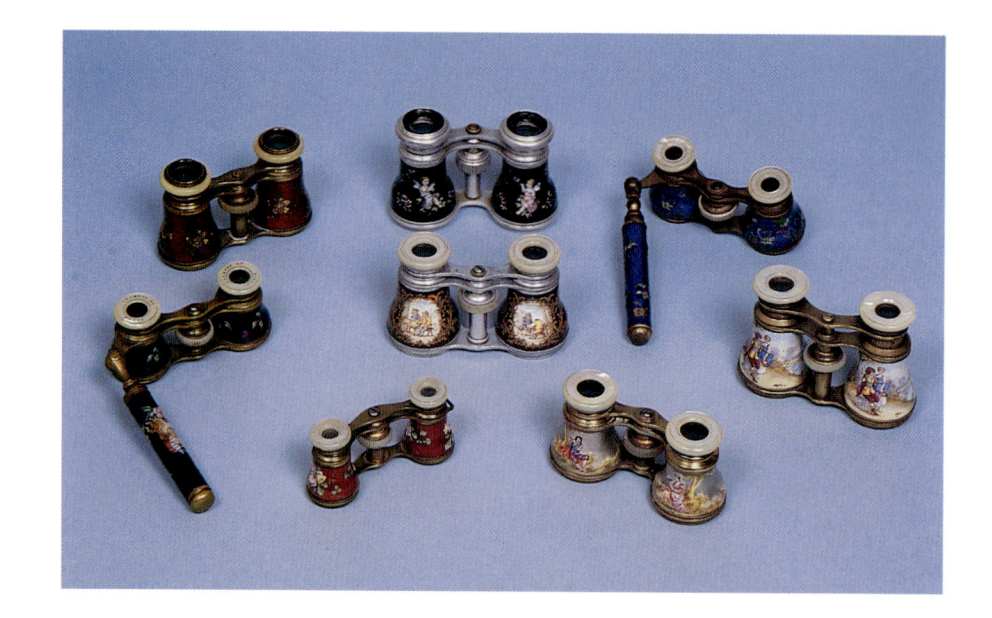

Figure R361. French opera glasses with (mostly) Austrian barrels.

Figure R362. Reticulated metal opera glasses.

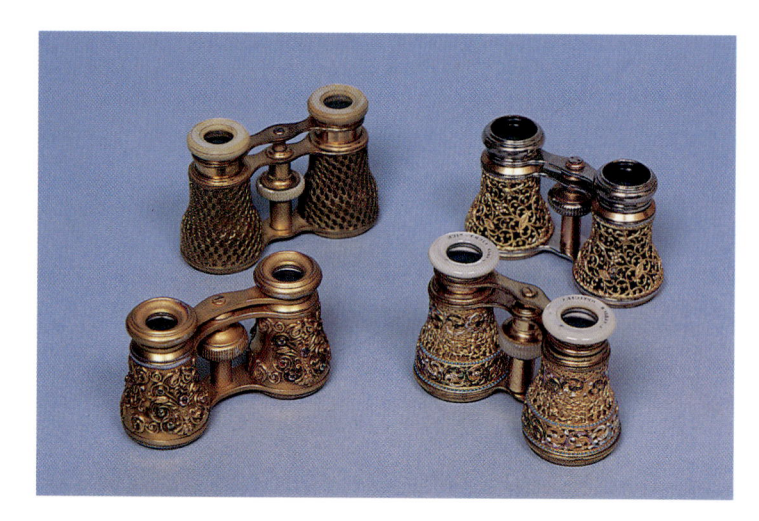

Figure R363. Opera glasses that fold flat.

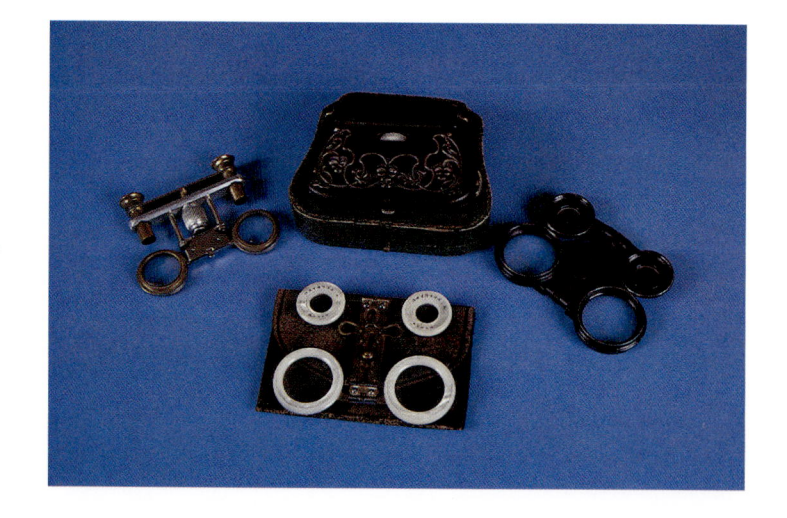

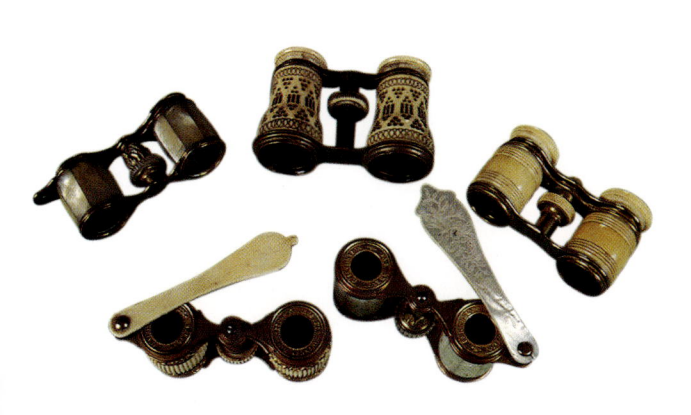

Figure R364. Cylindrical-shaped opera glasses (bone above).

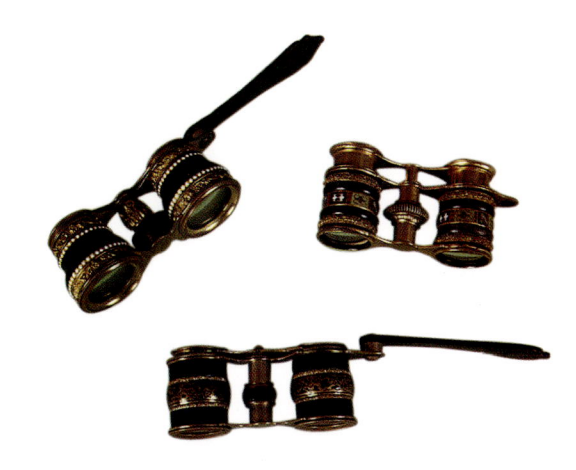

Figure R365. Cylindrical-shaped opera glasses.

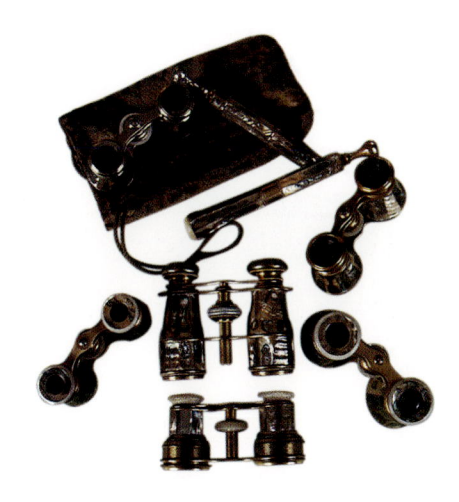

Figure R366. Abalone-clad opera glasses.

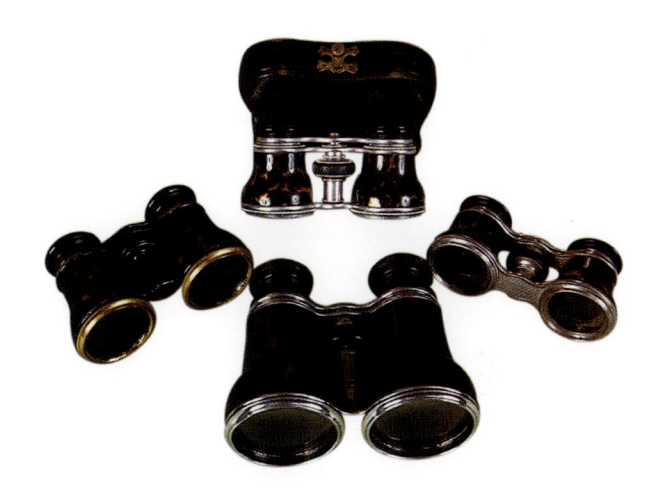

Figure R367. Tortoiseshell opera glasses.

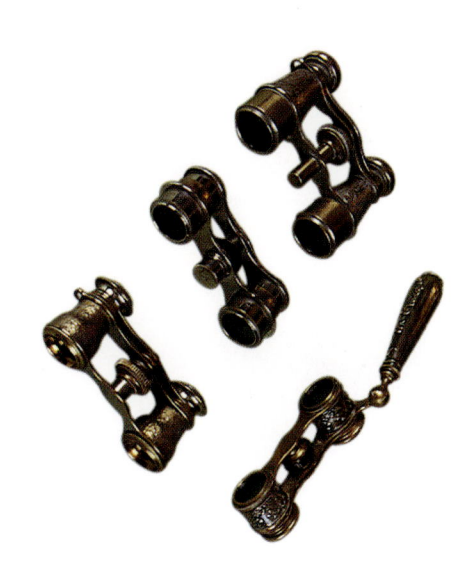

Figure R368. Brass and pewter opera glasses.

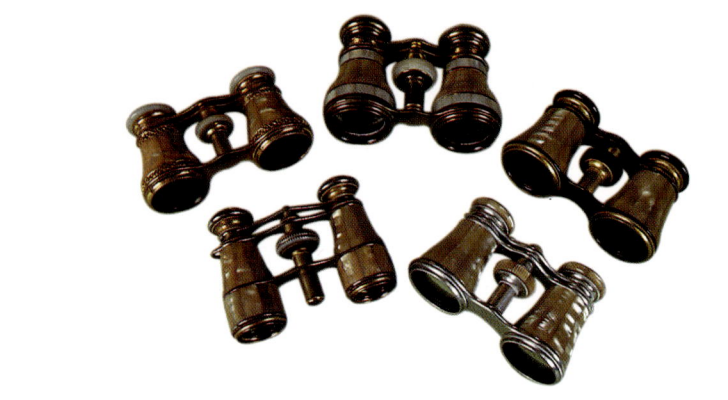

Figure R369. Sea snail opera glasses.

Figure R370. Black lip pearl opera glasses.

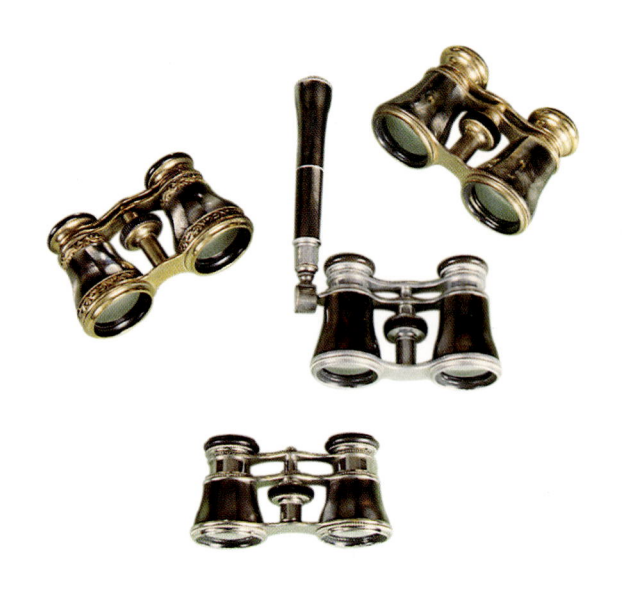

Figure R371. Embossed pewter opera glasses (3 above).

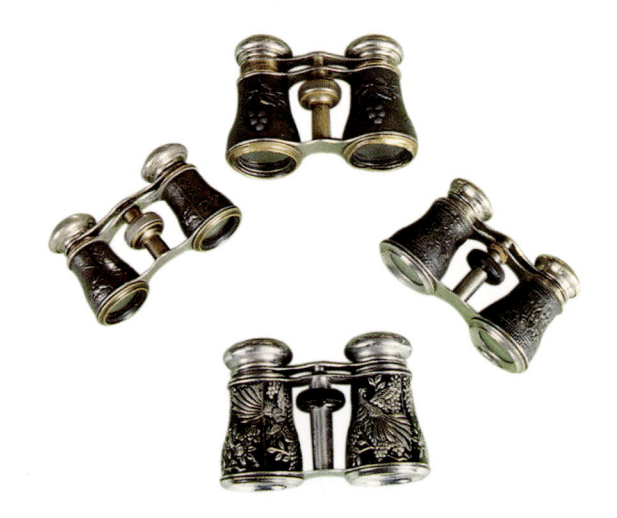

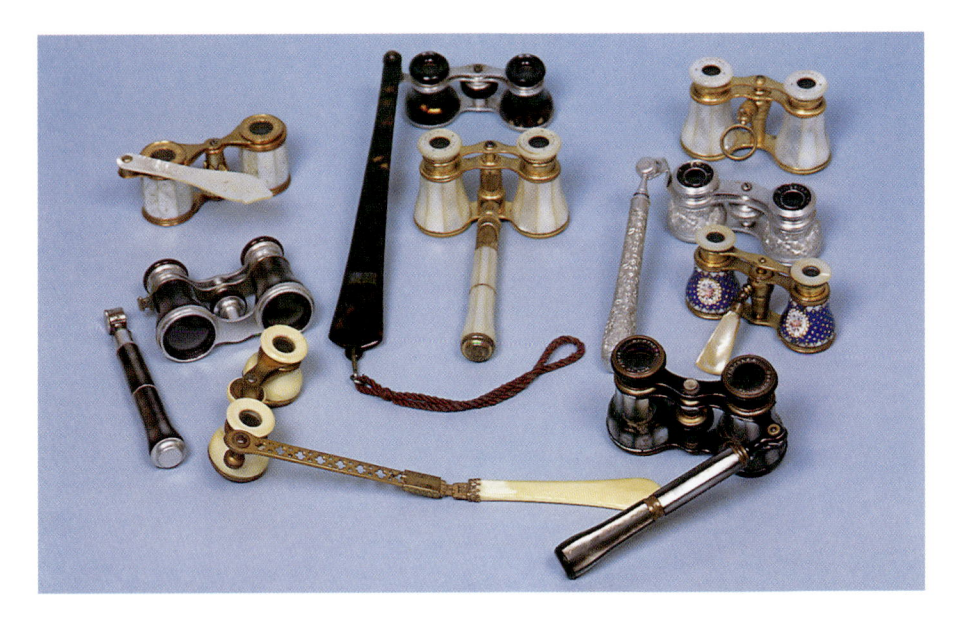

Figure R372. Opera glasses with various types of handles.

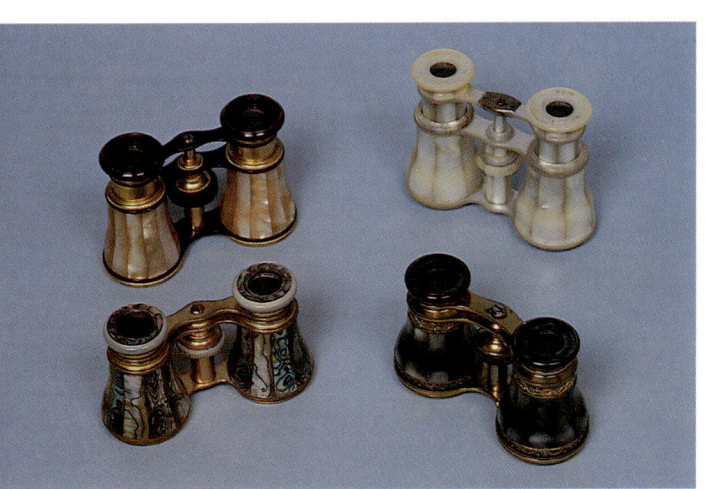

Figure R373. Opera glasses contrasting (clockwise from left) mother-of-pearl, sea snail, abalone, and black lip pearl.

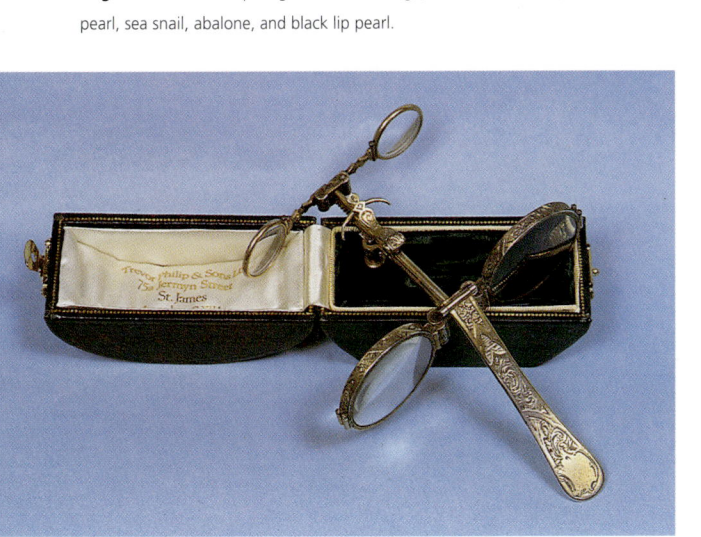

Figure R374. French field glass.

Figure R375. Silver-gilt French folding (automatic opening) opera glasses, circa 1890.

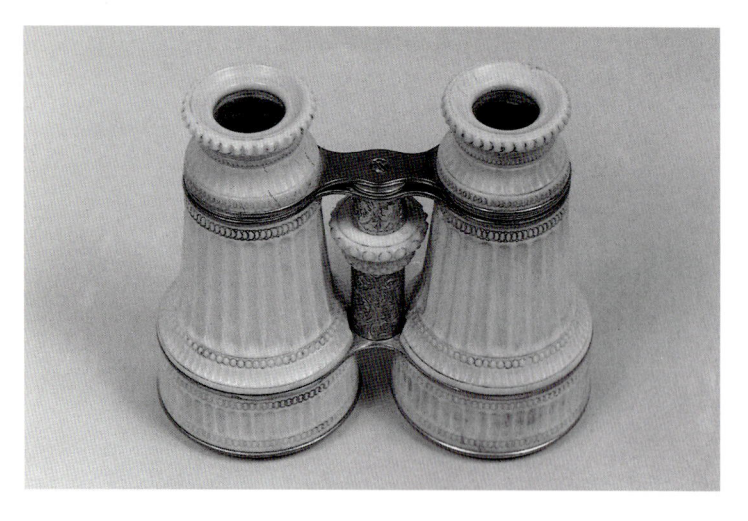

Figure R376. Carved ivory opera glasses, English circa 1890.

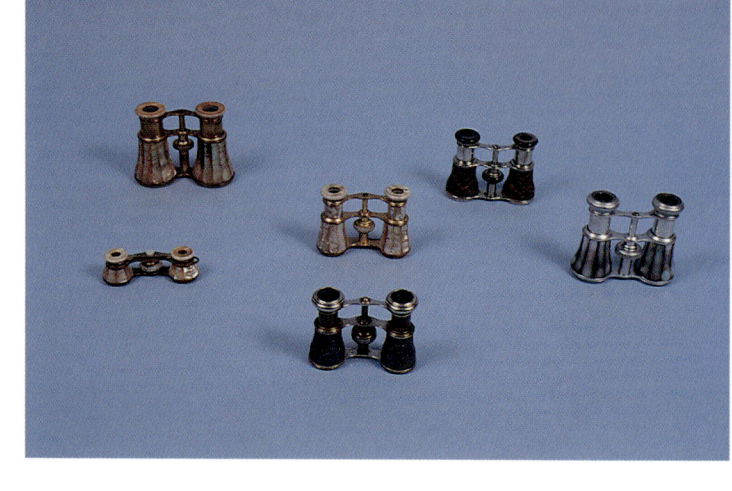

Figure C377. Opera glasses with various types, shapes, caps and barrels.

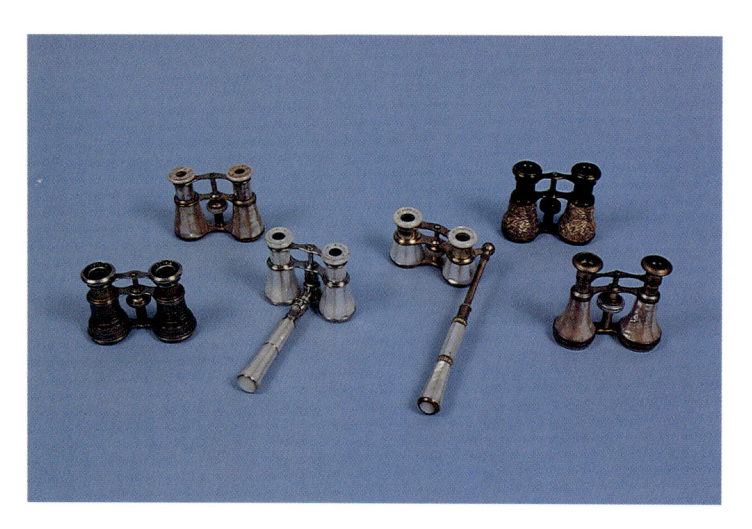

Figure C378. Various types of opera glasses (note trumpet shape and handles).

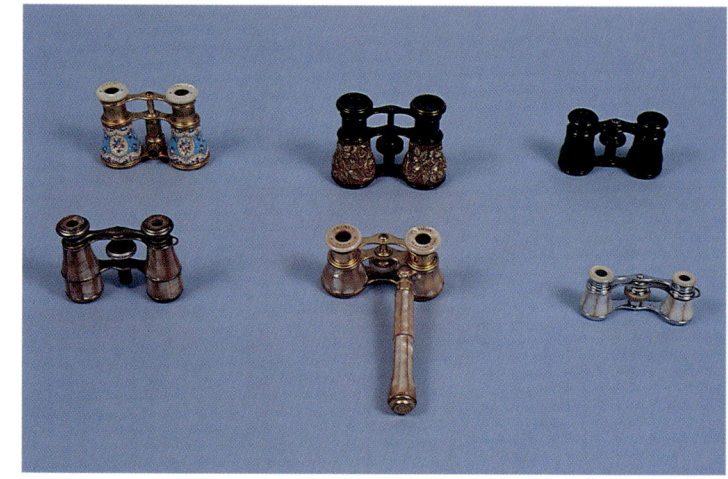

Figure C379. Various types of caps.

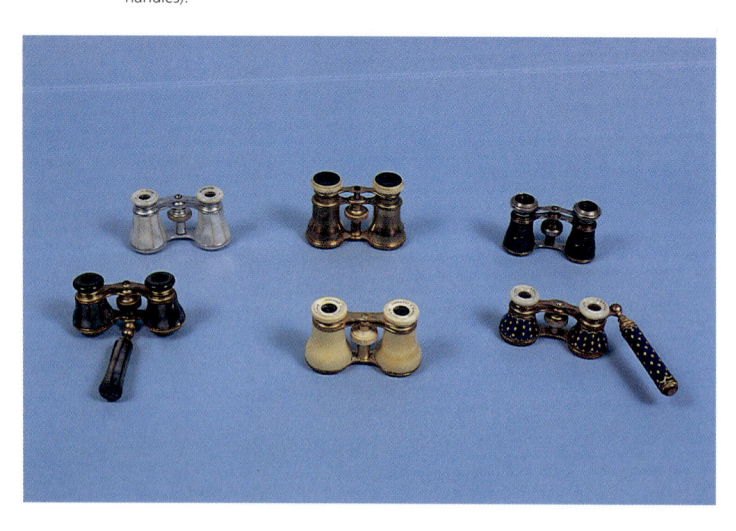

Figure C380. Variations.

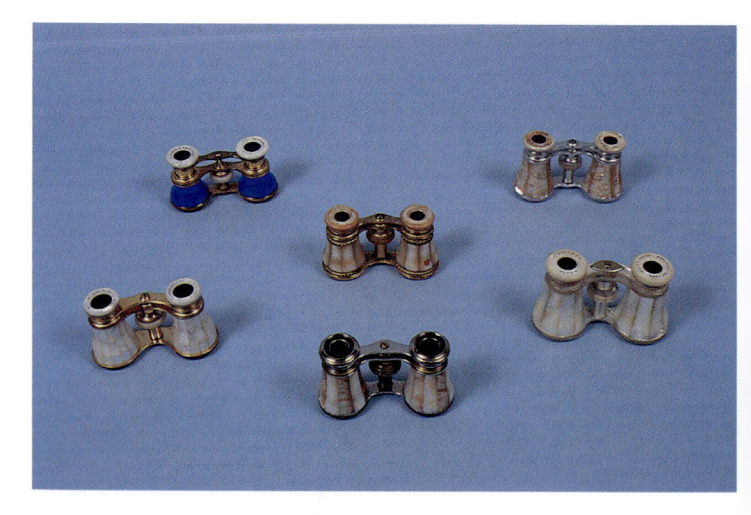

Figure C381. Note color differences.

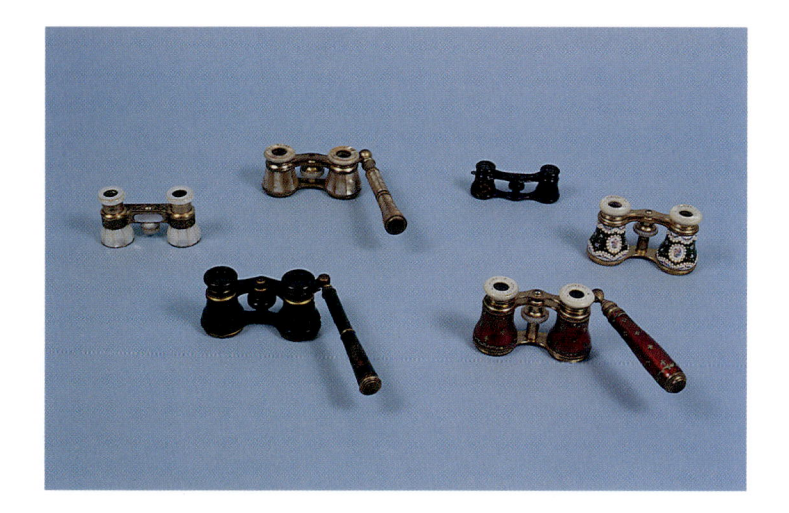

Figure C382. Beautiful colors, sizes, and shapes.

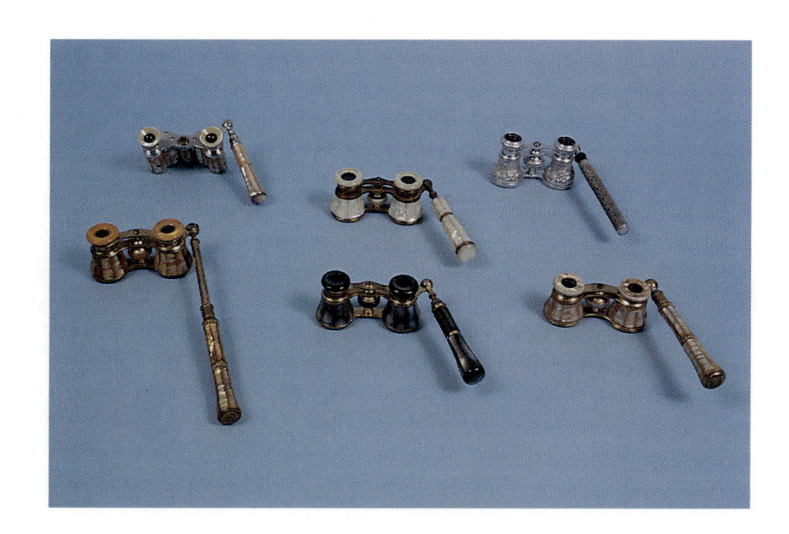

Figure C383. Variations in color, shape, and size.

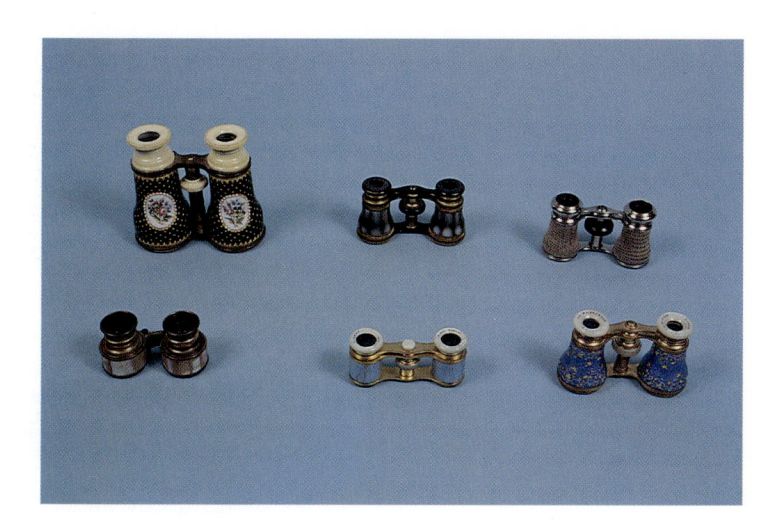

Figure C384. Further variations.

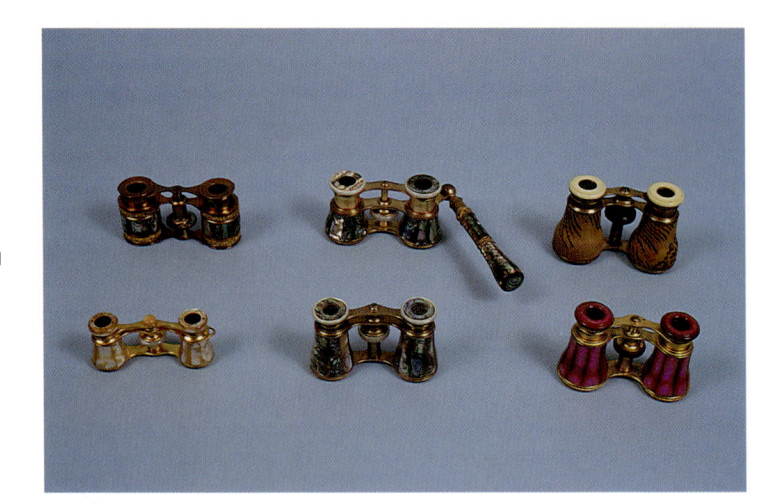

Figure C385. Purple-dyed mother-of-pearl and abalone.

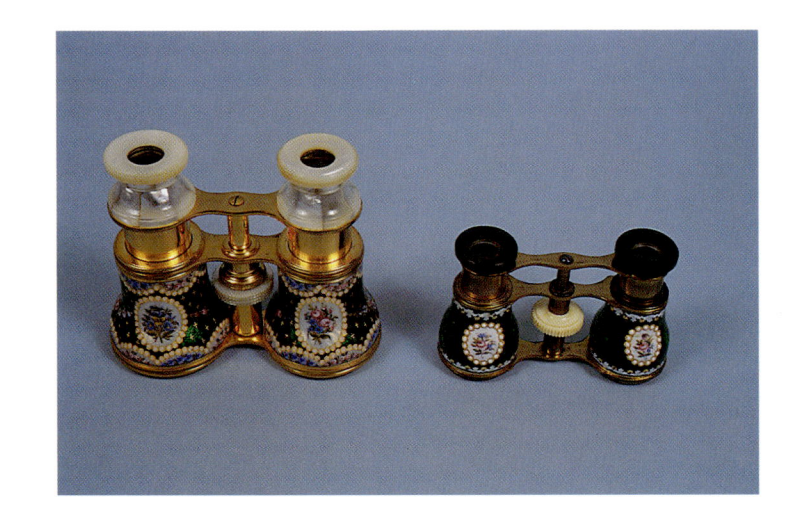

Figure C386. Size comparisons.

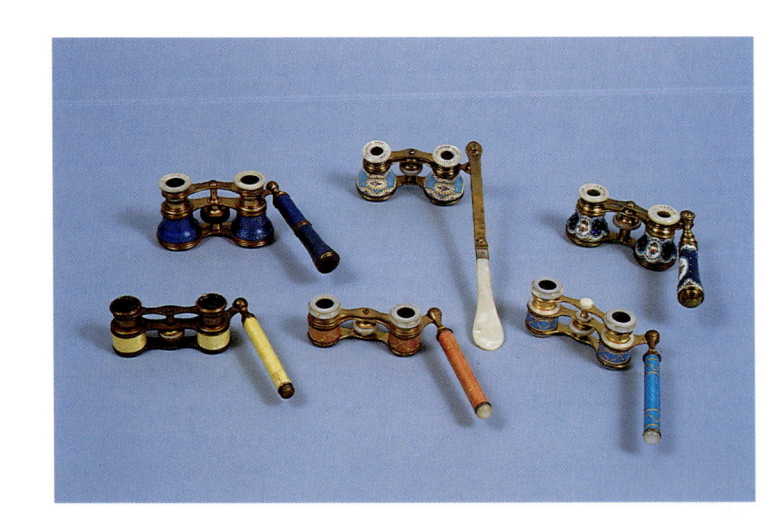

Figure C387. Various handle treatments and ages.

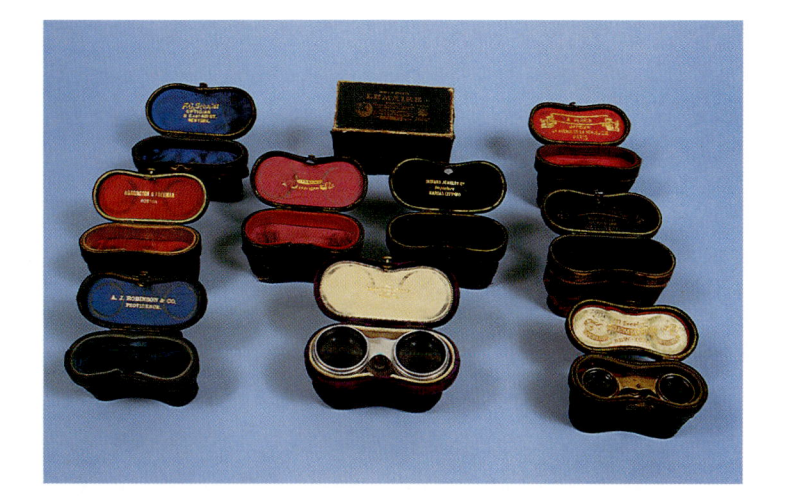

Figure C388. Demonstration of cases and one box (center).

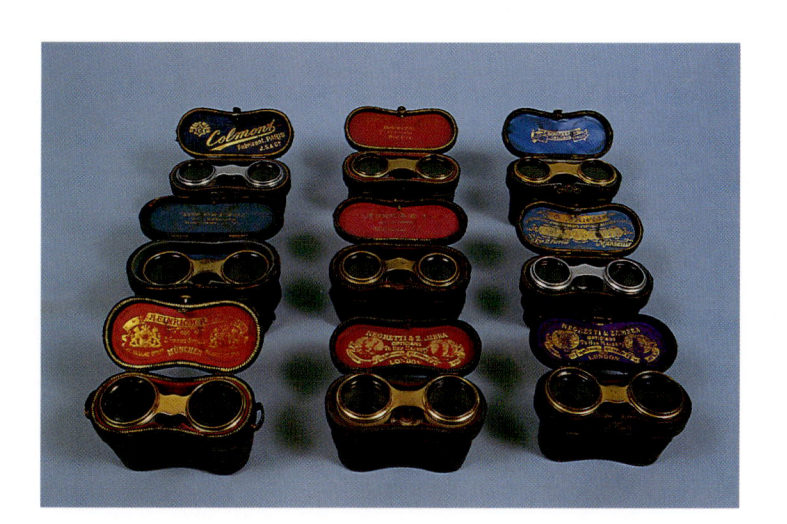

Figure C389. More cases and advertisements.

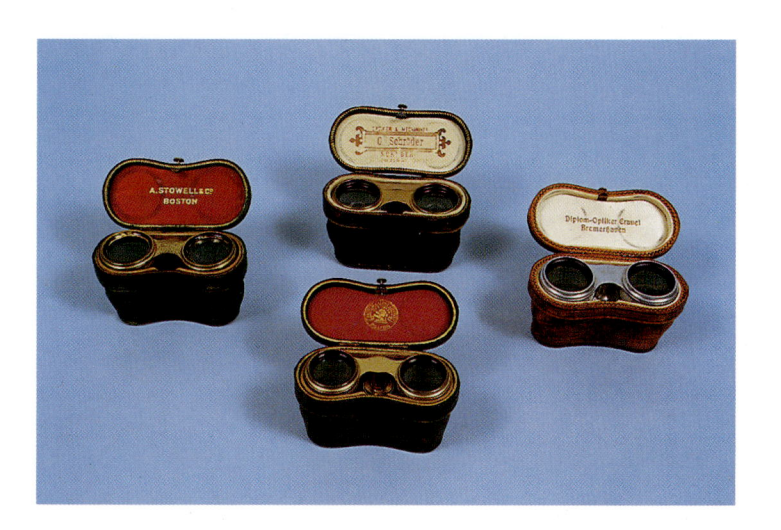

Figure C390. Different cases.

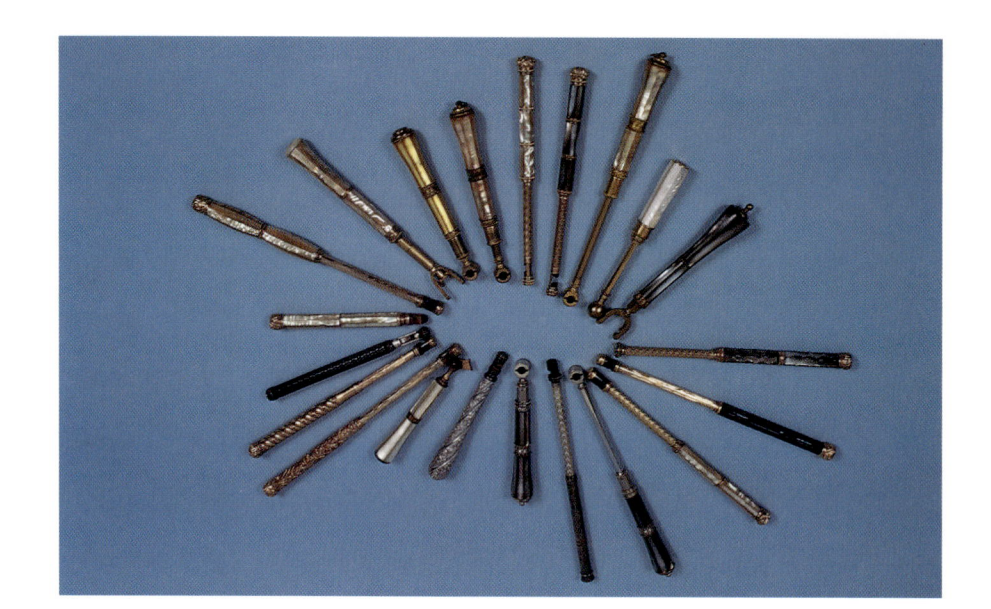

Figure C391. All separate handles.

Sources Consulted for Chapter 16

1. American Optical Company catalog, *Wellsworth Specialties, Opera Glasses* (circa 1890),11.
2. Anglo-American Optical Company catalog, pp. 230-246, London, n.d.
3. "Spectacles sold for 5,000 pounds," *Optician* 7(1990): October 12.
4. J. & W. E. Archbutt, catalog, series 2, *Field & Ordinary Opera Glasses* (London, n.d.), 15,16..
5. British Optical Association, Print from *Dioptric Review*, 1935.
6. George J. Bull, *Lunettes et Pince-nez* (Paris: G. Masson, 1889), 77.
7. Richard Corson, *Fashions in Eyeglasses* (London: Peter Owen Ltd., 1980).
8. T. H. Court and M. Von Rohr, "On the Development of Spectacles in London from the End of the Seventeenth Century," *Trans. Optical Soc.* 30, no. 1 (1928–1929):1–21
9. D. C. Davidson, *Spectacles, Lorgnettes and Monocles* Princes Risborough (Bucks): Shire Publications, 1989).
10. Audrey Davis and Mark Dreyfus *The Finest Instruments Ever Made* (Arlington, MA: Med. Hist. Publ. Assoc., 1986), 59.
11. J. M. Devriendt, "Spyglasses and Opera Glasses," *J. Oph. Antiques Int'l. Coll. Club*, January 1992.
12. C. Dewaord, Jr.,*De geschiedeni v Nole venckyker*. 1906.
13. Geneva Optical Company catalog, *Field Glasses* (Chicago, IL, circa 1922), 98–101.
14. Hudson, J.T., *Useful Remarks upon Spectacles, Lenses, and Opera-Glasses; with Hints to Spectacle Weares and Others...* (London: Joseph Thomas, Finch-Lane, Cornhill, 1840).
15. Henri C. King, "The History of the Telescope,"*British Ophthalmic International Antiques Collectors' Newsletter*, 1994.
16. A. Klotz, *Die Brille* (Stuttgart: Wuerttemberg. Landesbibliothek, 1988).
17. G. Kuehn and W. Rods, *Sieben Jahrhunderte Brillen* (Muenchen: Verlag R. Oldenbourg, 1968).
18. A. Kuisle, *Brillen, Glaeser, Fassungen, Herstellung* (Muenchen: Deutsches Museum, 1985).
19. Leon-Nicole, *Lunettes et Pince-nez* (Lyon, 1900[?]), 53–55
20. Pierre Marley, *Spectacles and Spyglasses*Paris: Hoebeke, 1988), 142–44).
21. William McAllister, *Catalogue* (Philadelphia, circa 1871), 43–46.
22. Merry Optical Company catalog, (Kansas City, MO, circa 1910), 205–211.
23. New Era Optical Company catalog, *Opera & Field Glasses* (Chicago, IL, circa 1940), 35–40.

24. Nitsche and Gunther catalog, *Field Glasses* (Rathenow, circa 1880), 795.
25. Nitsche & Guenther, *Haupt Katalog* (Rathenow:1900[?]), 660–715, 802.
26. Optico catalog, *Purse type, Prism, Opera, & Field Glasses* (Utrecht, circa 1939).
27. Hugh Orr, *Illustrated History of Early Spectacles* (London, 1985).
28. Benjamin Pike, Jr., *Catalogue #II* (New York: circa 1850), 174–176.
29. James W. Queen & Company catalog, *Ordinary Opera & Field Glasses* (Philadelphia, 18 February 1878), 42.
30. H. Sachs, H. *Das Staendebuch* (Frankfurt, 1568). Reprint Leipzig, 1934. Quoted by Kuisle in *Brillen, Glaeser, Fassungen, Herstellung* (Muenchen: Deutsches Museum, 1985).
31. Rienitz Sammlung, *Kulturgeschichte des Fernrohrs* Sears Roebuck & Co., catalogue, 1902, page 128 (Tubingen, 1985).
32. *Société des Lunetiers* (Paris, 1901), 102–103.
33. Spencer Optical Company, *Catalogue #17*, (New York, n.d.), 134–148.
34. J. Teunissen, "Optisch antiek IV," *Oculus* (Amsterdam) 45, no. 4(1983):17–21.
35. J. Teunissen, "Op zoek naar de oude brillen in Nederland," *Oculus* (Amsterdam) 52, no. 9 (1990):59.
36. Dr. Vineburg, picture of opera glasses in a flier, 1885–96, Albany, N.Y.
37. J. W. Waterer, *Leather in Life, Art, and Industry* (London: Faber & Faber, 1956).

17

Quizzing Glasses

Probably the first convex lens bound in a frame and embellished with a handle was the first quizzing glass. Time, usage, geography, and nationality changed its decoration and nomenclature to some extent. Basically, however, the quizzing glass consisted of a small lens encased in a frame with a short handle (Figure 392).

According to Richard Horne (quoting "The Art of Preserving Sight Unimpaired to an Extreme Old Age"—1821), the real old quizzing glass was actually a small mirror held in the hand and used to mischievously scrutinize objects to the rear of the person who held it. Saying that it was a relic of Hogarth's period, it was employed in the days of "Beau Nash and the Bath Chair Fops."[1]

We use the term *quizzer* (the familiar form) to discuss the quizzing glass now, but it has also been called lanstier, monocle, reading glass, prospect glass, or perspective glass. We recognize the beginning as a distinct optical form in the early eighteenth century in Europe and England. Such a cognizance came about because of the quizzer's great popularity at that time.

Uses

The main purpose of this optical device was to decorate oneself and impress others. Invariably, the quizzer was hung on a cord or tape that encircled the neck. This arrangement was convenient, as it was available for use at a moment's notice and was quite visible to others as well (Figure 393). Even as an article of fashion, it was used by men and women alike. The French incroyables were young foppish nobles who played with the quizzers in gesticulating ways (Figure 394). It was thought that their posturing would allow them recognition or notoriety. The quizzer was also sometimes fondled and caressed, much as the Greek worry beads are used today.

Some people did use quizzing glasses for vision correction. Pope Leo X, a known myope, is shown using a myopic lens in his portrait by Raphael Santi in 1517. Presbyopes likewise had legitimate claim to the medical necessity of quizzers. Most others, however, used them for the effect.

Lenses

While very few of the lenses were myopic, and therefore truly useful in distant vision, most were ground convex for close viewing or were plano for cosmetic effect only. These lenses were held with one hand before the eye while closing the other eye. Some individuals employed the quizzing glass as a monocle and did so until about 1825, when it became old-fashioned. It was then replaced by the monocle as we know it today.

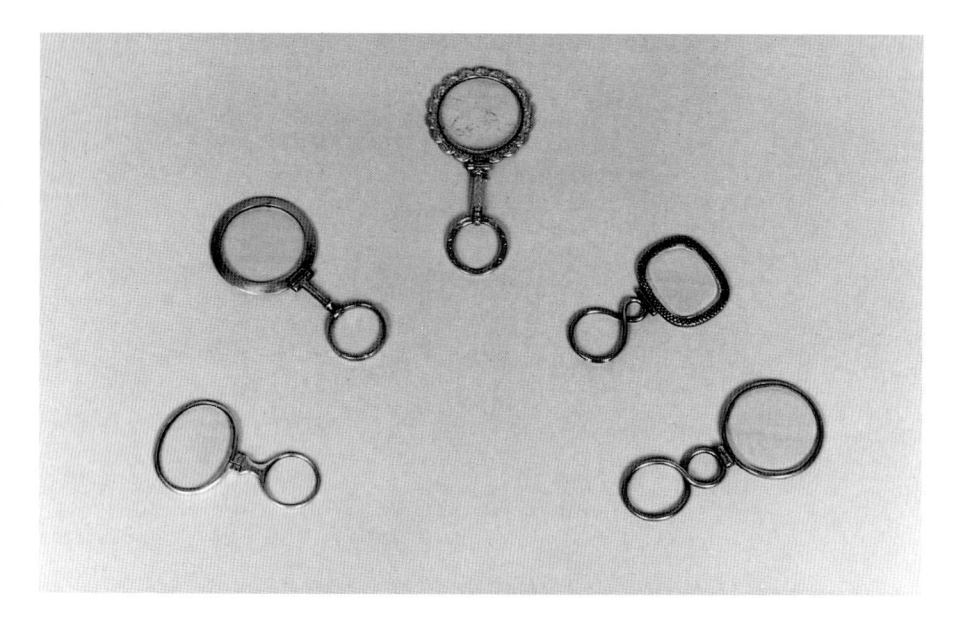

Figure 392. Group of English quizzing glasses with silver and gold handles circa 1800.

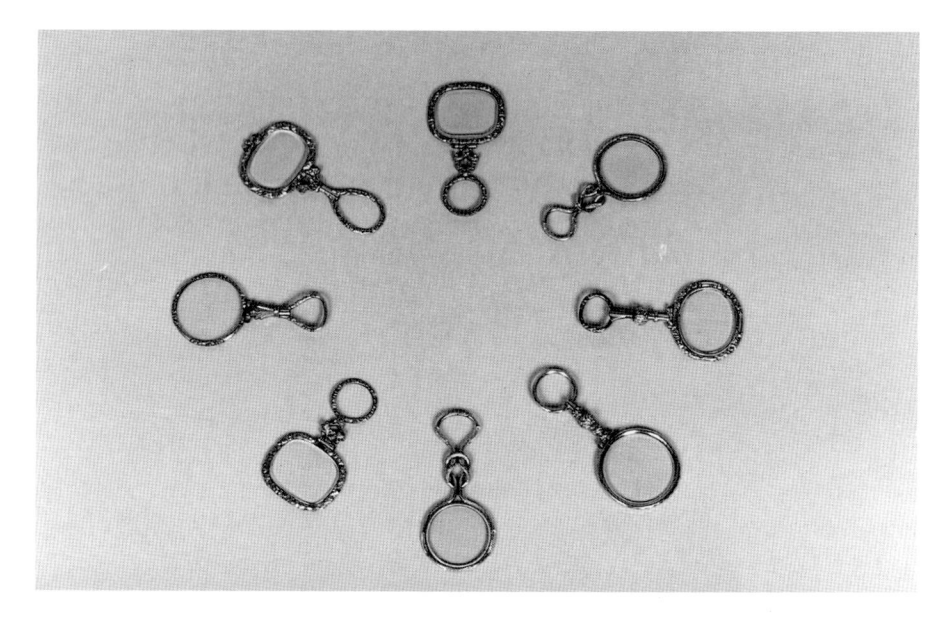

Figure 393. Group of English and French gold quizzing glasses.

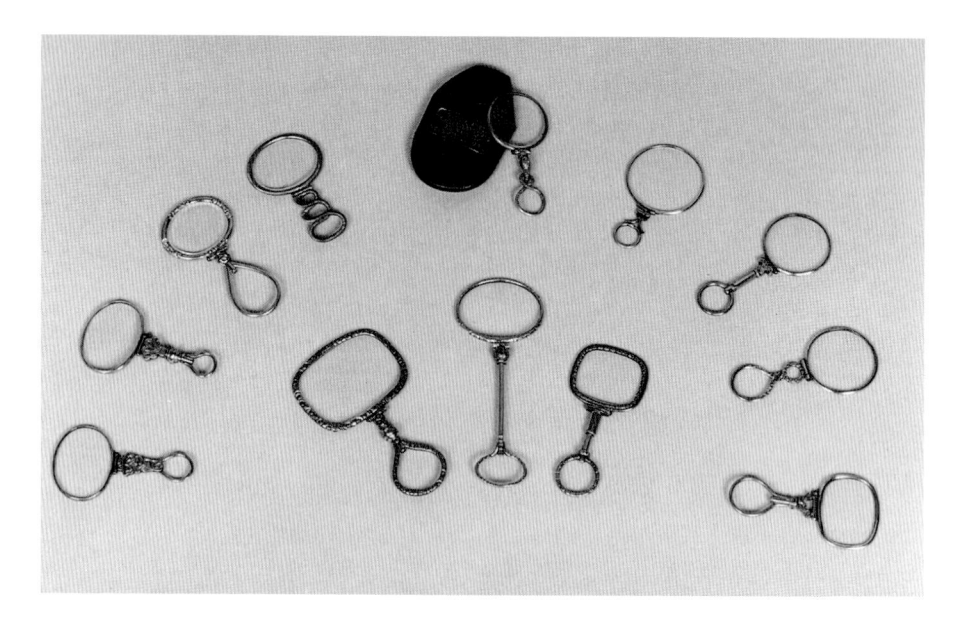

Figure 394. French quizzing glasses (center).

Shape

From the simple circle comes, in turn, oval, rectangular, square and square with round lenses, octagonal, and triangular shapes (Figure 395).[2]

Frames and Handles

Some quizzers were said to have been rimless—many of which were square. Most, however, had rims (frames). Frames were usually continuous, with their handles of the same material and decorated similarly. All designs imaginable were used to decorate these parts of the quizzer. Although early quizzers had relatively plain frames and handles made of wood, most of the later models were ornate, as the whole purpose of the article was to decorate. Those made of metal were of silver, gold, steel, or base metal. Polished steel embellished by pearls was popular with the incroyables.[3] When gold was employed, it often was merely coated on the base metal by one of several methods. Therefore, the purchaser of such an article should be aware of the possibility that it may not be solid gold. Other fashionable pieces were made of bone or tortoiseshell. Mother-of-pearl was also used and was sometimes inlaid with gold or silver designs. Others employed precious stones or colored glass for decoration.

Handles sported rings at their base. Some of the rings were rigid, while others rotated so that the quizzer would lie flat.

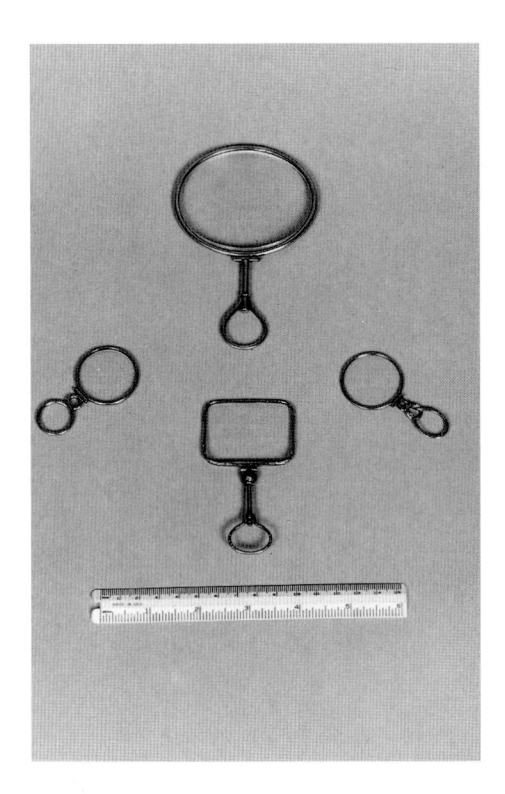

Figure 395. Rectangular, oval, and large-sized quizzing glasses.

Conclusion

Among the optical devices presented in this book, quizzers undeniably belong to the group used primarily for fashion purposes. These well-crafted and beautifully decorated articles were truly considered a statement in and of themselves.

Notes

1. Richard Horne, *Fraser's Magazine* (England, 1876).
2. Richard Corson, *Fashions in Eyeglasses* (London: Peter Owen, Ltd., 1967), 4, 7, 11–13, 15, 19, 24, 26, 30, 79–83, 114, 200.
3. Pierre Marley, *Spectacles and Spyglasses* (Paris: Hoebeke, 1988), 12, 13.

18

Optical Uses of Fans

In Europe, particularly in France in the 1600s, a large part of the social life consisted of observing others who attended the theater and other similar events. A blunt but appropriate term for this would be *spying*. One instrument used for this purpose was the ordinary prospect glass (small telescope) (Figure 396). Another was the jealousy-glass, similar to a periscope (Figure 397), with which observers surreptitiously viewed their subjects from a 90 degree angle. This "nosy" habit, however, began to be considered offensive to many, prompting numerous complaints by prominent socialites. Protests such as these did not, however, deter those bent on scrutinizing their objects of interest. To the contrary, such people were prompted to find ingenious ways to conceal their vision aids. Late in the 1700s, small telescopes were placed in women's fans so that women could inconspicuously peep at their subjects.[1]

Mostly, these small lorgnettes (or telescopes) were placed at the base of the fans and helped to act as the axis for rotation of the blades. Note the French brisé fan, made of horn, clouté with steel, showing a monocular set in the pivot (Figure 398). Many other types of fans have been found with small telescopes at their fulcrums and were used particularly on the Continent. Some of these fans opened to a full 360 degrees, and their popularity started with the Empire period (1803) (Figure 399). In general, they tended to be smaller in size than those previously used. Around 1820, these telescopes were replaced by small kaleidoscopes, which had become quite popular.

More simple use of the fan for observation employed a small mirror attached to the outside of the fan's main (protective) blade (or blades) (Figures 400 & 401). Not only was the fan decorative but it also allowed discreet ogling from various angles. One unusual type is the French/Spanish "flirtation fan" or *eventail cocarde*. The mirror is large, and the method of opening and closing is unique. This fan dates 1810 (Figures 402 & 403).

It was quite easy to work a hole (of various shapes) into the design of fan blades or ribs so that (open or closed) the fan could shield a woman's eyes and allow her to scan the area without being detected (Figure 404). When the fan was closed, the holes in the fan blades would line up to produce a pinhole effect (Figure 405).

A more complicated type of optical apparatus was installed in some fans. Lenses were placed in the two main fan blades so that they lined up together with similarly placed holes in the inside blades, thus forming a telescope (Figure 406). Given the crudeness of the lenses and the variation of their alignment in the fan blades, one can imagine that their accuracy was less than desirable.

Moving to the end of the nineteenth century, we find that women still needed fans and vision aids. Although binocular opera glasses had superseded other magnifiers for long distances, menus and theater programs still needed to be read. An ingenious combination of a fan and spectacle is shown in

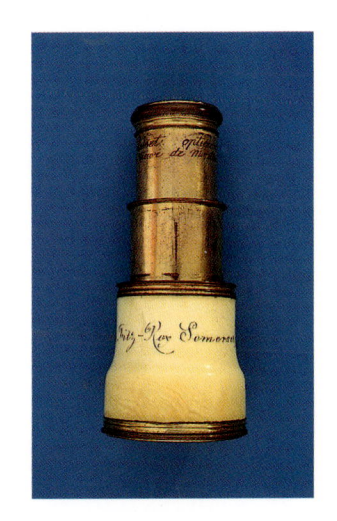

Figure 396. Prospect glass, French, ivory, and gilt.

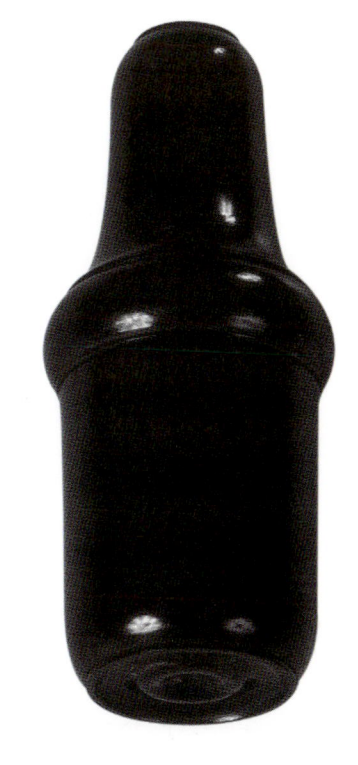

Figure 397. Jealousy glass, wood, in case.

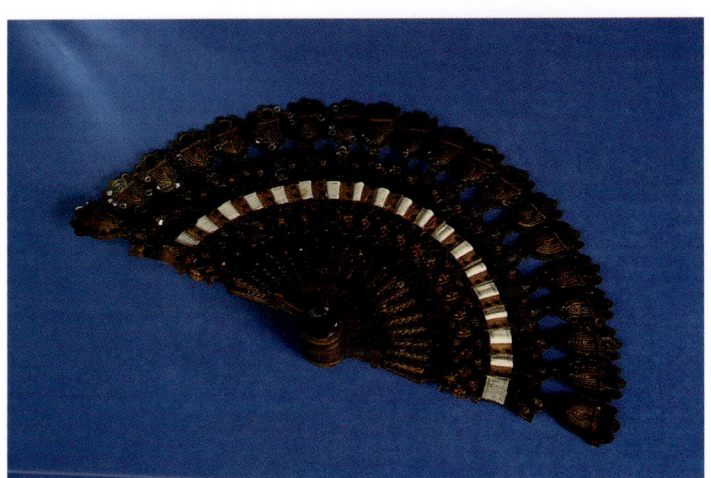

Figure 398. French brisé fan.

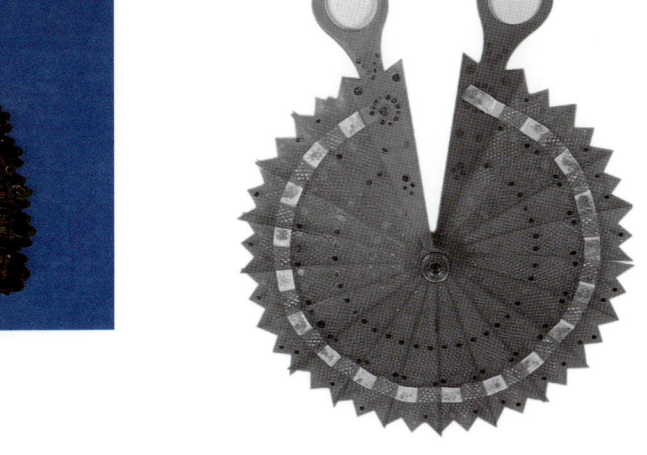

Figure 399. Cockade fan, French, circa 1790–1810, with quizzing glass in center fulcrum.

FANS 225

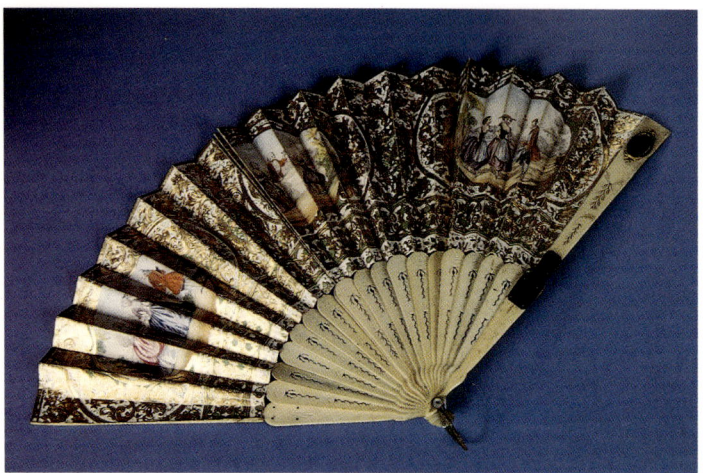

Figures 400 & 401. Fan with small mirror on main (outside) blade.

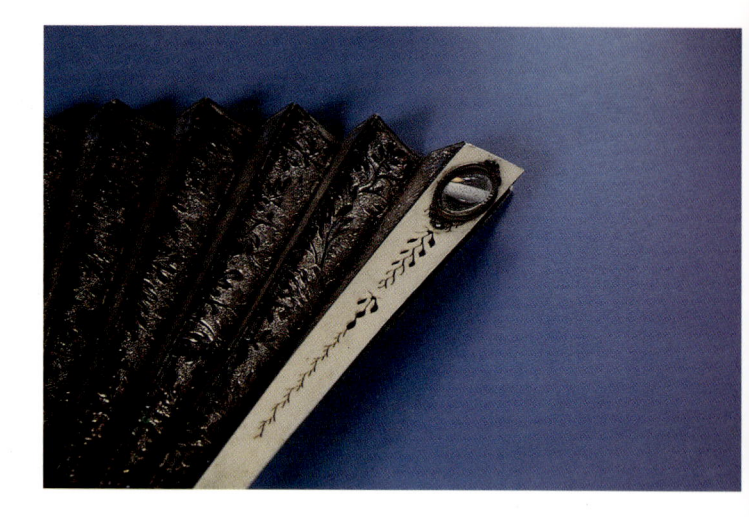

Figure 401.

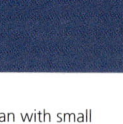

Figure 402. Eventail cocarde fan—closed.

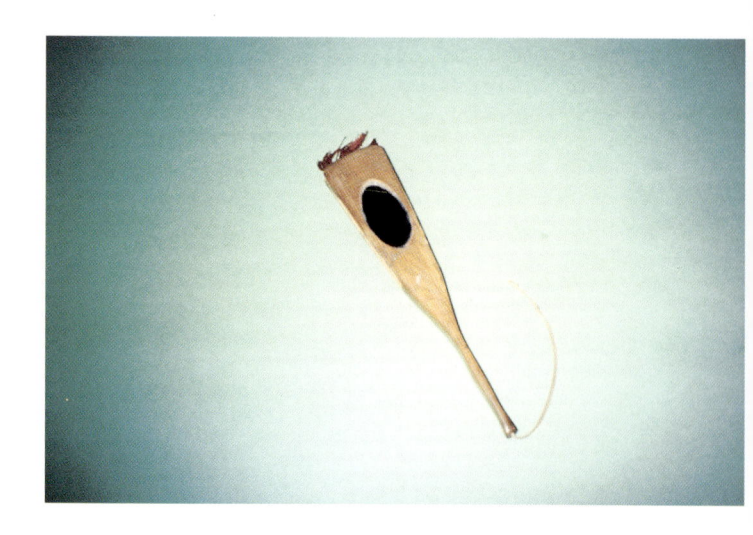

Figure 403. Eventail cocarde fan—open.

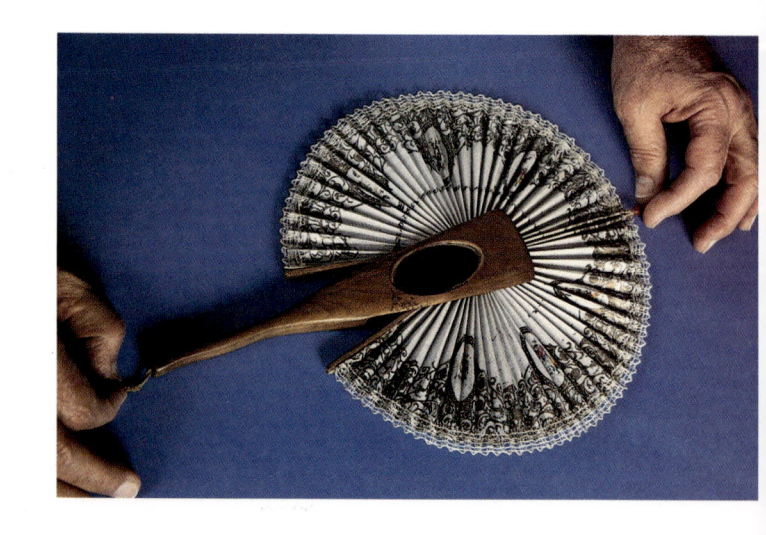

226 CHAPTER 18

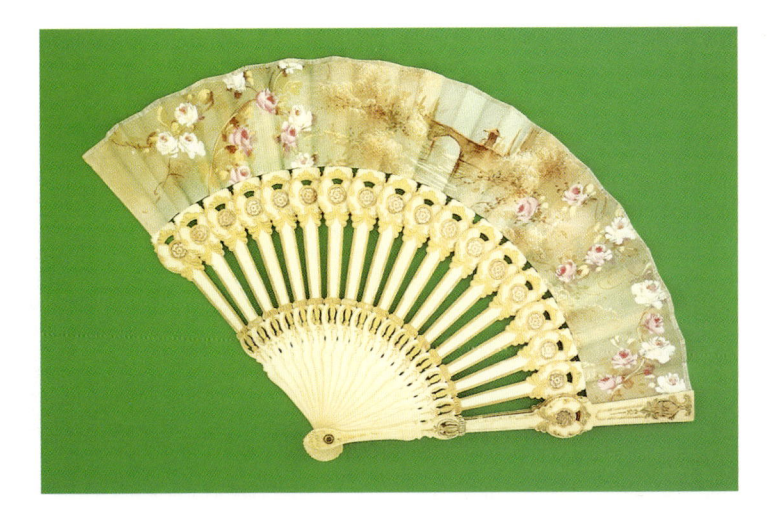

Figure 404. Peepholes in the blades of a woman's fan.

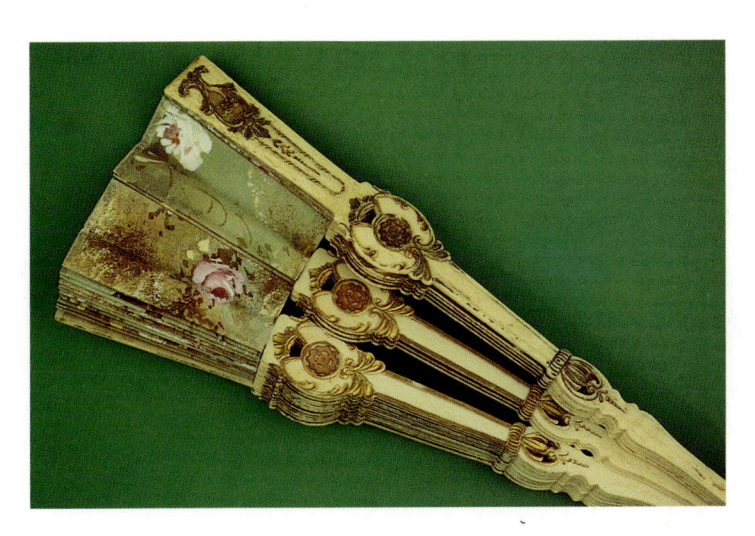

Figure 405. Demonstrating continuity of peepholes as fan is closed.

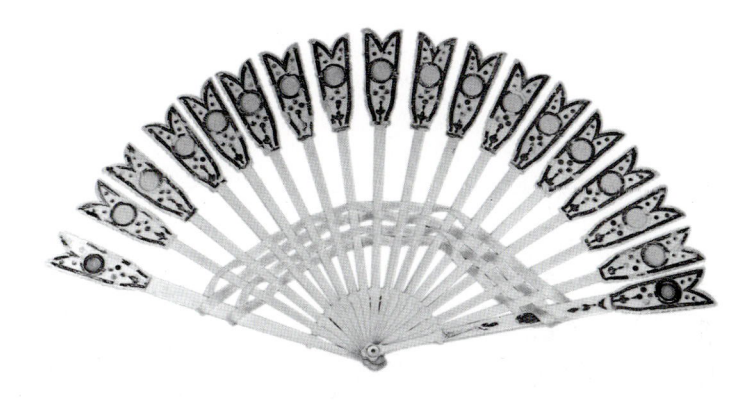

Figure 406. Fan blades line up to help form a small telescope. Note lenses on main fan blades.

FANS   **227**

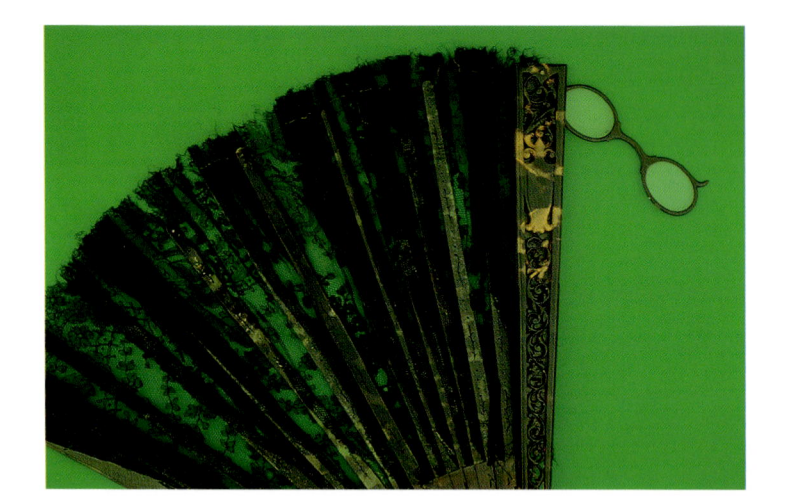

Figure 407. Tortoiseshell and lace fan with integral lorgnette circa 1890.

Figure 407. The fan is made of fine lace and is quite large, with blades and spectacle front made of tortoiseshell. It is housed in its own silk-lined and silk-covered box.

MacIver Percival, in *The Fan Book* (1920), provided the following details of fans fitted with optical devices:

> Perhaps the secret, or one of the secrets, of the fascination that fans have for so many of us is the light they throw on the ways and manners of the days when they were made. The Lorgnette Fan could only have had a vogue in a period when affectation was the "correct thing." It is to all appearance an ordinary small fan, with silk or gauze leaf ornamented with spangles or painting, the decoration finished with a rather heavy border round the top. Often this consists of interlaced ovals or circles in spangles, sometimes there is an applique of coarsish silk lace. If examined more closely, it will be noted that in this border several of the circles differ in appearance from the rest; the solid silk or skin has been cut away from the back of them, and they are transparent. It might be imagined that this is a feature in the scheme of decoration, but it is not so. These open-work circles are, as a matter of fact, 'peepholes', through which the owner, while pretending to screen her eyes with her fan from a risque scene in a play, or other sight which ought to have offended her modesty, but in reality only excited her interest, could see all that was going on. After all, it can only have been an affectation of affectation, because these fans were well known, and cannot have deceived any one by the ruse. There is another variety of the lorgnette fan which is rather different. The entire border consists of large open circles, and in one of the guards is fixed a magnifying glass. This kind of fan was intended for use by short-sighted people, or as a substitute for an opera glass. The idea was quite a good one.
>
> Both these kinds of fans were made at the end of the eighteenth century and the beginning of the nineteenth, and were decorated in exactly the same way as other fans of that period. The transparencies were sometimes of net, and sometimes of mica, glass, or gelatine. Lorgnette fans fitted with a glass were sometimes of the brise type made of pierced ivory. Still another kind of fan, in which the same idea is worked out, is one with an enormously enlarged head, in which is set instead of a rivet a small spy glass, which acts as a rivet. This kind of fan is ugly and clumsy, and must be considered as a freak. There were fans something of this kind in the seventeenth century. Uzanne in "The Fan," English translation, p. 67, quotes from Menagiana:—
>
> The open-work fans which the women carry when they go to the Porte Saint Bernard to breathe the fresh air on the bank of the river, and occasionally to look at the bathers, are called lorgnettes (opera glasses).
>
> This, however, may just as likely be meant satirically, and refer to the cut-work fans of vellum, which were then in ordinary use.

Once more, to quote from Uzanne ("The Fan," p. 91), the lorgnette or opera-glass fan was in use in 1759, as the following extract from the paper called "Necessaire" for that year proves:—

Curiosity being equal to the two sexes, and the ladies loving almost as well as ourselves to draw near to them such objects as appear interesting, a means of satisfying this desire without wounding modesty has been imagined. An opera-glass is set in the chief sticks of a fan, of which ladies may make use without compromising themselves, forming a sort of counter-battery, which they may oppose to the indiscreet opera-glasses of our "petit maitres."[2]

Conclusion

It is interesting that the need for such a practical instrument, coupled with the desire to be inconspicuous, could be designed into such a fashionable object. The innovative and artistic efforts in the making of these fans produced quite beautiful results.

Notes

1. Richard Corson, *Fashions in Eyeglasses* (London: Peter Owen, Ltd., 1980).
2. MacIver Percival, *The Fan Book* (London: T. Fisher Unwin Ltd., 1920), 169–175.

19

The Story of the Monocle

The history of the monocle (Figure 408) is like most objects, in that an individual or several scattered individuals had a need or an idea and used it for personal improvement. The popular period of the monocle's use dates from about 1270 to 1918. However, monocles are still available commercially today and can be purchased in many parts of the world.

Origins

We are not certain of the origin of the word *monocle*. Holtman states that the word came either from the Latin *monoculus*, meaning one-eyed, or from the fact that the single glass must be held with one hand before one eye.[1] Therefore, *monocle* could be a contraction of the Latin *manus* and *oculus*—a "manocel."

Our knowledge of the origins of the monocle (about 1270) comes mostly from paintings of individuals whom we know and can satisfactorily date. The development of the monocle started with a reading stone, which was placed into a frame and given a handle so that it could be held before the eye. The oldest picture of such a vision aid was found on a tombstone in the Maritius Rotunda in the cathedral of Konstanz. This sculpture, produced around 1270, shows a man holding a monocle with a handle in his left hand.[2]

Later pieces of art help chronicle the development and use of the monocle. A portrait of an individual known to be highly myopic (Pope Leo X), painted by Raphael Santi from Orbino in 1517, shows for the first time that the monocle could be used for the correction of myopia.[3] From the reflexes of the lens in the painting, there is no doubt that the lens was myopic. A portrait of Anna Dorethea Therbusch shows the eighteenth-century painter with a monocle fastened to a ribbon around her head. A portrait of Thomas Moore, probably dating 1810, shows the poet holding a monocle in his right hand. Evidence of the use of the monocle was also found in a lithograph by Boilly of 1821. The lithograph not only shows an individual using a monocle but also shows spectacles and scissors glasses. Often, drawings depicted foppish young men using a monocle, as shown in a caricature by the Englishman, Thomas McLean, of 1827. A caricature of Bismarck by Kikerikí also depicted the German chancellor using a monocle.[4] Beethoven had a silver monocle on a black cord and is said to have used it continually in the street.

It is probable that most of the early monocles were used to correct presbyopia. However, some were also used for myopia, as previously stated regarding the portrait of Pope Leo X. We know from documents of the optician J. H. Dobler of Berlin that only later during the eighteenth century was the monocle used more often for myopic correction. Although the first monocles were certainly used for corrective purposes, later ones were often worn purely as a matter of fashion in

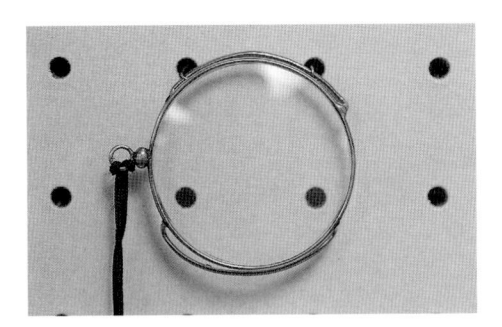

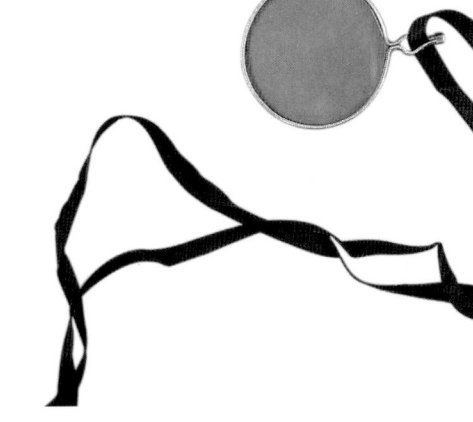

Figure 408. Monocle.

Figure 409. Monocle with small handle.

imitation of the aristocracy. In the upper classes of society, they were worn as affectations and were therefore thought to indicate a certain amount of arrogance. Additionally, though originally used by older men for presbyopic correction, monocles were later adopted by younger men to conform to the fashion of the time.

During the second half of the eighteenth century, the monocle became quite popular, especially in France. Its handle was perforated so that a string could be pulled through the hole and it could be hung from the neck. For some time, the monocle was more popular than spectacles because it was considered extremely elegant to look through a monocle to which a handle was attached (Figure 409).

The true monocle as we know it today was primarily developed by the German baron, Philipp von Stosch (1691–1757).[5] Von Stosch fashioned a string to the lens and then used the squeezing of the orbicularis muscle to hold it in place before the eye. He used this monocle mostly for near vision.

Modern Monocles

Von Stosch's modern monocle became widely used in German-speaking countries only at the beginning of the nineteenth century. This use was established by the Viennese optician, Johann Friedrich Voigtlander (1779–1859), who brought the monocle from England to Vienna at the beginning of the century and then produced the first of these devices. During the Congress of Vienna (1814–1815), the monocle was first used by diplomats. (In Germany, incidentally, the monocle was also called a "telescope" for quite a long period of time.)

A different opinion was expressed by Richard Corson,[6] who stated that Professor von Rohr dated the introduction of the monocle as differentiating from the quizzing glass in about 1806, though Corson admitted the date was speculative. Corson also stated that the monocle appeared to be of British origin and suggested that it originated on the stage. Through the attention thus attracted, the monocle was gradually taken up by British aristocracy. Sometimes the wearer carried two monocles: one for distance and the other for reading.

The monocle fad subsided for about ten years but then was revived about 1820. Monocles of various shapes (Figure 410)—round, oval, octagonal, square, and rectangular—and sizes and those of various materials—gold, silver, gold-plated (Figure 411), horn, and shell (Figure 412)—were seen in profusion. Corson stated that early monocle frames were often of solid gold and occasionally studded with diamonds.[7] This author however, who is an avid collector, has never seen any with more than a simple frame of gold, silver, or plated metal. Some rimless monocles had a hole for the cord (Figure 413). There was even one shown attached to the handle of a riding whip.

About that time, galleries—wires braised to the supporting metal frame—were added (Figure 414). One wire was placed above to engage the top lid, and one was placed below for the lower lid. The wires followed the arc of the frame about one

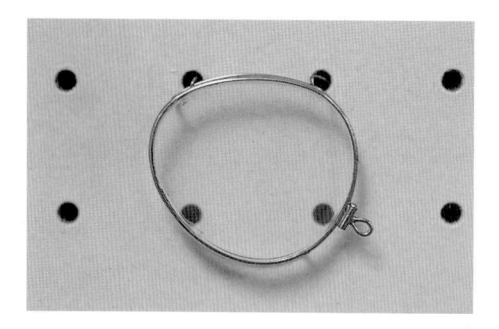

Figure 410. Monocle shaped to fit left eye.

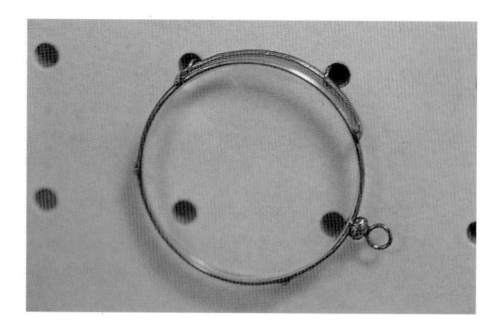

Figure 411. Gold-plated round monocle with galleries.

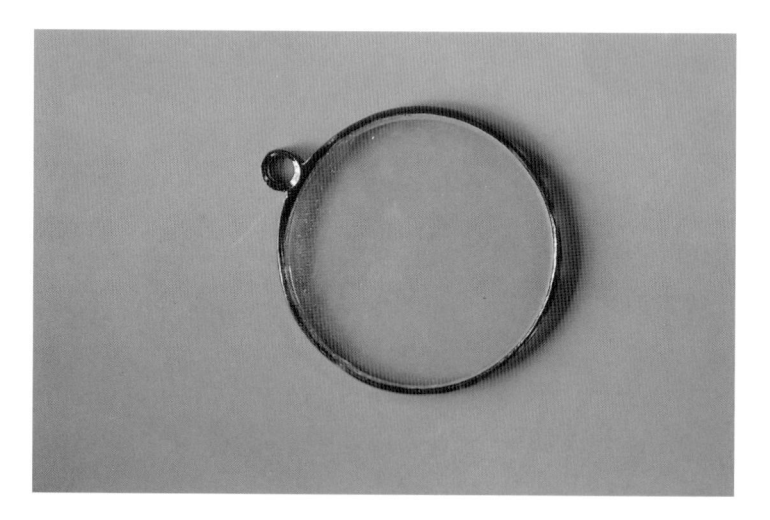

Figure 412. Tortoiseshell monocle.

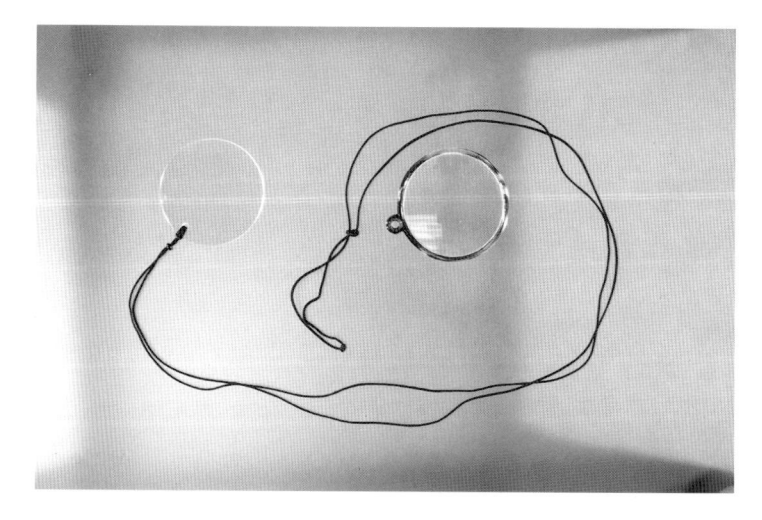

Figure 413. Rimless and tortoiseshell monocles with cords.

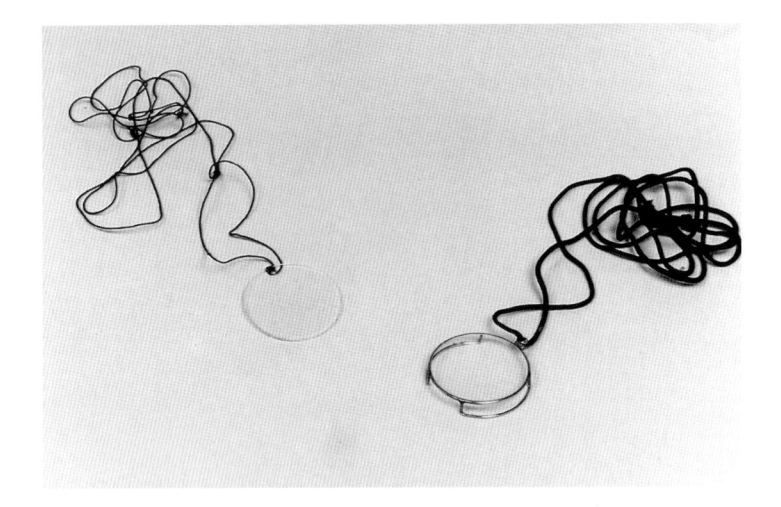

Figure 414. Rimless and gold monocles with cords. The monocle on the right exhibits galleries.

fourth of the circumference (90 degrees) and 5 millimeters to the rear. This allowed the orbicularis and eyelid skin to more easily hold the monocle in the eye socket and keep it away from the eyeball and eyelashes.

Many of the later models were mass produced. This mass production was commented on by Mr. Pitt Herbert in *An Eye on the Monocle*:

> They were worn with an air of conscious elegance and often one had the feeling the wearer was being a trifle foolish, an attitude which resulted to some extent from the fact that monocles frequently did not fit and kept dropping out of place. The orbit of the eye was too small, too large, or too shallow; the eyeballs or too much of the lashes rubbed against the lens. Obviously the mass production of monocles was anything but encouraging to fitting precision [Figure 415].

Comments by Physicians

The monocle was not accepted by the entire medical community, and through the years, there were several denunciations of its use:

1. An anonymous German treatise on glasses, published in Leipzeig in 1824, stated: "The monocle with which a single eye is used must be avoided because it disturbs the balance of binocular vision. However, grown up children of both sexes play with the monocle hanging it on the chest like the triumph of their science, or wearing it attached to the hat in front of the face. Numerous young people with normal vision use a monocle with a plain glass. It seems truly that they use this style of eyeglass to lend themselves an amiable air of impudence and to make themselves noticed. The style of our day does not tolerate healthy vision and demands that one appear to be or be half blind."

2. In the same year in London, Dr. Kitchiner wrote, "A single glass set in a smart ring is often used by trinket fanciers merely for fashion sake, by folks who have not the least defect in their sight and are not aware of the mischievous consequences of such irritations. This pernicious plaything will most assuredly in a very few years bring on an imperfect vision in one or both eyes."[8]

3. In Paris in 1847, the monocle again came under attack, this time by Magne in a work entitled *Hygiene du la Vue*: "In our day the lorgnon has dethroned spectacles. That is to say, a grotesque custom has been replaced by an even more grotesque one. Of a hundred persons who use this little square piece of glass which they hold in place only by making faces, 90 surely could do without it. The only result is that they make themselves vulnerable to myopia at the same

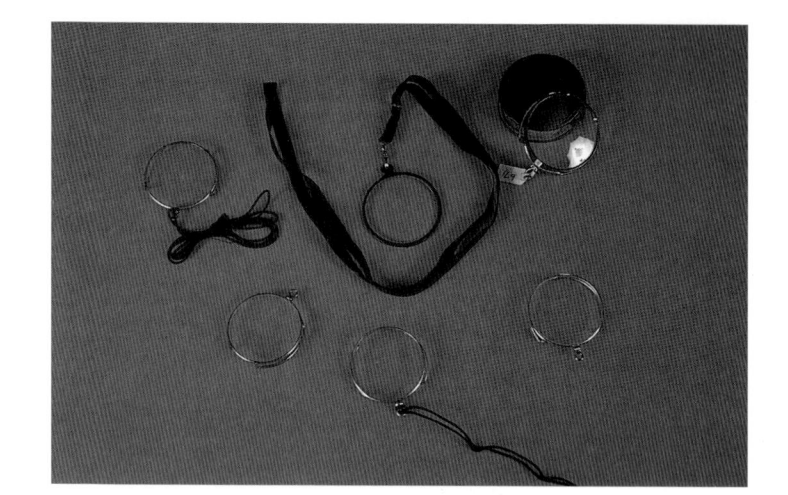

Figure 415. Group of monocles.

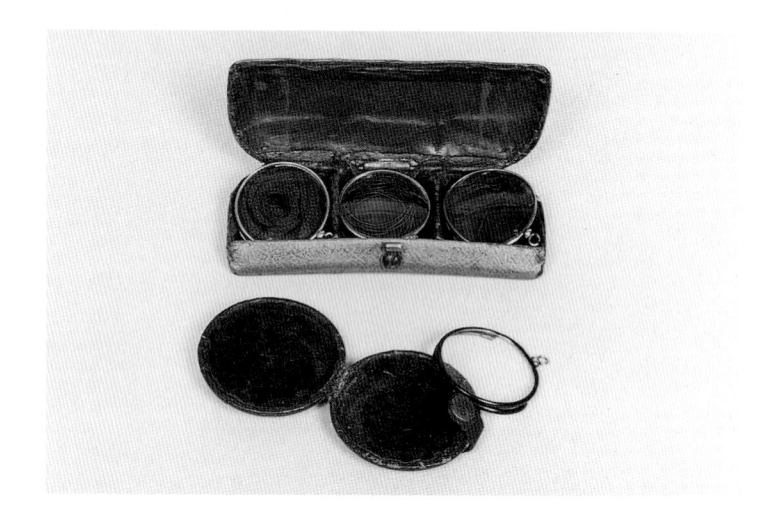

Figure 416. Monocles in cases. Top case holding three monocles is rare. Bottom tortoiseshell monocle with galleries is unusual.

time that they prematurely develop crow's feet, the despair of so many women."⁹ [Please note that Magne refers to square monocles. Although this author has never seen a square monocle, it may have been considered to be more popular than the round one.]

In Britain, the fad for the use of the monocle gradually faded. By 1830, only the hard core of monocle devotees were upholding its use. As a matter of fact, in 1826, Charles Dickens mercilessly ridiculed the monocle in his story "Little Dorrit." By the latter part of the nineteenth century, the monocle was still being used by the upper class of the British people and also in most parts of Germany.

In the United States, the monocle was introduced about 1880 but was not popular. It was used only by the social set.

Because of its German aura, it came into disrepute in the United States after World War I. Now it is found only in the entertainment media to define a character.

Monocle Cases

Monocles used mostly in England and the continent in the early 1900s were supposed to be impressive—clearly seen and used in public. Therefore, the small, round cases used to house these monocles were kept primarily at home. Similarly, the small leather slip-in cases with snaps at the top used to house oxford folding (pince-nez/lorgnettes) glasses were also kept at home. While in public, on the other hand, the owner of these glasses could impress his friends and acquaintances with his finery. (See Figure 416).

Conclusion

In the United Kingdom and on the Continent, the monocle is seldom found except with the older adherents of a previous era. Therefore, we bid farewell to this socially oriented and sometimes visually useful ocular adjunct.

Notes

1. W. H. Holtman, "A Short History of Spectacles," in W. Poulet, *Atlas on the History of Spectacles* (Germany, Bad Godesberg: Wayenborgh, 1978), xiv.
2. Richard Corson, *Fashions in Eyeglasses* (London: Peter Owen, Ltd., 1980).
3. Ibid.
4. Ibid.
5. Ibid.
6. Ibid.
7. Ibid.
8. Ibid.
9. Magne, *Hygiène du la Vue* (Paris, 1847).

Other Sources Consulted for Chapter 19

1. Dr. M. Von Rohr, *Eyes and Spectacles* (London: The Hatton Press, Limited, 1912).

20

Pince-Nez

Pince-nez, French for "pinch nose," is the name given to eyeglasses that do just that—pinch the nose. This is how they were held in place. The first glasses invented, made of two magnifying glasses with the handle ends riveted together (Figure 417), were probably used as pince-nez. They were described, however, as being "hung on the nose." The last type used was the Fits-U model from American Optical Company about 1915 (Figure 418). Some may remember their grandmothers using them as late as 1930. The advantage of their use for women was that they did not disturb the hair at a time when hairspray was not yet available.

Fitting

It is interesting to imagine the optician's task in fitting the various pince-nez to the face. Of course, the first riveted and hinged variety could be hung precariously on the nose if one had a hump in the middle (Figure 419). Otherwise, the glasses were pressed above or below the bony section. The former could not be employed for long, as it caused pain. Pressing the glasses on the lower part of the nose caused obstruction of the nasal passages, with accompanying voice changes and respiratory problems.

Later in the eighteenth century, pince-nez were therefore positioned on the superior part of the nose—attaching actually to the skin and subdermis. In this manner, nasal passages were not occluded. It was necessary, though, to have the lenses quite close to the lids, and sometimes lashes had to be cut. Ex-ophthalmic patients had a real problem (Figure 420).

Additionally, the pantoscopic angle, as well as the optical centers of each lens, had to be considered when applying the pince-nez. If cords were used, they dragged down one side; as a result, compensatory angling was needed. The patient needed lessons on how to apply his or her newly acquired glasses.

Developments

There were more patents for this style of eyewear than for any other prior to or since the pince-nez, as inventors made one attempt after another to find a more secure and comfortable method of holding eyeglasses to the nose.

In the sixteenth century, glasses were made of leather by the hundreds (Figure 421) and were held in place by "stuffing" them on the nose. Later, in the seventeenth (see Figure 58, Chapter 5) and eighteenth centuries, the slit bridge was employed, as it offered enough resiliency to grasp the nose and hold the glasses in position. These were made of bone, ivory, baleen (Figure 422), and various metals. Then around 1700, hinged eyeglasses, not unlike the riveted ones (Figure 423), were employed in a manner not only to clamp the nose but also to vary the pupillary distance according to need (Figure 424).[1]

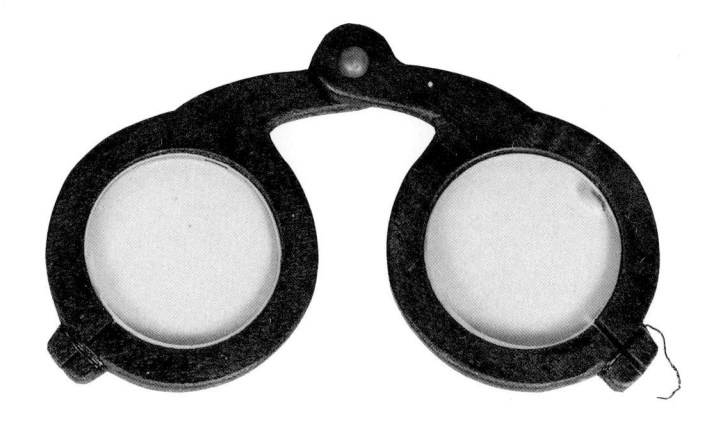

Figure 417. Riveted eyeglasses (reproduced) circa 1286.

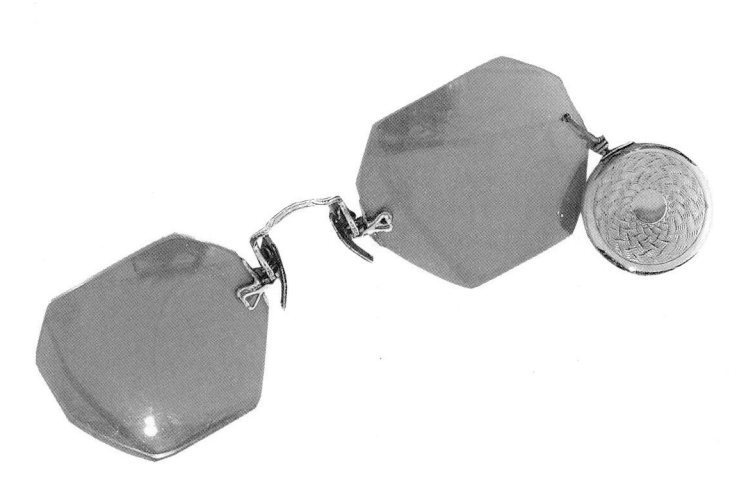

Figure 418. Fits-U model circa 1932.

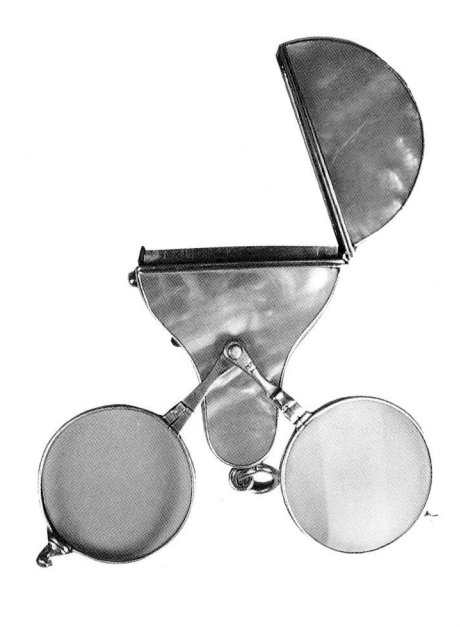

Figure 419. Silver-hinged pince-nez and mother-of-pearl and silver case circa 1650.

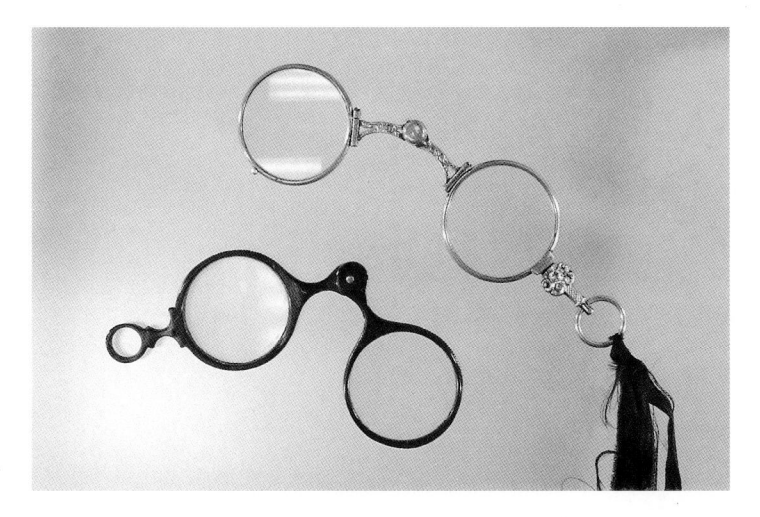

Figure 420. Riveted pince-nez in tortoiseshell and gold.

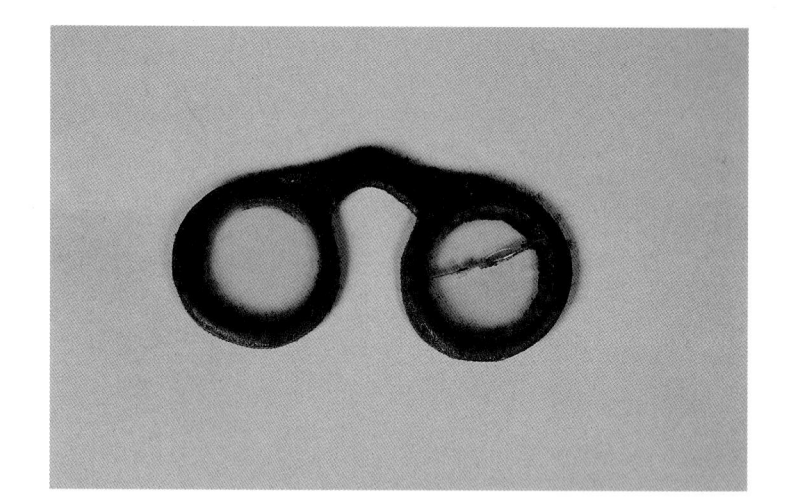

Figure 421. Ordinary leather eyeglasses circa 1600.

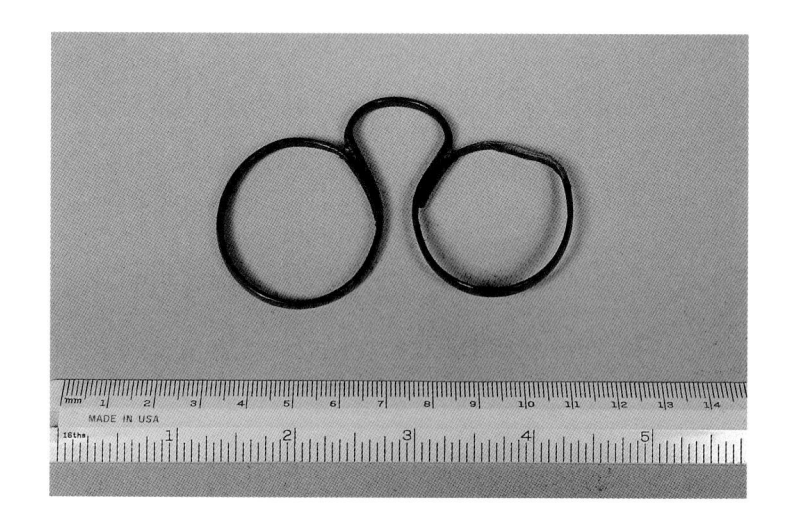

Figure 422. Baleen eyeglass frames.

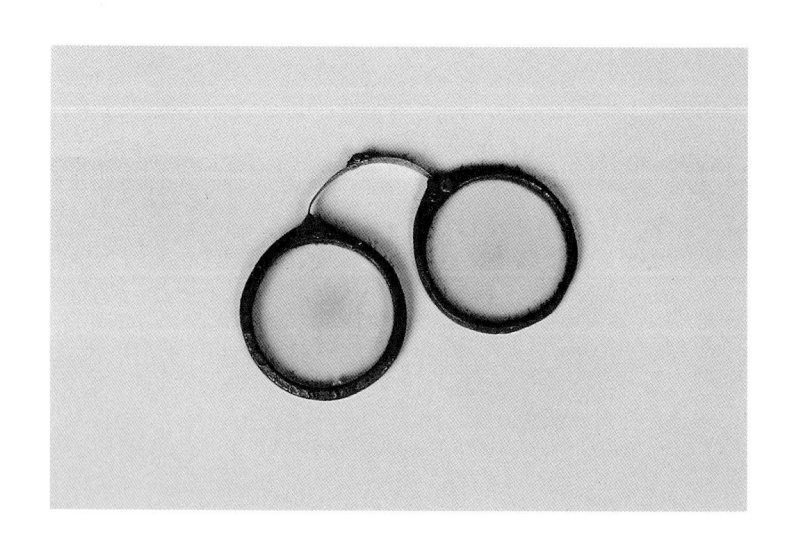

Figure 423. Leather rims, spring-bridge with central hinge, English circa 1700.

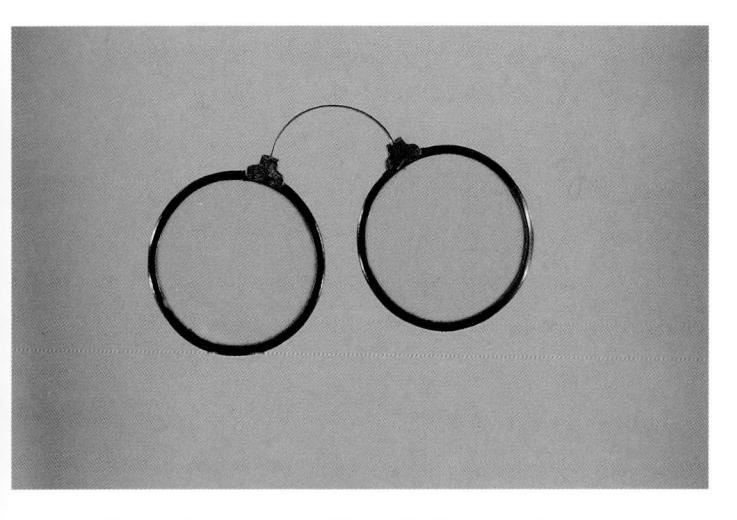

Figure 424. Later model of Figure 423 with tortoiseshell rims.

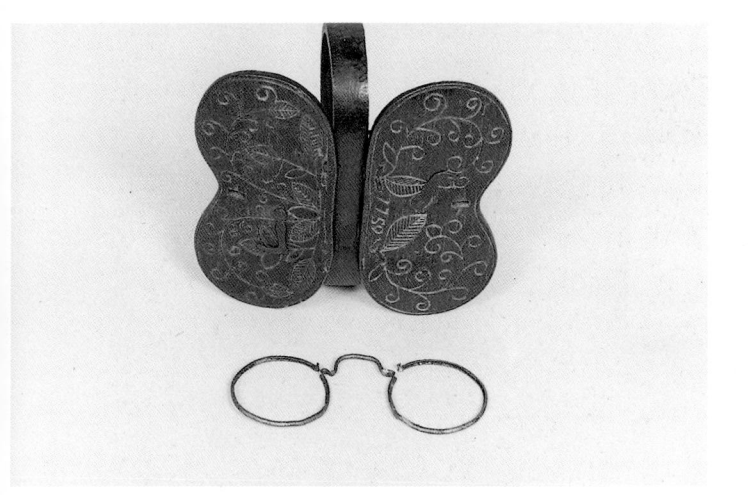

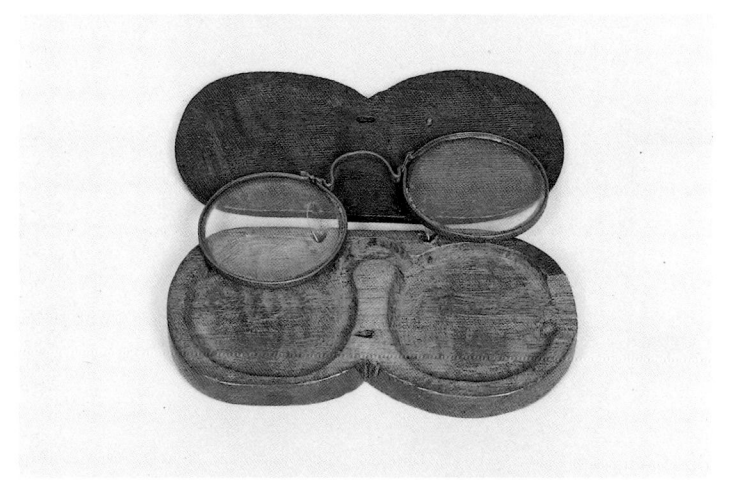

Figure 425. Typical Nuremberg eyeglasses in carved wooden case circa 1750.

Figure 426. Typical Nuremberg eyeglasses in double wooden case circa 1750.

The Musierwelle, a machine, was invented in the middle of the seventeenth century. Its double rollers were used to press a round wire into a flattened length, with a groove on one side and an embossed name or insignia on the other. This wire was used as the raw material for eyeglass makers, especially in Nuremberg, where they produced many pince-nez (Figures 425 & 426). Copper wire, which was sometimes silver plated, was used. In Belgium, brass was a favorite material. For cushioning and traction, the wire was wrapped with a silk thread in areas where the pince-nez rested on the nose. Many pince-nez have been recovered by digging in old privies and drainage canals.

Spring steel was used sometime later (Figure 427) and was even concealed in layers of baleen in a pair that the author has acquired. Baleen was used fairly often in European manufacture, and glasses of this material were recorded in portraits of men by Dürer and other artists.

When the steel spring was attached to rimless glasses, the glasses had to be scribed on the edge to secure the glasses to the nose (Figure 428). When a steel spring was fitted to a frame of wire, tortoiseshell, and later hard rubber or cellulose acetate, nose pads were attached to keep the pince-nez in place.

Whereas we have been discussing the use of spring steel as

Figure 427. Spring steel pince-nez.

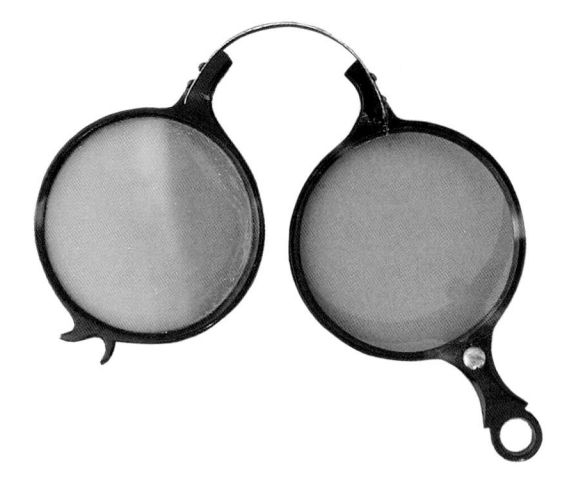

Figure 428. Rimless pince-nez, Belgian. Note the scribing on the nasal edges.

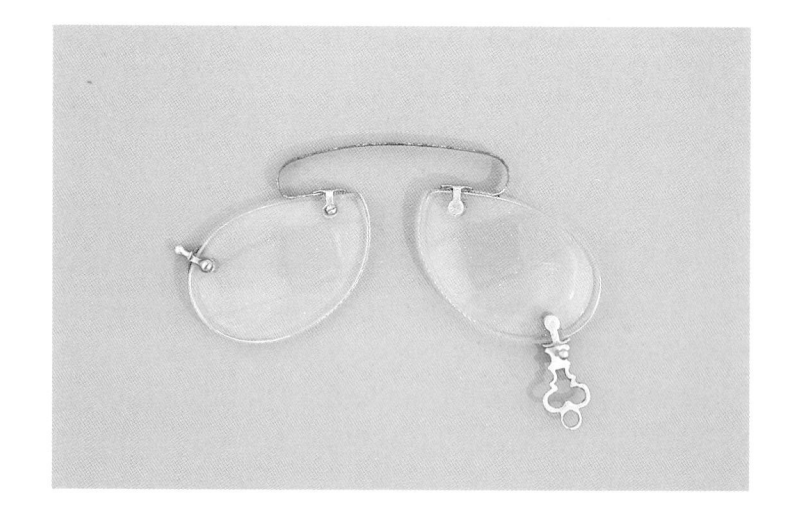

Figure 429. Various types of nose pads.

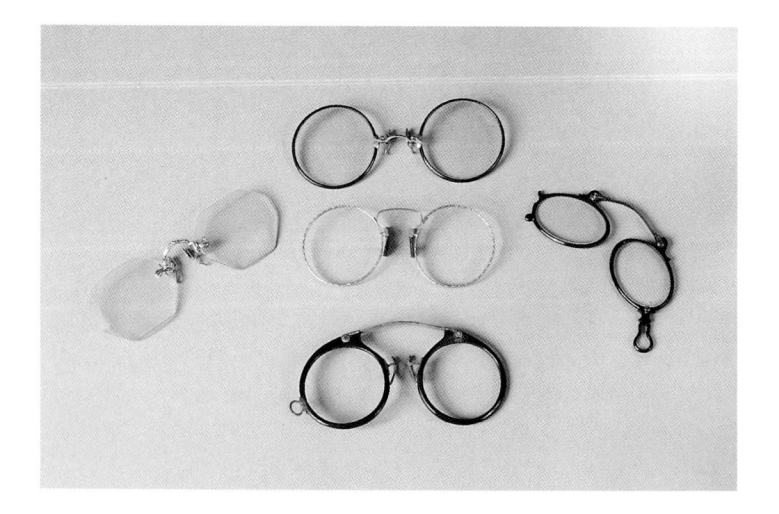

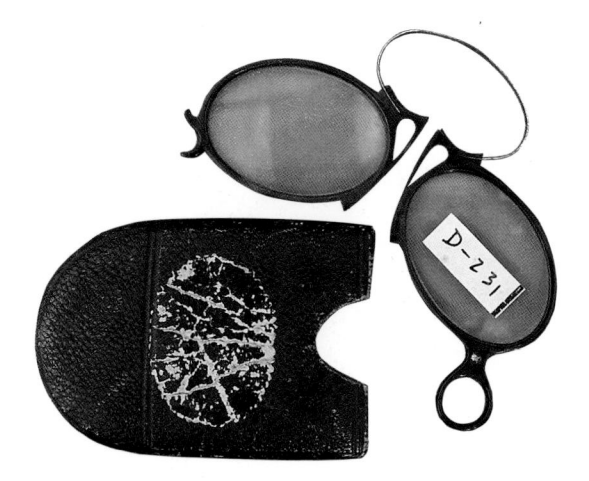

Figure 430. Tortoiseshell frames and integral nose pads.

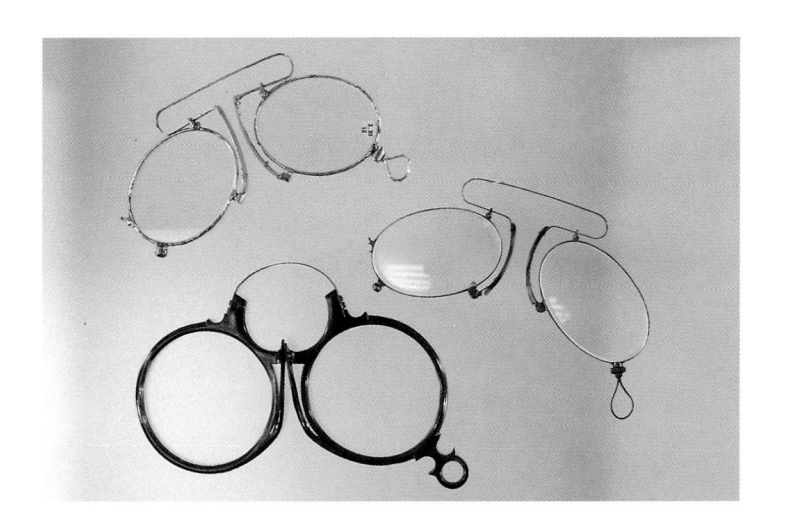

Figure 431. Various pince-nez and nose pads.

a bridge in pince-nez, this material was also placed in rimless models between the edge of the glass and the attachment to the bridge. These springs are almost flat, only about 1 to 1 ½ millimeters wide and perhaps 3 to 7 millimeters long. They may be used singly or in multiples. In position they act as do the flat layered springs on a buggy or automobile, as opposed to coiled springs. The advantage of these is that they cushion the glass against the bridge attachment. This forces the glass into position but allows just enough motion (or give) to keep the glass from breaking during normal wear, on-off tension, or sudden crashing against hard objects.

Nose pads improved patient comfort and were made of several different materials (Figures 429, 430, & 431). Tor-

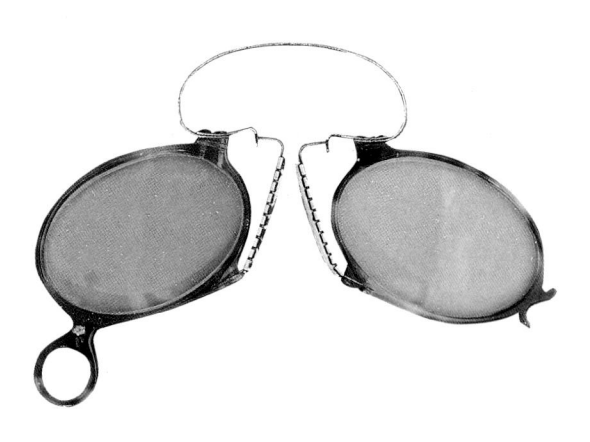

Figure 432. Cork nose pads.

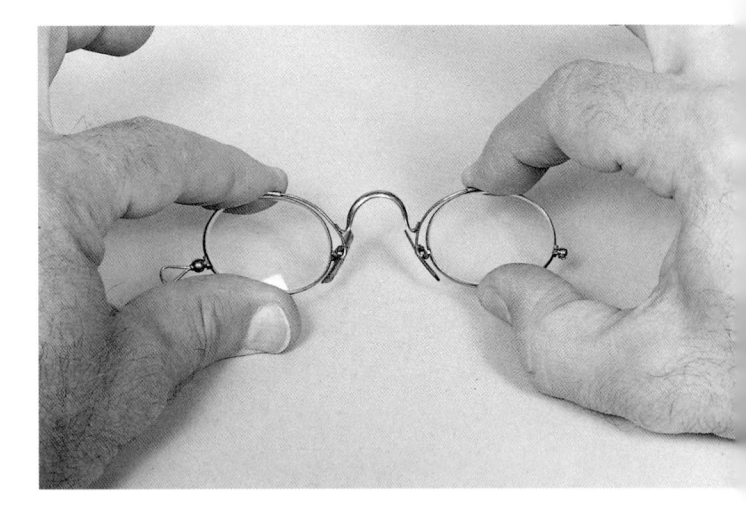

Figure 433. Leverage system of applying pince-nez.

Figure 434. Fun pince-nez with pinholes for viewing.

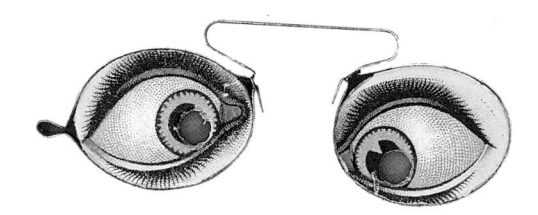

Figure 435. Coil springs combined with springed nose pads.

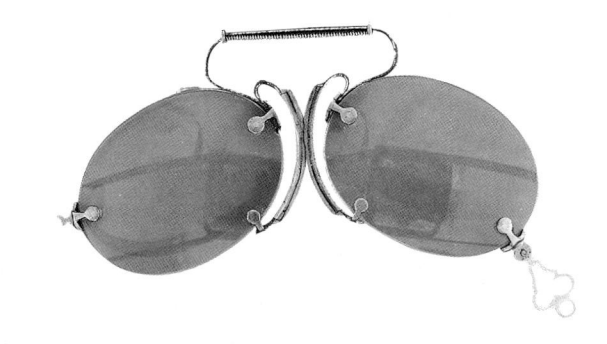

toiseshell liners were mounted on the nose guards with rough cut or corrugated surface so that no slippage would occur. Sharkskin-covered eye guards were also considered a valuable option, as found in the following 1911 advertisement from American Optical Company: "Few opticians realize what an ideal material the much despised creature furnishes for guard facings—The natural conformation of the surface, having minute corrugations, make it especially adaptable to eyeglass guards. Its peculiar property of holding on with a comfortable grip make it even more desirable than zylonite."

Cork became the most widely used method employed for improved friction on the nose and was used in a variety of methods in nose guard mountings (Figure 432). The advantages of cork were not only that it improved friction but also that it was softer and more comfortable against the nose. At one point, as many as eight cork pads were used on one bridge (or one nose).

A clever leverage system was also created (Figure 433). The nose pads could be opened prior to placing the eyeglasses on the nose by simply moving the eyeglasses (one lens in each hand) downward at the bridge while turning upward at the temporal area. This motion caused the lever mechanism to open the nose pads.

There was no lack of humor during this period either (Figure 434).

Spring mechanisms, which provided more pressure against the nose, began to appear (Figure 435). Coil springs working in conjunction with improved nose pads helped but didn't solve the retention problem (Figure 436). In July of 1882, George Bausch invented something called spring temples, which were built into the eyeglasses. When used, these fine wire springs pressed against the temple, securing the glasses to the face. They were really built-in cheaters, not unlike training wheels on a bicycle. These small attachments could be folded out of sight when the wearer was willing to take a chance and impress someone.

Several designs allowed a one-hand operation of the pince-nez (Figure 437). A bar was extended over the top of the bridge from the outer eyewire. When the eyeglass was held between the thumb and second finger, the forefinger could pull the bar downward, thereby opening the bridge area. Once in position, the release caused the spring tension in the bridge to again secure the eyeglass to the nose.

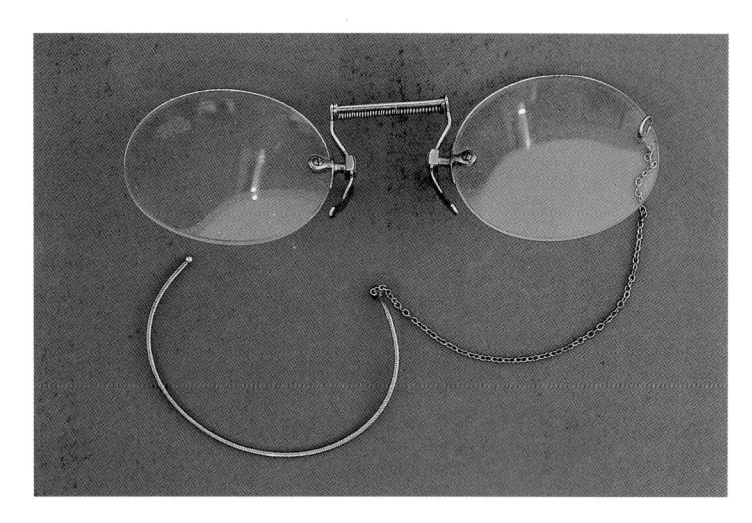

Figure 436. Coil springs combined with springed nose pads.

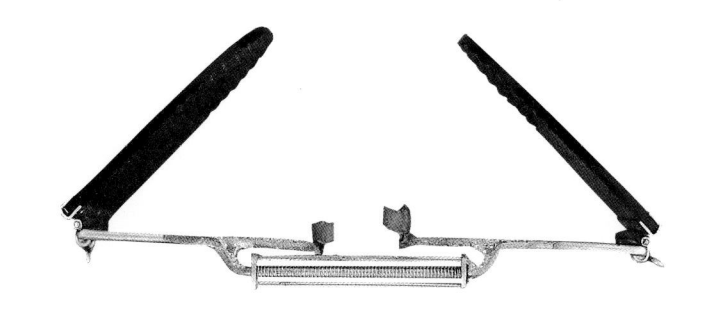

Figure 437. Unusual type of pince-nez.

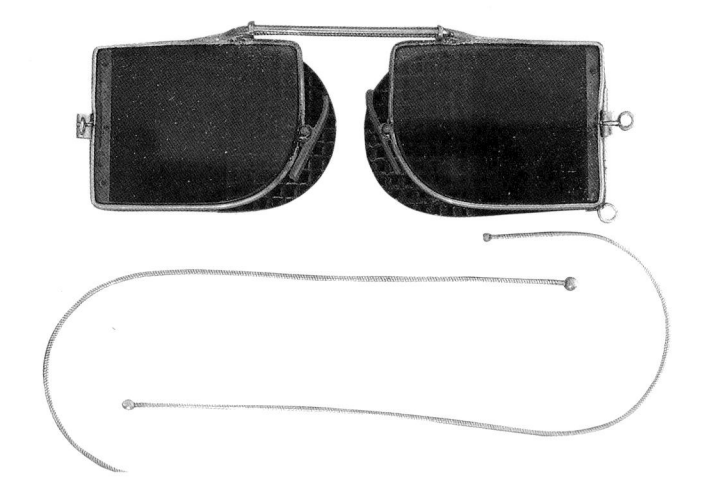

Figure 438. Pince-nez en suite with snap-on temples.

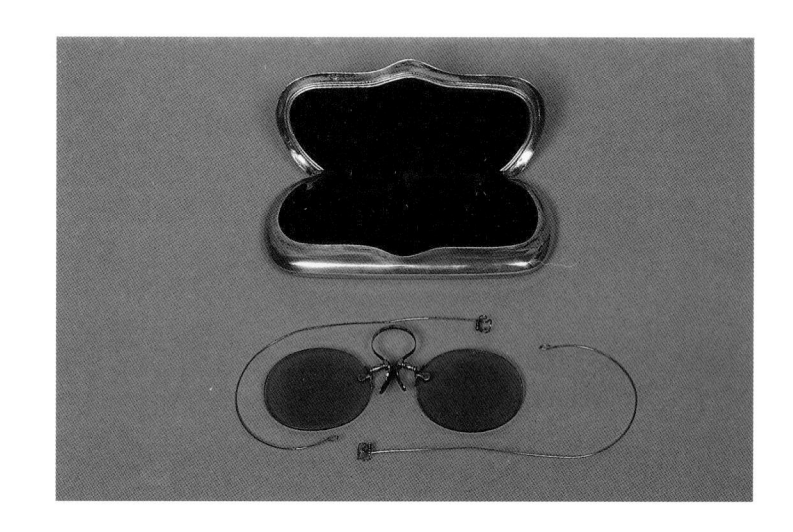

Figure 439. Rimless pince-nez en suite with snap-on temples.

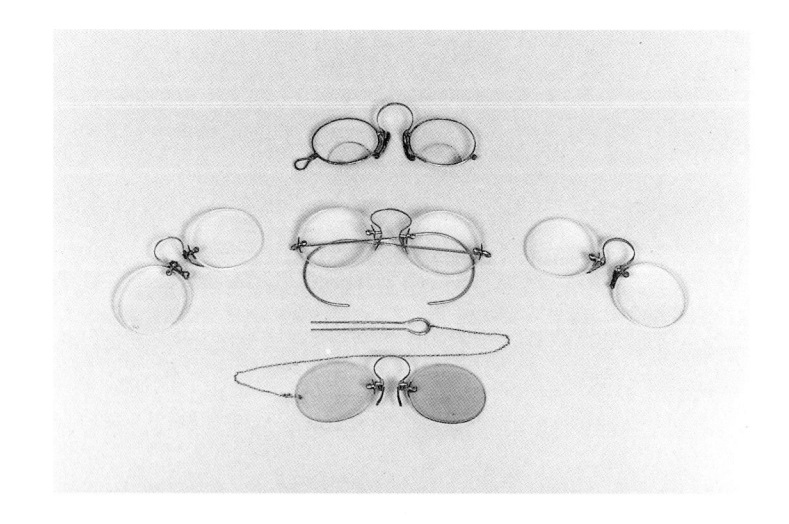

Figure 440. Combined pince-nez and riding bow spectacles (center).

244   CHAPTER 20

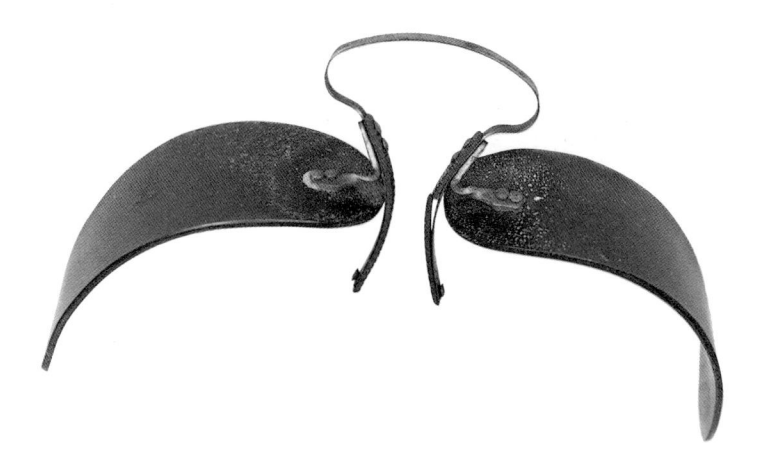

Figure 441. Curious pince-nez sun shield.

Manufacturers made temples that could snap onto the pince-nez, both with rims and rimless in style (Figures 438 & 439). Once again, the fainthearted could wear a fashionable eyeglass but be secure that it would not crash to the floor.

One manufacturer made a pince-nez "spectacle" that had full riding temples built into the design (Figure 440). These were an Australian model, the Mahtsorf, and were designed for the rough Australian back country "beyond the black stump," according to Fleming.[2] Since the pince-nez had a habit of falling off, this design was apparently the solution.

There was yet another curious design in 1912. The British designed an unusual pince-nez mounting called the Achilles. A one-piece wire with inshell pads was used in conjunction with predrilled rimless lenses so that the entire assembly could be sprung together using no screws and then taken apart in the same manner by optician or wearer. The need for this style was derived from the many British who were spread around the British Empire. Since opticians were not available in many areas, spare lenses were carried to repair breakage on the spot.

Another most unusual design is the pince-nez eye shields (Figure 441). These shields act as a ledge above the eye—a large overgrown eyebrow—or perhaps like the peak of a cap!

Because pince-nez were so popular, manufacturers wanted to make it easier for opticians to fit patients. They therefore provided sets with a variety of bridge sizes, pupillary distances, etc., to use as trial fits. Some of these sets are illustrated in Figures 442–445.

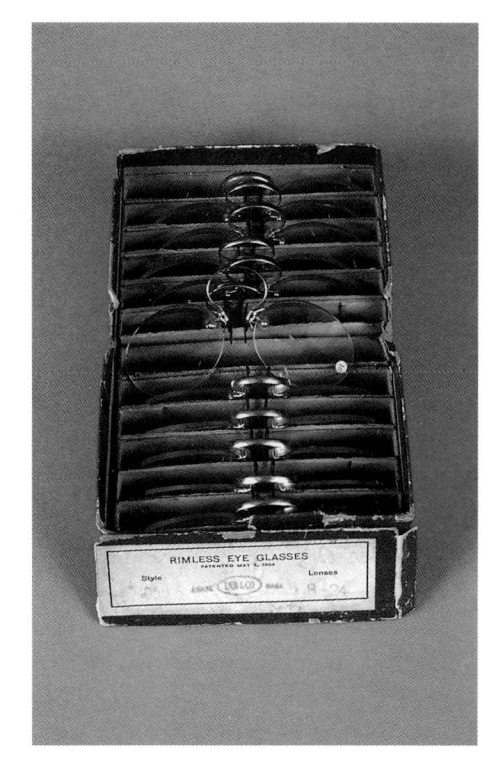

Figure 442. Pince-nez fitting set circa 1870.

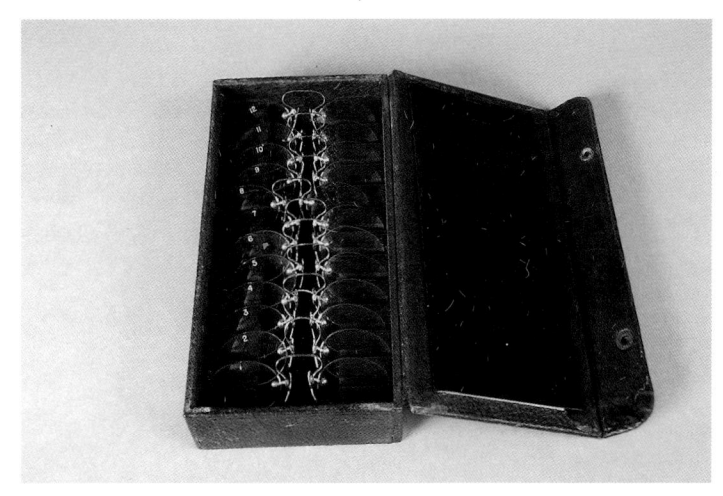

Figure 443. Pince-nez fitting set circa 1880.

PINCE-NEZ 245

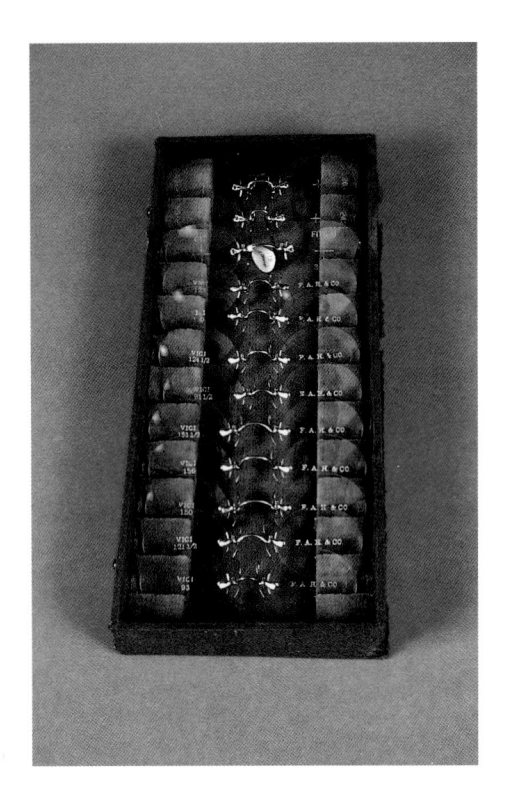

Figure 444. Pince-nez fitting set circa 1900.

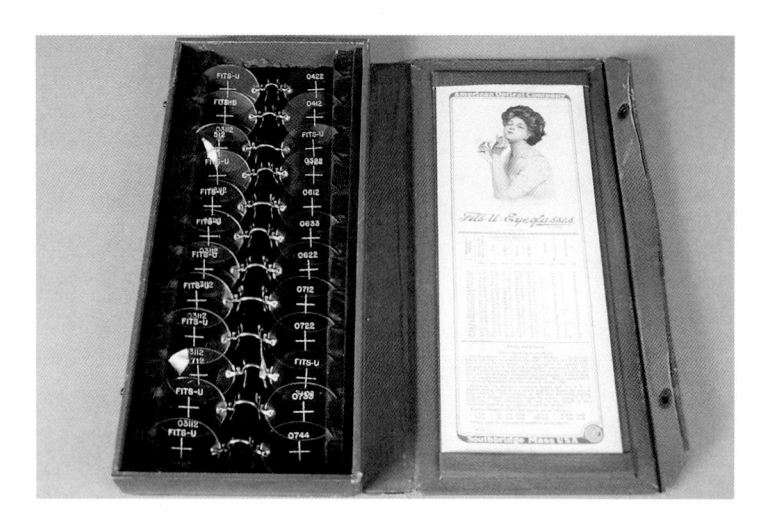

Figure 445. Another pince-nez fitting set circa 1900.

Bar-Springs

Upon the discovery of astigmatism in the early nineteenth century, cylindrical lenses were placed into pince-nez, but their rotation by the inherent mode of placement on the nose made accurate astigmatism angle setting a rare occurrence. Therefore, the bar-spring, or astigmatic clip was invented to correct this problem (Figure 446). A bar connecting the two lenses kept the lenses from rotating, and some variation was afforded in how the glasses might be placed on the nose. This was accomplished by hooking a separate bar to each lens and having the lenses slide back and forth against each other for attachment. These glasses were always accompanied by a coil spring mounted around the bars to maintain pressure against the nose (Figure 447). By keeping the lenses in steady rotary relationship to each other, the astigmatism angle was stabilized. Several varieties of the astigmatic clip were produced to meet demand for proper correction of astigmatism (Figures 448 & 449).

About 1900, when small, coiled steel springs were employed to mobilize each nose pad (finger-piece mounts), the pince-nez bridge was rigid. Thus, astigmatism as well as pupillary distance were normalized. Bar-springs were no longer needed.

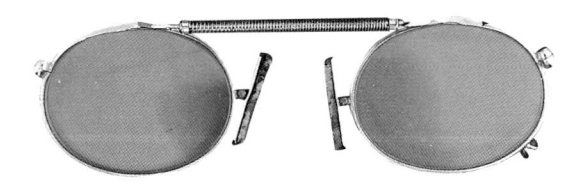

Figure 446. Typical bar-spring pince-nez circa 1890.

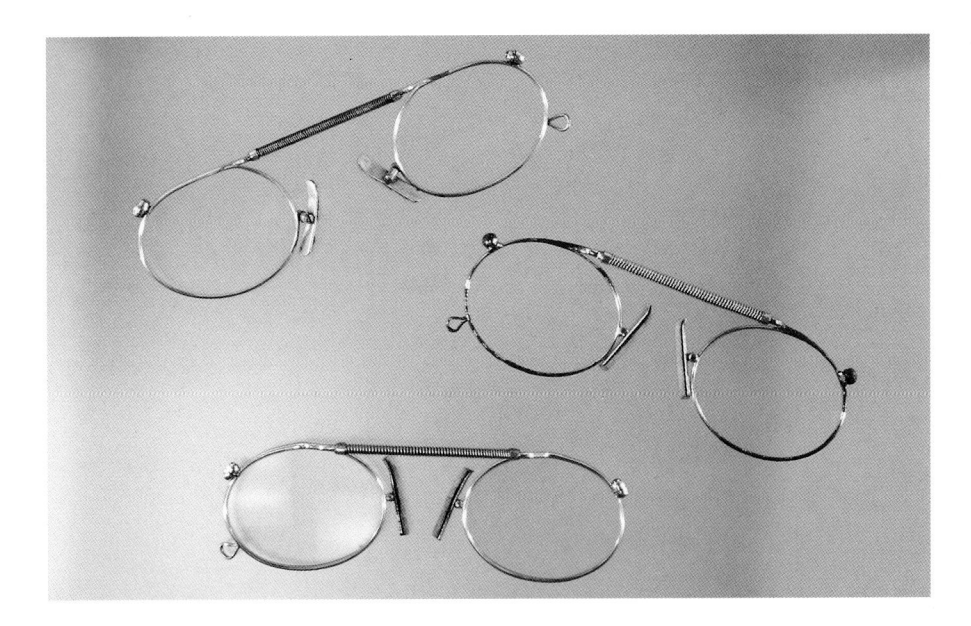

Figure 447. Other examples of a typical bar-spring pince-nez circa 1890.

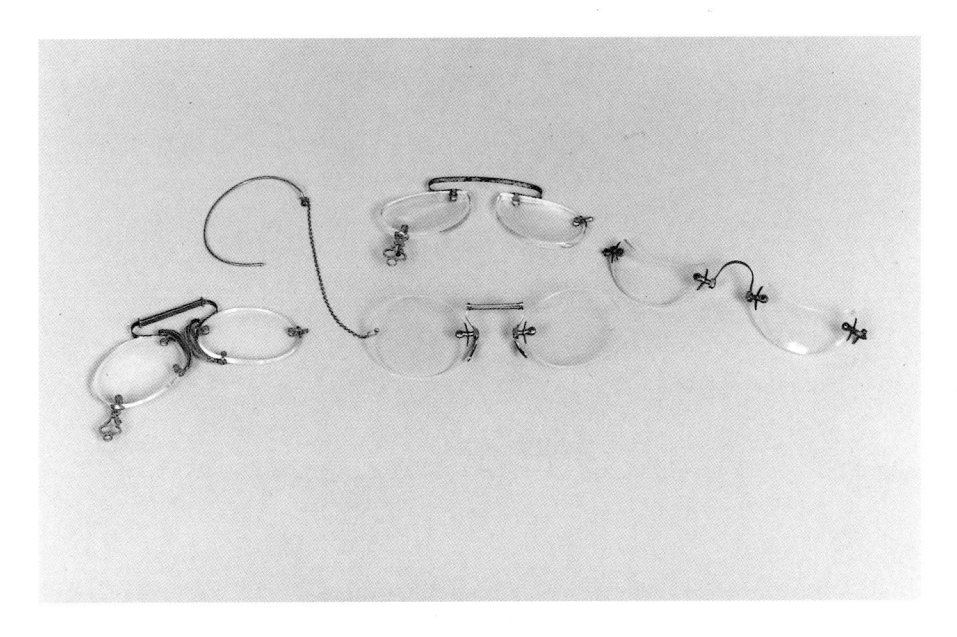

Figure 448. From left: bar-spring, bar-spring, rimless pince-nez, preacher's ½-glass pince-nez.

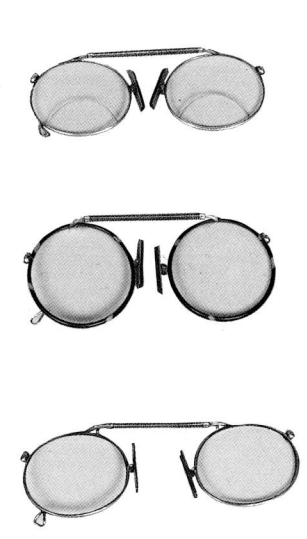

Figure 449. Three bar-spring types.

PINCE-NEZ 247

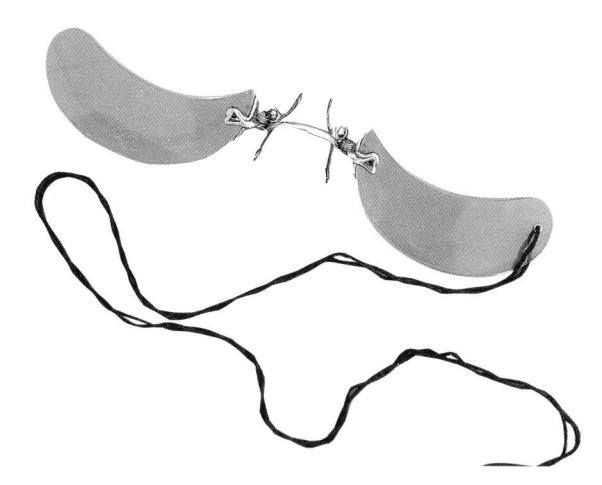

Figure 450. Speaker's ½-glass pince-nez with cord.

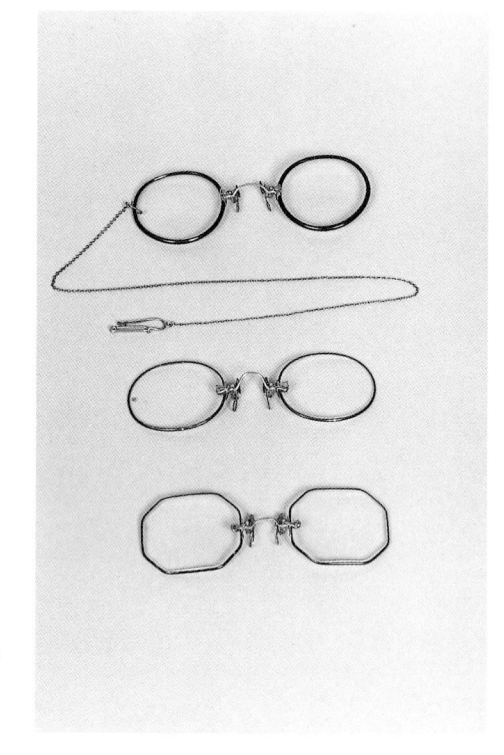

Figure 451. Three pince-nez with tortoiseshell rims; top example has a chain to attach to a lapel or dress with a pin.

Figure 452. British pince-nez with ear wire attached.

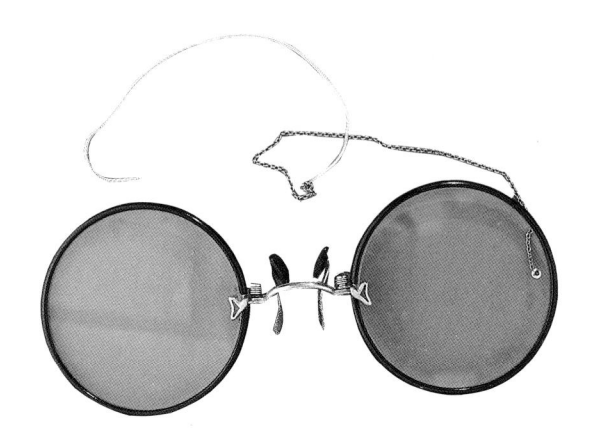

Figure 453. American pince-nez with hairpin attached.

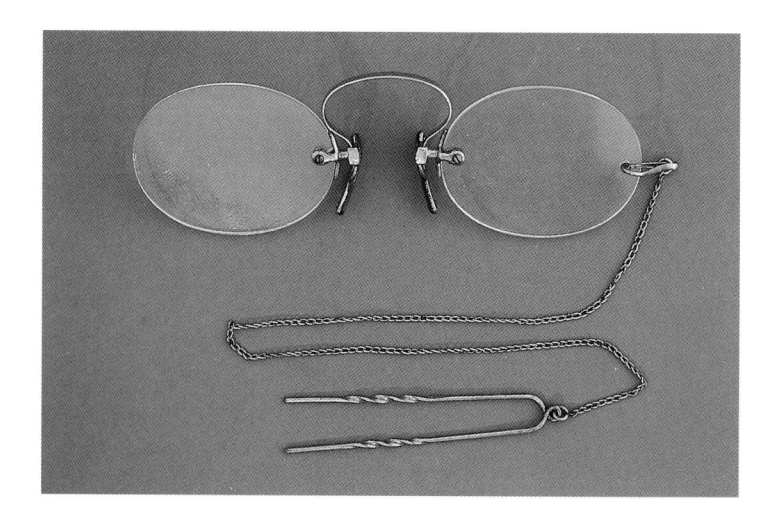

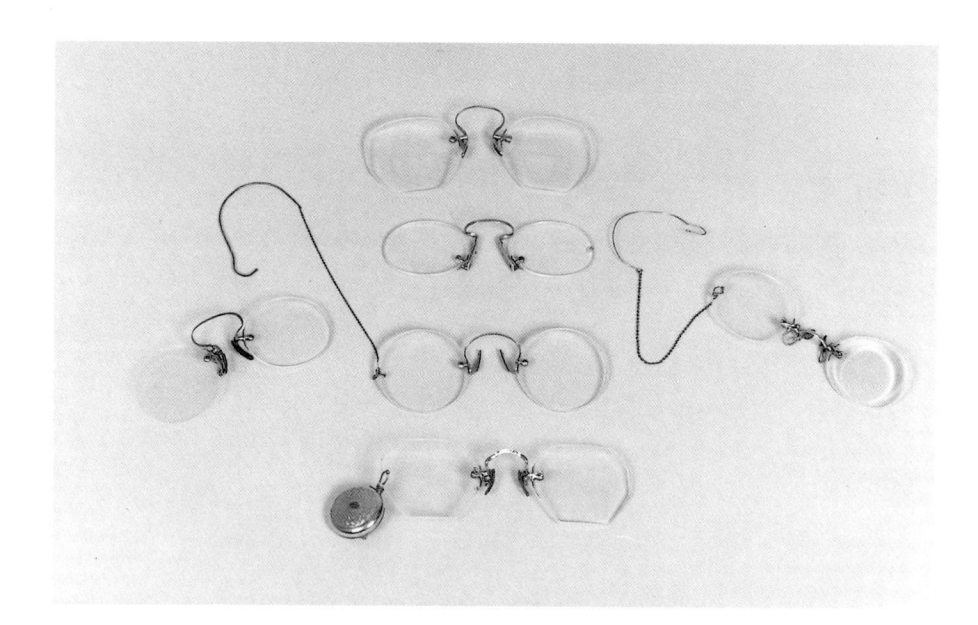

Figure 454. Group of rimless pince-nez. A chain in a reel is attached to the example on the bottom.

Adjuncts to Pince-Nez

Those small eyeglasses were anything but securely fastened to the face. Therefore, many ways of keeping them from falling and breaking were devised.

A simple cord or tape was attached to the small loop on the side of the frame in most cases (Figure 450). Rimless models, which started about 1825, had holes drilled in the edge of the glass. Cords, or possibly fine chains, were attached. The cords were either hung from the neck or attached to the dress or suit lapel (Figure 451). Chains were attached to formed ear wires (Figure 452) for men and women, as well as hairpins for women (Figure 453). By 1915, a small, gold chain-reeling mechanism could be purchased to reel up the chain and eyeglasses. The "automatic" reel was spring loaded and worked much like a window shade, as it could be extended to the desired length, and a catch would prevent it from returning (Figure 454). As so often is the case with window shades, some of the more cheaply made automatic reels would occasionally break and quickly reel in the chain—and eyeglasses—sharply whipping the glasses from the face, thus creating some embarrassment. It must not have been too bad, as (templeless) eyeglasses survived another 15 years. Fancy evening models were available, and some chains' cases were made of enamel, silver, gold, or platinum, embellished with jewels (Figure 455).

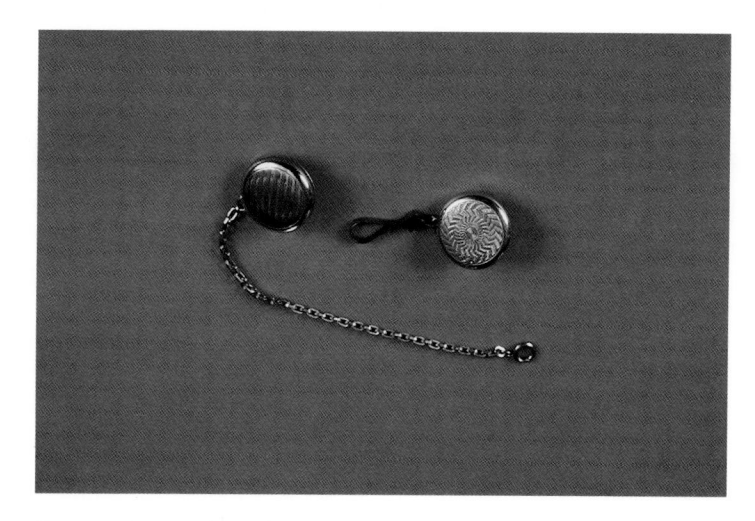

Figure 455. Fancy chain reel cases.

PINCE-NEZ 249

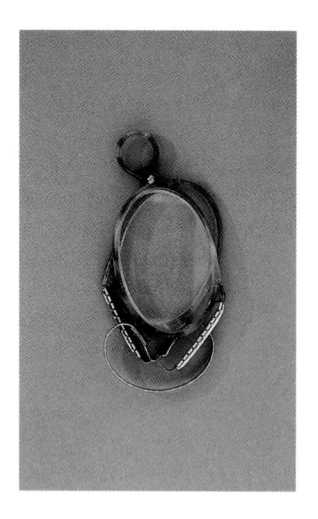

Figure 456. Tortoiseshell folded pince-nez.

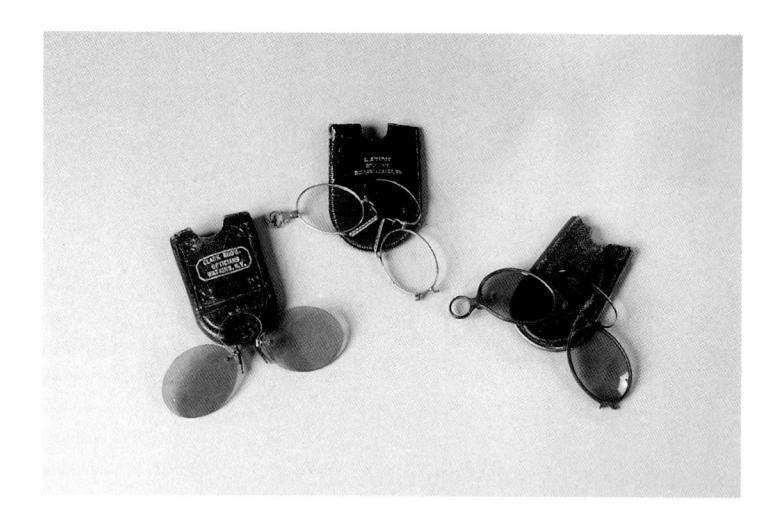

Figure 457. Folding pince-nez and their cases.

Figure 458. Group of pince-nez sunshades.

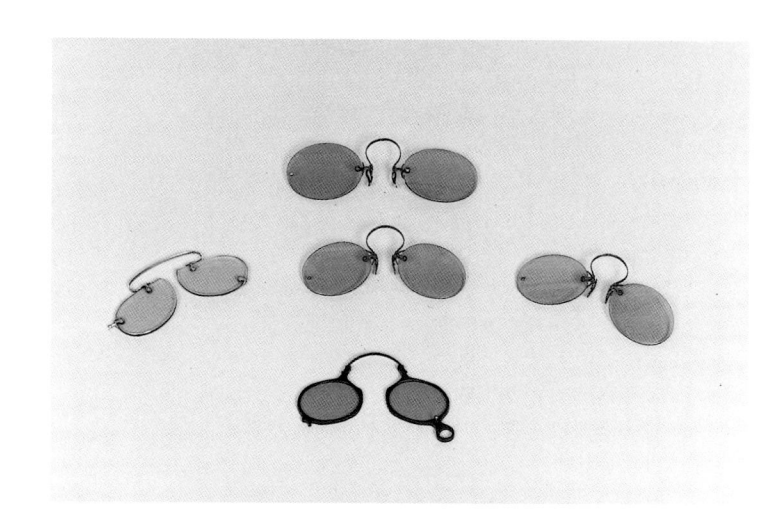

Figure 459. Another group of pince-nez sunshades.

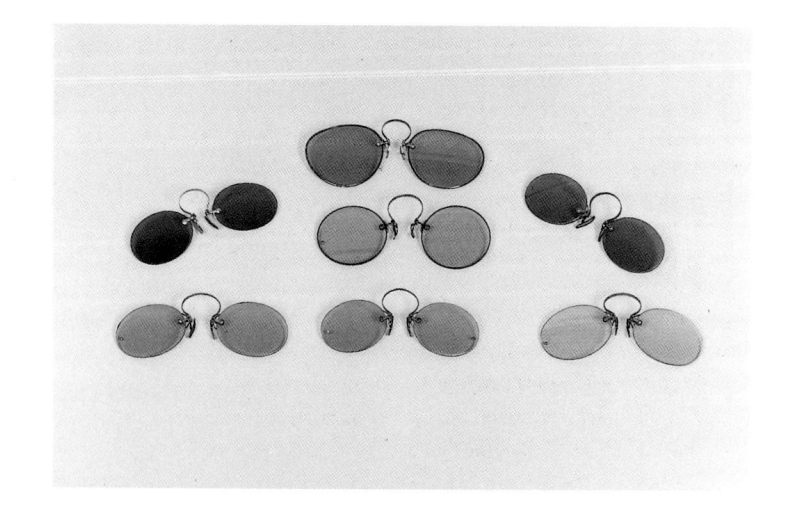

250 CHAPTER 20

Many models of pince-nez were designed to fold together when not in use (Figure 456). They could be hung from the neck, placed in a pocket, or placed in a case (Figure 457).

Pince-nez were also used as sunglasses (Figure 458), though the lenses were small. Blue lenses were supposed to be specific for relief in the exanthematous conditions exhibiting skin rash with conjunctivitis. Smoked glass was used in models of the 1800s as well as in pince-nez of the 1890s to 1910s (Figure 459). Yellow colors for the lenses were supposed to help clear the vision during fog or haze and were much in demand by hunters.

John M. Young gives us the following both instructive and amusing account regarding pince-nez:

> Although the pince-nez began in France in 1840, Bausch and Lomb introduced theirs in the United States at about 1855.... The advantage of the pince-nez was that they would fold, one lens over the other, which made for easy storage in the pocket or purse. In fact, they were often called "folders."
>
> These became popular for a variety of reasons. Due to the Industrial Revolution, eyeglasses were quite inexpensive which put the pince-nez within reach of almost everyone. Some people had other reasons, however, as many people wore non-prescription or plano lenses in their pince-nez eyeglasses. The following was written by just such an individual who wrote to an English magazine called "Answers" in 1898:
>
>> Apart from the fact that certain faces are improved by glasses, a pair can be made to render the wearer real service. I find them of most use during discussion, either at home or at the Debating Club. When I am fumbling with them, I gain several valuable seconds in which to collect my thoughts and no one notices the pause. If I need longer grace, I dexterously allow the obstinate things to fall from my nose. Nervous people should certainly take to eye-glasses; they cover a good deal of bashfulness. They act as a kind of shield. You feel something like a man who, from the interior of his house, is conducting a controversy with a man on the pavement. Through glasses, you can look a man full in the face, when without them you would from pure nervousness avoid his glance.
>
> Part of what made eyeglasses popular is some of the fancy accessories which one could purchase for them. The accessories were necessary due to the overwhelming need to keep them from hitting the floor. It becomes all too obvious that the nose alone is not a secure point of attachment.

> Black silk ribbon was most often seen but included were black and white ribbon, cord, braided cord, gimp gilt cords, gold chains and platinum chains. Chains could be attached to gold hairpins, gold ear loops (which would fit snugly around the ear as temples did), gold pins and gold snaps to affix to the belt or button hole. The snap was most often used with the long black ribbon or cord generally worn by men.[3]

The following is an interesting discourse on the ribbon from the *Literary Digest*, May 1916:

> We are becoming reconciled to the individuals who disregard the wisdom of nature in giving them a nose, eyes, and a mouth of more or less comeliness, artistically disposed about their expanse of face, and who distort and conceal the same with the aid of tortoise-shell, or imitation tortoise-shell, spectacles. But even yet we have not all of us learned to pass, without shying, an individual adorned with a black ribbon flowing from his eye-glasses. Somehow we miss his long hair. And yet, it is quite true that this form of ornament is being ever more widely affected. In this, as in all manner of personal adornment, there is a chic about it that only the initiate may attain. It will be worthwhile for all those who are contemplating the adoption of this form of depravity to listen to the wit and wisdom of this experienced New-Yorker. He writes:
>
>> I can quite appreciate the feeling of heart-failure described by your correspondent when his own or another's eyeglasses fall off. I had the same sensation until, a few years ago, I took to wearing a ribbon attached to my glasses. Since, the ribbon has saved my nerves, as the glasses have saved my eyes.
>>
>> It is a curious fact and worthy of note that the manner in which the ribbon is worn makes a vast difference in the appearance of the wearer. Because of this difference the wearer of the glasses-ribbon has a sort of Protean equipment. With the ribbon behind his ear he looks neat and businesslike; with the ribbon hanging down he at once takes on a learned and distinguished air, and his nose is accentuated. When I am looking at pictures or listening to music I do not understand, or asking for credit, or serving on the jury, I always wear my ribbon down.
>>
>> The wearing of the ribbon hanging down is not without its drawbacks. At first it tickles you and makes you want to laugh on the right side of your face. Then too, when the wind is blowing athwart your face it has a way of getting in your mouth, and thus interfering with your conversation.
>>
>> At first, when partaking of a highball, I had to put the ribbon

up behind my ear, and for that reason wore it so most of the time, but now I can drink anything, except water and milk, without regard to the ribbon, and even without my glasses, for that matter.

If the ribbon is free to fly about, care must be used when smoking a cigar. I once burned off a ribbon in a second when it chanced to light on the burning end of a cigar. At first the beginner will find that he often will catch the ribbon on the buttons of his right coat-sleeve. Then his glasses will be jerked off, and he will lose his dignity and his temper at the same time, to the unholy joy of those who chance to see him.

Notwithstanding all these disadvantages I have pointed out, I believe the man who once wears a glasses-ribbon will continue to do so, except, perhaps, if he buys a pair of those so-called library-glasses and goes about looking like Horace Walpole.

With such a variety to choose from, the use of pince-nez flourished. Nearly everyone was soon wearing some type of pince-nez. In 1913, William Hemmingway wrote this account after an optician had completed fitting a pair of pince-nez to his nose:

> "Oh-ow!" I exclaimed. "They'll give me cramps in the eyelids: The eyelashes are brushing them." "Oh, well," he advised patiently as one who had traversed the ground a thousand times before—"take a pair of scissors and trim your eyelashes short."[4]

Fits-U

In 1893, Jules Cottet, a Frenchman living in the quaint town of Morez-du-Jura in France, patented the finger-piece eyeglass, which was to become the next rage in fashion and eventually replace the pince-nez in this regard. Cottet patented the device in France, England, and the United States but lost interest and sold the patent to a London wholesale optical dealer who eventually sold it to an American jobber. After several years, the patent was purchased by American Optical Company, who did little with it. The following is Fleming's account of what happened thereafter:

> One day Jack Hardin of Hardy Optical (Chicago) was visiting American Optical—looking for something new. AO let him look around the sample drawers and Jack got hold of this seemingly useless finger piece mounting. Here was something worth attempting to improve. Every detail of the original unsalable model was changed—the "Fits U"

mountings burst on the business. I have never known any mounting which had such an instant success and the "Boston" (pince-nez) style gradually lost popularity.

The Fits-U was at first a rimless mounting that contained a solid bridge. Attached to either side of the bridge were movable nose guards operated by the thumb and forefinger through two tiny spring loaded protrusions, or finger-pieces. When squeezed between thumb and forefinger, the nose pads would open, allowing the eyeglasses to be placed on the nose.

The principal differences between the pince-nez and the Fits-U were slight. The pince-nez had a spring bridge, while the Fits-U was solid. The Fits-U had tiny protrusions in front of the bridge with which the eyeglasses could be placed upon the nose. The pince-nez had no such appendage, although a variety of other concoctions had been tried. Features advertised for the Fits-U were: "Don't have to touch lenses to put on." "Solid bridge so astigmatism axis stays correct." "Put on, take off with one hand." "Both rocking and rigid guards [nose pads] available."

Amoptico, Nov. 1910.[5]

The following is an interesting testimonial to the Fits-U from Camaguey, Cuba, in June 1916:

> A few days ago a patient of ours fell and had the misfortune to break her nose. A short time before the accident she had bought a pair of . . . Fits-U eyeglasses, . . . but at the time of which we happened to write happened to have them in her hand bag. The Fits-U guards served as splints, and the nose knit in the most satisfactory manner, being perfectly straight, and now the glasses stay on even as before, if possible. We strongly recommend Fits-U Finger Piece Mountings in all cases of broken noses.
> Very truely [sic] yours
> Anderson Bros.

The Fits-U, or finger-piece eyeglasses were a continuing attempt of humanity to retain corrective lenses upon the face without the aid of temples, which had now been available for two centuries. The finger-piece eyeglasses replaced the pince-nez but were never able to change the direction of this fading fashion. By 1935, few could be found in use. This did not deter the advocates of templeless glasses, however.

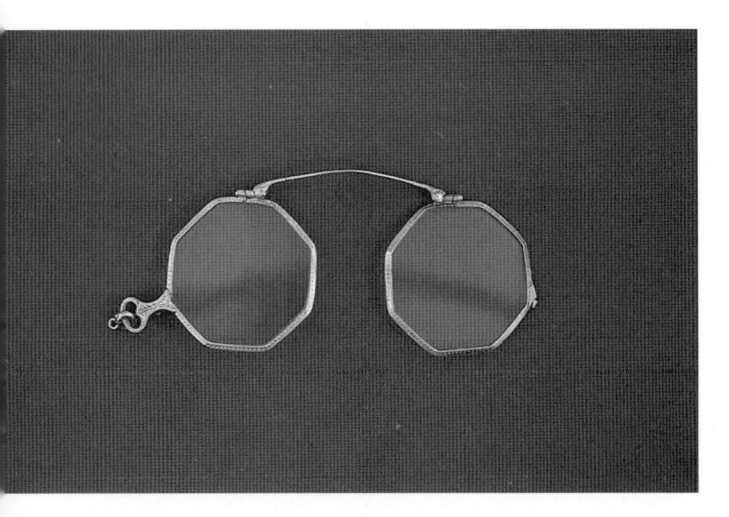

Figure 460. Octagonal-shaped oxford.

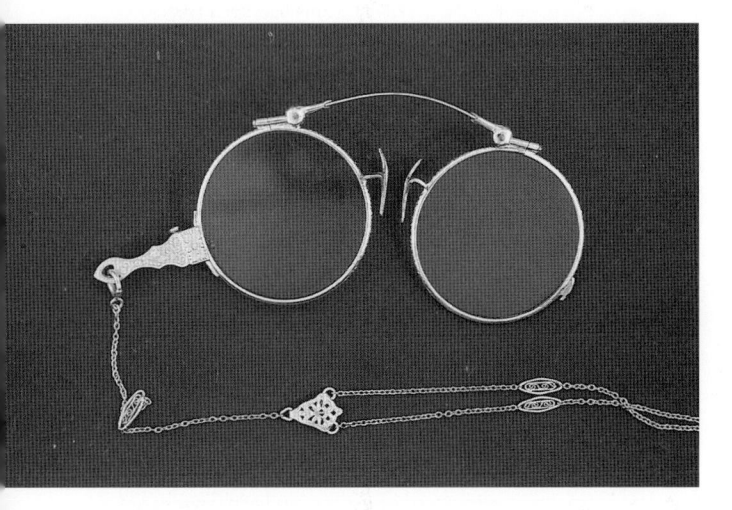

Figure 461. Gold oxford and chain.

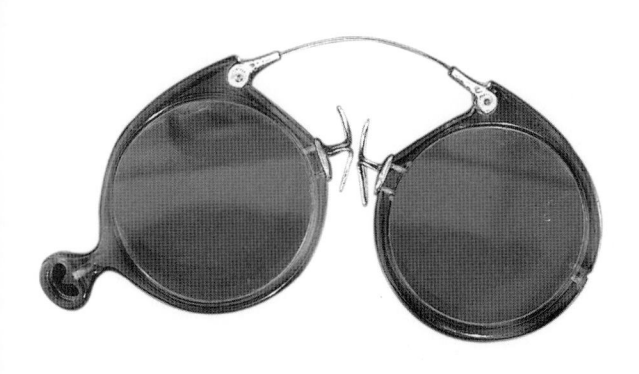

Figure 462. Tortoiseshell oxford.

Oxford

The oxford became the next eyeglass fashion fad and was first seen in the streets of New York in 1910. The best definition of an oxford is a pair of eyeglasses that look like pince-nez but have a somewhat larger eye size and a long, bowed bar connecting the two eye wires. At the point of connection, the brow bar pivots on the eye wire, and an internal coil spring at each pivot point retains pressure on the nose sufficient (one would hope) to hold the eyeglasses on the nose. The oxford could be folded, one lens over the other, much like the early pince-nez. Unlike the finger-piece mounting, the oxford could not maintain good axis alignment of a cylinder correction and, in this sense, was also much like the early pince-nez. Some were vocal about this possibly detrimental aspect to good vision:

> One rule should . . . be unexceptional: Abolish eyeglasses and order only spectacles. All useful lenses have optical centers, and it is only by means of the temple-pieces of spectacles, curved behind the ears, that accurate and constant adjustments are possible. . . . The worst of fashions is that of the sillies who dangle a long black ribbon from one side of their eyeglasses which displaces the axes of the astigmatism of the lenses from 20 to 30 degrees according to several quick changing conditions, the movements of the head, the weight of the ribbon, the slippage of the springs, etc.—an optical farce.
> Dr. George M. Gould, 1921.

The oxford persisted into the thirties and became a popular choice (Figure 460). Colorful ribbons as well as the standard black ribbon and cord adorned this device.

During the twenties, much of the population was enjoying a more affluent life than before. This was especially true of the United States, where the growth of industry had created many new jobs, at least until the stock market crash in 1929. For this reason, many of the fashionable oxfords sported 14-karat yellow and white gold (Figure 461), genuine tortoiseshell rim liners, and fancy filigree handles. Some were engraved over the entire body of the eyeglass frame. Both genuine tortoiseshell (Figure 462) and zyl were used in this product. Toward the end of this fashion cycle, aluminum oxfords of different colors could also be found.

PINCE-NEZ

In 1930, American Optical introduced an oxford called the Z-fold. This design allowed the lenses to be folded on top of each other through the use of a hinged brow bar. Looking down on the top of the eyeglasses as they were about halfway through the fold, one would see the letter *Z* being formed, hence the name.

The Hutten Oxford

The following article was written by E. P. Hutten in the *Optical Journal Review*, dated January 15, 1942:

> The Oxford eye glass was originally made in 1910 in Geoffrey & Co.'s factory on Park Place in New York City. A journeyman named McDougall and the writer had worked on a frame which had flat nose-guards. This frame folded but was not popular, due to the fact that few could hold it on their nose. Then a frame with offset guards was made, but because the nose-guards projected beyond the plane of the lenses, it could not fold, the guards preventing one lens from passing over the other.
>
> It was recognized by all interested that if a frame of this type could be so constructed as to allow the folding of the left lens over the right and then, by pressing a button in the handle, thereby release the left lens and make it open automatically, a frame of great utility would be had.
>
> After a great many suggestions had been received and differently shaped guards had been tried, the thought of how the guards would have to be made in order to pass each other came simultaneously to Mr. McDougall and myself, while we were experimenting with the working model. After comparing our thoughts, which were identical we made a pair of offset guards and attached them to the rims—and the Oxford was perfected.
>
> The frame, as originally made with the flat guards, was intended for masculine use, to be worn with a flat black silk ribbon around the neck, so that a man would have his glasses handy and always with him, the ribbon being long enough to allow for the glasses to be put in the vest pocket. However, when the offset guards were perfected it was realized that a beautiful and useful eye glass could be made which would be worn by both men and women. Women soon realized that the Oxford was a wonderful improvement over the lorgnon of Marie Antoinette's period, as the Oxford could be held on the nose, giving the wearer the free use of the hands, and that fact, if none other, made the Oxford most popular for feminine use.
>
> Oxfords were originally made only in 14 Kt. yellow gold and sold at retail for $18.00 a pair. The optical trade felt in the beginning that the price, which was considered extremely high, would kill the sale. In fact one Fifth Ave. optician said to the writer, "Hutten, you're crazy. No one will pay $18. for an eye glass." But the writer, being in the jewelry business and having sold lorgnons for many times this price, knew different. After being assured that the price was not high and would not interfere with the sale, the Fifth Ave. optician purchased a few frames for a trial and, being successful in disposing of them quickly, he next placed an order for 50 pair. These were also sold quickly; another order for 50 pair was placed, and then lots of 100 pairs were regular orders from this firm.
>
> The usefulness and convenience of the Oxford for women soon made other style handles and material necessary. The first shell Oxford was brought out in 1914. White gold was being used in jewelry, and that metal, in 15 Kt. soon became extremely popular in Oxfords. Then platinum, and platinum and diamonds were introduced into the line, and while $18.00 per pair was thought high in the beginning, frames of special design made in platinum and diamonds were sold as high as $700.00 and $800.00 per pair, and later even higher.
>
> Feeling that there was patent value in the construction of the Oxford, the writer applied for and received a patent. However, the frame was soon copied, and I then instituted a suit for infringement. After about a year and a half, the patent was declared invalid. Appeal was taken to the higher court but it upheld the lower court, and the way for general manufacture was thus opened.
>
> Thousands of Oxfords have been made and sold in the past 30 years and are still very popular for women's use. The Hutten Oxford became standard, and other manufacturers would use the phrase "As good as Hutten's," having in mind the workmanship, adjustability and comfort of our Oxford.[6]

The oxford fad disappeared as the quest for "eyeglasses" gave way to spectacles, which were also beginning to offer fashion appeal to the wearer. The oxford was survived only by an occasional lorgnette and the monocle.

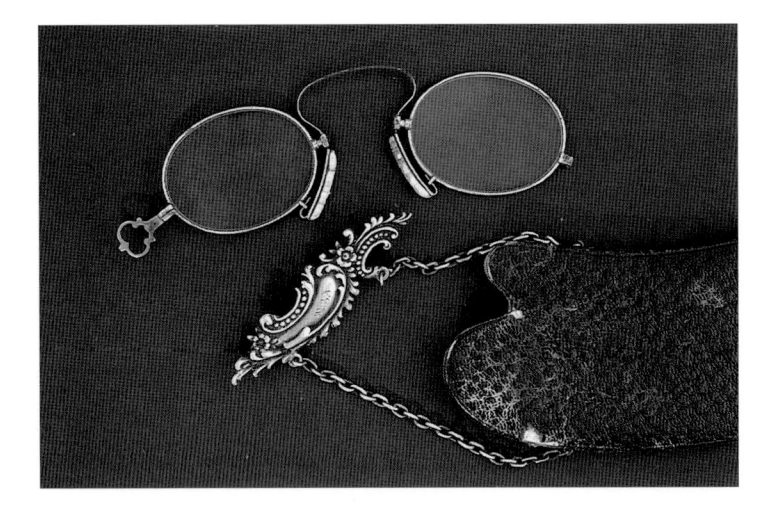

Figure 463. Pin-on chatelain type of case for pince-nez.

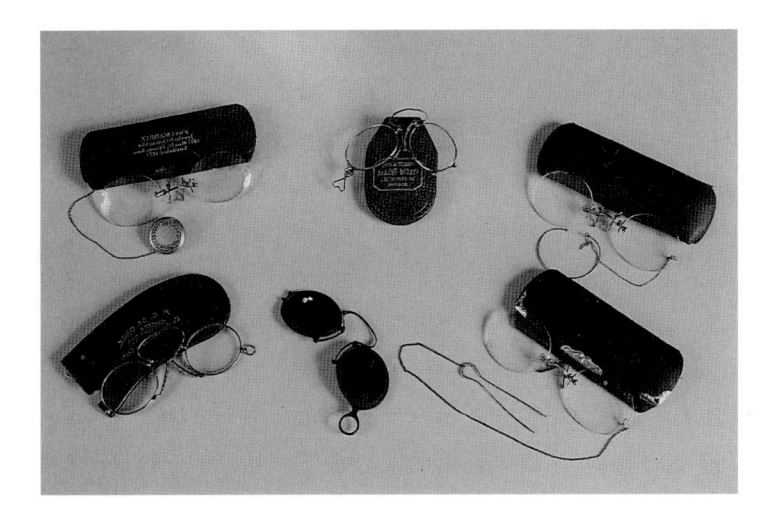

Figure 464. Group of pince-nez with cases, chains, etc.

Pince-Nez Cases

Cases for pince-nez were not popular since these vision aids were taken off and put on so frequently. Some pin-on and chatelain varieties are found (Figure 463), a few being small leather pouches as seen in previous illustrations. Mostly, though, pince-nez were delivered to the patient in snap-shut envelope cases, commonly used for spectacles with temples (Figure 464). Aluminum (Figure 465) and leather-covered cases were typical (Figures 466 & 467), but those made of carved wood (Figure 468) were especially decorative.

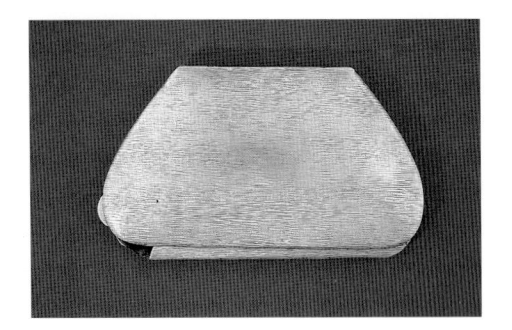

Figure 465. Aluminum pince-nez case.

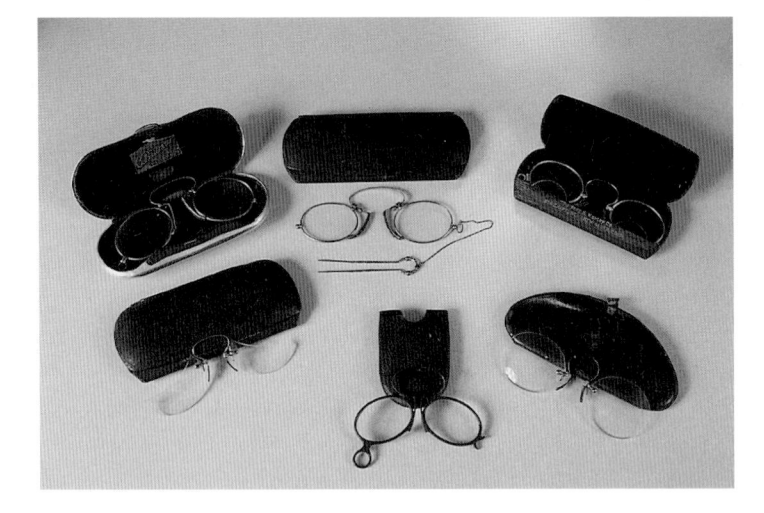

Figure 466. Group of pince-nez and leather cases.

Figure 467. Another group of pince-nez and leather cases.

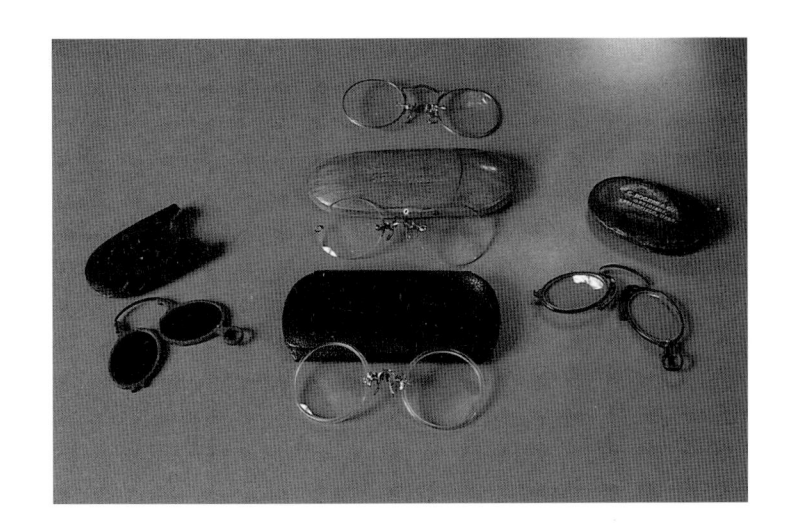

Figure 468. Wooden pince-nez case

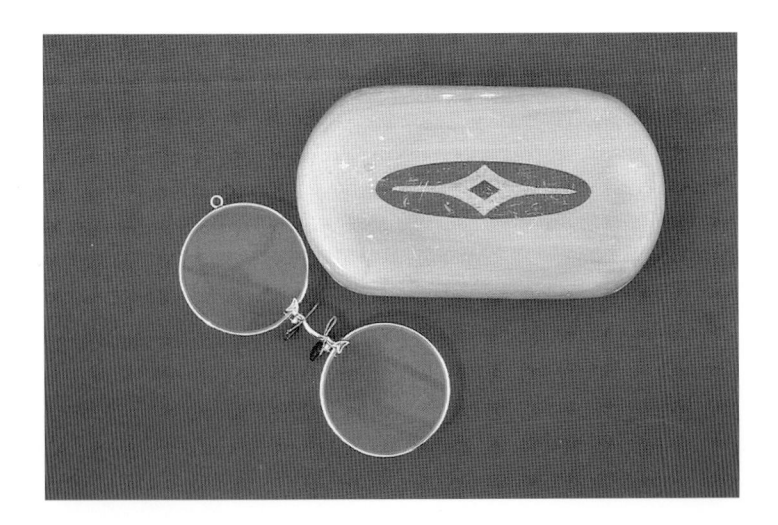

Conclusion

Despite all the improvements and their small size to reduce weight, pince-nez could not be used over long periods of time. This fact, of course, contributed to their demise—around 1930.

Notes

1. Anita Kuisle, *Brillen* (Munich: Deutsches Museum, 1985), 56–60.
2. Robert J. Fleming, *The Ophthalmic Trade and Industry since 1900* (London, 1958).
3. John M. Young, *The History of Eyewear* (Southbridge, Massachusetts: Optical Heritage Museum, 1985), 71–82.
4. Quoted in Young, op. cit., p. 78.
5. Quoted in Young, op. cit.
6. E. P. Hutten, *Optical Journal Review*, January 15, 1942, 97.

Other Sources Consulted for Chapter 20

1. George Bull, *Lunettes et pince-nez* (Paris: S. Masson, 1889), 65.

21

Bifocals

The Invention of Bifocals

It is now well past the two hundredth anniversary of the death of Benjamin Franklin, who is usually credited with the invention of the bifocal. This journeyman printer and son of a Boston tallow chandler and soap boiler was entirely self-made. He was known as an intellectual as well as a businessman, and during his younger days, he had been an importer of goods (including optical). He was a printer of *Poor Richard's Almanac* and, despite his marital status, was known somewhat as a roué. By the time Franklin was appointed as one of three commissioners to the French court in September of 1776, he was in his seventies and a widower. Yet he very well may have been the most successful ambassador to France that we have had from the United States. But what Franklin did most was to invent. In addition to the bifocal, he devised many other practical gadgets, which, interestingly enough, were done for the good of all rather than for personal gain. In *Our Ophthalmic Heritage*, written in 1967, Charles Snyder states:

> Others got rich from the ideas, not Franklin. Several of his inventions, or gadgets as they are sometimes termed, were to him simply devices to make life easier for him—his book hook, his letter copier, his chair ladder are examples. And in his mind his double spectacles were in this category, only another thing to make life easier for an old man—another thing to be freely shared with all old men so that their lives might be made easier.[1]

The scholarly discourse and intellectually analytical article on the invention of bifocals by John R. Levene (Memphis, Tennessee)[2] supported the fact that the invention was attributed to Franklin, while others for various reasons should be given some recognition.

Although many along the historical path have doubted his invention of the bifocal, Franklin finally obtained his just due when Charles Letocha recorded his latest findings.[3] Dr. Letocha pointed out that the letter of John Fenno, editor of *The Gazette of the United States*, documents that Franklin did, in fact, invent bifocals—not in 1784, as originally thought, but perhaps 50 years earlier. He supports this in his article, "The Invention and Early Manufacture of Bifocals," where he presents the Whatley letters. Of particular interest is an excerpt from a letter by Dr. Franklin to George Whatley:

> ... Finding this change troublesome [from distance spectacles to near spectacles], and not always sufficiently ready, I had the glasses cut and half of each kind associated in the same circle. By this means, as I wear my spectacles constantly, I have only to move my eyes up or down, as I want to see distinctly far or near, the proper glasses being always ready. This I find more particularly convenient since my being in France, the glasses that serve me best at table to see what I eat not being the best to see the faces of those on the other side of the table who speak to me; and when one's

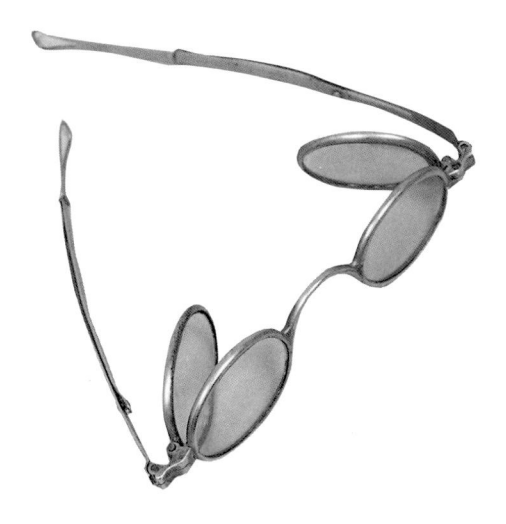

Figure 469. Hinged near glass circa 1797.

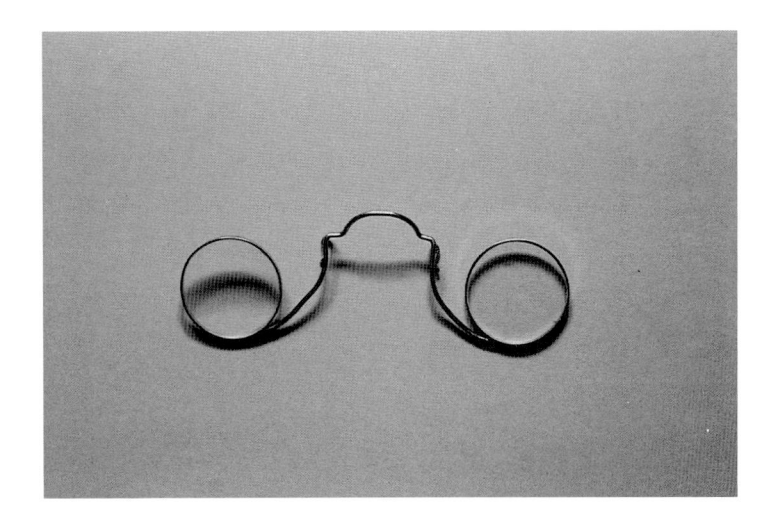

Figure 470. Early hang-on reading addition.

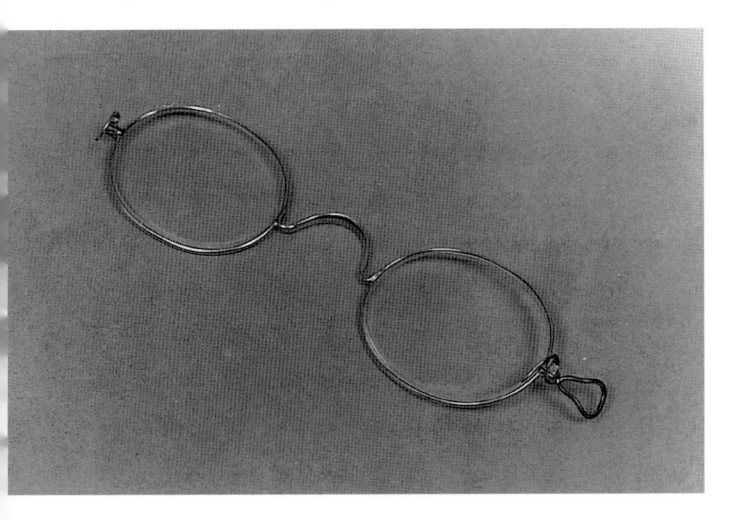

Figure 471. Later hang-on reading addition.

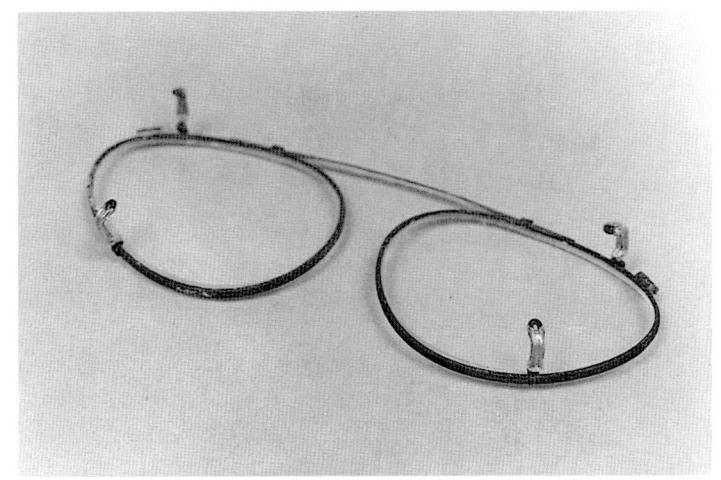

Figure 472. Twentieth-century clip-on.

ears are not well accustomed to the sounds of a language, a sight of the movements in the features of him that speaks helps to explain; so that I understand French better by the help of my spectacles.[4]

Dr. Letocha follows with, "In reading these letters carefully, it would appear that the double spectacles were truly Franklin's invention."

The Development of Bifocals

Obviously, before bifocals were used, individuals used two pairs of spectacles, one for close and one for distance. The inconvenience of this arrangement led to the universal adoption of the bifocal.

Several attempts to obviate bifocals were made only after it was shown that they were clinically convenient. One such attempt was John Richardson's English patent in 1797 (Figure 469). A separate glass hinged to the side of the temple rotated behind the regular spectacle distance glass, and that was used for near. Other attempts included the hang-on addition on the front of the distance spectacle (Figures 470 & 471) and the clip-on of the twentieth century (Figure 472).

The actual bifocal, of course, started with the invention of Dr. Franklin (Figure 473). Franklin's distance glass and near glass were cut horizontally and placed into the same frame. This resulted in a visible horizontal line separating the distance glass above from the close prescription below. The Franklin bifocal was still being made in the late nineteenth century.

BIFOCALS **259**

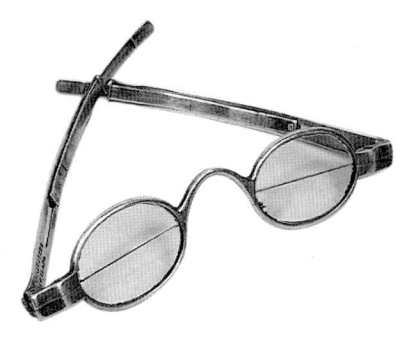

Figure 473. An early Franklin bifocal.

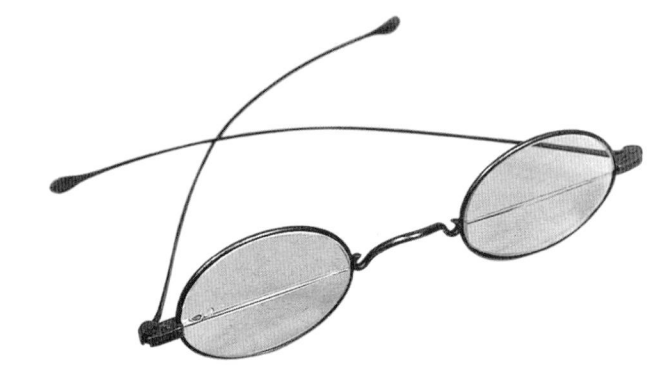

Figure 474. American Franklin bifocal circa 1885.

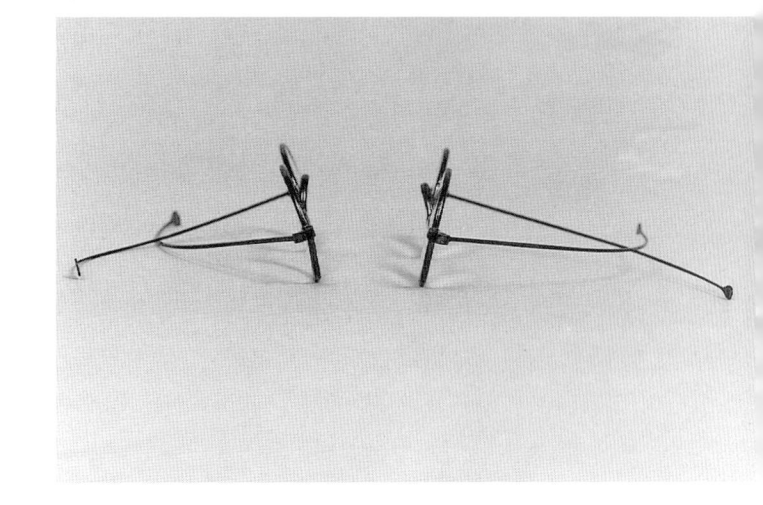

Figure 475. American Franklin bifocal with pantoscopic angle below.

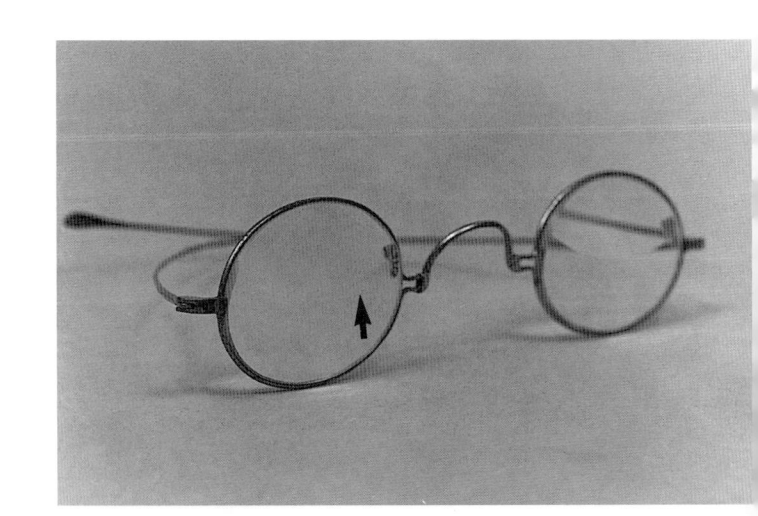

Figure 476. Solid up-curved bifocal (arrow indicates bifocal).

260   CHAPTER 21

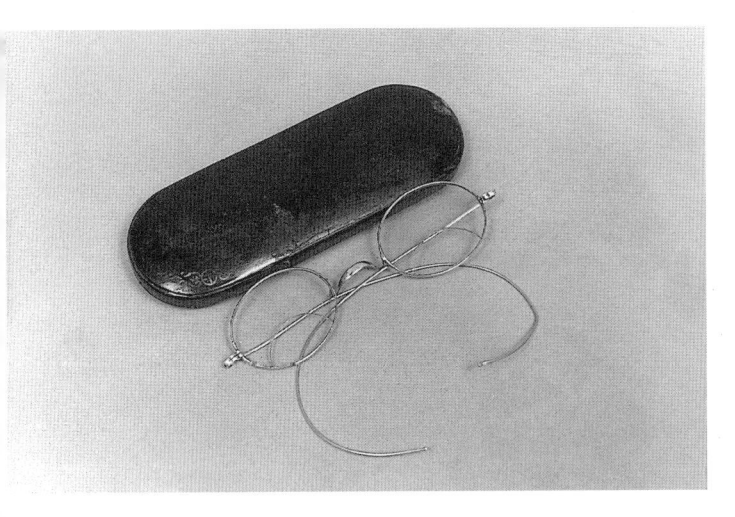

Figure 477. Perfection bifocal.

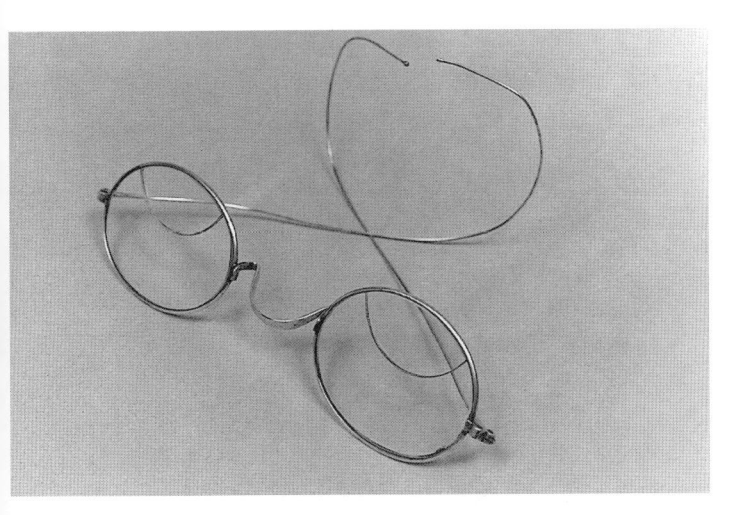

Figure 478. Cement bifocal.

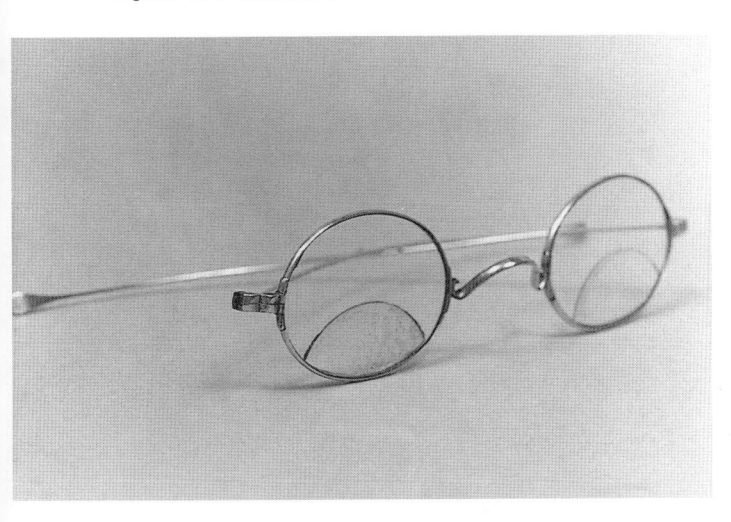

Figure 479. Cement bifocal showing imperfections.

Note the blued steel frame (American) (Figure 474), with both straight and angled lower pantoscopic angle (Figure 475). Following this in 1836, there was an attempt to make the bifocal less obvious with the design of the solid up-curve bifocal (Figure 476). To make this bifocal, the upper part of a reading (or near) prescription was ground away (slabbed off) until it was weakened down to the necessary prescription for good distance. This certainly facilitated invisibility, but it had a terribly distracting problem. The strong prismatic effect that the user experienced while going from the distance to the close prescription was so severe that it was intolerable.

The Perfection Bifocal

In 1888, August Morck invented the perfection bifocal (Figure 477) a Franklin type of bifocal wherein the top was curved instead of being a horizontal line.[5] The two pieces of glass used to form the bifocal were placed together using a tongue and groove technique and sometimes were cemented together. The lenses had good optical qualities but had the disadvantage of a Franklin bifocal: the dividing line filled up with dirt, and unless the bifocal was very skillfully manufactured, many times it came apart.

The Cement Bifocal

The invention of the cement bifocal (Figure 478) has been variously attributed to Dr. George M. Gould, George W. Wells (1885), and August Morck (1888) (previously mentioned).[6] This bifocal was made by cementing a very small, thin wafer of glass to the back surface of a distance prescription. The shape of this wafer, used for close vision, was sometimes that of an arc (like a modern Ultex) or a round disc (like the present kryptok). This bifocal had good optical qualities when it was new and constructed correctly. However, it had several disadvantages (Figure 479):

1. It, too, accumulated dirt at the junction of the two pieces of glass.
2. The cement tended to melt in hot weather, and the wafer would slide around.
3. The cement would crystallize in cold weather.
4. The wafer would tend to break off and get lost.

BIFOCALS 261

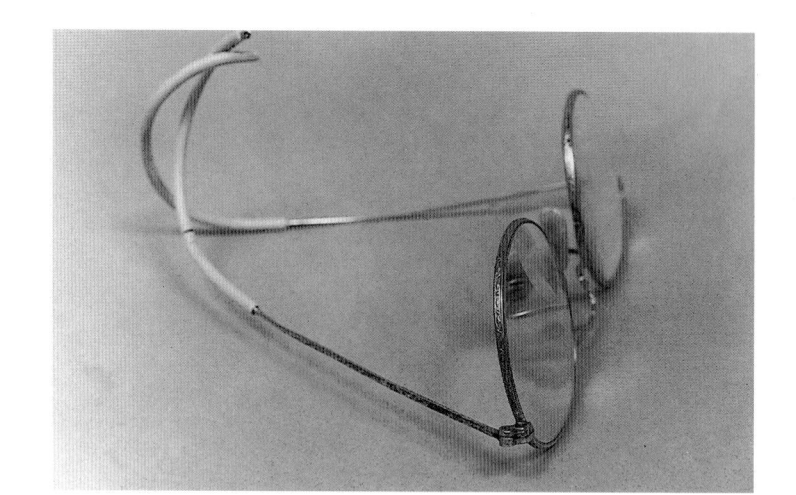

Figure 480. Kryptok bifocal.

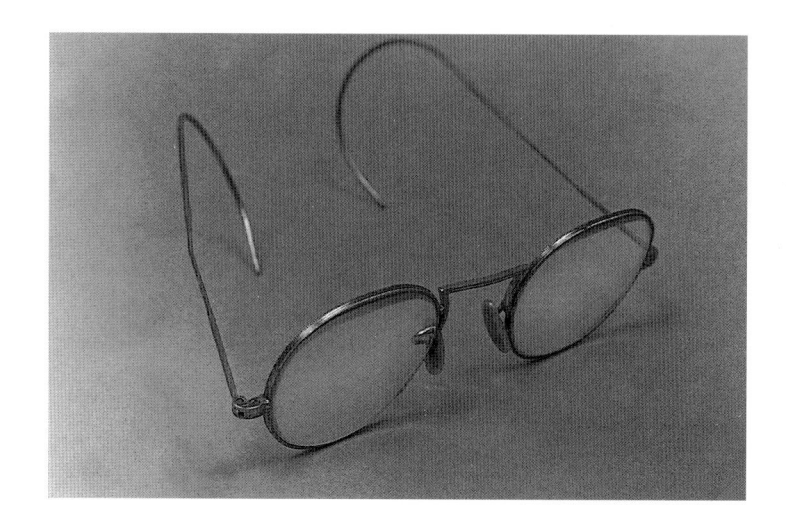

Figure 481. Straight-top bifocal.

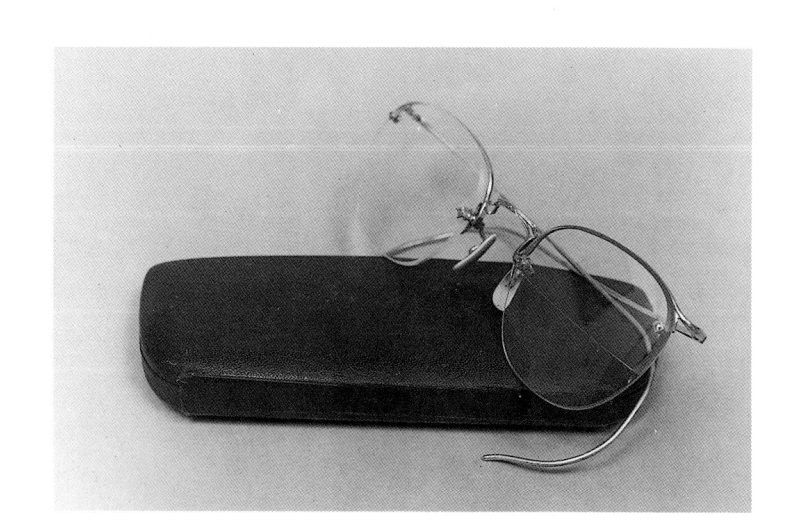

Figure 482. Executive bifocal.

The Optifex Bifocal

This is a cement type of bifocal, improved only in the fact that the wafer was ground extremely thin, making it far less visible. However, this thin grind caused easy chipping and detachment when the cement was not properly applied.

Cemented Kryptok

This lens was invented by John L. Borsch of Philadelphia in 1899. Although it is different from the kryptok fused bifocal, the two are sometimes confused. With the cemented kryptok, two types of glass were used—flint and crown, both with the same radius and curvature. This lens was made by grinding a small depression in the front surface of the distance-vision portion of a crown glass lens. A small disc of flint glass was cemented into this depression. This facilitated better close vision. The flint glass, in turn, was held in place by a curved wafer (cover glass) of crown glass, which was cemented over the front surface of both the distance and the flint glass piece. Since this was a little thicker than the ordinary glass lens, it did hold the flint glass wafer in place and was very good optically. However, because of the difficulty of manufacturing it, this lens was quite expensive.

Fused Bifocals

Kryptok In 1908, John L. Borsch, Jr. (see above) patented a new type of bifocal similar to the cemented kryptok. In the new lens, a disc of flint glass was placed in a ground-out front section of a crown glass lens. The two pieces were heated to over 1,000 degrees Fahrenheit, allowing them to be fused. Upon cooling, both front and back surfaces of this lens blank could be ground to the necessary prescription. Of course, the strength of the flint glass section could be varied to meet the needs of the bifocal (Figure 480) Although this bifocal was rather small, it was a practical optical instrument and relatively inexpensive. This made it a very successful and popular model, thereby superseding the cement bifocal and making it obsolete.

Other Fused Bifocals In 1939, J. H. Hammon patented a fused, multifocal lens, later to be called the panoptic lens. It had a curved top, with the bottom two thirds being teardrop shaped. Another of the fused bifocals had a straight top shape,

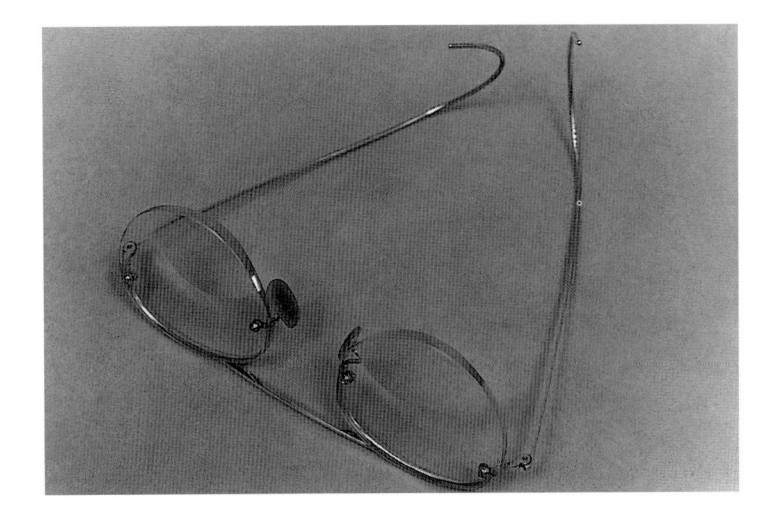

Figure 483. The Ultex bifocal.

with top linear measurements of 26, 28, and 35 millimeters in length. The bottom portion of this bifocal also had a rounded, oval shape (Figure 481).

Following this, the executive bifocal was developed (Figure 482). It was essentially a one-piece bifocal, but the near section was ground in the lower half, creating a quite prominent horizontal nick or line between the upper and lower halves. Although this bifocal was made of only one piece, it strongly resembled the Franklin bifocal and carried the same cosmetic objections in that it had a clearly visible small shelf separating the two halves.

The Ultex One-piece Bifocal

The Ultex one-piece bifocal lens (Figure 483) was ground from a single piece of hard crown glass of low dispersion power. As two pieces of glass were not approximated, there was very little indication of chromatic or spherical aberration. The position of the near segment occupied approximately one quarter of the lower portion of the lens and arched from nasal to temporal, with a spherical top to this segment.

"Invisible" Bifocals

The "easy-vue" was the first type of invisible bifocal to be foisted upon the public. It was essentially a fused kryptok bifocal wherein the edges of the round segment were fused together so that there was no visible dividing line. However,

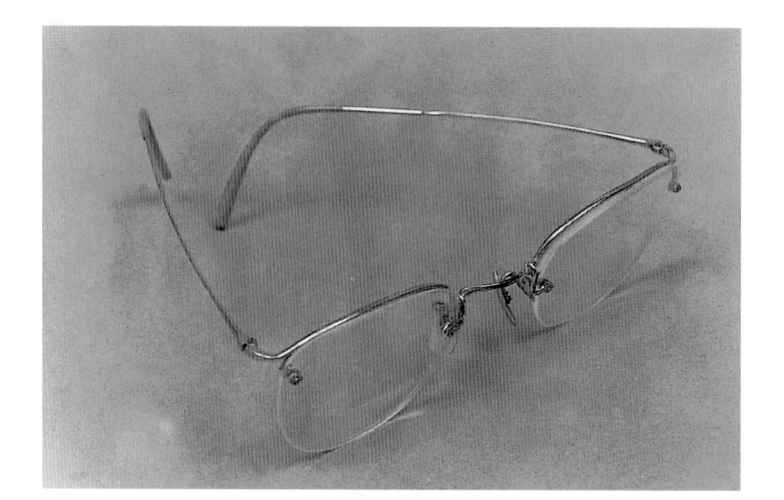

Figure 484. Panoptik trifocal.

the area where these two pieces of glass were fused was easily seen and, in fact, converted a sharp line of demarcation to an area of fuzzy vision. Although it was a little less visible as a bifocal than an ordinary kryptok and therefore more cosmetically acceptable, it was, of course, less acceptable optically.

Progressive Bifocals or Trifocals

The next bifocals developed were what we call progressive bifocals, a series of lenses produced by various manufacturers with an increased amount of bifocal strength, starting from the center of the lens and increasing as it approaches the inferior, or lower, part of the lens edge. The advantage is that the bifocal segment is truly invisible to the observer and has a progressive strength. The disadvantage of this lens is that the areas to the right and left of this central progressive increase in strength are quite blurry, and the wearer must learn to avoid these distorted areas of vision. However, once the individual learns how to use them, these glasses are quite effective in facilitating good vision. Furthermore, since these lenses are made from one piece of glass, they avoid the aberrations otherwise seen in a two-piece fused bifocal. Several companies have put out their own version of this type of bifocal, some with fewer aberrations than others.

Trifocals

Hawkins, an Englishman, invented trifocals in the year 1800.[7] Trifocals were used to give an intermediate, or arm's length, focusing area for those who needed it in their work or hobbies. The lens consists of a larger upper area for distance vision, a smaller intermediate area for arm's length vision, and finally a bifocal or reading section larger than the intermediate section. There are six trifocals available: the Ultex, Widesite, Univis, Executive, Panoptik, and the two-segment Panoptik (Figure 484)

Specialized bifocals and trifocals are available for vocational and special uses. One in particular is called a baseball, wherein the bifocal is set in its usual manner, but the upper part of the distance vision is ground to an intermediate vision. This is useful for individuals such as librarians who have to look at upper shelves and mechanics who have to work on their backs under automobiles.

Conclusion

Quite a progression in development has occurred in bifocals from Ben Franklin's first invention to the modern-day versions. It is interesting to note that for over 200 years, we have been improving on and benefiting from that original concept of a man who freely shared his invention of bifocals.

Notes

1. Charles Snyder, *Our Ophthalmic Heritage* (Boston: Little, Brown, & Co., 1967).
2. John R. Levene, *Clinical Refraction and Visual Science* (Boston: Butterworth's, 1977).

3. Charles E. Letocha, M.D. "The Invention and Early Manufacture of Bifocals," *Survey of Ophthalmology*, Vol. 35, No. 3, Nov./Dec. 1990.
4. Ibid.
5. Theo E. Obrig, *Modern Ophthalmic Lenses and Optical Glass* (Chilton, N.Y., 1935).
6. W. L. Bugbee, Jr., and Sr., *Bifocals* (Indianapolis: One Piece Bifocal Lens Company, 1921).
7. Ibid.

Other Sources Consulted for Chapter 21

1. A. G. Bennett, *The Optician,* July 21, 1972, pp. 6–11.
2. M. Bentzon and A. H. Emerson, "Improvements in Bifocal Lenses and Their Manufacture, and in Apparatus to Be Employed in the Said Manufacture", Brit. Pat. 28,823 (1904).
3. H. A. Courmettes, "Bifocal Lens and Method for Making the Same", US Pat. 1,160,383 (1915).
4. S. A. Emerson, "Some Recent Improvements in Modern Ophthalmic Lenses", *Trans. Opt. Soc.* 27(1925/6): 1-8.
5. W. E. Hardy, "John Hamer Sutcliffe, A Great Champion of Ophthalmics", *The Optician* 141(1961): 33-34.
6. H. Newbold and W. R. Williams, "Improvements in Bifocal Lenses and Apparatus for Their Manufacture", Brit. Pat. 5,441 (1912).
7. C. P. Reynolds, "Benjamin Franklin," *Gourmet Magazine*, April 1990, p. 100.
8. J. H. Sutcliffe, "Improvements in and Relating to Lenses for Spectacles or Eyeglasses and in Methods of an Apparatus for Manufacturing the Same", Brit. Pat. 6,263 (1900).
9. United Kingdom Optical Company Limited, E. Culver, and F. B. Watson, "Improvements to Fused Bifocal Lenses", Brit. Pat. 255,941 (1926).
10. Dr. M. Von Rohr, *Eyes and Spectacles* (London: The Hatton Press, Ltd., 1912).

22

Eyeshades for Invalids

In Victorian times, it was the treatment of choice for many chronic diseases to give the patient "the airs," that is, to expose the patient to fresh air, sunlight, and gentle breezes to help him or her recover from such conditions as tuberculosis, paralyses, end-stage infections, and severe trauma. As no other therapies were available, this mild physiotherapy or solartherapy was understandably helpful, as it provided the time needed for the body to recover naturally. It also served as a needed psychological boost for the patient. We must remember that in those times, many of the recovery hospitals, and indeed residences, were not exactly the antiseptic (note the word derivation) havens of an ideal sort for recovery. Even today, nosocomial infections are a factor we must guard against. Noxious odors insult the psyche, while sweet flowery breezes buoy it to aid in the will to recover.

Being outside on a balcony or terrace while in the recumbent position exposed the eyes to direct rays of the sun. Besides colored lenses, which were not comfortable over a long period of time, eyeshades were employed. They were particularly useful in cases of inflammatory eye diseases. No doubt they were made for the privileged set, as they were well constructed of fine materials and could be nicely decorated. As the shaded area was designed to cover only the face, the author concludes that the shades had to be frequently adjusted in position to be effective. This activity indicated personal attendance.

Several examples of these eyeshades have come into the author's possession, one portable and others more permanent (Figure 485). Neither are of such a size or weight that they could not be easily carried. The shades weigh one half pound and one pound, respectively. When deployed, an iron base (Figure 486) was designed to keep the shade in position, even in a fair breeze. The portable one is housed in a leather, gold-embossed case—2 × 5 × 16 centimeters (Figure 487)—while the others (Figure 488) are in a gilded, brass pylon—8 centimeters at the base, 2.5 centimeters at the top, and 24 centimeters high—except for one huge example 64 centimeters high.

The portable example is supported by a foldable cross of two rigid brass straps, 15 centimeters long, that act as a base (Figure 489). A brass tube, 1.5 centimeters in diameter and 14 centimeters long, telescoping to 36 centimeters, screws tightly to the center of this base. At the top of the tube, a rotating and hinged smaller tube allows the shade to be wedged in and positioned exactly. The shade itself is really a 360-degree black fan, made of silk, 25.5 centimeters in diameter. It is accordion pleated and therefore self-sustaining without ribs when it is radially unfolded. The silk is sewn to its two supporting brass plates by black thread. All this is very nicely constructed to tolerance and is quite firm. It is a true example of engineering and machining, fitting precisely together and housed in its red morocco leather case.

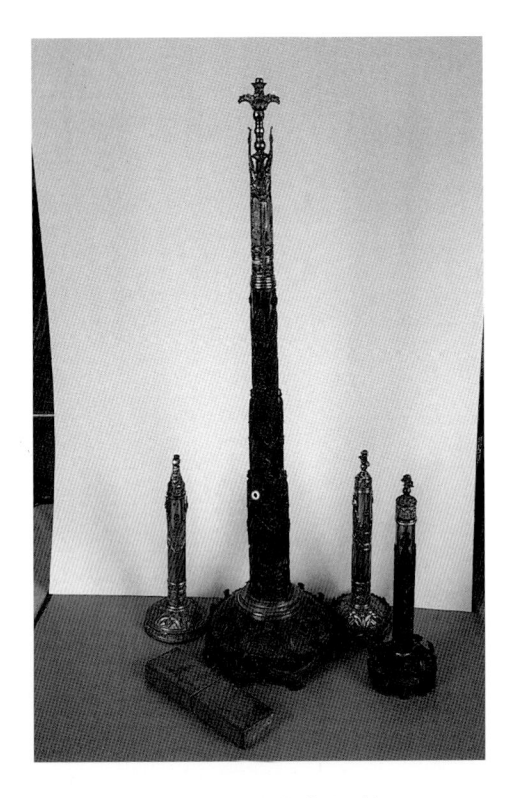

Figure 485. Group of eyeshades for invalids.

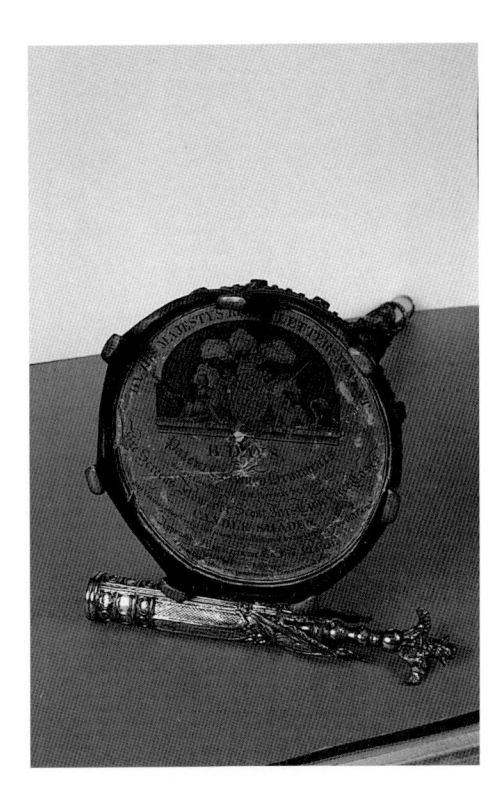

Figure 486. Iron base, covered with advertisement.

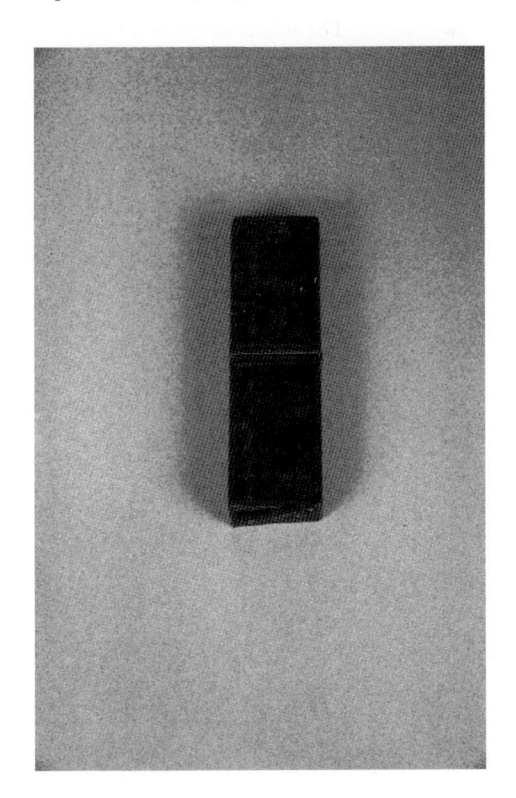

Figure 487. Morocco leather carrying case for portable shade.

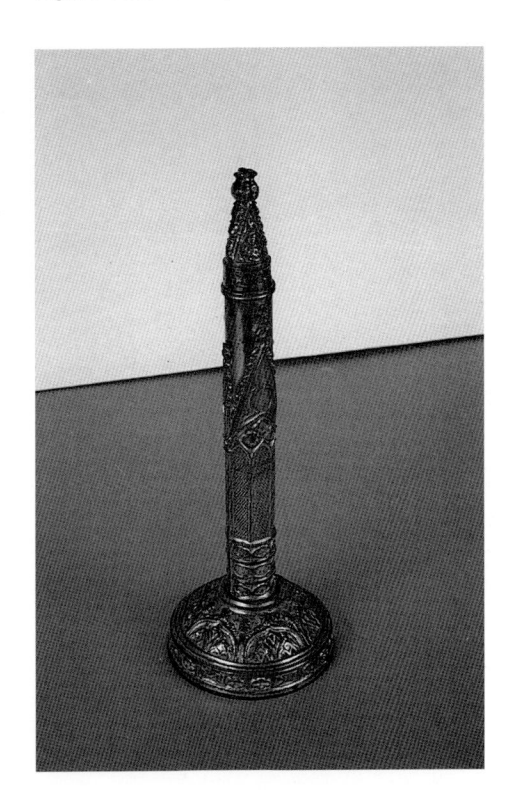

Figure 488. Pylon type of shade holder.

EYESHADES FOR INVALIDS

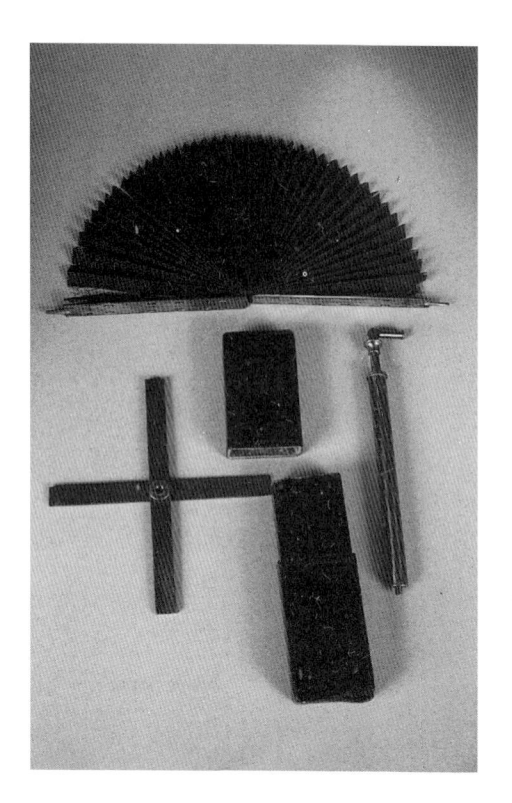

Figure 489. The parts of the portable eyeshade.

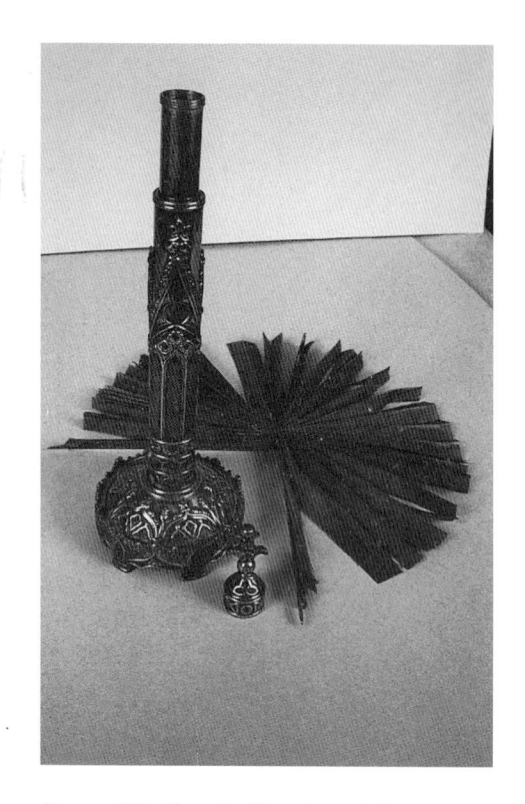

Figure 490. The parts of the pylon eyeshade—note splits in delicate black silk.

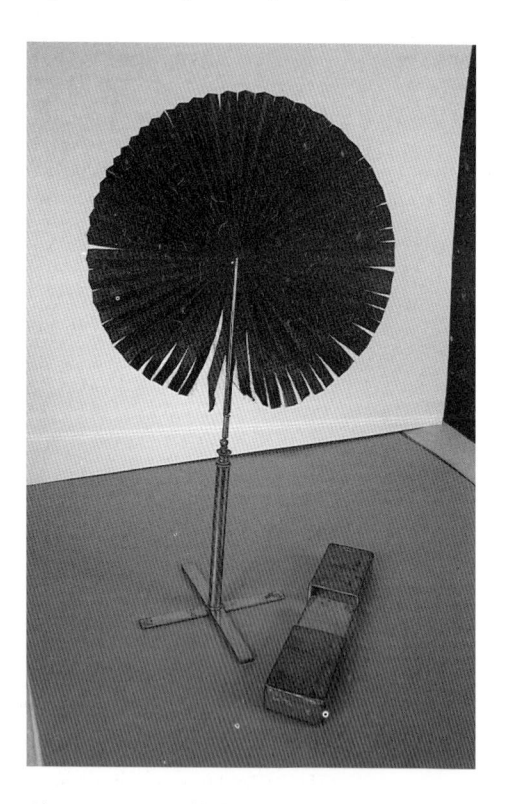

Figure 491. Portable shade ready for use.

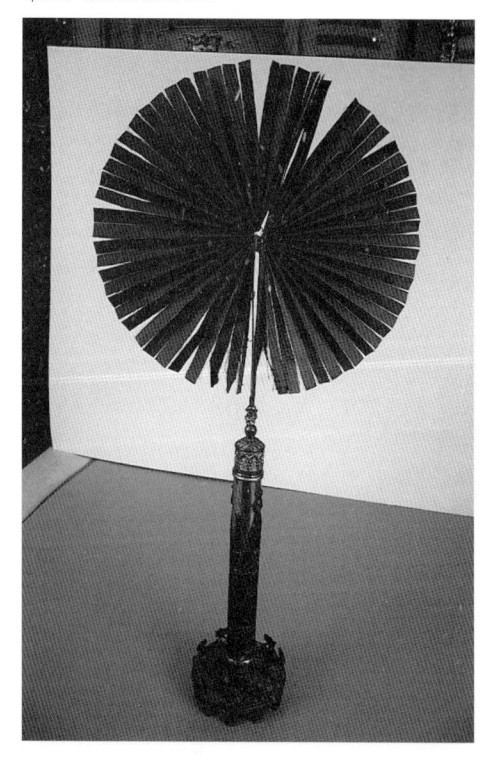

Figure 492. Pylon shade ready for use.

The other examples (Figure 490) show the style of decoration *tout ensemble*, more fancy but still utilitarian. They have round, permanent weighted bases for brass tubes, lavishly decorated with applied brass overlay. This is embossed with Gothic-style arches, topped with a fleur-de-lis shaped pediment with ball, and with an armorial. The armorial shows a lion rampant, a lyre, three oak leaves vertically, and three horizontally. All this is surrounded by "Honi Soit Qui Mal"— no doubt for *honi soit qui mal y pense*—evil to those who think evil. This round plaque is flanked by two deerlike animals (one is a unicorn) and beneath it a banner proclaiming, "Dieu Et Mon Droit." Over the plaque is a crown, and topping it all, embossed is "Day's Patent." What a letdown to Victorian commercialism.

To make this worse, on the end of the telescopic section of the central pylon tube is a cast brass piece—an armorial similar to that previously described but with the four quadrants showing a lion rampant, a fish, a fleur-de-lis and a Maltese cross. In place of "Honi Soit Qui Mal" is "Day's Patent."

Unscrewing the top of the brass tube exposes the two brass plates with pointed ends. These plates support the black silk, accordion-pleated fan in the same manner as the portable version. Also, the fan size is exactly the same, and indeed, side-by-side comparison of the fans' brass supporting plates indicates very close similarities of construction. The fans may have been made by the same person.

When removed from the tube of the permanent example, the fan is expanded to 360 degrees (Figures 491 & 492). The ends of the brass plates are wedged into a hole at the top of the fancy pediment. It is thus in a rigid position that cannot be rotated or angled easily, as with the portable piece. The whole assembled height of this piece is 36 centimeters, extended another 12 centimeters by one telescoping tube section. Dates of these pieces are estimated 1840.

Conclusion

And so we see that by examining these relics, we gain insight into some of the everyday problems of a bygone era 150 years ago. We find that such problems were addressed and solved in a practical, and occasionally grandiose, manner.

23

Lenses for Sun, Glare and Related Eye Protection

Perhaps the earliest, most primitive sun/glare protection known today is the Eskimo slit or pinhole "snow shield" (see Figure 506, Chapter 24). These lenses were adapted centuries before 1287 (the official year of spectacle invention) and have been used and produced ever since. Details of their construction are considered in Chapter 24 of this book.

In another part of the world, Roman Emperor Nero is described as observing games at the Colosseum through an emerald held in his hand. There is speculation as to whether the jewel was used as a sunglass, for ostentatious purposes, or as a mirror to observe those behind him (possibly to avoid attack).

Chinese spectacles, as noted by Marco Polo on his first voyage in 1271, were furnished with plano lenses (no power) and came in (almost) clear, tea shade, and dark colors (Figure 493). All lenses were made of mined crystal, mostly from Mongolia. The Chinese names were *ai-tai*, or *tcha-chi*, and Caucasians call it "tea stone."

Otto Rasmussen's remarks (1908) clarify the Chinese use and beliefs of these spectacles:

> ... any middle-aged Wang, feeling that his eyes were bothering him, bought over the counter a pair of, say, "tortoiseshell-monkey-fish-scale-ink" for distance, and "brass-40 years-water" for reading. The ink shade would be a light smoke tint, suitable for the hot, brilliant summers of China, coupled with the light yellow loess soil of the coastal areas. If Wang was rich he might get a smarter pair of tortoiseshell with high filigreed bridge; pure, unblemished tea-crystals—the colour of that beverage without milk. They would cost at least twenty-five pounds. These were the most expensive spectacles one could buy.

It was the visit of a young Chinese woman that started my inquiry many years ago. She asked me for "medicine glasses" ("Yoh-shui Yen-ching"). If I had not lived in China from childhood, I might have been sceptical. She explained: "My sight is good. I can see clearly, and have no pain, but in early summer I get pink eye regularly. My doctor told me to get 'medicine glasses.' The native city is too far. I am afraid of the soldiers. Can you help me?"

The superstitious ancients, lacking scientific knowledge, held that rock crystal contained a sort of solidified "medicine." Light passing through was supposed to pick up particles and deposit them on the eye surface. The Tea-Crystal was best of all.

Acting in this belief, any Chinese who could afford the high price of all crystals generally (and not many poor people could), apart from the costly tea colour, wore them to guard against pink eye and other epidemics. The question arises: Did they do any good? Of course they did, but not

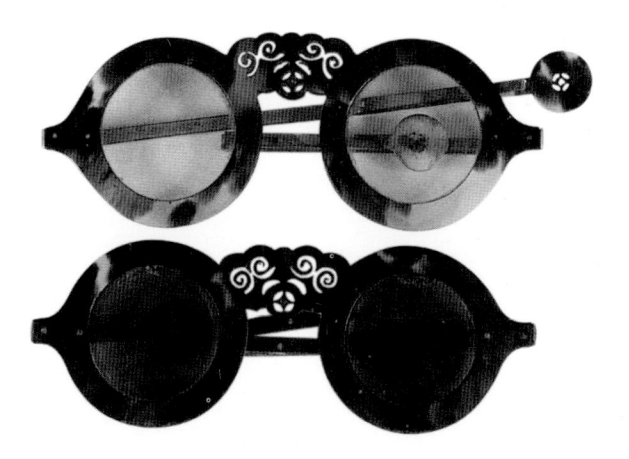

Figure 493. Clear and dark tea-stone Chinese spectacles.

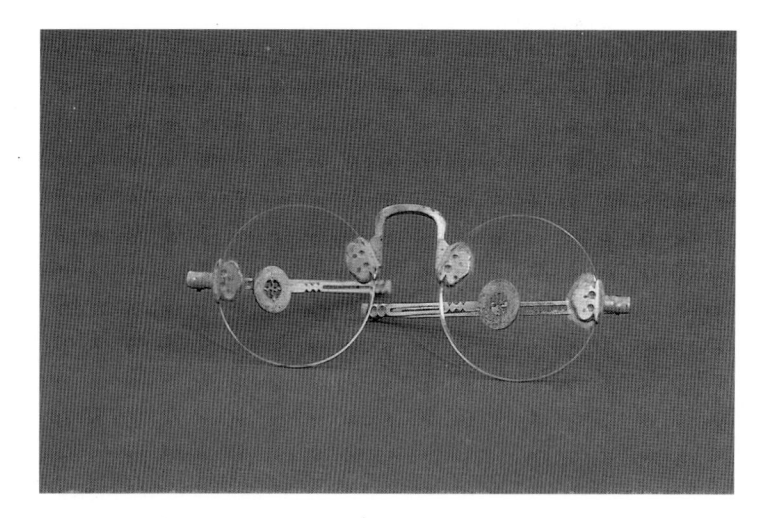

Figure 494. Large, clear crystal Chinese spectacles.

for the reasons given. As will be described later, crystals always feel cooler than the surrounding atmosphere, cooler than glass, as most people know. Native spectacles were always made very large because they rested on the cheeks and not on the nose [Figure 494]. Consequently the presence of these large slabs of cool crystal near the eyes, not only kept out the strong light, but also kept down the temperature. They were at once a defense from the sun and a cold compress. We have similar methods, get the same results, but have a better explanation.[1]

Because of the impurities of glass, the original spectacle lenses (1287 and following) had a light greenish hue, bubbles, and imperfections. Aside from this, no record of colored lenses is available until 1561, when Jarius Aucott advocated the use of green glass in spectacles lenses as being of "great public utility and benefit."

Then in 1623 Daca de Valdes in his book, *Uso de los Antoios*, had a spectacles maker in one of his dialogues speak of light yellow, dark yellow, red, green, and blue lenses. The spectacles maker especially recommends the light yellow and blue lenses.[2]

Our next recorded reference to colored lenses in the literature is in 1672, when Richard Pierson of London recommended the use of blue glass as being superior to green.[3] The author gave no reason for this superiority.

A rainbow of colors for ophthalmic lenses was available in the 1700s in Europe (Figure 495). The lenses were described as "yellow-green, meadow-green, sea green, light blue, deep blue, yellow, violet, wine-colored and pink."[4] Smoked (grey) lenses were used in London in 1767.

Amber lenses were patented in England by George and Elias Solomons in 1832. King George IV granted this royal patent (Figures 496 & 497).

In 1854, Robert Hunt of England found that sunlight passed through a plano blue lens and then, when focused on a compass needle, could magnetize the needle. No other colored lens accomplished this. Therefore, the blue lens became immensely popular in the 1800s (Figure 498). It was believed to have some mysterious power.

Then in 1871, General A. J. Pleasanton of Philadelphia demonstrated that sunlight filtered through a dark blue glass was stimulating to plant and animal life. If such was the case, many concluded, it would also be stimulating to the eye. Therefore, we see many blue lenses in glasses from this era (Figure 499). In Germany, they were described as the rage. Perhaps they do give the irritated eye some protection during exanthematous diseases, but their other attributes have not been harnessed in the twentieth century.

SUNGLASSES

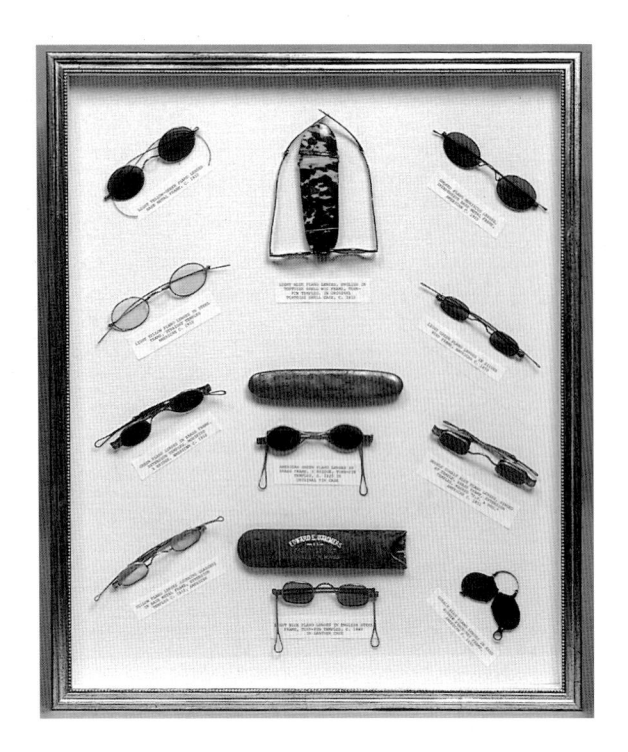

Figure 495. Variety of colors offered in early spectacles.

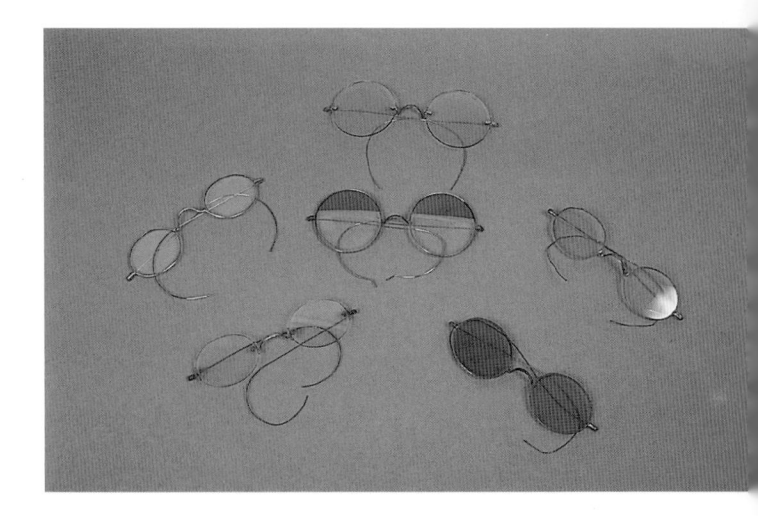

Figure 496. Amber lenses.

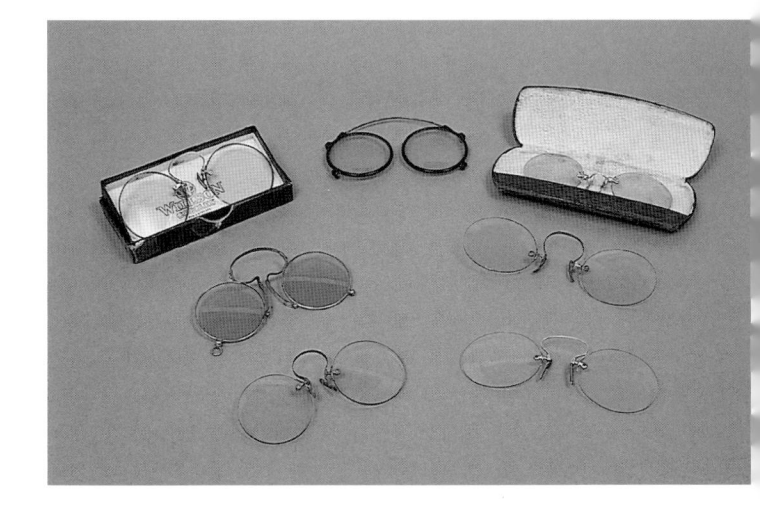

Figure 497. Pince-nez with amber lenses.

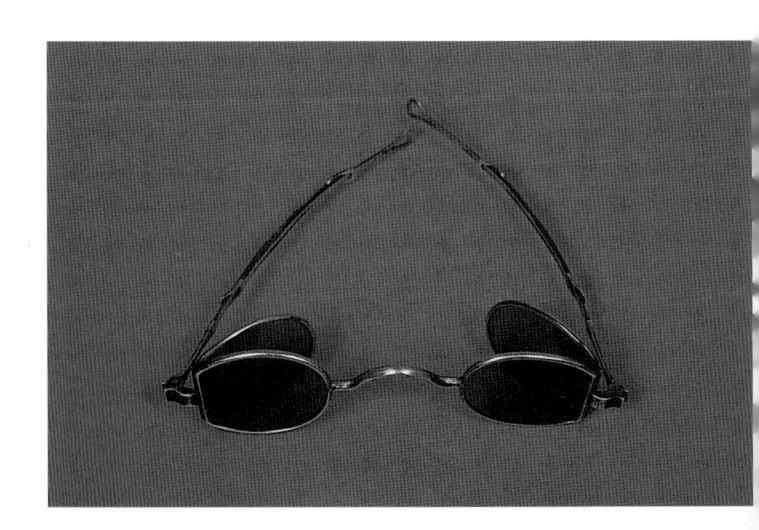

Figure 498. Silver spectacles, double blue lenses.

272   CHAPTER 23

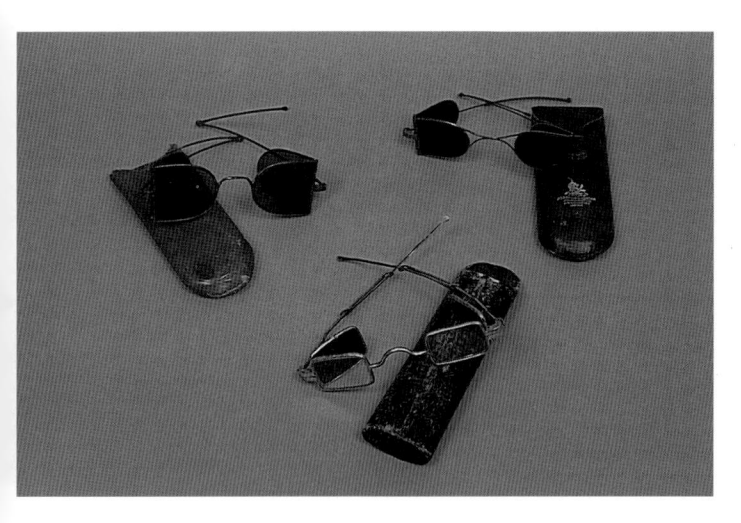

Figure 499. Blue lenses circa 1870.

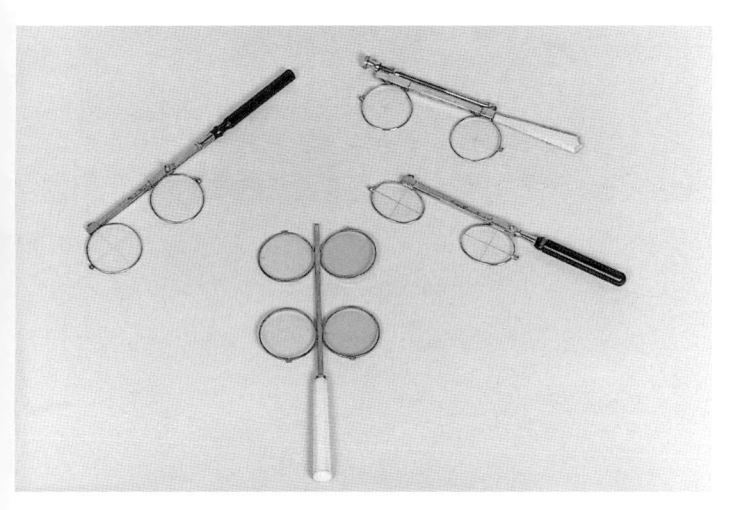

Figure 500. Softlite lens demonstrator, center, below.

A unique ultraviolet-absorbing lens was invented in 1871 by Brachet and Gesell. It was colored by salts of uranium. Then T. A. Wilson produced his pink arundel lens in 1872.

Others to work on ultraviolet absorbing lenses were Dr. Fieuzel of Paris and, when he died, his associate, Dr. Leon Fargier, who completed the work. A yellow-green or "chloris green" or "Phillis-aleaf" lens resulted. This was accomplished in 1880.

Five years later, Dr. William Thompson of Philadelphia, an ophthalmologist, suggested amethyst-tinted lenses for sensitive eyes. This color glass was obtained from old window panes that had turned amethyst from exposure to the sun. Heat will bleach these lenses, but amethyst-colored lenses obtained by adding manganese oxide to white glass will hold their color if heated.

Dr. Otto Hallauer of Bern, Switzerland, produced a smoky green glass that was very soothing. This glass was used for many years, starting in 1905. This is the same Dr. Hallauer who founded the Ophthalmic Museum at the University of Bern Medical School by donating his extensive ophthalmic collection.

Another greenish yellow glass containing uranium was produced in Germany in 1907 by Doctors Schauz and Stockhausen. The doctors made this glass in Dresden and called it Euphos.

In 1913 in England, Sir William Crookes produced a glass that absorbed both the ultraviolet and the infrared rays of the sun. This glass is called the Crookes glass and is possibly still used by some of the older practicing ophthalmologists. Originally, the color was sage green, though now it is brownish grey. The latter of these does not filter out infrared rays. It has, of course, been superseded by more modern lenses.

After World War I, pink softlite lenses, designed by Martin Singer's father, came into vogue (Figure 500). They were made in the United States by the Bausch and Lomb Optical Company. Several shades were available. Bausch and Lomb also sold Ray Ban (green) lenses, and G 15 and G 30, which were grey.

American Optical Company produced the Cruxite (Figure 501) (pink) and True-Color (grey) lenses as sun protectors.

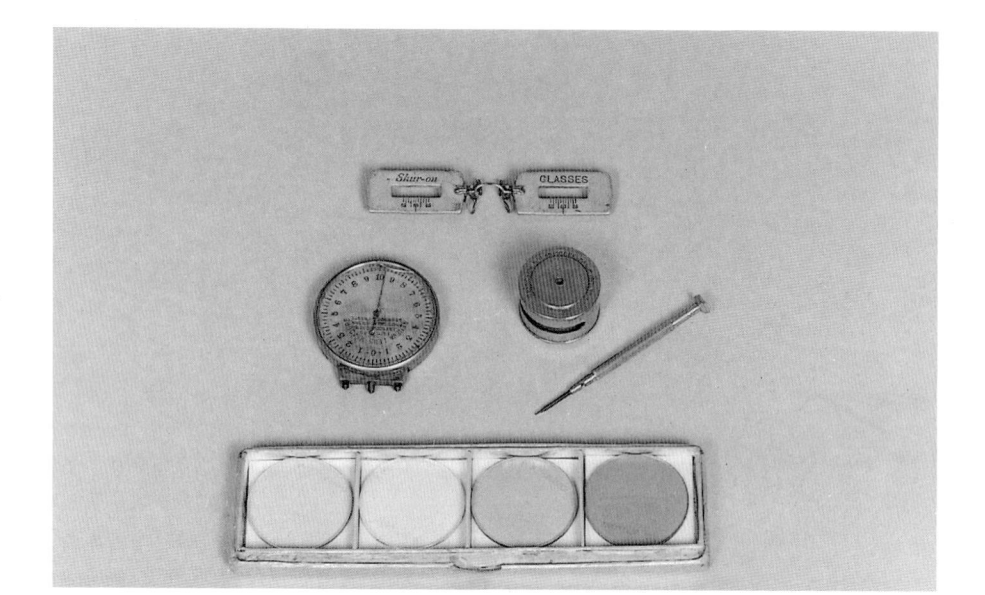

Figure 501. Cruxite lens demonstrator set, below.

Coloring of Glass Lenses

Various metallic oxides, when added to crown glass, will produce a glass of different colors. These oxides have been identified and purified over the years. Originally, however, mixed chemicals with impurities supplied optical glass with its color.

The following table indicates colors produced by their oxide additives:

>   Blue—cobalt oxide
>   Brown—cerium
>   Green—chrome oxide and ferrous iron oxide
>   Red—gold oxide
>   Salmon pink—didymium
>   Yellow—silver oxide and uranium
>   Violet—manganese oxide

Ferrous oxide is the most useful additive in the manufacture of colored glass lenses, as it increases the absorption of ultraviolet and infrared spectrum rays. It also facilitates heat absorption. It does, however, with its green color, disturb the normal transmission of the visible spectrum.

Claude Lorraine Filters

In the middle of the nineteenth century, one method of passive amusement was to view landscapes and the sky from various perspectives. Claude Lorraine devised dark glass filters to further augment the illusion and produce a great variety of colors. When using the filters, combinations of colors could be obtained.[5]

The use of the darkest filter was recommended when viewing the eclipse. Today, such an activity is deemed dangerous as it risks destruction of the macula.

The author has procured an example of these filters (Figure 502), circa 1848, which has three filters: brown, almost royal blue, and a dark reddish-purple. Each filter is set in a horn bezel, the handles of which are joined by a pin so that they can rotate. They are contained in a cover handle of tortoiseshell. The whole is 2 ½ inches in length, and each lens is one inch in diameter.

A description and picture of a similar filter set containing six filters is found in the catalog *Pike's Scientific and Medical Instruments* (Vol. II, p. 193). Each lens is not named by color but is described as "a variety of different colored glasses about one inch in diameter. . . . "[6] (price $1.50 to $3.00).

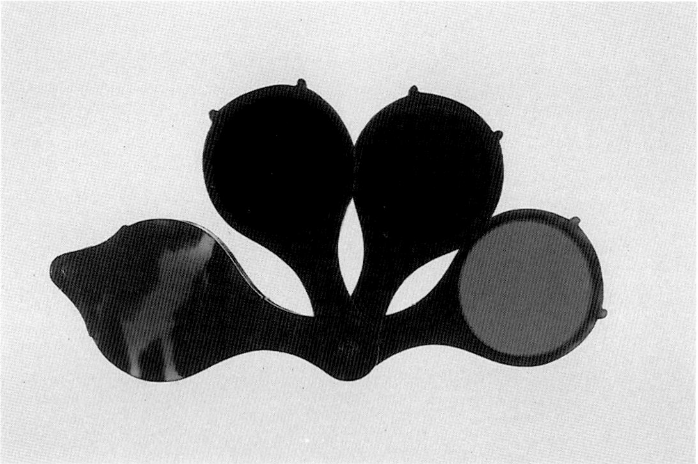

Figure 502. Claude Lorraine filters.

In the supplement to *Pike's Scientific and Medical Instruments* (Vol. I, p. 373) is a description of the Claude Lorraine Mirror:

> I don't know whether it was the invention of the famous Italian artist, who was in landscape paintings what Landseer is in the representation of animals, or whether the mirror was so called because, like Claude Lorraine, it is said to improve upon nature; but, at all events, it is a great curiosity. Its construction is the same with the ordinary looking glass, except that jet is used in place of quicksilver, and it is intended to reflect only the inanimate world. The Claude Lorraine mirror derives its value from the principle that all objects are more beautiful in miniature, which renders their defects less apparent; for the unsightly strikes the eye with immediate pain, while that which is perfect grows upon us more gradually. With this mirror, you frame for yourself, as it were, little landscapes at every turn, in which the sky is softer, the grass richer, and the feelings more graceful than anything you can see without it.[7]

These mirrors are mounted in neat embossed morocco cases, from 4 × 5 ¾ inches to 6 × 7 inches ($2.50 to $6.00).

Deborah Jean Warner, curator, history of astronomy, National Museum of History and Technology, provided the following article on the landscape mirror and glass:

In 1769 the poet Thomas Gray (1716–1771) heralded the beginning of the romantic age in England with a walking tour through the Lake District. While marveling over natural beauties he felt had never before been appreciated by artists, he had frequent recourse to a mirror to focus and frame particular views.

On the ascent of the hill above Appleby the thick hanging wood and the only reaches of the Eden (rapid, clear, and full as ever) winding below with views of the castle and town gave much employment to the mirror. . . . From hence I got to the "Parsonage" a little before sunset, and saw in my glass a picture, that if I could transmit to you, and fix it in all the softness of its living colours, would fairly sell for a thousand pounds.

The mirror was described more fully by William Mason, who published Gray's "Journal in the Lakes" in 1775: "Mr. Gray carried usually with him on these tours a Plano-Convex Mirror of about four inches in diameter on a black foil, and bound up like a pocket book. A glass of this sort is perhaps the best and most convenient substitute for a camera obscura, of anything that has hitherto been invented, and may be had of any optician."

Gray's landscape mirror was made of clear glass backed with dark foil. Others recommended dark foil mirrors for sunny days and silver-backed ones for cloudy or gloomy days. By the end of the eighteenth century landscape mirrors were regularly made of black glass or obsidian.

These mirrors were widely used in England by those in

search of picturesque beauty. They reduced the variety of natural colors to shades of a monotone and their convex surface enhanced the perspective lines.

In the late eighteenth century landscape mirrors were often associated with Thomas Gray. In 1787 the London instrument maker George Adams advertised "Black convex glass mirrors (recommended by Gray the poet)." A few years later Peter Crosthwaite, "Master of the Celebrated Museum" at Keswick, and dealer in maps and landscapes of the Lake District, advertised "Gray's Landscape Glasses."

In the nineteenth century, however, the landscape mirror for an unknown reason came to be associated with the French painter Claude Lorraine (1600-1682), although it is almost certain that he never used such a mirror. In 1856, for example, a Philadelphia firm advertised:

Claude Lorraine or Landscape Mirror. A pleasing and beautiful instrument for viewing clouds, landscapes, &c.; particularly adapted for use in the country and at the sea-shore. As the Mirror condenses or diminishes the view into a true perspective effect, the instrument is invaluable to the artist, and a very desirable companion for the tourist. The Mirror produces, instantaneously, the most charming reflection of scenery, buildings, &c. $2.25 to $6.00.

The paintings of Claude Lorraine were immensely pleasing to the romantic eye. Again and again in the late eighteenth and nineteenth centuries natural views were compared with those drawn by Claude, and would-be artists, professional as well as amateur, were encouraged to copy his style. The English painter and engraver John Burnet (1784–1868), for example, in his instructive "Landscape Painting in Oil Colours" refers to "the great master of aerial perspective, Claude Lorraine, the skies of whose landscapes are so captivating, both those of evening and midday.... The sun, being often placed near the point of sight, make both the emanation of the light and the receding of the several lines converge to the same focus." A Claude Lorraine sunrise or sunset, with the sun at the perspective vanishing point would, of course, be blinding if viewed directly. However, reflected in a dark mirror it can be enjoyed with safety. The mirror could also be used for viewing sunspots and solar eclipses.

Another optical device actually quite different from the Claude Lorraine mirror, but often confused with it, is the Claude Lorraine glass. Like the mirrors, the glasses were widely advertised by optical instrument dealers throughout the nineteenth century. According to the 1856 *Illustrated Descriptive Catalogue* issued by Benjamin Pike Jr., of New York, the Claude Lorraine glass

"consists of a variety of different colored glasses, about one inch in diameter, mounted in horn frame and turning on one centre, for producing a great variety of colors and showing their combination; it also will be found both pleasing and useful for viewing eclipses, clouds, landscapes, &c. Price $1.50 to $3.00."[8]

While optical filters had long been known, appreciation for the way they enhanced the views of land, sea, and sky soared during the nineteenth century. In 1789 the writer William Gilpin (1724–1804), in one of his many lessons on viewing and capturing on paper the beauty of a picturesque landscape, advised the use of this instrument and explained its name: "The only picturesque glasses are those, which the artists call Claude Lorraine glasses. They are combined of two or three different colours; and if the hues are well sorted, they give the objects of nature a soft, mellow tinge, like the colouring of that master."

Contemporary literary references to these Claude Lorraine glasses are sufficiently numerous to suggest that they were indeed widely known [Figure 503]. In an English play of 1798, for example, the heroine viewing the landscape through her gold-tinted Claude Lorraine glass exclaims, "How gorgeously glowing!"; then changing to the dark glass, "How gloomily glaring!"; and finally the blue glass, "How frigidly frozen!" A quarter of a century later, in Sir Walter Scott's *Redgauntlet*, Alan Fairford wrote to Darsie Latimer: "Didst ever see what artists call a Claude Lorraine glass, which spreads its own particular hue over the whole landscape which you see it through? Thou beholdest ordinary events just through such a medium."

Apparently the landscape mirror and the landscape glass were first widely used in England in the middle of the eighteenth century. It seems likely that both instruments came to be linked with Claude Lorraine simply because they showed landscape as it was in many of Claude's paintings.[9]

Conclusion

The information in this chapter applies to ordinary sunglasses for everyday and general use by civilians. Insight on the various colors available and the chemicals used in their

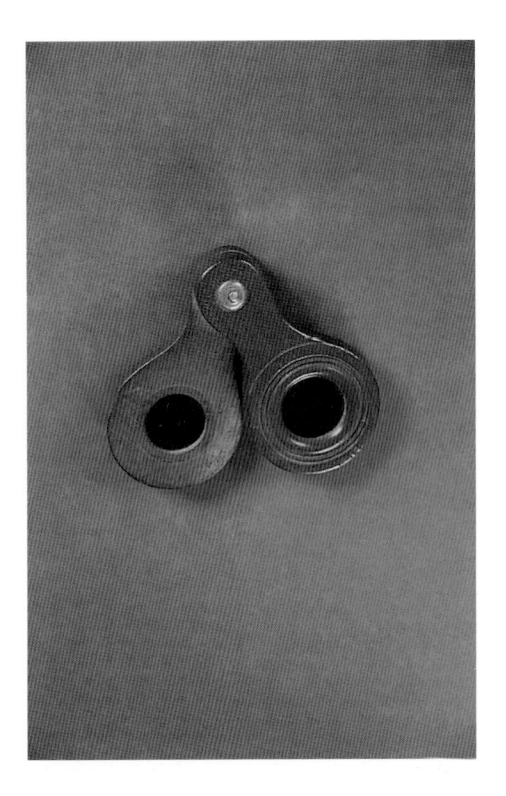

Figure 503. Claude Lorraine filters.

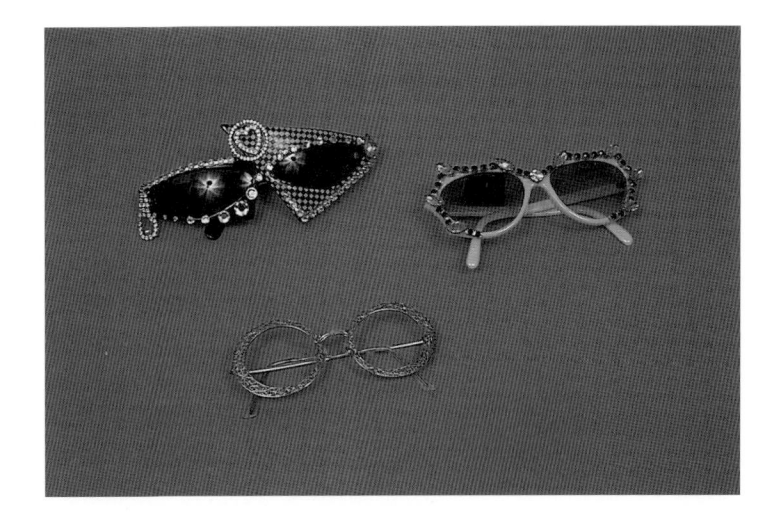

Figures 504 & 505. Some modern sunshades.

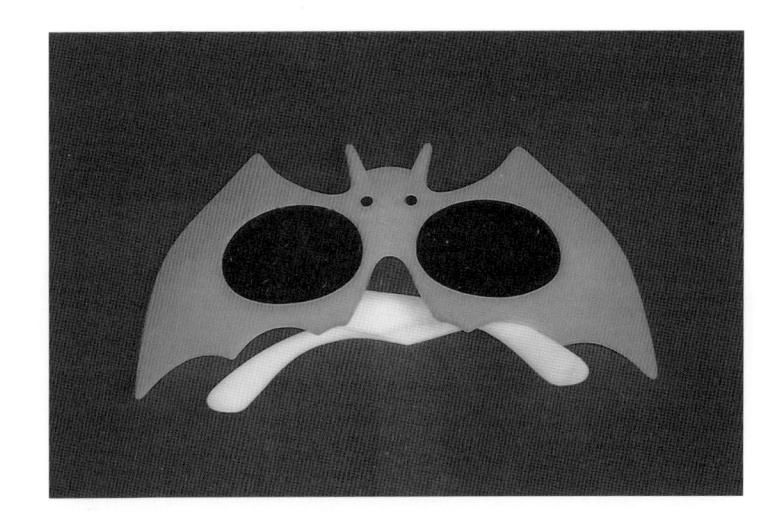

Figure 505.

production was included, but only those lenses used to reduce light intensity as a whole were considered (Figures 504 & 505). Industrial and protective lenses are discussed in Chapter 25.

Notes
1. Otto Durham Rasmussen, *Chinese Eyesight and Spectacles* (Tonbridge, England: Tonbridge Free Press, Ltd., 1915–1949)
2. Daca de Valdes, *Uso de los Antoios* (Perez, 1623).
3. Theo Obrig, *Modern Ophthalmic Lenses* (New York: The Chilton Co., 1935), 40 ff.
4. Ibid.
5. Pierre Marley, *Spectacles* (Paris: Hoebeke, 1988), 12.
6. *Pike's Scientific and Medical Instruments*, Vol. I & II, pp. 193, 373.
7. Ibid.
8. Ibid.
9. Deborah Warner, "Antiques," p. 158.

Other Sources Consulted for Chapter 23
1. J. T. Hudson, "On Coloured Shades and Lenses," in *Useful Remarks upon Spectacles, Lenses, and Opera-Glasses; with Hints to Spectacle Wearers and Others....* (London: Joseph Thomas, Finch-Lane, Cornhill, 1840), 25.
2. Casey A. Wood, "The First Scientific Work on Spectacles," *Annals of Medical History*, p. 150.

24

Eskimo Shades

Little has been recorded regarding the development, manufacture, and use of Eskimo shades—this microcosm in the realm of eyewear. Most of us are cognizant that there is such a thing as snowblindness and that protection of the eyes is needed from glare in areas where snow and ice predominate. Today, protective goggles are available against glare and wind when skiing, ice skating, and the like. Primitive peoples, however, had no materials for protective, dark, or reflective lenses. Their ingenuity of making do with the materials at hand, nevertheless, provided ample protection. The American Academy of Ophthalmology Foundation Museum has one pair of Eskimo shades dating about 1750 (Figure 506). However, conjecture is that they were made long before that time. These shades are still being made and used today.

The author has seen one of pair of bone shades reputed to be from the Punic Culture (A.D. 1000), excavated on Gambel, St. Lawrence Island, Alaska (courtesy Dr. Gilbert Blass Cohen).

Territory

The areas inhabited by Eskimos are in the northern parts of Canada, Alaska, the islands of the Bering sea, and parts of Russia as well as Labrador and Greenland. Eskimos' subsistence depends on the seasons, the weather, and the ability to hunt and fish. The ice and snow of the harsh winters subject the Eskimos to a great deal of glare. The Eskimos still, however, must obtain food and therefore must have protection for their eyes.

Materials

Protection from ice and snow is partly provided by a fringe of fur on the edge of the Eskimo's parka or head covering. Direct frontal glare is repelled by a slab of wood (Figure 507), bone (Figure 508), ivory, baleen (Figure 509), or hoof (Figure 517)—used over the eyes. All materials must be dried, fixed, and stabilized before use. All organic shreds must be meticulously removed by mechanical means, boiling, or drying in the sun. This material is then carved to fit the face in a frontal curve to keep sidelight out as well (Figure 510). The slab is additionally carved to fit the nose and is held onto the head with a leather thong from a reindeer, seal, or other animal. (Please note that the materials used would not stick to the skin in the frozen state.) For further protection, the inside is usually stained black (Figure 511).

To see through this slab, the Eskimo carves a horizontal slit (Figure 512), allowing side as well as lateral vision, limiting glare, working as a stenopaic slit, and offering protection from the wind. How ingenious! Some Eskimos have made pinholes in their material rather than slits. Whereas the slits are about 3 millimeters high and 5 centimeters long, the pinholes are about 8 millimeters round.

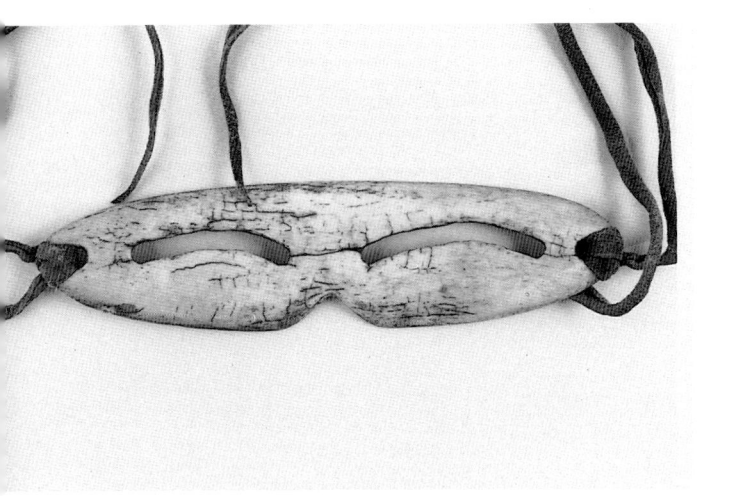

Figure 506. Eskimo shades circa 1750.

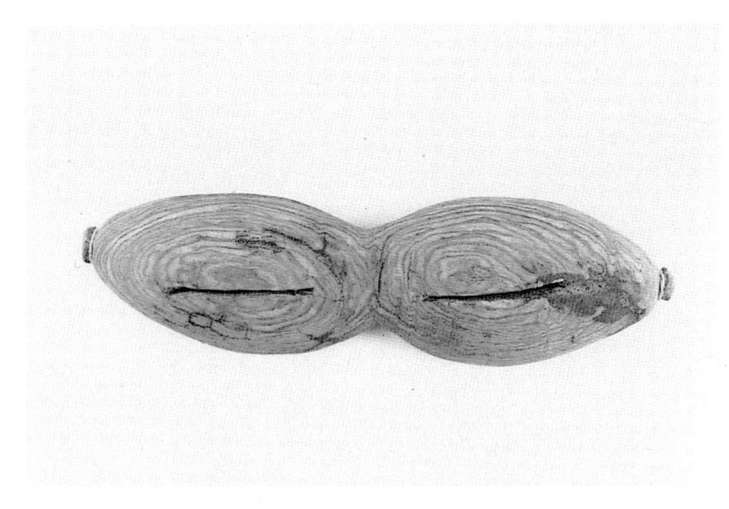

Figure 507. Wooden carved Eskimo eyeshade.

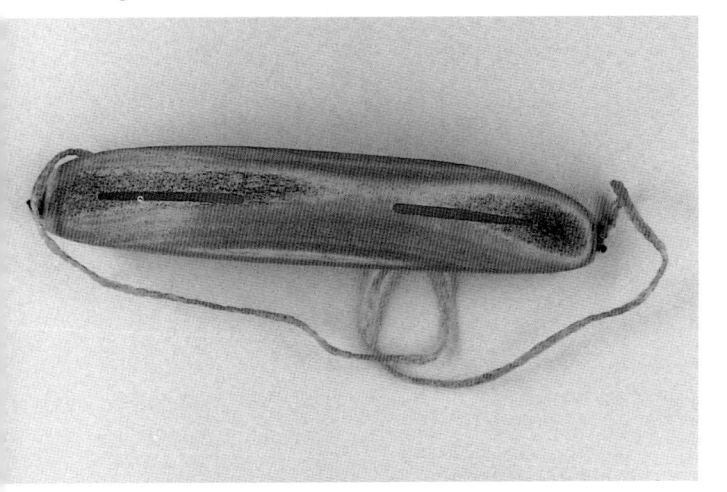

Figure 508. Bone Eskimo eyeshade.

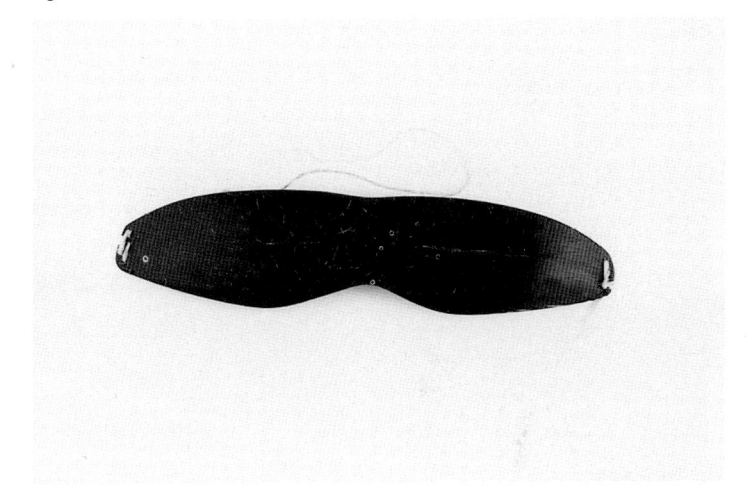

Figure 509. Baleen Eskimo eyeshade.

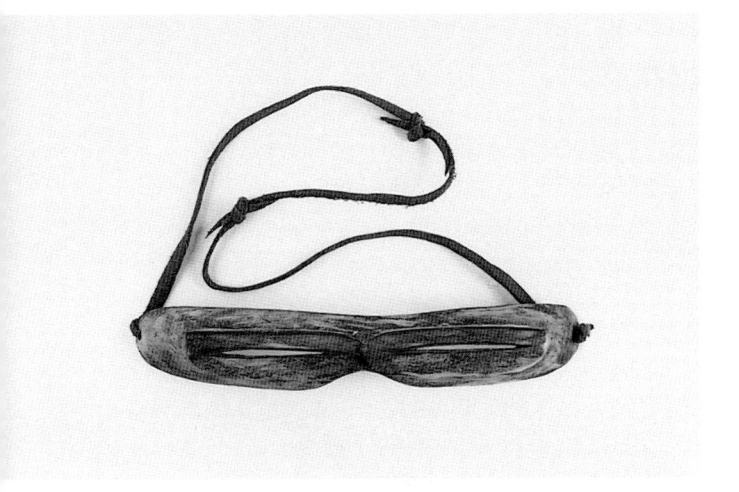

Figure 510. Recessed eye slits to keep out wind and snow.

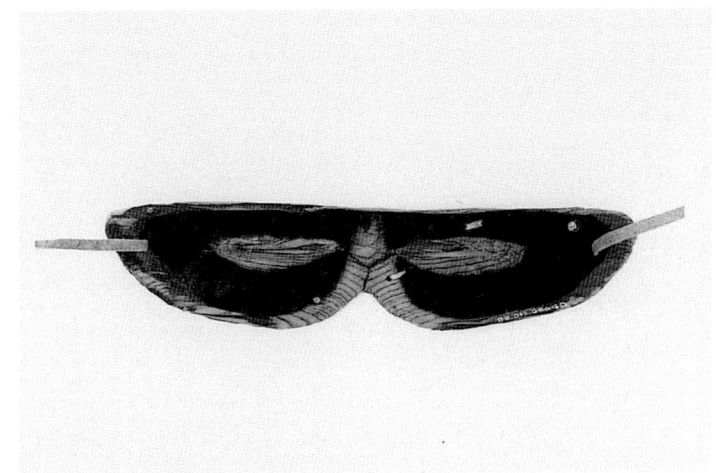

Figure 511. Blackened inside of eyeshade.

ESKIMO SHADES **279**

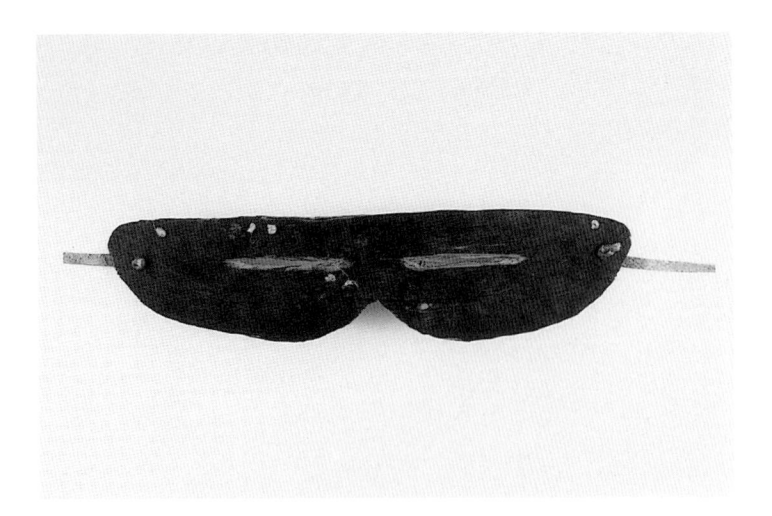

Figure 512. Typical horizontal slit in Eskimo eyeshade.

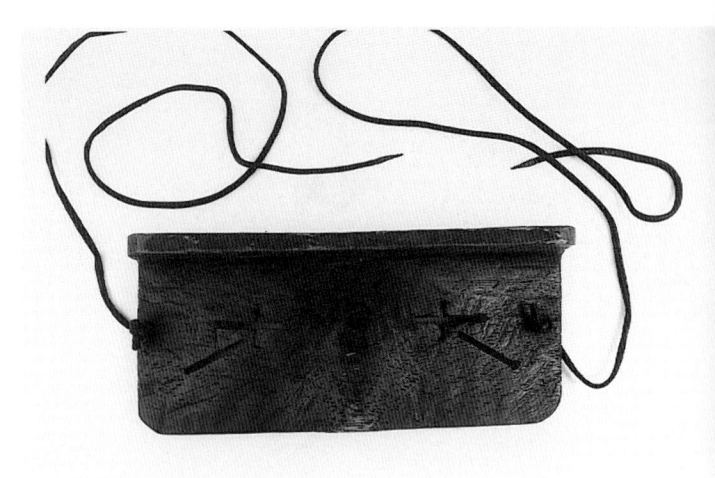

Figure 513. Eskimo shade with additional peak (frontal view).

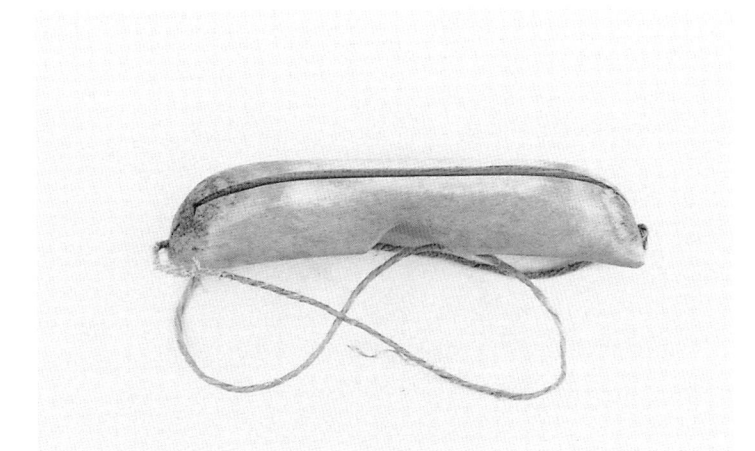

Figure 514. Continuous slit across the face.

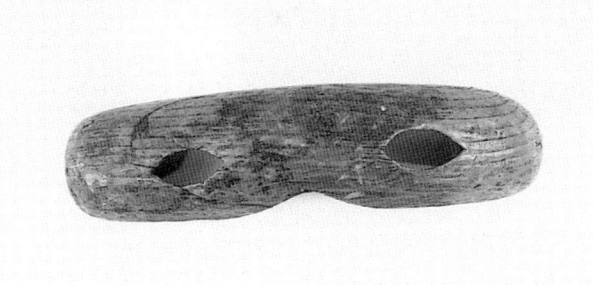

Figure 515. Oval eye openings.

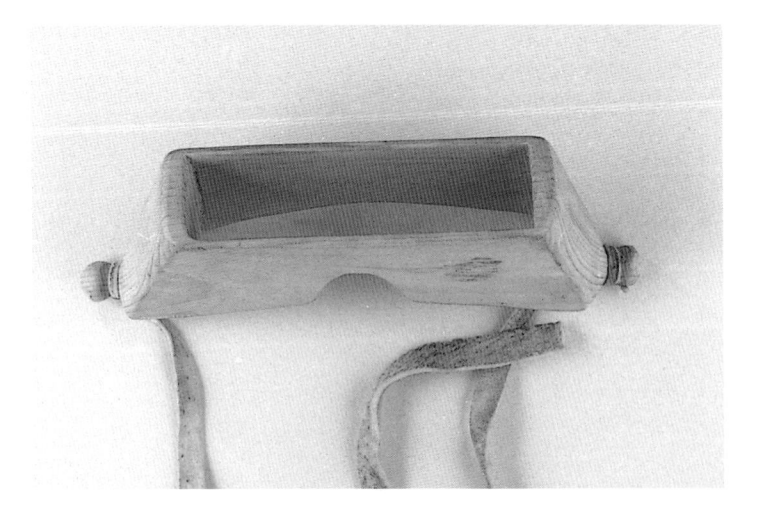

Figure 516. Boxlike Eskimo eyeshade.

Variations

The author has seen one quite large pair of shades made of wood that extends to the forehead and consists of a ledge or peak at the top to further shade the eyes (Figure 513). The slit of another pair extends completely across the face (Figure 514). One has the slits curved upward, while another has no slits but has oval openings for the eyes (Figure 515). The pair shown in Figure 513, made of black wood, contains not only a peak but also crosses for the eye slits, allowing up-and-down vision as well. An unusual variety is made like a hollow box, with a cutout for the nose (Figure 516).

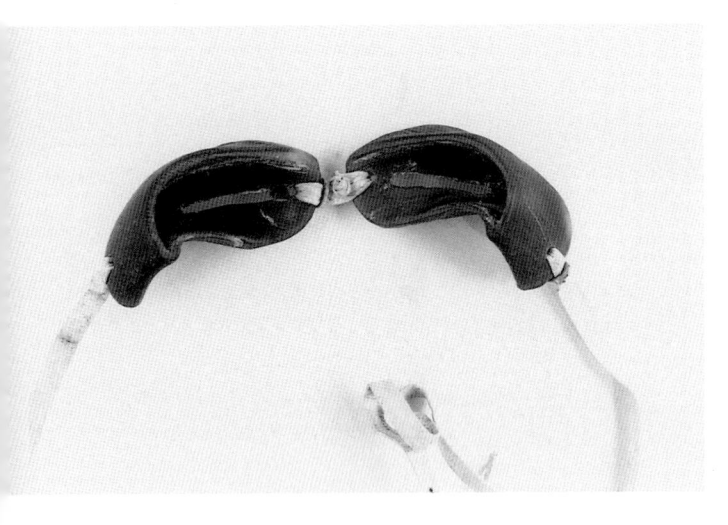

Figure 517. Eskimo eyeshade fashioned from animal hoof.

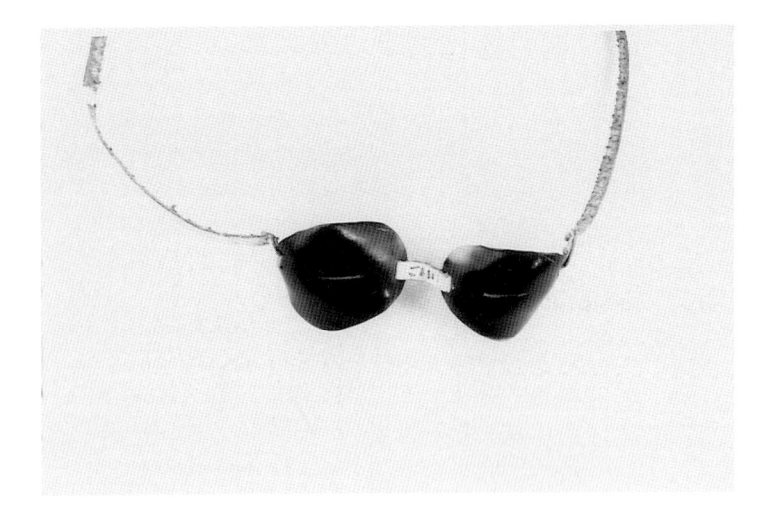

Figure 518. Eskimo eyeshade fashioned from baleen.

Individual Eye Covers

A precisely correct size hoof from an animal (usually reindeer) can be split and carved to make individual cups to cover each eye (Figure 517). A slit is then made to see through. The cups are joined over the nose to form a bridge with a leather thong, with another thong that ties around the back of the head.

Cups like this have also been fashioned of baleen (Figure 518). Since baleen and hoofs are naturally dark, no coloration is needed.

Decoration

Scrimshanders have been attacking ivory, bone, and tooth for many years.[1] The Eskimos are no different. They decorate their glasses with lines, spots, curves, etc., using incision and blackening with carbon. Wax holds the carbon in place.

Dating

Eskimo sunshades are still being carved today, mostly for the tourism trade or as an art form. However, ancient examples of these artifacts are difficult to date. As the shades are dug up (or worked up if a "placer mining" technique is used), the years of origin are determined by the types and forms of artifacts accompanying them, such as bone needles and pottery shards. The depth in the earth in which the shades are found is also a determining factor. The deeper, of course, the older the artifact.

Attempts to carbon date sunshades have not been successful, as their composition does not lend itself to the accuracy of this determination. Additionally, a large piece of material is needed for analysis, and using this may destroy a major part of the object.

Following is a description of another process used to date artifacts from an article by M. J. Aitken and S. J. Fleming of the Research Laboratory for Archaeology and the History of Art:

AUTHENTICITY TESTS BY THERMOLUMINESCENCE

Introduction Thermoluminescence (hereafter referred to as "TL") is a phenomenon exhibited to varying degrees by many minerals. It is the emission of light when a substance is heated; this light is additional to ordinary red-hot glow and usually occurs at a less elevated temperature. It represents the release of energy which has been stored as trapped electrons in the crystal lattice of the mineral. This stored energy is acquired by absorption from any nuclear (or ionizing) radiation to which the mineral may have been exposed; consequently the amount of TL observed (measured with a very sensitive photo-multiplier) is proportional to the overall dose of radiation which has been received.

In terracotta and most types of pottery there are mineral constituents (e.g. quartz) that have this property of accumulating TL and they receive a small but significant dosage of nuclear radiation which over thousands of years adds up to an appreciable total. This dosage comes from radioactive impurities (a few parts per million of uranium and thorium, a few per cent of potassium) in the clay of the object itself, and also, but to a lesser extent, from the radioactive impurities in the surroundings; cosmic rays also make a small contribution.

Heating to above 500 degrees C removes the geologically accumulated thermoluminescence and consequently the firing of the clay sets the "thermoluminescent clock" to zero. Thereafter the TL grows with time. The growth is also dependent on the particular TL constituents in a given sample as well as on the radiation dose-rate as explained above. By laboratory measurements the TL carried by a sample can be expressed as an "accumulated radiation dose." This is determined by exposing the sample to radiation from an artificial radioisotope and finding the amount of radiation required to induce a level of TL equal to the "natural" TL carried by the sample.

By measuring the amounts of uranium, thorium and potassium present in the sample and taking a typical value for the contribution from the burial soil, the radiation dose received by the fragment each year can be estimated. The age is then directly obtained as: Age = Accumulated Radiation Dose/Dose per year.

Applicability   The first essential is that the object to be tested was made from clay by firing to 500 degrees C or higher. The method measures the years that have elapsed since firing and if the object has been reheated (to 300 degrees C or more) subsequently, it is the latter that is dated. In some cases it is possible to determine whether or not this has been so.

The method is applicable to terracotta and earthenware etc., but not, at the moment, to very hard fabrics such as porcelain.

If an object has been subjected to X-ray, y-ray or neutron examination it may not be possible to obtain a conclusive result. Where there is the possibility that such exposure may have occurred, the object should not be submitted for testing without special consultation.

Sample Taking   Ideally the sample should be a lump at least 5 millimetres thick and 10 or 20 millimetres across. Such a sample is usually obtainable from a terracotta statue for instance—by means of a pair of pliers or a hacksaw.

For smaller objects where this cruder treatment is not permissible, a sample can be obtained by means of drilling a small hole two or three millimetres across and a few millimetres deep in an unobtrusive place (using a 1/16" Glazemaster tungsten drill type U, for instance). *It is important to discard the first millimetre, to carry out the drilling in subdued bulb light, to exclude daylight and fluorescent light from the room, and to put the powder into a container which is kept dark. Whenever possible the drilling is done at the Laboratory or at any rate by a member of the Laboratory staff.*

The advantage of having a lump rather than a powder is that the age can be determined to narrower limits. As a general rule, when the expected age if authentic is less than twice the expected age if imitative, it is essential to have a lump. On the other hand if the former is more than five times the latter then a drilled sample is adequate (as long as the light restrictions are observed).

If the object has suffered restoration it should be borne in mind that the component parts may be of differing antiquity. It may then be necessary to sample in several places, and in some cases the situation may be too complex for testing to be practical. The Laboratory reserves the right to decline to test an object when the circumstances are ambiguous for this reason, or for any other reason, and to use its discretion as to the most suitable region for sampling.

Accuracy   In the absence of knowledge of the burial conditions it is not possible to obtain the age to better then +/- 25% even when a lump is available. When only a drilled sample is available, and for various established technical limitations, the accuracy obtainable may be worse.

There is an additional limitation (due to "spurious" TL) in dealing with recent samples and whether or not these considerations are applicable to material of the last four or five centuries depends on individual circumstances.

The method is an absolute one and it does not rely on comparison with other objects of the same type.[2]

Numerous methods have been used to date these and other artifacts, but obviously these tests are not done by the average collector. They are performed by trained scientists/archaeologists. The means by which these experts obtain dates of origin are time consuming and expensive. This, coupled with the knowledge/expertise required to date objects, sometimes prevents the collector from ever gaining true and accurate information regarding his find.

Obtaining Specimens

Being on the spot where such objects are excavated would, of course, be ideal in adding to one's collection. Few of us, however, have the time, connections, or willingness, to participate in such activities. We are therefore forced to rely upon local individuals who sell artifacts or lore in Eskimo country, or on dealers in remote areas who make their living buying and selling these relics. Antique stores, flea markets, auctions, and the like are also possible places for finds. When artifacts are found away from the areas of origin, the prices are considerably higher. However, guarantees of authenticity are offered (and should be obtained).

Conclusion

Through the necessity of ocular protection, Eskimo shades were developed and perfected using primitive but effective methods and materials. Even in isolation, with no past experience and with limited supplies, Eskimos used techniques that were most useful. We salute them for their ingenuity.

Notes

1. Pierre Marley, *Spectacles* (Paris: Hoebeke, 1988), 116.
2. M. J. Aitken and S. J. Fleming, "Authenticity Tests by Thermoluminescence," *Research Laboratory for Archaeology*, February, 1971.

25

Industrial and Protective Goggles and Spectacles

The realities of life in the eighteenth century entailed economic choices much as in modern times. When traveling on a stagecoach, the comfortable, clean seats inside cost more than the outside seats or clinging to the "rails" on the outside. To protect one's eyes from the dust, rocks, and sunlight, "railroad" glasses were used (Figure 519). These were glasses with side pieces whose lenses were rather thick and colored. About 50 to 75 years later, a very sophisticated version appeared—double D-shaped lenses, some sporting thick plates of Brazilian pebble (Figure 520). These were advertised by John Browning as being "shot proof."

During manufacturing and other commercial pursuits, the eyes needed protection. Figures 521, 522, and 523 show types of spectacles used for this purpose. Robert Fulton (1765–1815) invented the steam engine. When this power source was fitted to the railroad, despite obvious transport advantages, it posed threats to the health of the eye. Engineers had to peer into the distance while traveling at great speed, and eyes were pummeled with bugs, cinders, and smoke. Cinders also attacked the eyes of the train's firemen and even the passengers. To protect against this, goggles were made, many with green or grey lenses with blued wire gauze all around, padded near the face. These two eyepieces were joined (for a bridge) with a cord. Longer cords were used for temples (Figures 524 & 525). Goggles were sold in small tin boxes that were oval, tear-shaped, or square. Some had fixed wire bridges and temples (Figure 526). Stone masons' eyes were protected with cups of wire gauze arranged similarly (Figure 527).

Aviators, when flying airplanes unprotected by a cabin, needed goggles to protect their eyes from the wind and airborne debris (Figure 528). These goggles were plastic lenses without refractive power and were set in a leather frame that fit tightly to the face (Figure 529). This allowed vision to either side for a 180-degree visual field (Figure 530). Some were made en suite with a helmet.

Automobile drivers and motorcycle riders also can benefit from protective eyewear. Many styles have been devised, and there was previously a great exhibition of them at the American Optical Company Museum in Southbridge, Massachusetts (Figures 531–535).

While riding in a pack of horses at a speed of about 60 miles per hour, it is necessary for racing jockeys to protect their eyes. Appropriate goggles have been designed for this purpose (Figure 536).

Divers have a unique need for eye protection. This need, coupled with the negation of refraction of the cornea by the immersion in water, led to the early invention of specific lenses. As early as 1331, pearl divers used tortoiseshell transparent cups to maintain underwater vision. These cups were also described by Leonardo da Vinci about 1490, drawn by the

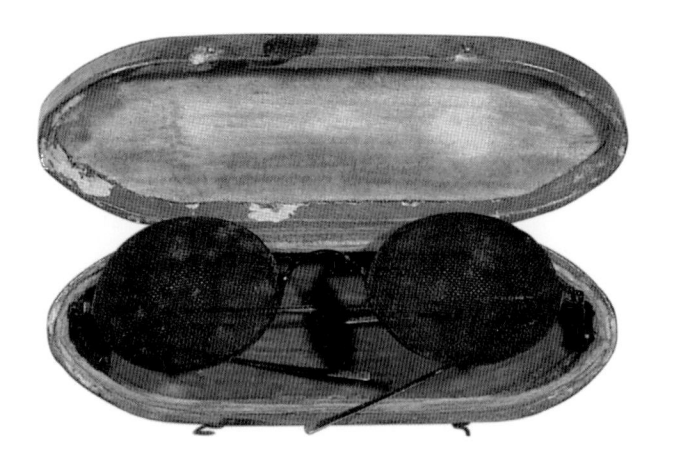

Figure 519. Early railroad glasses circa 1750.

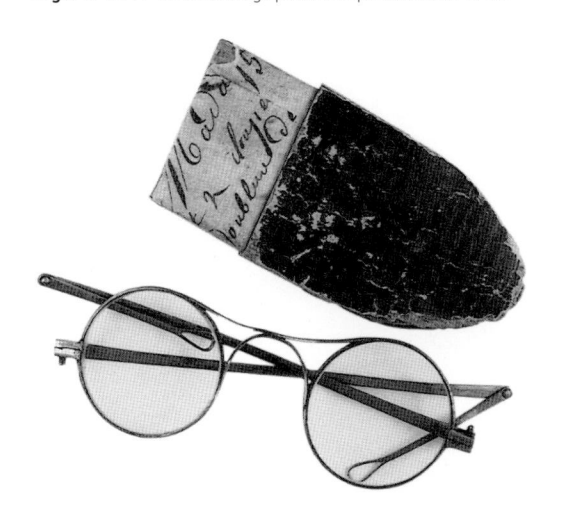

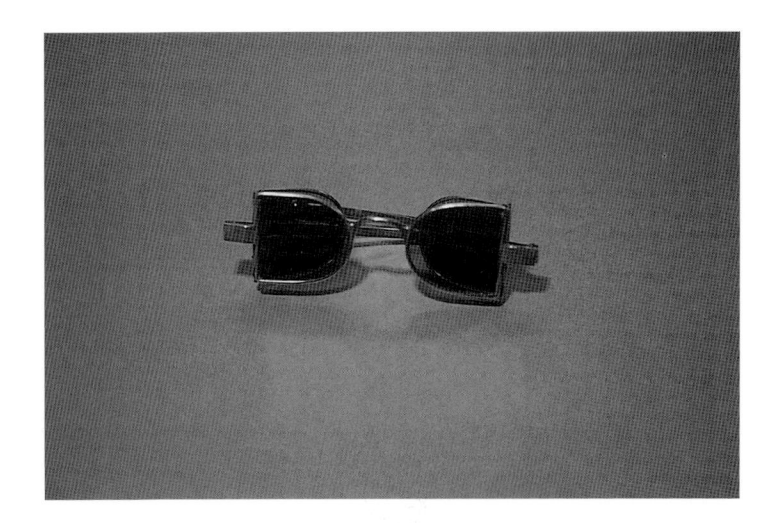

Figure 520. Double-D railroad glasses.

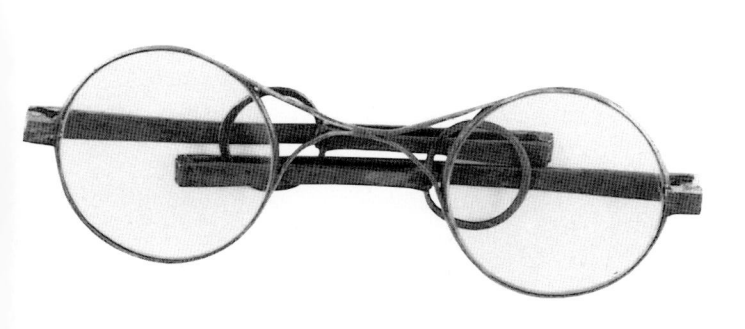

Figure 521. French X-bridge protective spectacles circa 1750.

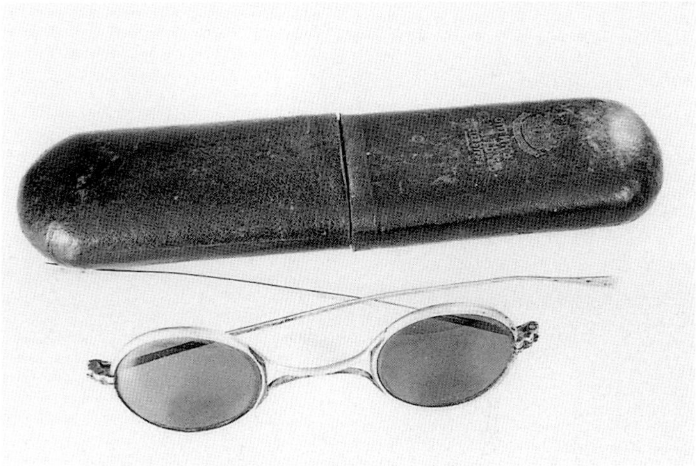

Figure 522. English X-bridge protective spectacles.

Figure 523. English X-bridge protective spectacles.

PROTECTIVE SPECTACLES 285

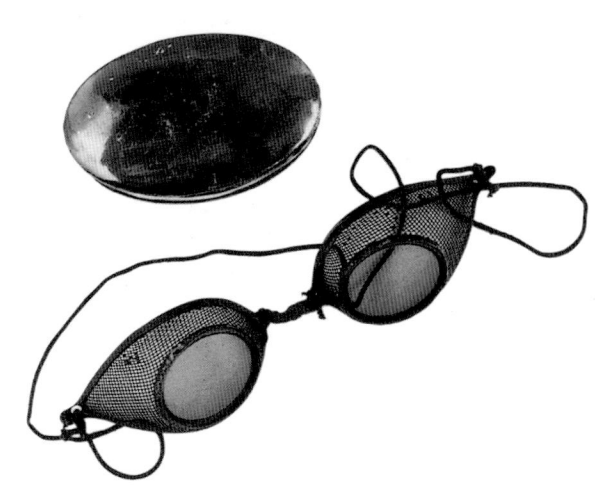

Figure 524. Protective spectacles with gauze wire shades and oval case.

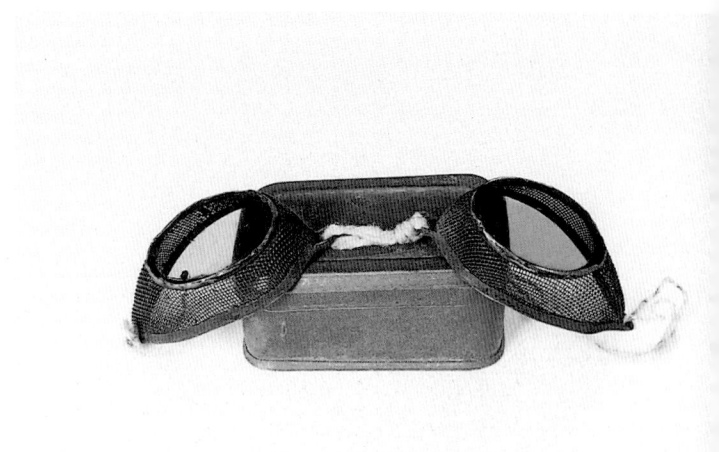

Figure 525. Protective spectacles with gauze wire shades and rectangular case.

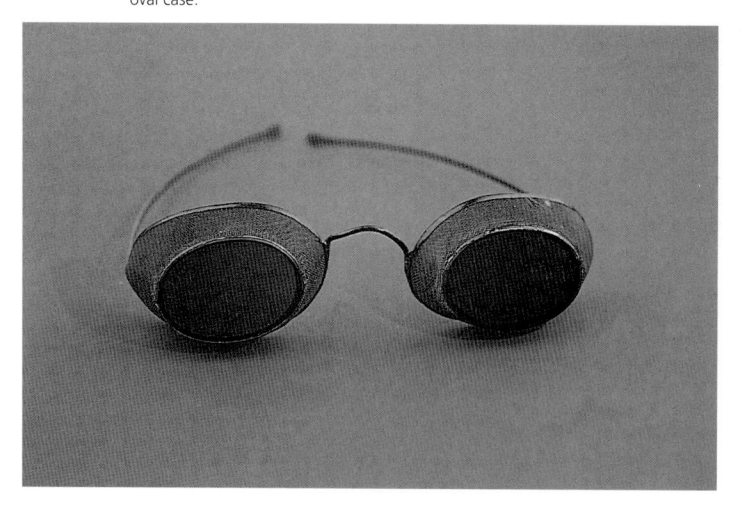

Figure 526. Protective spectacles with gauze wire shades.

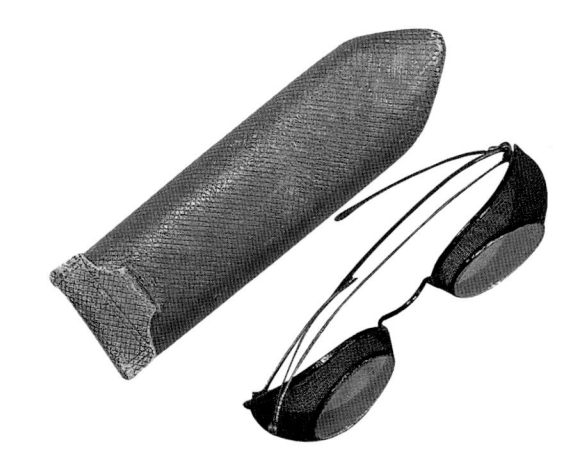

Figure 527. Stone mason's spectacles.

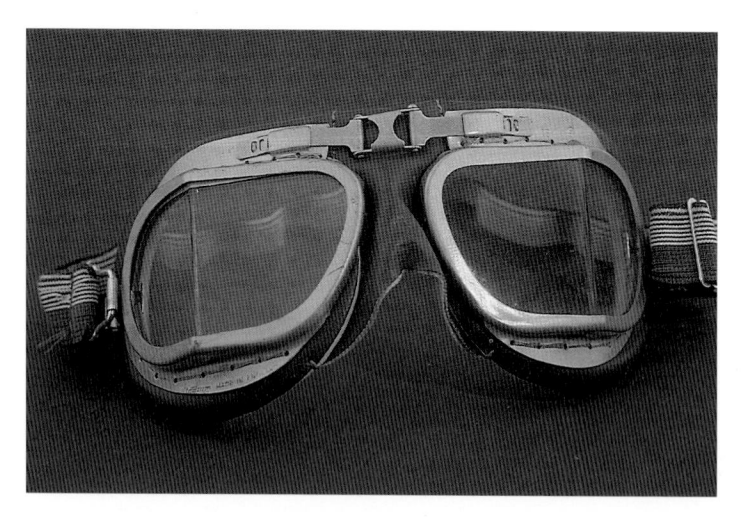

Figure 528. Aviator's goggles.

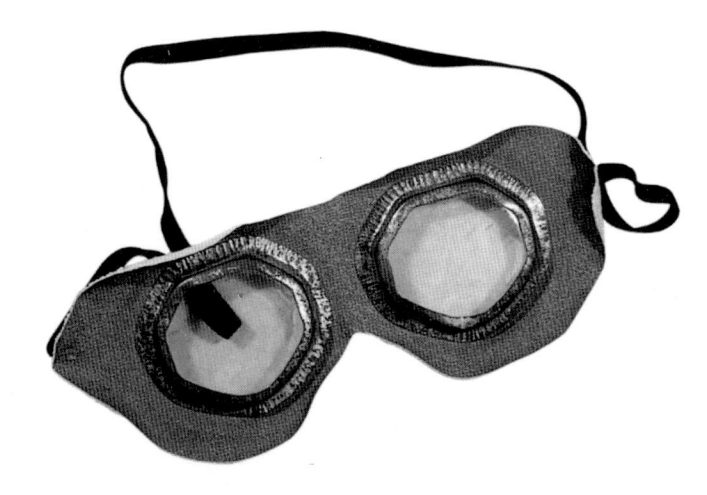

Figure 529. Aviator's goggles.

286 CHAPTER 25

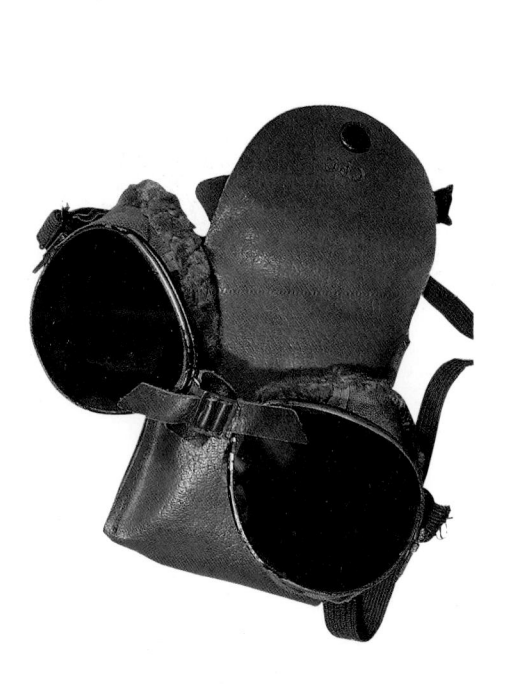

Figure 530. Aviator's goggles.

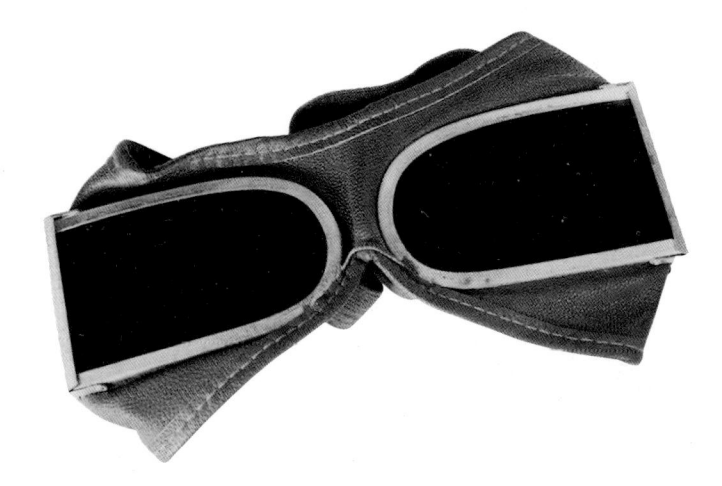

Figure 531. Automobile driving goggles.

Figure 532. Antiglare driving goggles.

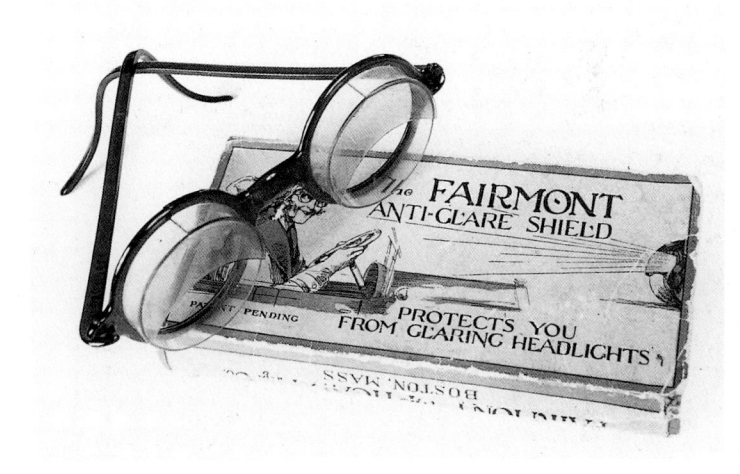

Figure 533. German pressed-tin glass case.

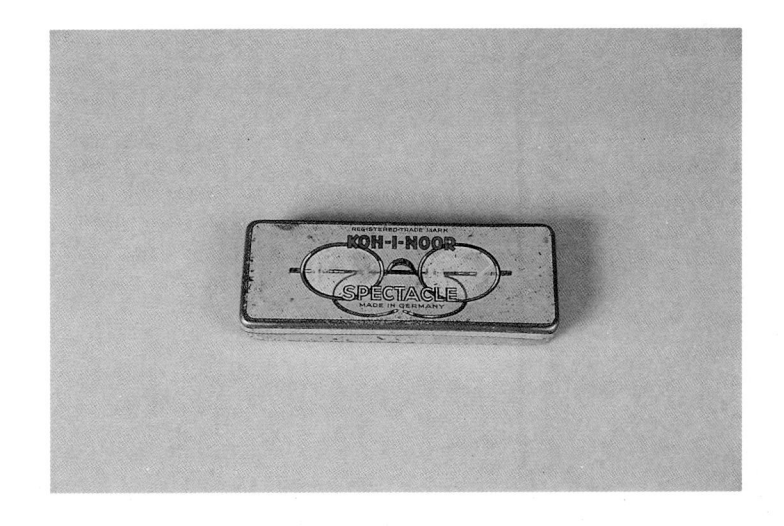

PROTECTIVE SPECTACLES

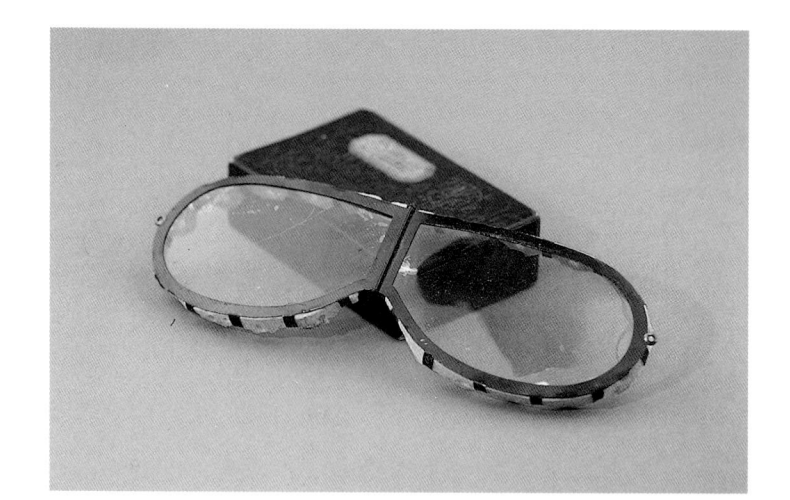

Figure 534. Driving goggles.

Figure 535. Willson / Albex / American Optical goggles.

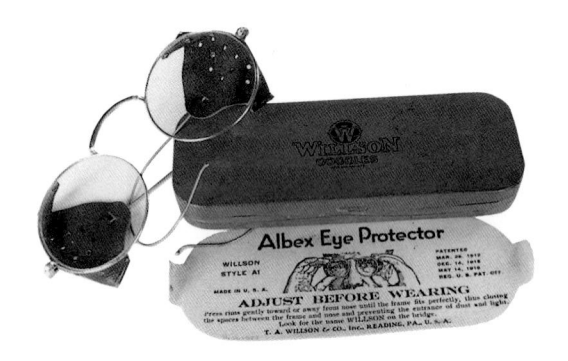

Figure 536. Jockey's protective shield.

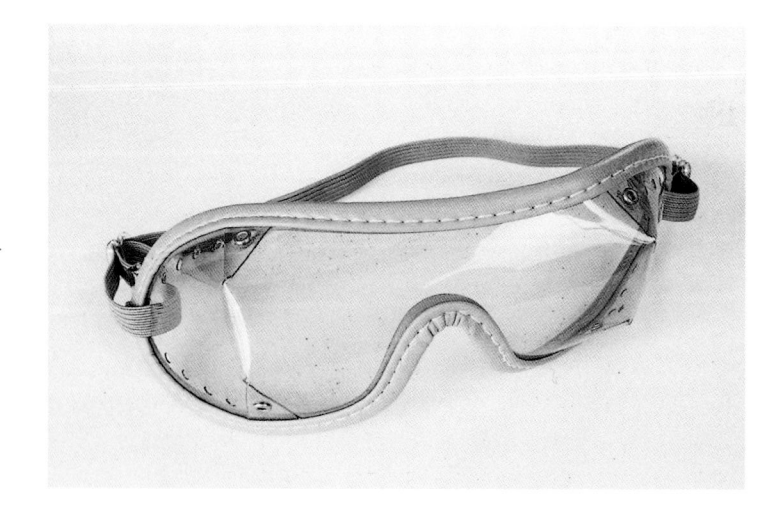

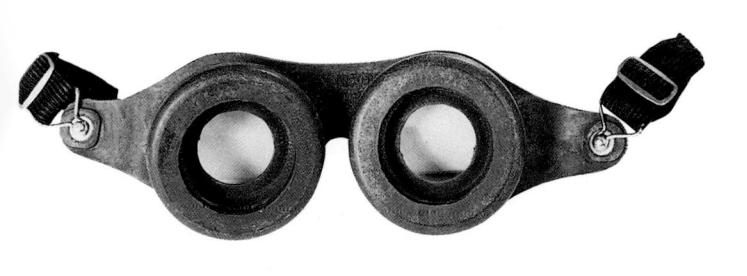

Figure 537. Diver's goggles.

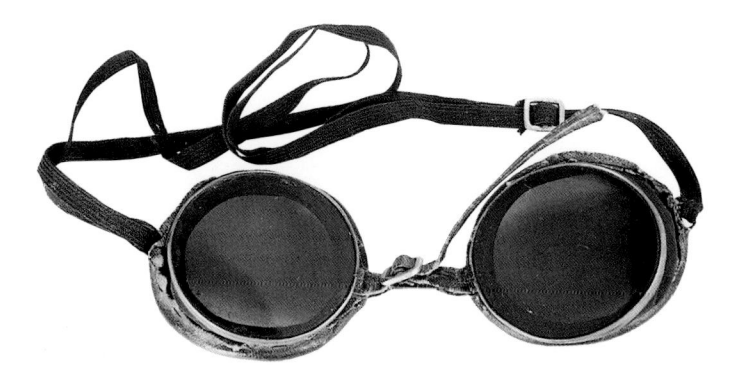

Figures 538–541. Examples of industrial goggles with dark lenses.

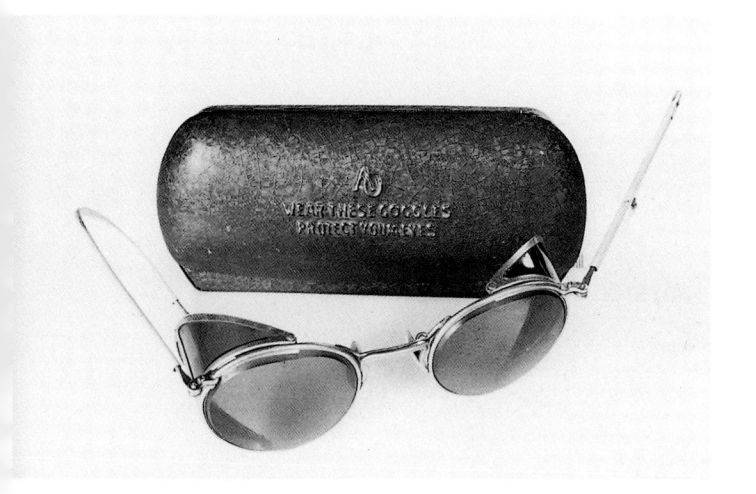

Figure 539.

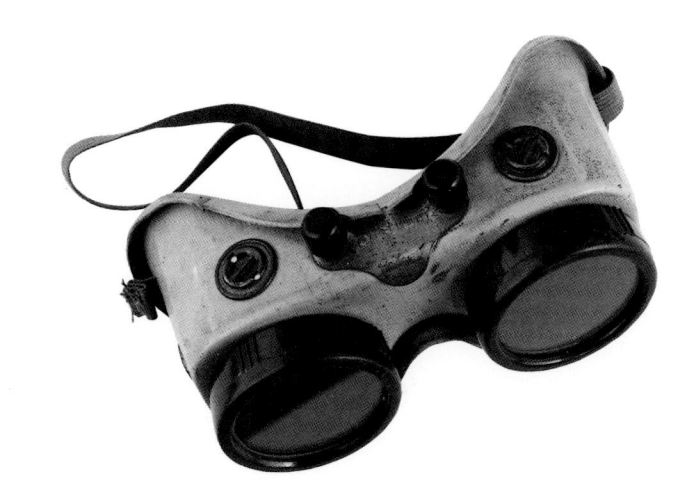

Figure 540.

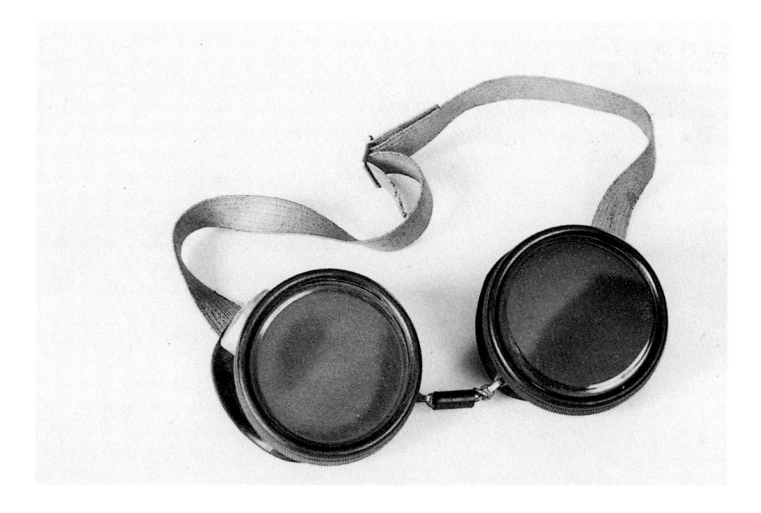

Figure 541.

Dutch artist Jan van Straet. A new lens was described in 1870 by R.E. Dudgeon. Other, more modern lenses have since been devised (Figure 537).

Spectacles or goggles made for protection of the eyes and adnexa against mechanical or radiation injury are called industrial or shatterproof glasses. Some lenses are clear and some are dark, particularly those used to prevent ultraviolet injury (flash burn) during welding of metals (Figures 538–543). Some lenses are plain (no prescription), while others, such as those used for scuba divers, have a ground-in prescription. Some lenses are plastic, while others are glass. Cobalt blue lenses are used for ironworkers who are stationed at smelters.

PROTECTIVE SPECTACLES 289

Figure 542. Example of nonrefractive lenses.

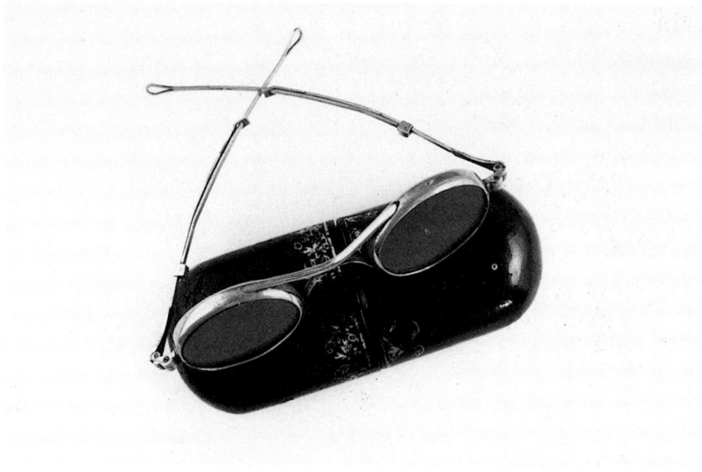

Figure 543. Example of industrial goggles with clear lenses.

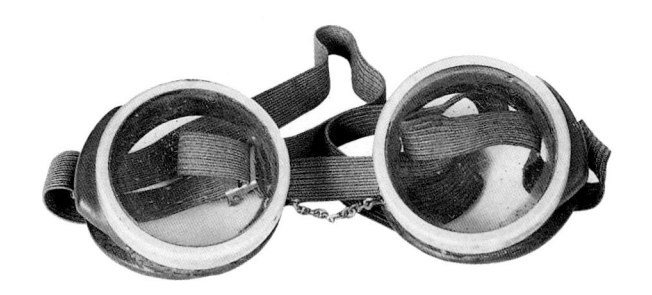

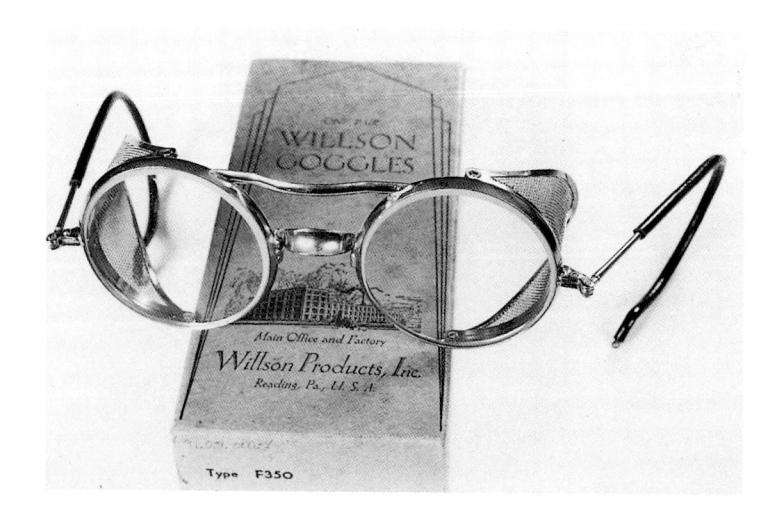

Figure 544. Shatterproof industrial glasses.

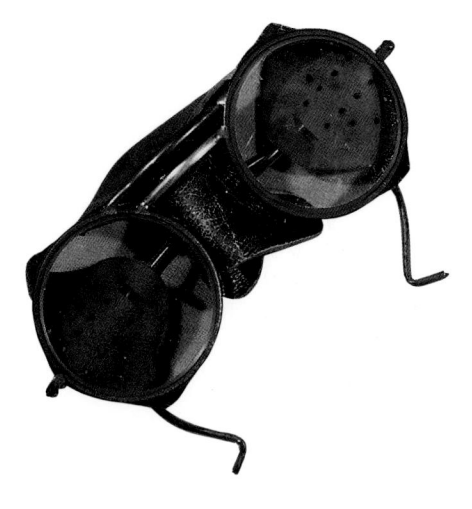

Figure 545. Laminated industrial glasses.

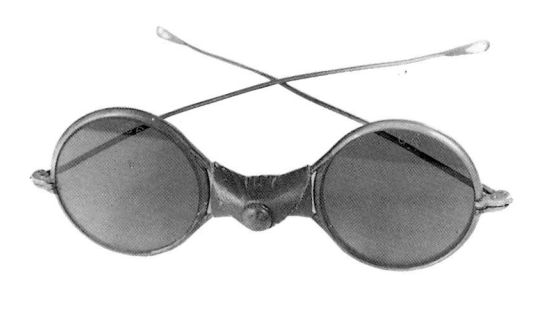

Figure 546. Heavy spectacles with leather nose guard.

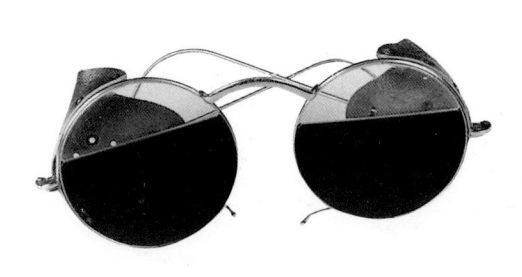

Figure 547. Clear lenses above; dark below.

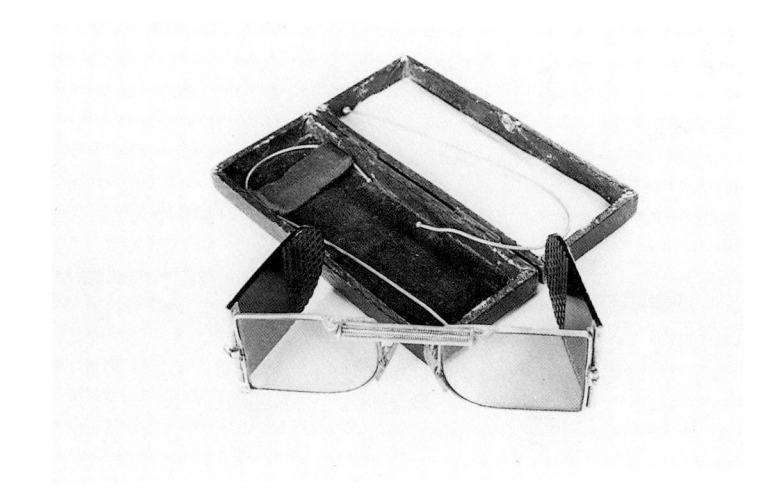

Figure 548. Bar-spring, detachable wire temples with side guards as temples.

The nonshatterable lenses are also known under names such as splinter-proof, shatterproof, safety glass, Triplex, Salvoc, Splinternil, and Motex.[1] These lenses are particularly robust to withstand the rigors of work-related accidents (Figure 544).

The process of laminating lenses to make them shatterproof began in 1912 (Figure 545), but the laminating materials usually discolor after several years. Additionally, these lenses are thicker and heavier than ordinary lenses. Around 1930, lamination with cellulose acetate began and was an improvement.[2]

A variety of protective eyewear, illustrative of the types needed, made and used is presented in Figures 546–557.

Truly useful lenses that are additionally protective are now made of case-hardened glass, polymethyl esthers, or polycarbonate plastic (Figures 558 & 559).

By U.S. law, all spectacles dispensed in the United States today must be made of safety glass—to the extent that each lens must pass the "ball drop" test. A $5/8$-inch, 8.6 ounce metal ball must be dropped from 50 inches onto the lens without breaking it.

PROTECTIVE SPECTACLES

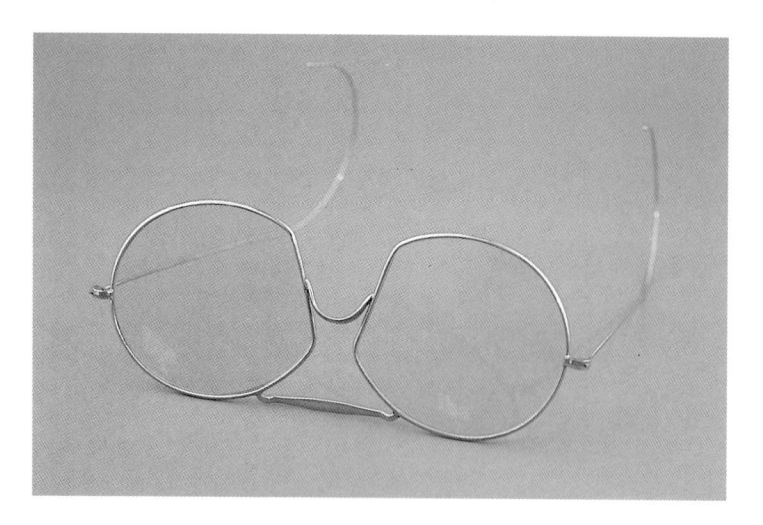

Figure 549. Lightweight protective spectacles.

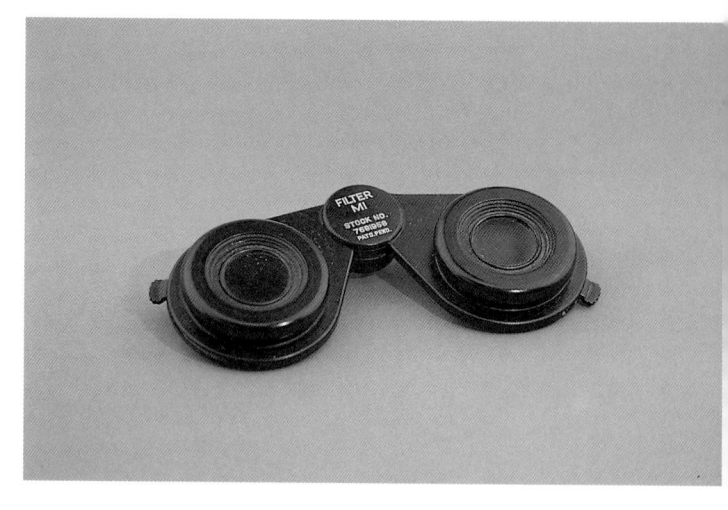

Figure 550. WW II U.S. Navy Polaroid rotating lenses.

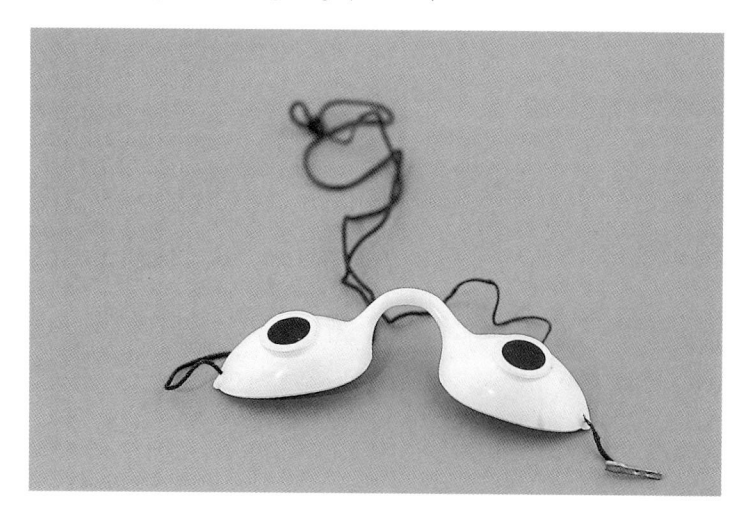

Figure 551. Woman's lid protection from sunburn.

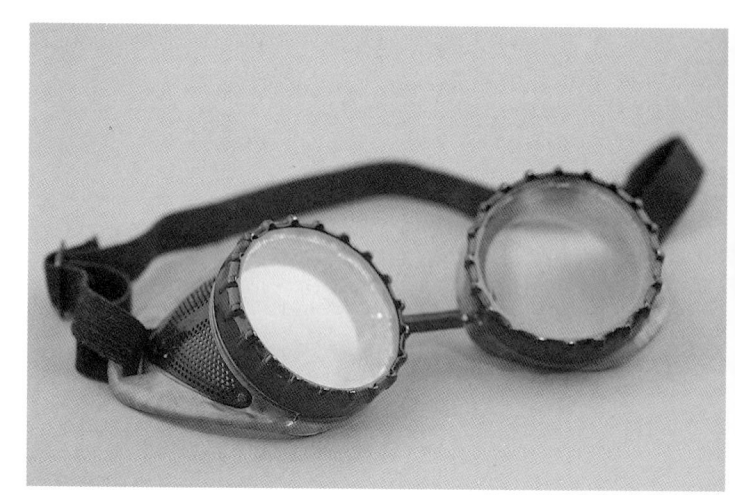

Figure 552. Grinder's glasses.

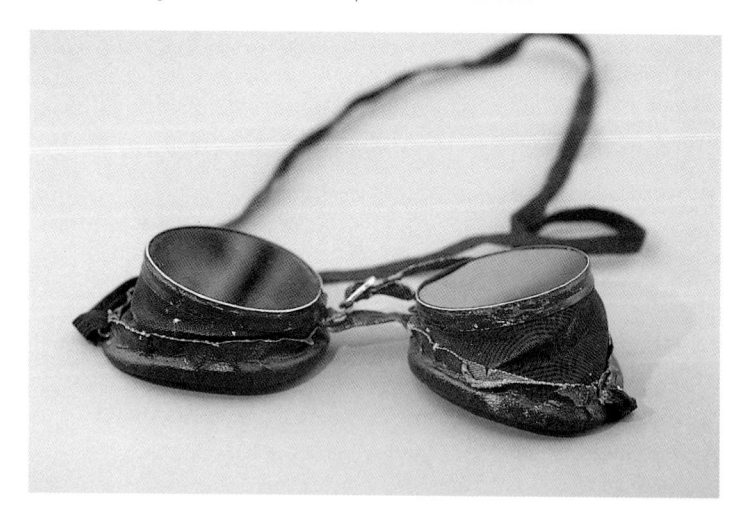

Figure 553. Welder's goggles.

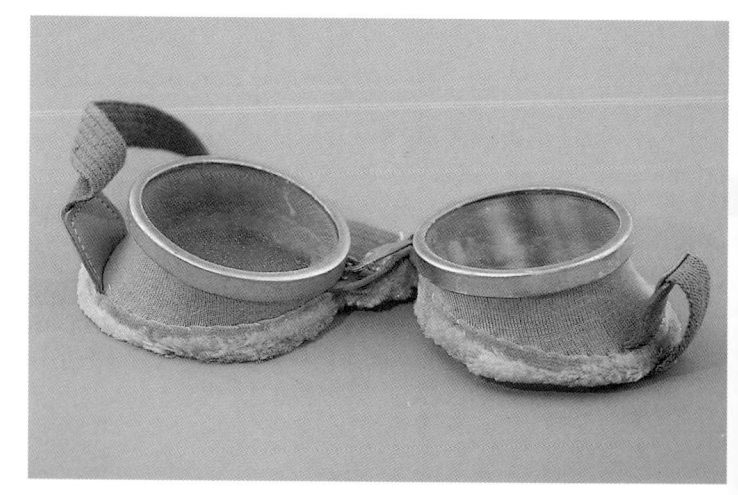

Figure 554. Glare and projectile protection.

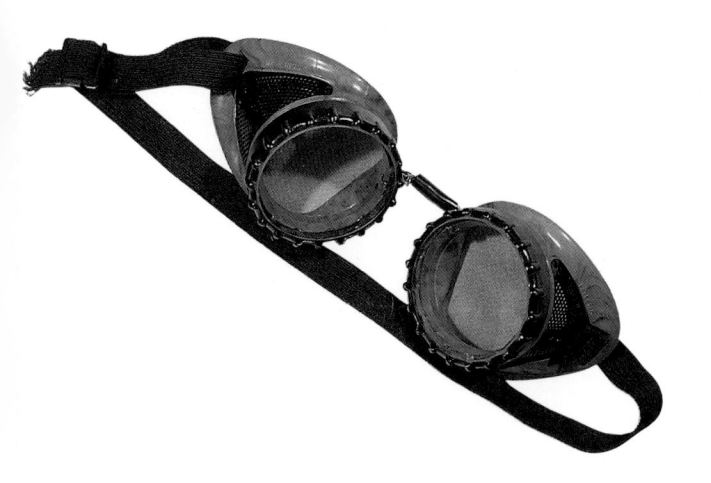

Figure 555. Typical shop protection.

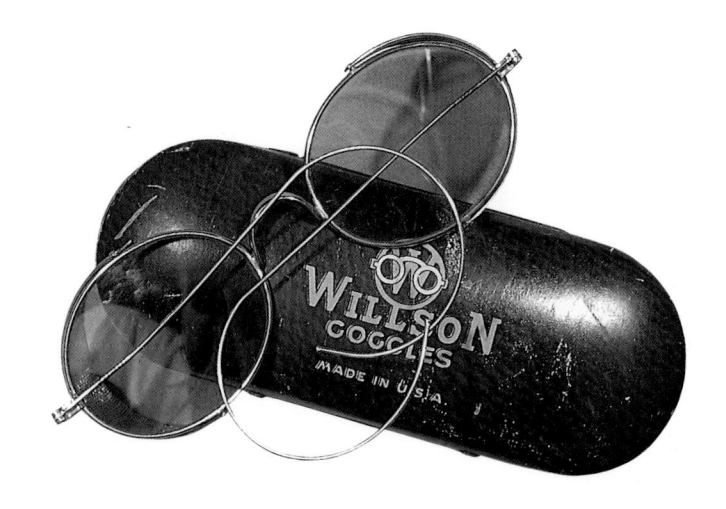

Figure 556. The famous Willson brand.

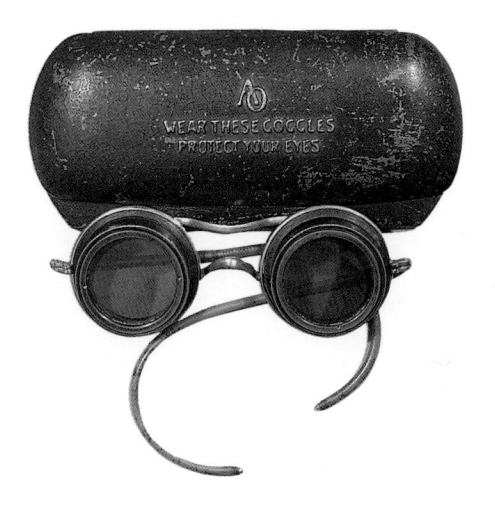

Figure 557. American Optical type of goggles circa 1930.

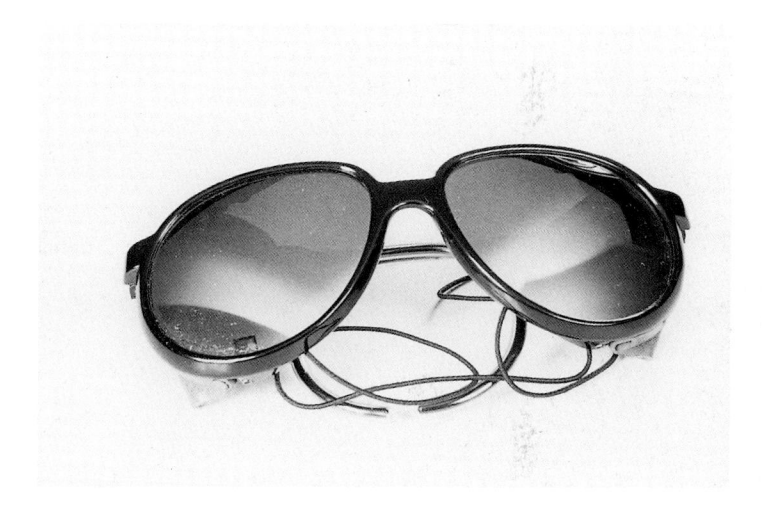

Figures 558–559. Modern protective glasses.

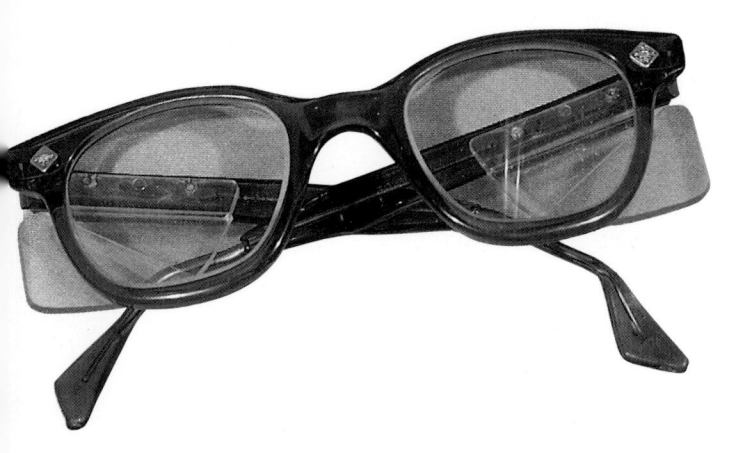

Figure 559.

PROTECTIVE SPECTACLES 293

Conclusion

As technology and industry have progressed through the centuries, so has the need for protective eyewear. Certainly, as further developments evolve in these fields, we will see still more changes in this optical apparatus.

Notes

1. Theo Obrig, *Modern Ophthalmic Lenses* (New York: The Chilton Co., 1935).
2. Duke-Elder. *System of Ophthalmology,* Vols. XIV & V (St. Louis: C.V. Mosby & Co., 1965).

Other Sources Consulted for Chapter 25

1. D. C. Davidson, *Spectacles, Lorgnettes and Monocles* (United Kingdom: Shire Publications, 1989).
2. R. J. S. MacGregor, *Collecting Ophthalmic Antiques* (United Kingdom: Ophthalmic Antiques International Collectors Club, 1992).

26

Shooting Glasses

Vision aids intended to increase human acuity (visual and psychological) are known from the crystal glasses of the early Chinese to the infrared night vision telescopes of the modern military forces. Glasses for hunters and sharpshooters fit somewhere in this history.

Amber-colored glasses allow greater penetration of vision in foggy or misty conditions. For many years, automobile companies have produced bright amber headlights to more efficiently penetrate fog and aid the driver. As amber (yellow-orange) is near the short-wavelength end of the spectrum, it is logical to assume that object brightness would increase and the dispersion of the edge discrimination of the object would be less than if a long-wavelength colored lens were used. Hunters and sharpshooters down through the ages have noticed this and have used amber colored lenses in their glasses (Figure 560) Various shades of this color can be found, which may include personal preference, use for different conditions, or perhaps merely ease of manufacture. Light yellow-green color is also used in these spectacles, as well as some reds and blues (Figures 561 & 562). Precious little can be found in texts or articles on this subject of vision aids. Only the offerings in existing old catalogs give true verification.[1]

Although European and Eastern sportsmen used amber-colored lenses in their spectacles, these lenses were never as popular there as in the United States. Typical American shooting (or gunning) glasses (Figure 563) had coated steel frames, with oval, amber lenses—2.5 × 3.5 centimeters, with the center 1 centimeter clear and the periphery frosted. These were produced from about 1880 to 1910.

Varieties

Variations in the lenses include a frosted periphery white glass with an amber (sometimes red) center circle (Figure 564). Also, glasses with various shades of amber in the center clear circle are seen, as well as spectacles that have no frosting (Figure 565). The author has one pair with no lens color—only peripheral frosting and rectangular clear areas. The frosting is intended to keep the hunter's attention on the prey and away from distractions. Medium or light blue colored lenses are infrequently seen, as are light green or olive-blue lenses.

Early frames (circa 1880) had quadrangular lenses, hump (crank) bridges, and straight temples. Mostly, there are C-bridges with straight springy temples, but also wire temples to fit behind the ears are seen (Figure 565) The author has a pair with 2 ½-centimeter round lenses.

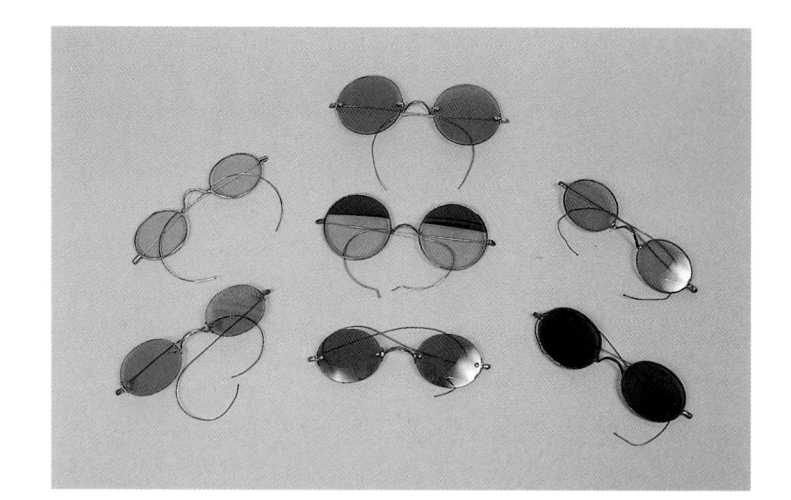

Figure 560. Amber glasses—various shades.

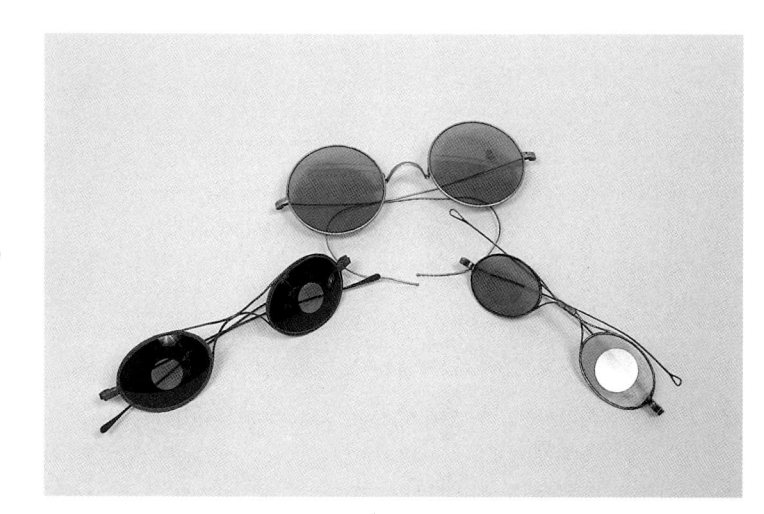

Figure 561. Blue lenses, including two shooting types.

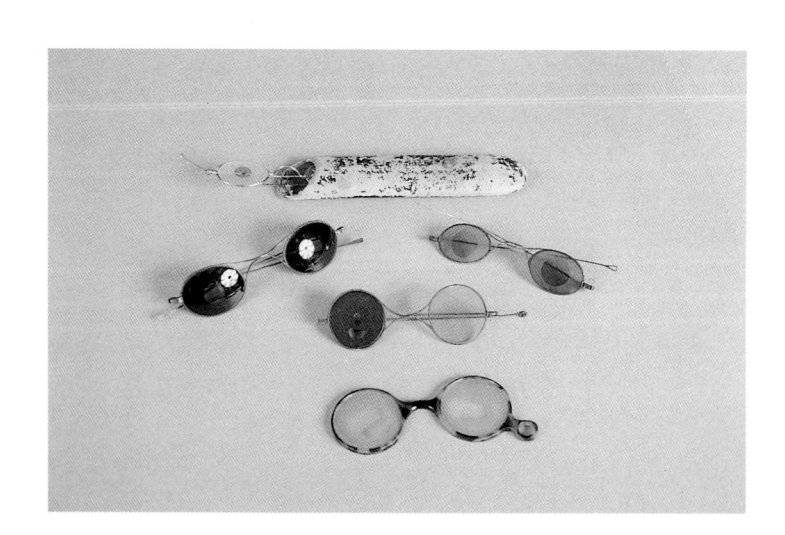

Figure 562. Additional amber and blue lenses.

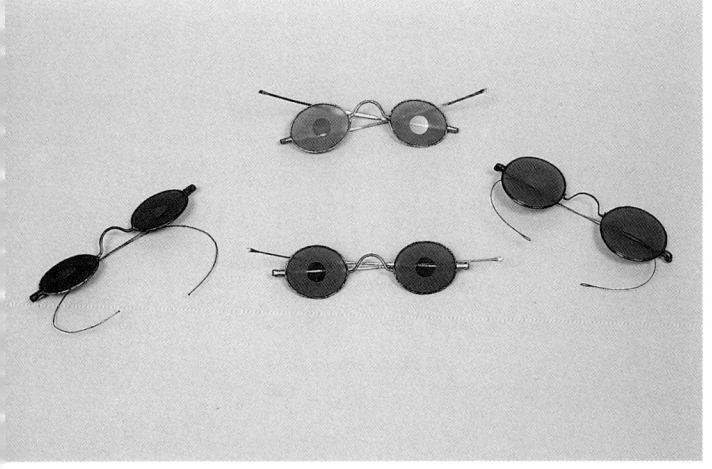

Figure 563. Typical U.S. shooting glasses.

Figure 564. Variations.

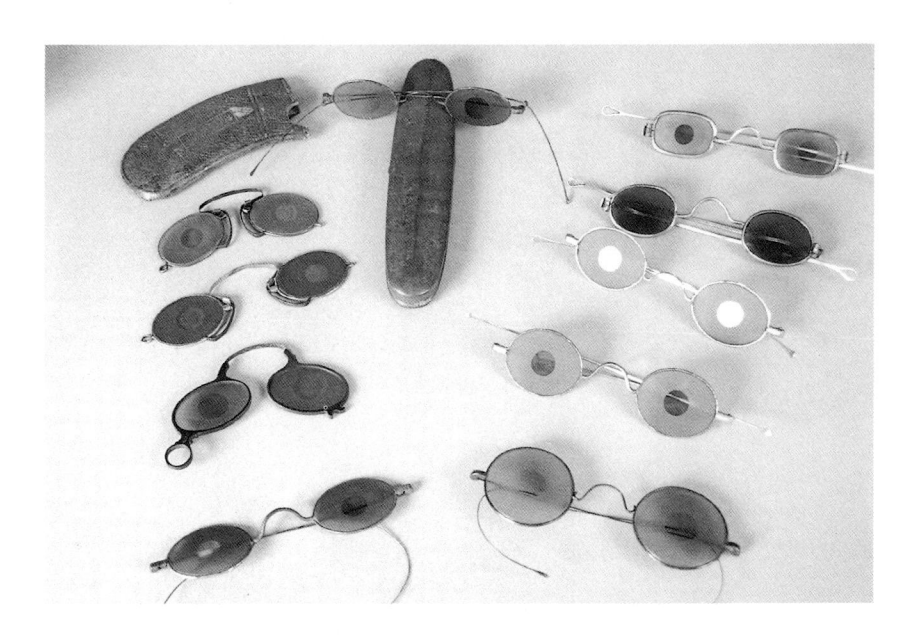

Figure 565. Crank and C-bridges, straight and wire temples. Some pince nez.

SHOOTING GLASSES **297**

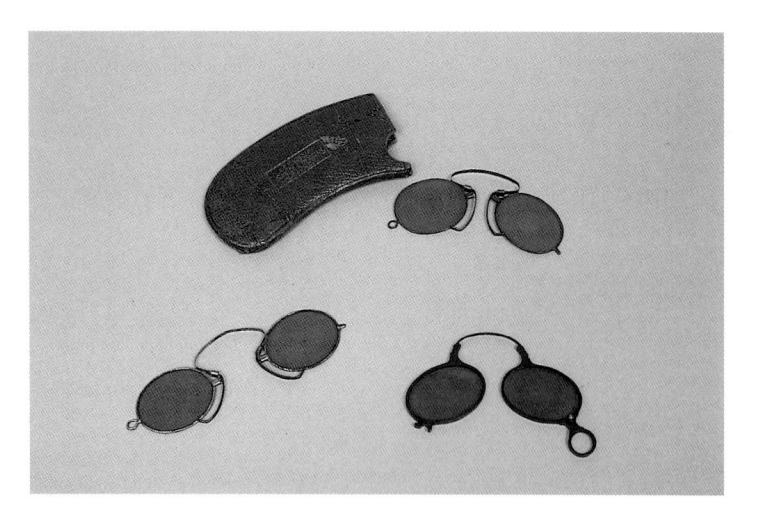

Figure 566. Pince-nez shooting glasses.

Pince-Nez

Surprisingly, there are a variety of pince-nez shooting glasses (Figure 566). These glasses started with simple hard rubber and spring-bridge types (circa 1890), and went through 1910–1915, when gold and plated spring-bridges predominated. When coil-spring (finger-piece) mechanisms started in the 1920s, even these were used on shooting glasses.

Other Types

The author has a pair of blued-steel, K-bridge shooting spectacles, with light blue lenses and black periphery to a one-centimeter aperture in the center (Figure 561, left)

Certain oddities exist in this area, such as a pair with a K-bridge, blued-steel frame and blue lenses, but with frosting, as well as a pair of amber round clip-ons (Figure 567). Often mistaken for use after retinal detachment surgery or for correction of crossed eyes is a pair of spectacles of blued steel, with straight temples and X-bridge (upper pair in Figure 568).

Figure 567. Amber round clip-ons (above).

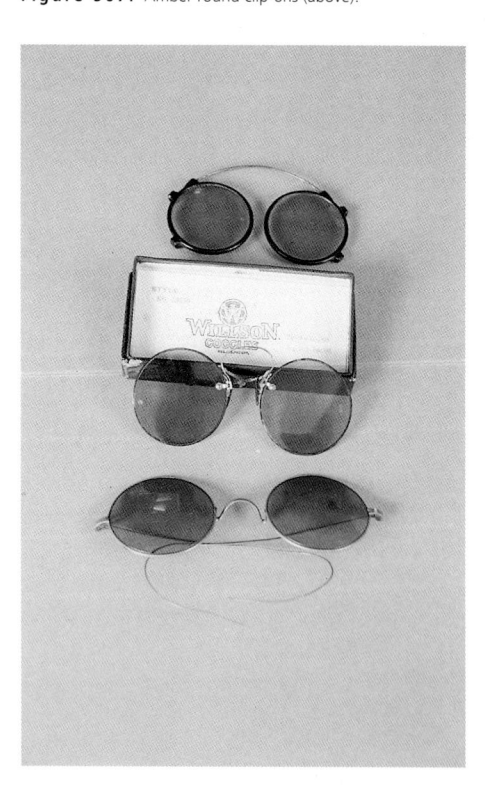

Figure 568. Target spectacles (above and below).

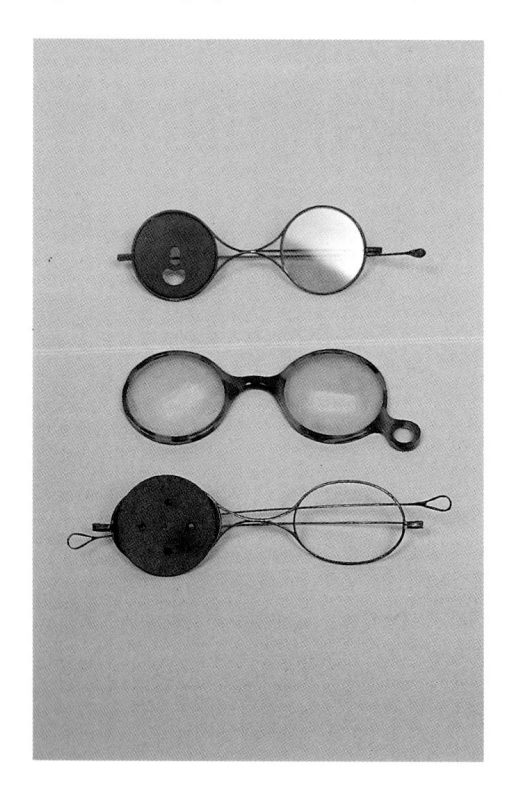

298   CHAPTER 26

Lenses are 2 ½ centimeters round, one being light blue and the other of opaque hard rubber with a vertical ovoid perforation centrally and a bean-shaped perforation below that. They are made for target shooting, apparently.

W. Poulet (Vol. I, pp. 240ff) shows several types of shooting glasses with various apertures, diaphragms, covering plates, and side-vision protection.[2] He pictures only one pair with tea-colored lenses. It is interesting that a vision aid used primarily for sport has been produced in so many varieties (Figure 569).

Notes

1. American Optical Company catalog, circa 1912, pp. 189, 190; Spencer Optical Company, Catalog #17, 1914, pp. 79, 86.
2. W. Poulet, *Atlas on the History of Spectacles,* Vol. I. Translated by Frederick Blodi. (Bad Godeberg, Germany: Wayenborgh, 1978), 240, 241, 242.

Other Sources Consulted for Chapter 26

1. J. Wm. Rosenthal, personal collection.

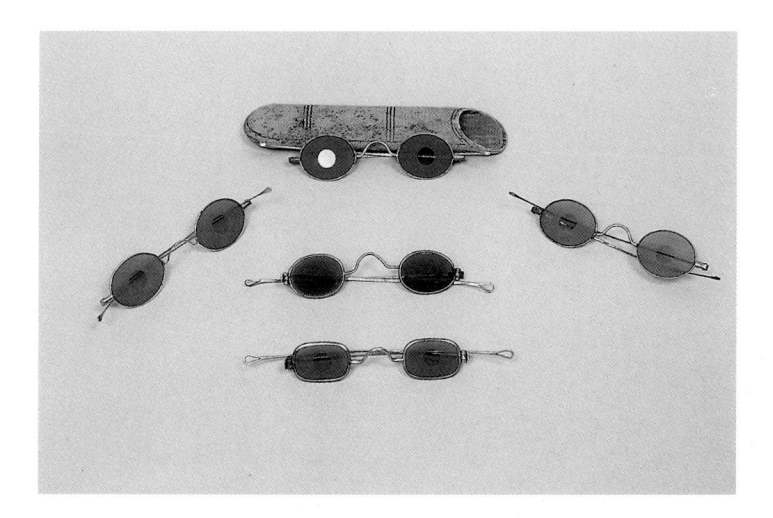

Figure 569. Varieties of shooting glasses.

27

Specialized Spectacles

Although other sections of this book discuss at length glasses that were conceived for particular purposes, some spectacles were made for such narrow usage that a mere short description will suffice for completeness and identification only. Even so, glasses will be found, as two pairs in the author's collection, that cannot be assigned to a specific purpose (Figure 570).

Prism Glasses

Most common amongst prism glasses are horizontally oriented prisms for patients with large extraocular muscle imbalances (Figure 571).[1] One specific type of horizontal prism is placed in a frame with a very small pupillary distance. This is designed for use by individuals who do very close and detailed work over a protracted period of time—watchmakers (Figure 572), for instance. Watchmakers also employ a jeweler's loup attached to their regular spectacles. Orthoscopic spectacles are another variety.

A horizontal prism attached to one spectacle lens is used for people with hemianopia to obtain greater side vision. A similar result is obtained by placing a small mirror nasally or temporally on the spectacle frame and at the correct reflective angle (Figure 571, bottom 3).

Vertical prisms used for correction of muscle imbalance are ordinarily so small that it is necessary only to decenter the prescription lens to obtain orthophoria. Strong bilateral, vertically placed prisms are used by invalids who are recumbent and need to read without having to continually depress the eye direction (Figure 573).

Adaptation Spectacles

Photographic developers or those who develop or read X-ray films need to maintain their dark adaptation even when they are outside the darkroom performing everyday tasks. Therefore, to avoid the 10 to 30 minutes needed for this adaptation, red glass filter goggles are available.

Others who may use this appliance are night drivers, aviators, and those who do fluoroscopy.

Industrial Radiation

Workers who blow glass or peer into vats of molten glass or metal have special goggles available to protect them from the offending wavelengths of light that come their way. Likewise, welders need to wear goggles or shields to keep the ultraviolet rays from producing what is known in the trade as flash burn—really a type of severe concentrated sunburn of the eyelids and cornea (Figure 574).

Oxygen-Administration Glasses

Spectacle frames have been designed to help administer

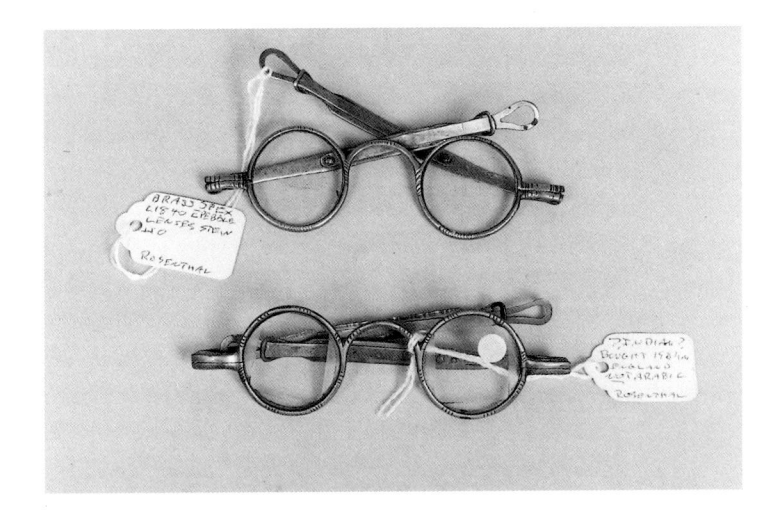

Figure 570. Spectacles with ill-defined purpose.

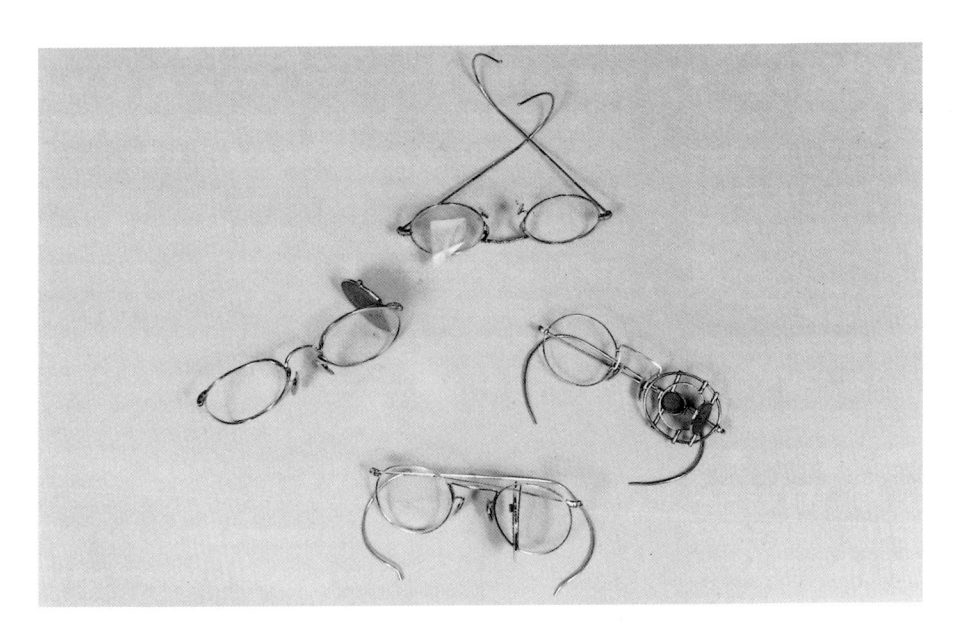

Figure 571. Mirror frames for use by hemianopic patients.

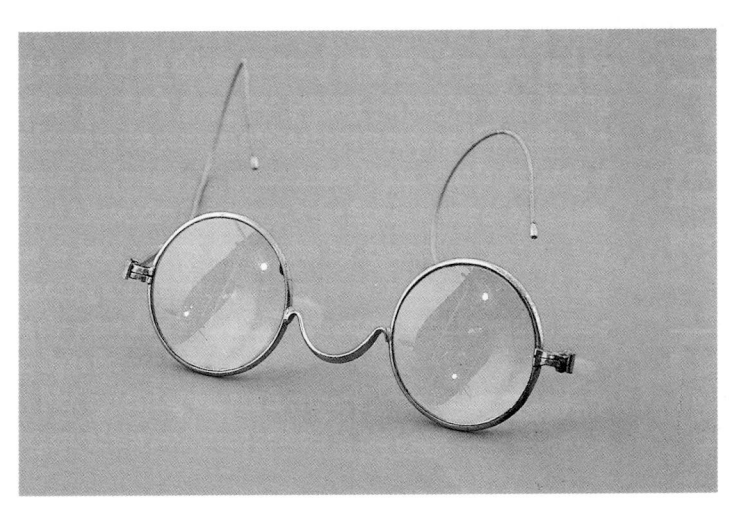

Figure 572. Watchmaker's glasses.

SPECIALIZED SPECTACLES

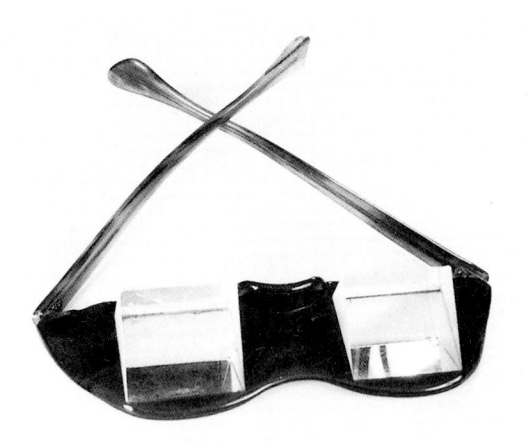

Figure 573. Recumbent patient prism spectacles.

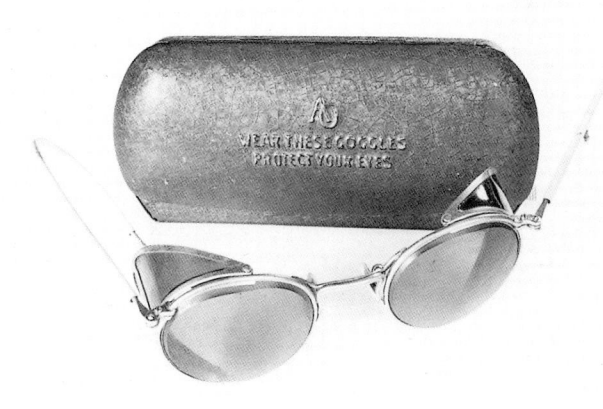

Figure 574. Welder's goggles.

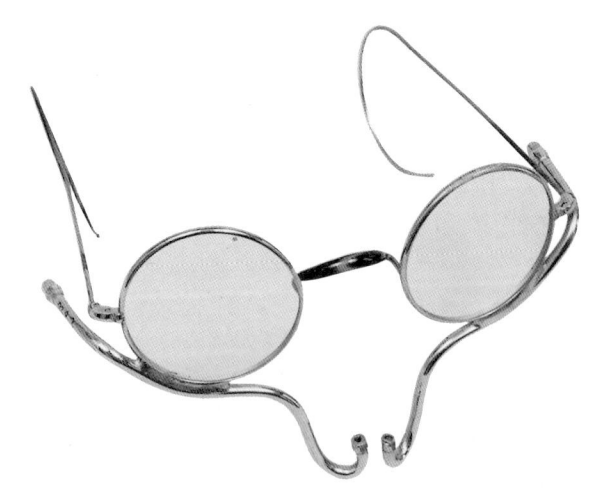

Figure 575. Oxygen-administration spectacles.

oxygen (mostly) to patients (Figure 575). These frames are made of a base metal and have a small tube attached with openings directed to the nostrils, and the temporal ends are fitted for oxygen tube application. No doubt they were used before the invention of disposable nasal tubes.

Vocational Lenses

We have the single lens for distance and near, in several sizes. Each refractionist has his or her favorite shaped bifocal for designated jobs. The same may be said of trifocals. It is not necessary at this point to delve into the bifocal-trifocal history or note the design with multiple lenses (see Chapter 21). Invisible trifocals (or continuous vision lenses) serve from distance to near.

Individuals who need a middle distance focus at a high level (librarians, mechanics, electricians, etc.) can get a regular bifocal and a segment placed at the top of the lens. This is sometimes called a "baseball."

Desk and computer workers need a lens that is mostly bifocal, with only the top 10 percent available for distance viewing. Just the opposite applies for golfers, who need to see the ball during a shot without the bifocal's interfering.

Trifocals work well for the intermediate needs of the older computer operator or the organ or piano artist, as well as other musicians. Other artists in painting and sculpture have similar needs, as does the drafter. Larger trifocals, such as the executive type, do well for the dentist and surgeon.

Half glasses (lower half) for ametropic but presbyopic orators, desk workers, etc., have been used for years. Fairly recently, however, reverse half glasses (myopic above and no glass below) have proven useful for myopic presbyopes.

Aniseikonic lenses have been made by American Optical and are mentioned here for completeness' sake.

Reversible Glasses

In the second decade of the twentieth century, a convenient invention was brought to light. Spectacle frames with a C-bridge that was fixed exteriorly but hinged on the nasal side allowed the frame to be used right side up, or the opposite. Lenses were round.

Add to this a temple, solid near the front and cable to the rear, with the cable end rotating on its long axis. The lenses are usually reading prescription.

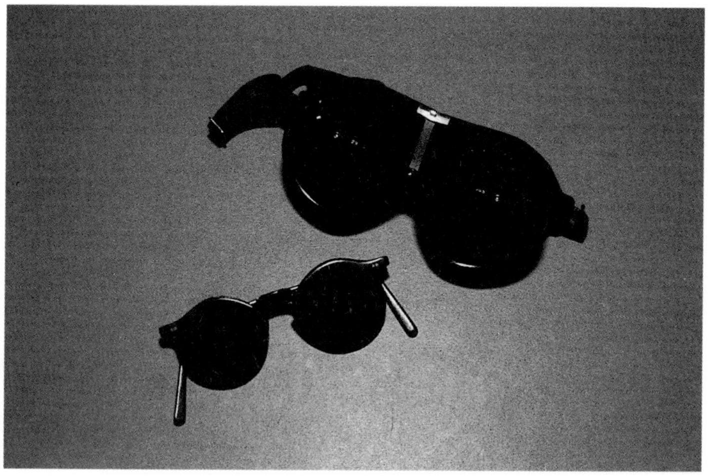

Figure 576. Pinhole spectacles for patient's with retinal detachment.

This arrangement allowed people with equal presbyopia (most individuals) the convenience of laying their glasses down without worrying about how they retrieved them, as gravity automatically oriented the frames to the face, with either hand or eye being used.

Some individuals, unfortunately, have one eye with very poor vision. Again, when they retrieve these glasses, any way that the glasses are placed on the face allows good vision.

Pinhole Glasses

Glasses with bilateral opaque lenses of bilateral pinholes were designed in the 1940s for patients who had undergone recent retinal detachment surgery (Figure 576). They were made of black plastic and usually had side shields. Some were quite large to accommodate an eye bandage. Some had a rotary disc with a choice of various size pinholes. A modern spectacle with multiple pinholes was a recent fad, as it was advertised as the universal lens and as having other advantages.

Occlusion Glasses

To facilitate the development of vision in a crossed eye of a child, occlusion of the uncrossed (better) eye is sometimes used. An occlusive (opaque) lens is placed before the better eye and a side occluder added to discourage peeping. This is used during the orthoptic training period and can be changed from one eye to the other.

Diplopia

In cases not correctable by surgery or prisms, diplopia is often intolerable to the patient. Obvious relief is found in occlusion of one eye. This is easily accomplished by many types of occluders—clip-on, clamp-on to the back of the lens, and even adhesive tape on the lens.

Etiology of this symptom can be from diabetes mellitus, multiple sclerosis, hypertension, brain tumor or hemorrhage, cranial nerve disease or trauma, syphilis, or orbital trauma.

Because many patients desire to change from one eye to the other, a glasses frame has been designed with an occluder lens hinged at the bridge so that it can swing over either eye.

Crutch Glasses

Wires attached to the rear of a glass frame may be anchored at one or both ends, either above or below. Those attached above are contoured to the upper lid and are positioned to accept the skin of the upper lid. Thus, the lid can be supported and opened in those patients who have ptosis.

For entropion, where surgery is contraindicated, or even as a temporary measure where the patient's skin is sensitive to adhesive tape, the entropion crutch frame is another modality to be considered. These wires, attached to the lower nose pads and arching parallel to the lower frame, will engage the lower lid and prevent it from turning in. Thus, the lashes do not rub on the cornea or conjunctiva.

Frames for Facial Disfigurement

Unfortunate patients with craniofacial dysostosis or tumors of the naso-frontal area or the like need to have glasses frames with a large or unusually shaped bridge to be comfortable. These may be seen in modern frames. Even at the time that wig glasses in tortoiseshell were used (circa 1850), large bridges to fit cases of rhinophyma were designed.

Cases of nasal deformity from nasal fracture, facial carcinoma, and similar conditions can have special glasses frames fitted. Theses glasses are made with plastic, flesh-colored shells fitted to shield, cover, or fill in the deformity. This is done with surgical consultation. Some patients are missing the pinna from one or both ears. To allow the spectacle fronts to stay in place, elastic can be used instead of the temple pieces. This, of course, reaches around the head. The short temple pieces in tortoiseshell-fashioned wig glasses of the seventeenth and eighteenth centuries functioned similarly but were designed for a different reason. Modern frames used by women in the beauty parlor while under the hair dryer also have abbreviated temples that press in the temporal fossa and keep the glasses in position. The temples therefore do not heat up and burn the wearer.

For persons with facial features that cannot be adequately fitted by ordinary frames, one may find (a) frames with one eye wire higher than the other, (b) a bridge designed to thrust the frame away from the eyes, (c) a frame designed to bring the lenses closer to the eyes, and (d) frames made to be supported by the cheeks or forehead if the nose is too sensitive.

Other Special Glasses

Before the availability of artificial tears and ointments to the practitioner's armamentarium, it was occasionally necessary to prescribe clear or moist chambers for the protection of those with dry eye due to keratitis sicca or Soëgren's syndrome. Use of this protection also excluded dust and drafts. These moisture-including membranes were often attached to spectacle frames for convenience and to obviate the use of facial adhesives. They are infrequently found today.

Another unusual type of glasses is sometimes found. Certain clubs or fraternal organizations had (or have) initiation ceremonies wherein the newcomer is blindfolded with a solid

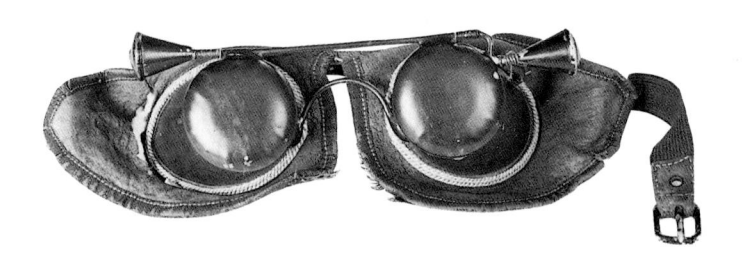

Figure 577. Fraternal induction goggles.

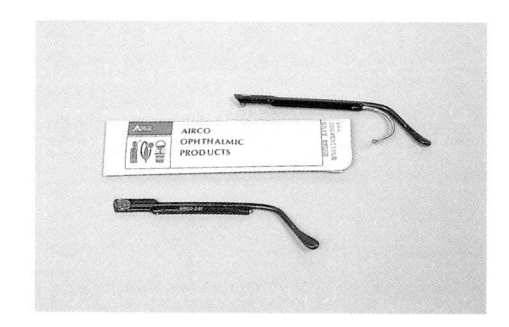

Figure 578. Combination spatula and cable temples.

metal goggle. Apparently, the initiate is afforded the opportunity to peek occasionally, as each eye has a trapdoor arrangement to facilitate vision by rotating a side knob (Figure 577).

For persons who like spatula temples but occasionally need cable temples, a combination is available (Figure 578).

In the late 1800s some individuals believed that spectacles could gather electrical (static?) impulses and to insure that they were transmitted to their body, the inside of the spatula-shaped steel temples were fitted with a 1- to 2-millimeter round contact of a soft metal. They thusly felt invigorated.

Conclusion

Numerous varieties of special spectacles have been produced to aid in extenuating circumstances. It is fortunate for those in need to have these ingenious inventions available to them (Figure 579).

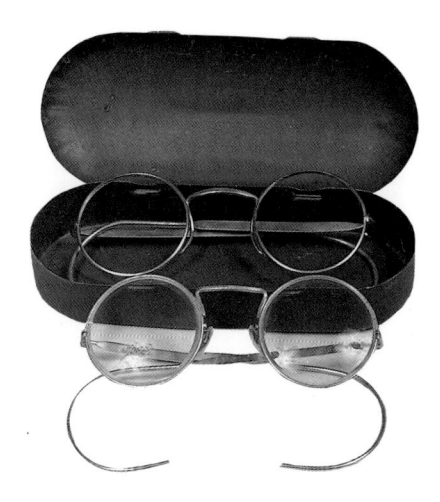

Figure 579. Gas mask glasses, British circa 1940.

Notes
1. *Rare Visual Aids*. The Kono Manufacturing Company, Woodside, N.Y., 1952.

Other Sources Consulted for Chapter 27
1. S. Duke-Elder, *System of Ophthalmology*, Vol. V, p. 703. (London: Henry Kimpton, 1965).

28

Makeup Spectacles

Of all the "interesting" customs of the human race, makeup application has certainly endured through time. Along legions of sometimes mystical and sophisticated modalities, (mostly) women have continued to enhance their given facial being with cosmetics.

A portion of these individuals, particularly presbyopes, have difficulty focusing their eyes closely on their physiognomy, so that vision aids are brought into play. Magnifying mirrors, although helpful, do not always supply sufficient detail for the job at hand. Additional magnification and focusing can be supplied by spectacles that work well when most of the facial cosmetics are applied but become an obstruction where eye makeup is concerned.

Voila! The invention of makeup or cosmetic spectacle frames came into existence. These frames, made originally by (or for) that great optic concern, Revlon, have been copied several times. Essentially, they are frames that allow individually hinged lenses to be raised or lowered so that vision is afforded by one eye while the other eye is "made up." The eyebrow, as well as lids and lashes, can be exposed to plucking, embellishment, eye shadow, liner, mascara, etc. Fortunes have been made thusly, and not exclusively by cosmetic corporations.

Some of these frames are made of metal (Figure 580) and others of plastic (Figures 581 & 582). Some are constructed so that the lenses can be raised above the field of action, where others may be lowered. Lenses moving from side to side have apparently been avoided because of positioning problems of the hand applying the makeup. As not much variation has evolved in this type of spectacle, we must assume that the present types available have been sufficient.

And so we see another example where spectacles bring much delight and satisfaction to those on both sides of the lenses.

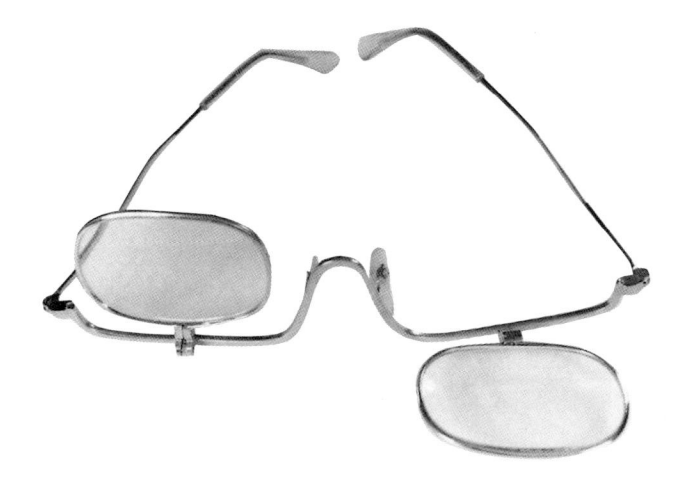

Figure 580. Metal makeup spectacles.

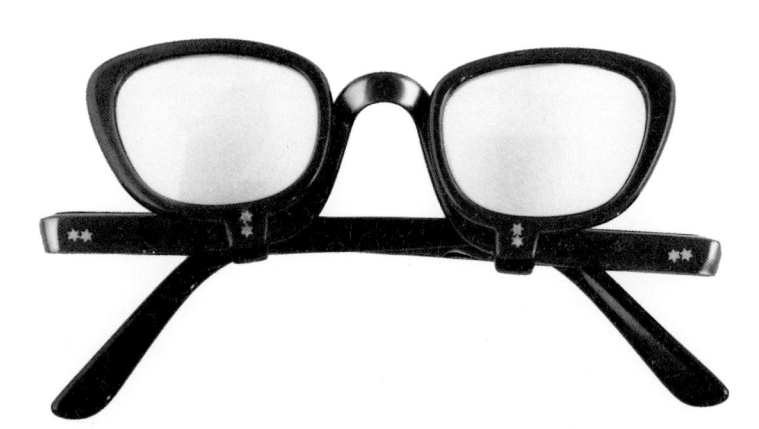

Figure 581. Plastic makeup spectacles.

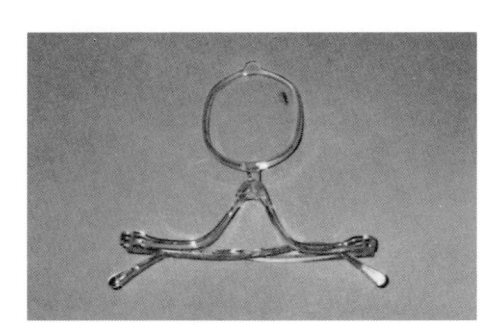

Figure 582. Plastic monocular variety.

MAKEUP SPECTACLES

29

Trial Lenses and Frames

In the eighteenth century, the patient individually chose his or her own spectacles, usually offered by an itinerant peddler. Such spectacles were of inferior quality in frame and lens grinding, having been turned out by the dozens per day in sweat shops by ignorant and untrained workers. It is not astounding, then, that most ophthalmologists of 150 years ago believed that spectacles weakened the eyes and advised against their use.

The trial method of glass fitting originated about 1690. At that time, lenses were placed in leather belts to be held before the eye. The lenses chosen thusly were removed from the belt and placed in rims for the patient. Later, lenses were put into wooden or metal holders for patient viewing. To this day, prism bars are handy in office use.

The charlatan William Rowley (1743–1806) was the first to recommend spectacle use. However, it took the authority of Donders (1864) and George Fronmuller (1843) to change the attitude of rank-and-file ophthalmologists so that they would espouse the use of these optical aids.[1] Until that time, there was no ophthalmological refractionist. Fronmuller pointed out that prescribing glasses on the basis of age was unscientific. Each patient, he said, deserved a history, examination for eye disease, and then an examination with trial frames and lenses for the best visual result.

The Optometer

William Porterfield (1683–1760) invented the optometer (Figure 583),[2] which was useful for measuring sight, but it was not until about 1850 that its use became widespread in the United States and England and on the Continent.

Well-constructed models in wood, brass, hard rubber, etc. were found in ophthalmologists' offices. However, optical companies sent cheaply constructed models directly to patients through the mail to encourage them to measure their own sight at home (Figures 584–587). Measurements thusly obtained were returned to these companies, and glasses were sent via mail to the patients. One could imagine that results were usually not ideal.

Trial Lens Sets

The use of trial sets and frames began in Germany in 1843. Sets of lenses were encased in horn or tortoiseshell holders (Figures 588 & 589). Since that time, many styles have been designed and used (Figure 590). Various sets of trial lenses and frames have been available—from the 40 pairs of sphericals and 24 pairs of cylinders in the 1924 American Optical Company catalog to the 12 pairs available in a retinoscopy set (Figure 591) designed and boxed for traveling use.[3] Of course, cases for these sets were tailor-made (manufactured) to each type of set

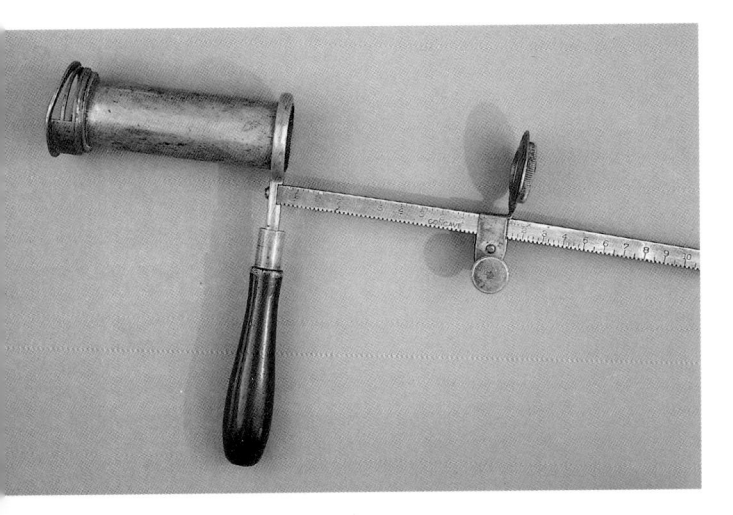

Figure 583. Brass optometer circa 1800, courtesy American Academy of Ophthalmology Museum.

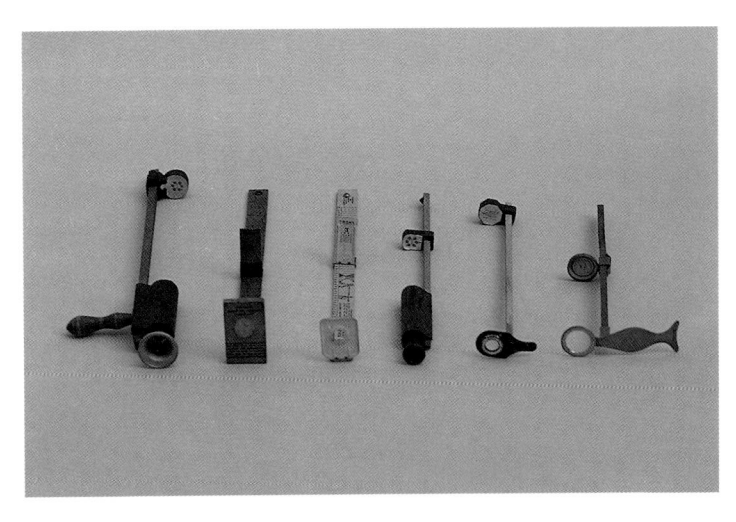

Figure 584. Group of wood-based optometers, courtesy W.H. Marshall, M.D.

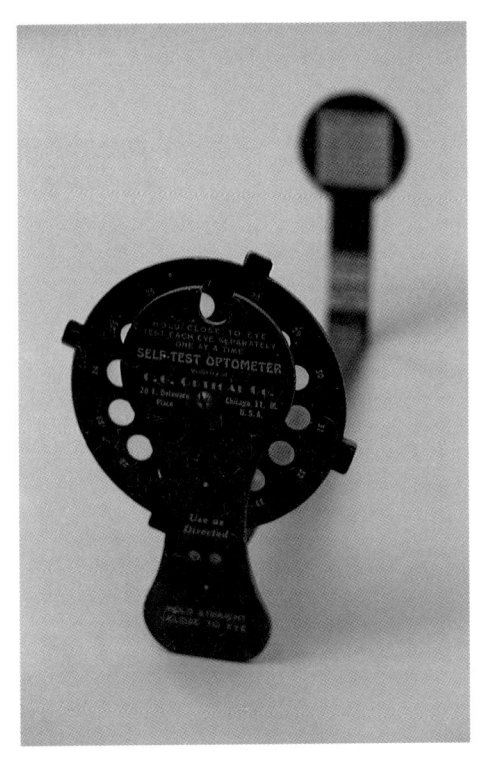

Figure 585. Self-test optometer, courtesy W.H. Marshall, M.D.

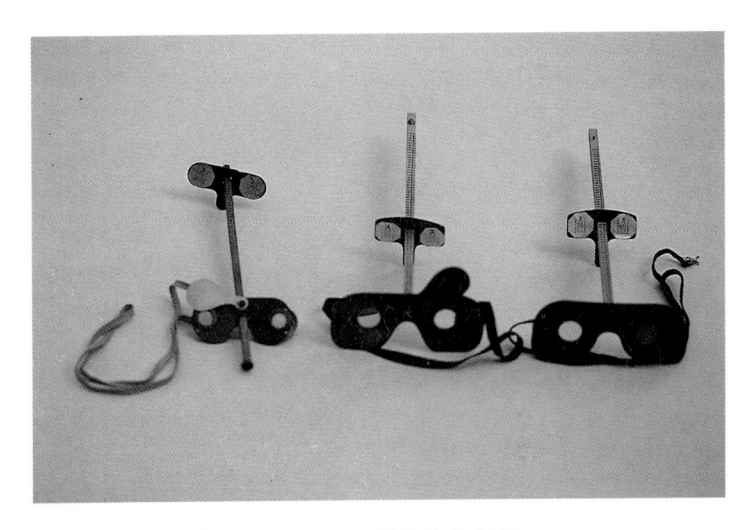

Figure 586. Binocular optometers, courtesy W.H. Marshall, M.D.

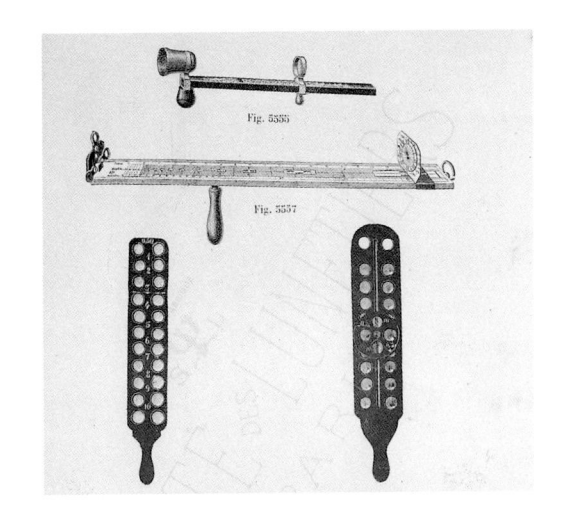

Figure 587. Figures 5555 and 5557 (above) are optometers; Figures 5567 and 5568 (below) are lens bars.

TRIAL LENSES AND FRAMES

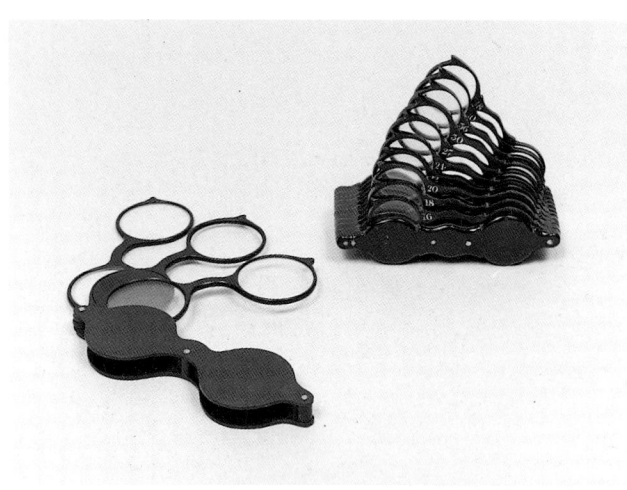

Figure 588. Cased trial lenses.

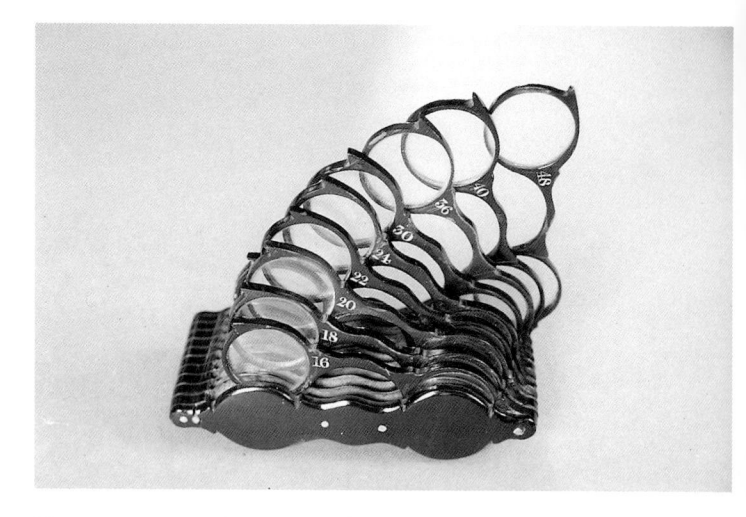

Figure 589. Tortoiseshell set of trial spectacles.

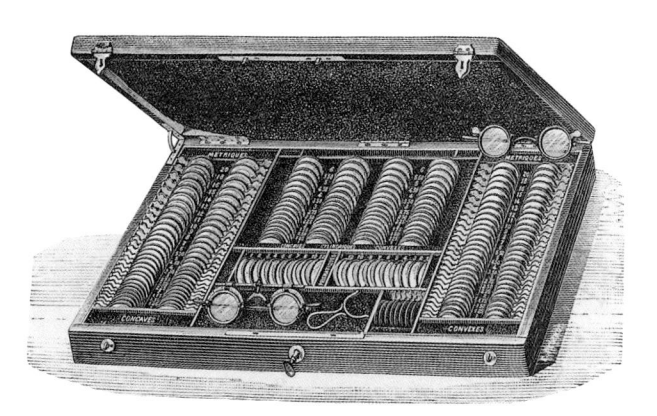

Figure 590. Trial lens set circa 1920.

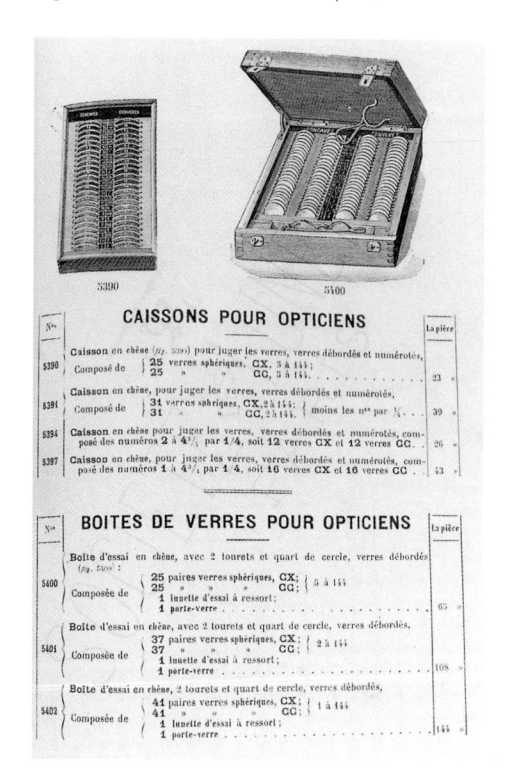

Figure 591. Retinoscopy lens set.

310   CHAPTER 29

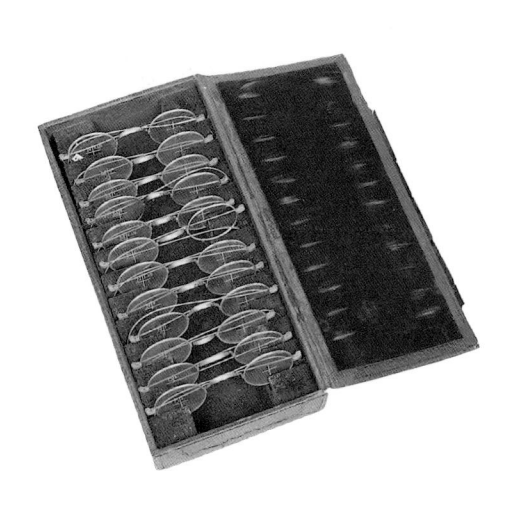

Figure 592. Set of C-bridge fitting spectacles.

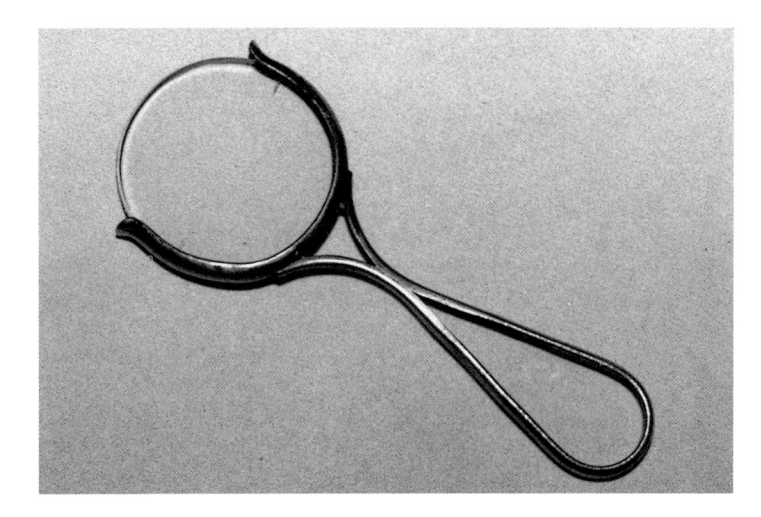

Figure 593. Rimless trial lens in holder.

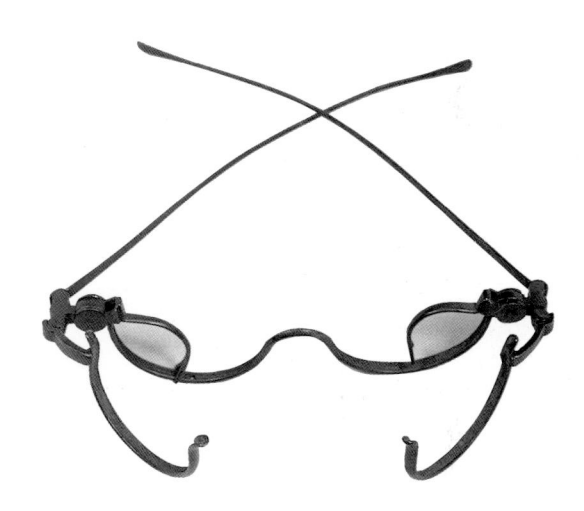

Figure 594. Steel trial frames for rimless lenses. English, circa 1885.

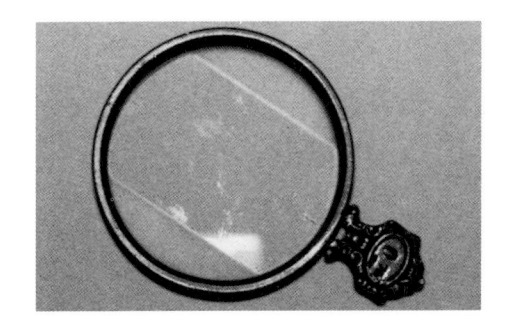

Figure 595. Trial lens from set circa 1890.

for stationary office use and transportable models. Cases for the latter were made to close and sported a handle. The trays that held the lenses, in both types of cases, were of wood (oak or mahogany) or were covered with velvet. A case could be used flat or ordered with a support in the back to raise it at an angle. Some cases were integral with an entire piece of furniture, with convenient drawers and a pullout writing surface. These could be obtained in wood or metal. Auxiliary lenses were also housed in the case, such as prisms, red glass, Maddox rod, and frosted.

Fitting cases for eyeglasses (pince-nez—see Chapter 20) and spectacles (C-bridge) containing a dozen assorted sizes of bridge, lens, temple, and pupillary distance were also available (Figure 592). The notable Fits-U style is a prime example.

Early trial lens sets afforded the glass lenses little protection. The lenses were rimless and were easily broken if dropped (Figures 593 & 594). Later sets encased the glass lenses in a metal frame of various designs, some specifically to fit the trial frame that was purchased with the lens set (Figure 595). Brass

TRIAL LENSES AND FRAMES 311

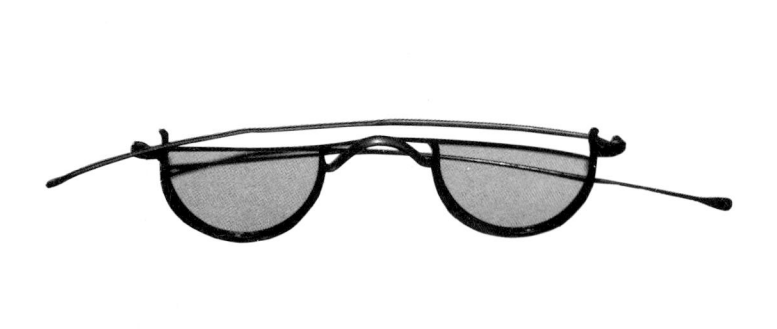

Figure 596. Simple trial frame holds one lens over each eye.

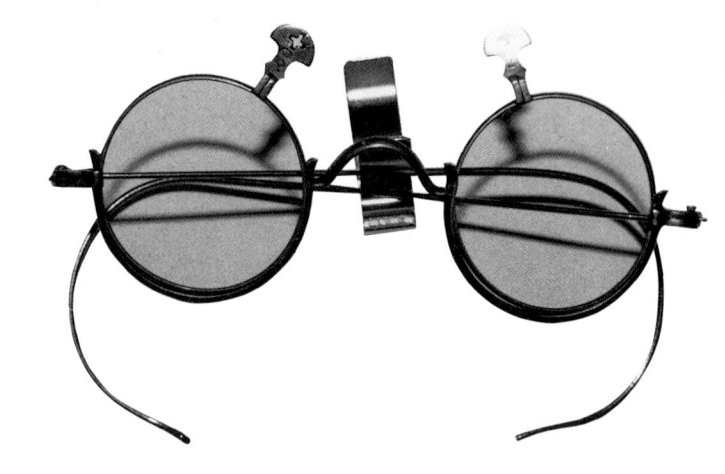

Figure 597. Simple trial frame with cable temples.

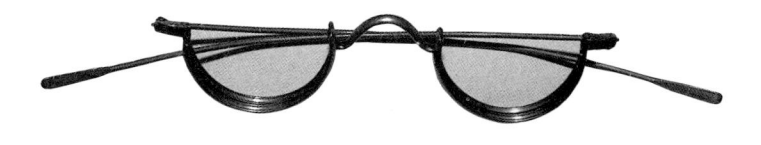

Figure 598. Double trial frame holder.

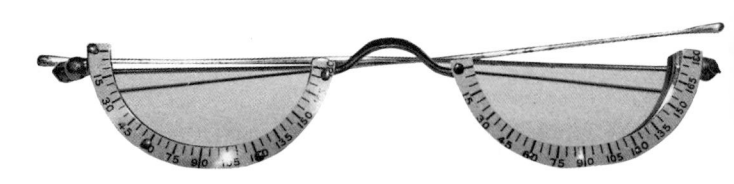

Figure 599. Double trial frame with astigmatism angle markers.

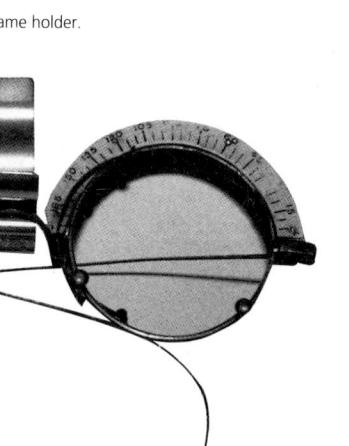

Figure 600. Double trial frame with astigmatism markings above.

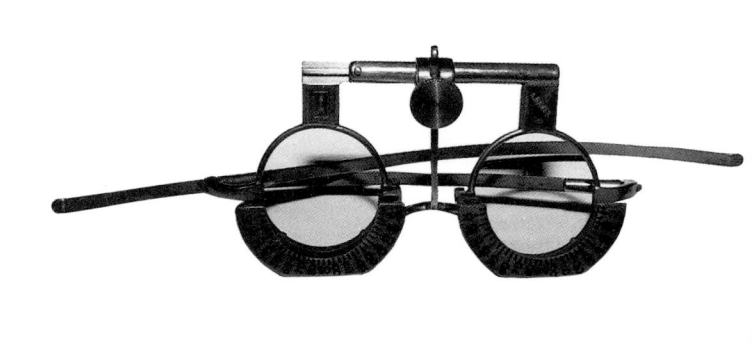

Figure 601. Adjustable trial frame.

312 CHAPTER 29

rims denoted the minus lenses, and white (silver-colored, nickel, or chromium-plated) rims indicated the plus series. Tabs attached to the rims made it easier to grasp each lens with a plus or minus perforation afforded to indicate the lens series. A more sophisticated set also had the lens power stamped on the tab.

Currently, collectors find trial sets available for purchase as a result of use of the more popular phoropter. Such sets are often incomplete because of loss of lenses, breakage, and use of the plus series for magnifying glasses. The latter may be offered by antique dealers trying to utilize parts of an otherwise unmarketable item.

Trial-Frame Design

Originally trial frames were simply made to hold one trial lens in front of each eye (Figures 596 & 597). Temples were straight metal with a C-bridge and had eye wires, U-shaped, with a central trough to accommodate the trial lens. Later, additional lenses could be accommodated with spring clips or troughs in front of or behind the trial frame body (Figures 598, 599, & 600). As the frames became more sophisticated, these lens holders could be rotated individually with a screw mechanism for each eye. Astigmatism angles could thusly be adjusted.

The bridge itself became a mechanism so that it could be raised or lowered and adjusted front and rear (Figure 601) to accommodate individual facial features.

Pupillary distance accuracy was obtained by a screw mechanism above the brow that "hung" the whole eye-wire mechanism and lenses from above (Figures 602 & 603).

A screw adjustment on each temple piece near the hinge could alter the lens's pantoscopic angle. Telescoping or extending the temples could accommodate larger or smaller size individuals (Figure 604). Some temples had cable temples, others spatulas that bent behind the ears.

Measurements

The metal parts of many frames were embossed with increments of measure, such as the pupillary distance, astigmatism angle, and temple length. Later, white plastic with up to ⅛-inch distances and five-degree angles were placed on the metal frame skeletons so that they could be more easily seen in a darkened room.

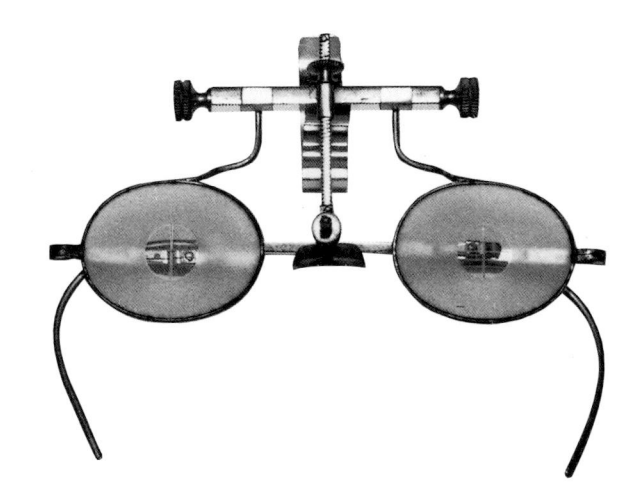

Figure 602. Adjustable trial frame circa 1880 for P.D. measurement..

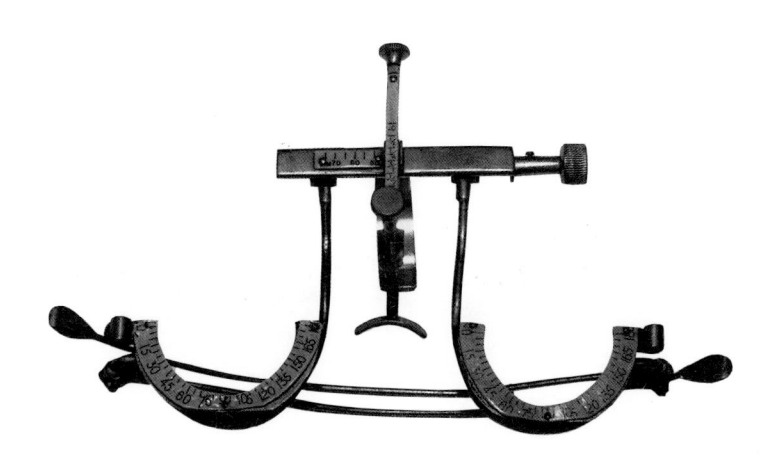

Figure 603. Trial frame, adjustable pupillary distance, bridge, straight temple.

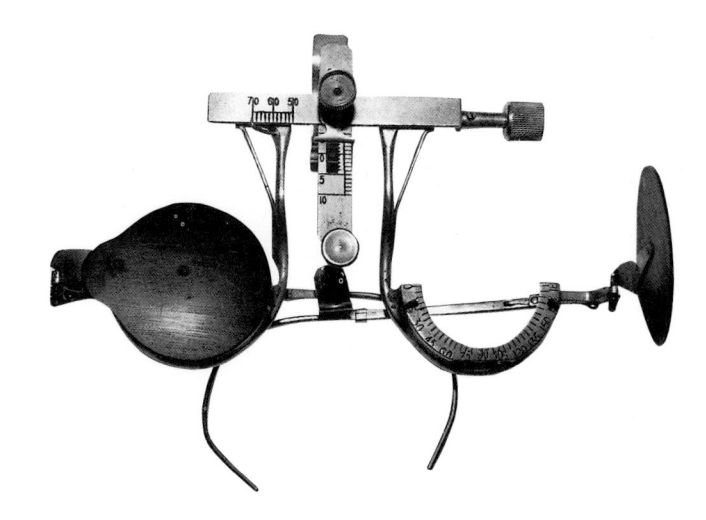

Figure 604. Trial frame, adjustable, with eye covers, cable temples.

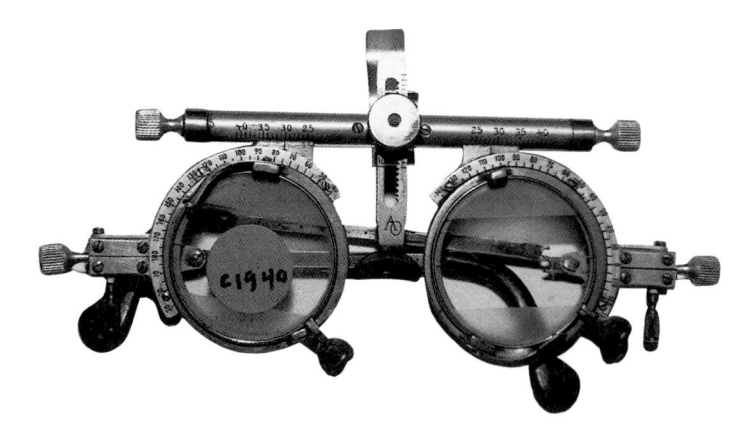

Figure 605. American Optical frame, rotating bridge pad.

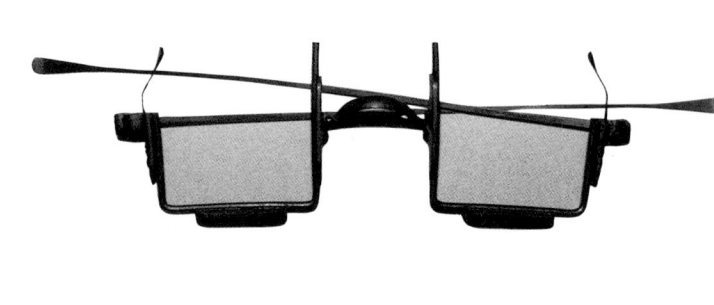

Figure 606. Trial frames to accept prisms.

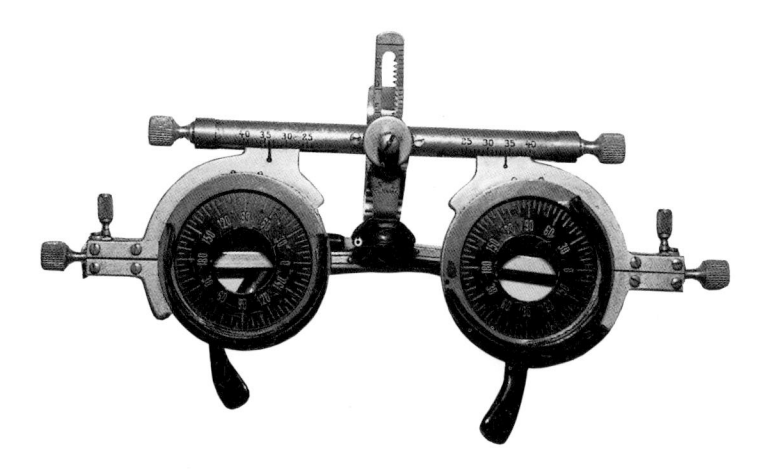

Figure 607. Fully adjustable trial frame.

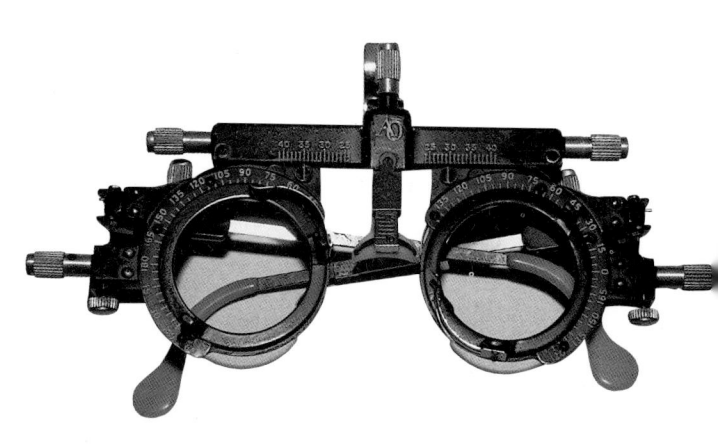

Figure 608. American Optical trial frame.

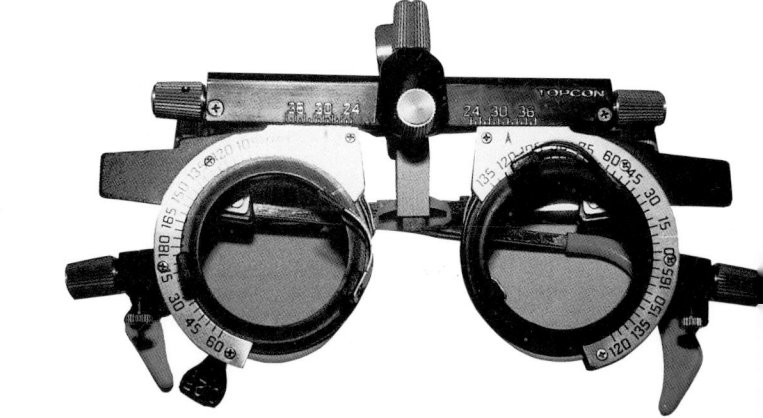

Figure 609. Topcon trial frame.

314 CHAPTER 29

Whole pieces of the frame were later made of plastic, which was lighter in weight than metal. Some frames even allowed bridge height to be ascertained, and comfortable rotating bridge pads were added (Figure 605). Temple measurements to the quarter inch were added for comfort.

Unusual Styles

Mechanisms that allowed each face to be fit individually produced grotesque frame styles before engineering sanity brought the frames into a more reasonable form. Still, each optical company and many ophthalmologists designed and produced their own trial frame version.

One frame is made only to receive square prism lenses (Figure 606), and the eye wire is U-shaped with 90-degree angles below and flanges to hold the lenses (American Optical Company, circa 1910). Another frame (U.S., circa 1895) is designed only to measure pupillary distance (Figure 602), and is fitted with permanent trial lenses 1 inch × 1 3/8 inches. These lenses are frosted, except for the center 3/8-inch, which itself is incised with crossed lines to mark the center. A "P.D. stick" bar with handle and two center marked lenses attached—one adjustable—was patented and available. Please refer to the illustrations to note other styles (Figure 607).

Companies that offered trial frames include American Optical Company (Figure 608), Bausch and Lomb, probably Shuron (although the author has no marked examples of their production), and Topcon (Figure 609). Many trial frames are unmarked, and others are marked only "PAT. APPLIED FOR," possibly with a manufacture date.

Conclusion

At the time the trial frames and case were used for refraction, the process was tedious and slow—as difficult for the patient to determine whether a certain lens was "good or bad" as it was for the ophthalmologist. These days, with the use of modern phoropters, which include all lenses in a trial case, the process is much more rapid and accurate. Automatic refracters also aid in this process.

Notes

1. Duke-Elder, *System of Ophthalmology*. Vol. V. (St. Louis: C. V. Mosby and Company, 1965), 832.
2. Elisabeth Bennion, *Antique Medical Instruments* (Berkeley: University of California Press, 1979), 148.
3. American Optical Company catalog, 1924, pp. 230–259.

30

Telescopic Operating Loupes

Jacques Daviel performed the first intracapsular cataract extraction (accidentally) in 1747. Since that time, and with the use of Albert von Graefe's preliminary iridectomy, magnification during operative procedures has proved to be most useful. Although binocular opera glasses were in use in 1823, it was not until at least 50 years later that they were adapted to operating-room use.

At first, simple magnifying lenses were used, and later the compound variety were utilized. The lenses were not fully telescopic until about 1910. It was then that the Zeiss Company (Jena) produced small telescopes for subnormal vision aids that were adapted for operating-room use (Figure 610). These were fine, small (about 1 centimeter in diameter), light, with great optics and a most useful focal distance of about 12 inches. They were designed like spectacles, with a C-bridge and cable temples.

Later, other companies and nations attempted to imitate these loupes. The British manufacturers Keeler and Hamblin (Figure 611) are two, and the Neitz Company of Japan is another (Figure 612). All of these products were delivered in a wooden box covered with black leather or plastic and lined with cushioned silk.

The Beebe Loupe

The Beebe loupe is a type of skeleton binocular using the telescopic principle with no tubes supporting the lenses. However, a pair of small square lenses is set into a holder 2 ½ to 3 inches in front of the physician's eyeglass bridge. One set was attached to a headband (Figure 613, center), but others were (a) attached to the bridge in a slot and could be flipped up, (b) set into special glasses with a centrally ground bifocal (Figure 614), (c) set into a trial pair of glasses to receive any lens needed from a trial set (American Optical Company), or (d) attached to a special frame with plano (protective) lenses and an adjustable pupillary distance (Bausch and Lomb Optical Company) (Figure 615).

In the 1940s, larger loupes were used. They were attached to a headband and set at the end of a black-funnel shaped piece of plastic. The purpose was probably to concentrate the surgeon's attention, vis-a-vis his vision, on the surgical area.

A headband-mounted loupe is used today for medical and many nonmedical purposes (Figure 616).

Currently, surgeons wear shields during surgery to protect against blood hitting the face and possibly transmitting AIDS or other diseases. Fortunately, we are now able to utilize floor- and ceiling-mounted operating telescopes, which offer surgeons (and patients) benefits not possible with the previously used devices.

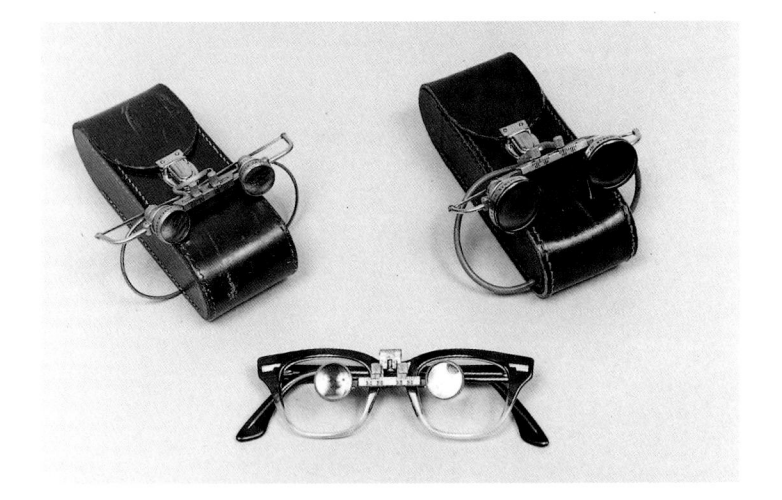

Figure 610. Zeiss loupes.

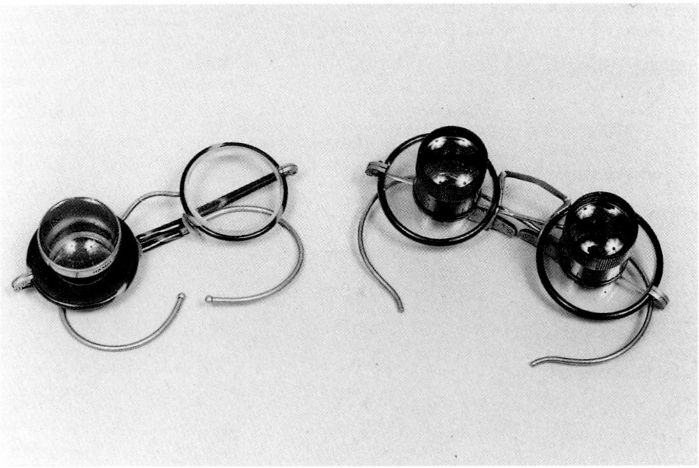

Figure 611. Hamblin loupe, left.

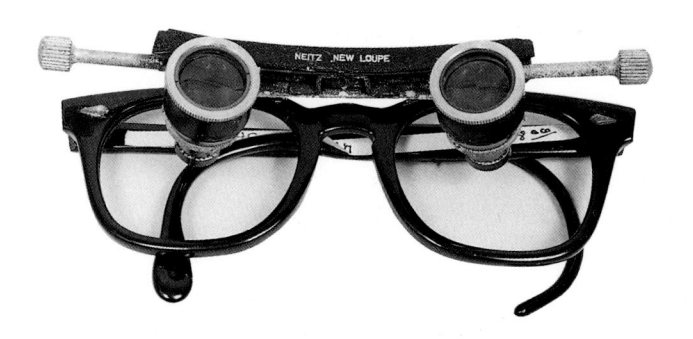

Figure 612. Neitz loupe.

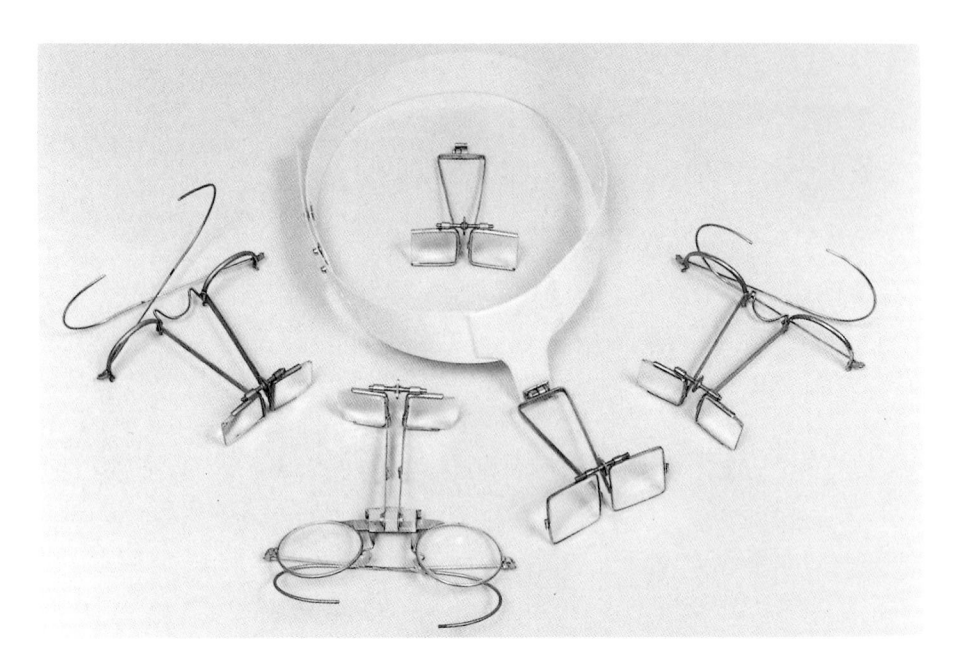

Figure 613. Types of Beebe loupes.

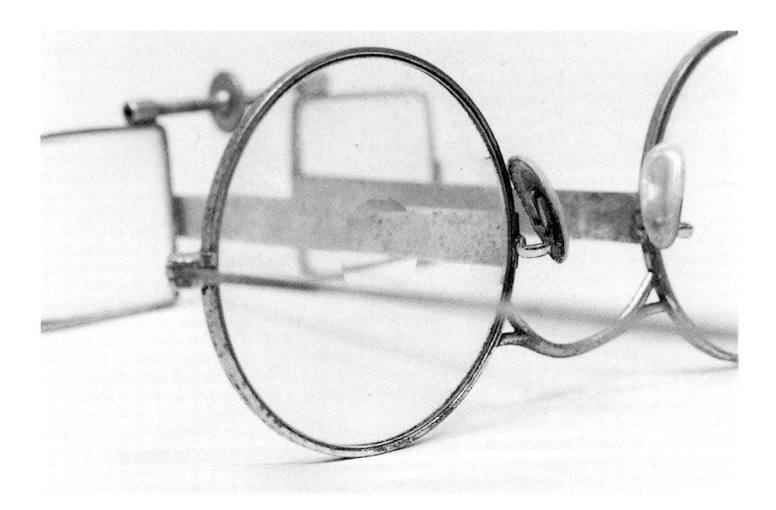

Figure 614. Type of Beebe loupes with centrally ground bifocal.

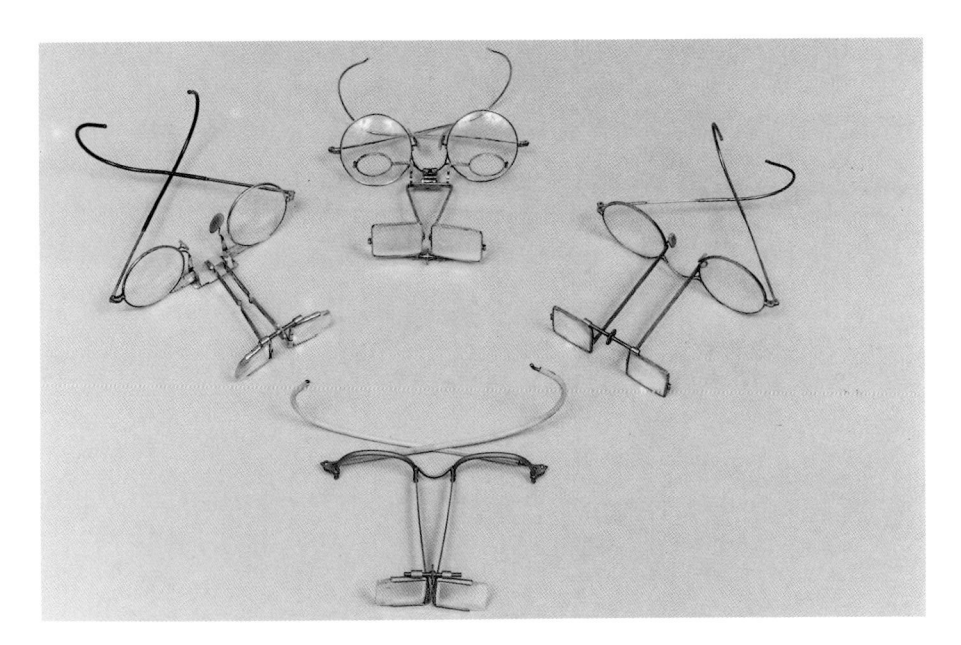

Figure 615. Various Beebe loupes.

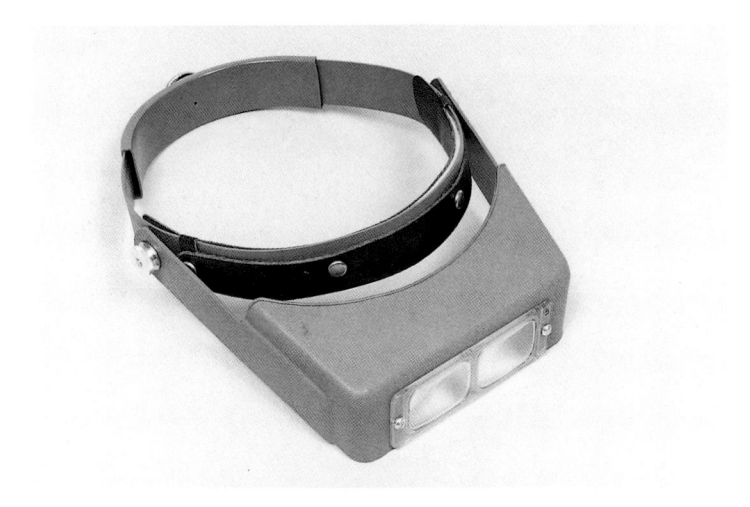

Figure 616. Common head loupe used 1980 to present.

OPERATING LOUPES   319

31

Spectacles Cases

When spectacles were first produced, they were made for individuals on a one-to-one basis and were considered valuable possessions. Because they needed protection when not in use, the eyeglass case was born. At first these cases were rather crude, but as time went on, they were made more decorative. Their beauty was representative of the owner's knowledge, education, and social status.

Early cases were made of brass, wood, horn, tortoiseshell, and leather, reflecting the same taste as containers for other common, useful products of the age (Figure 617). The cases were shaped to fit the spectacles, such as a teardrop shape for riveted spectacles and an oblong flat shape for Nuremburg spectacles (Figure 618). Some wood cases were carved on the inside for specific spectacles and on the outside to meet the demands of the owner.

When gold, silver, and shagreen cases were produced, they were lined with silk and other cloth (velvet, cotton). Even fur was reportedly used for that purpose. Some regularly used books had a thick cover made with a recess to accommodate a pair of spectacles. Very few of these actually remain (perhaps a dozen in the world), and they are mostly in museums. They date from the fifteenth century.

The 1600s

Cases from the 1600s were usually hand-carved wood with wire-loop hinges and brass hooks with staple catches. They came mostly from Northern Europe and are of the clamshell variety.

The 1700s

When steel frames emerged in the early and mid-1700s, steel cases were made for them. Some cases were clamshell and others flip-top (Figure 619). Most were lined, but such does not remain to be seen today. Although the author has a gold-washed Benjamin Martin set of glasses, the set came without a case. A case in the author's possession for a similar set retains large areas of its former gilt decoration.

The clamshell cases close with a pushbutton catch (Figure 620), while the flip-top can close either with a pushbutton catch or with friction on extensions inside the lid (Figure 621). Steel spectacles fit snugly inside the cases, and it is understood that many of the spectacles and cases may not be the original partners—breakage, substitutions and commerce being what they are. Further description can be found in Chapter 10. By the late 1700s, cases were narrower as spectacles were made smaller and production became more sophisticated (Figure 618).

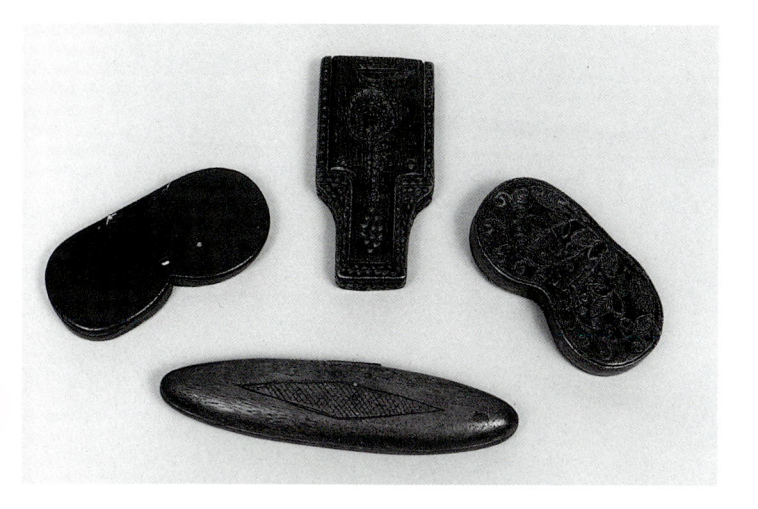

Figure 617. Carved wooden eyeglass cases circa 1700.

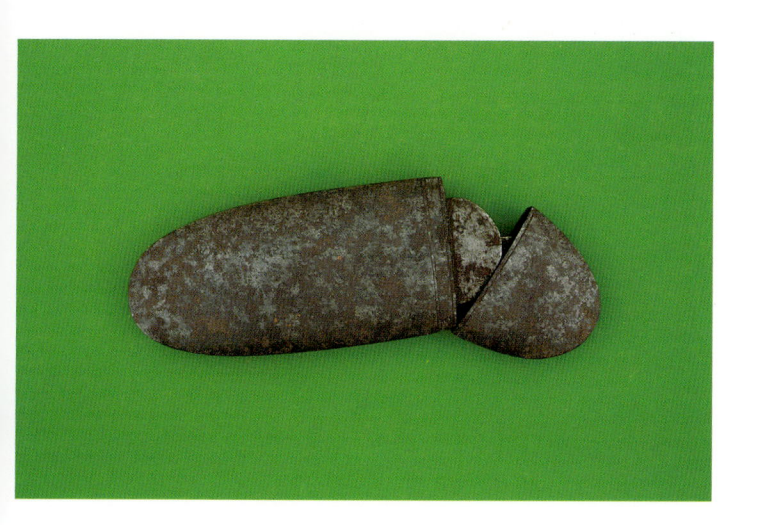

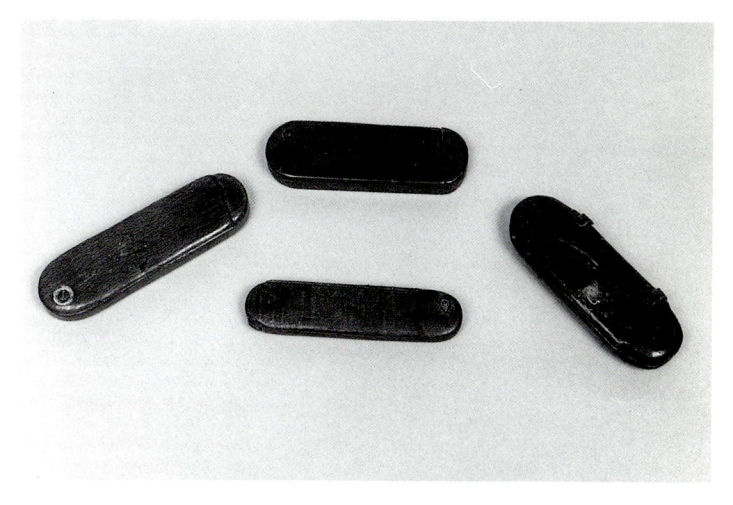

Figure 618. Oblong wooden eyeglass cases.

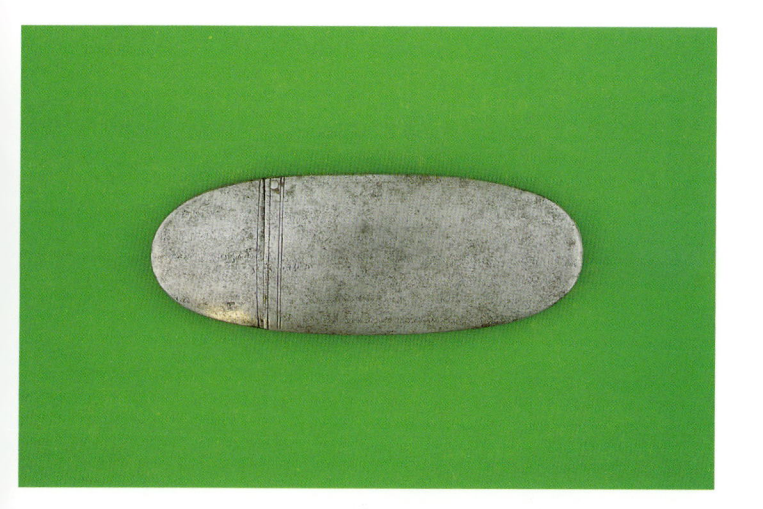

Figure 619. Flip-top steel spectacles case circa 1750.

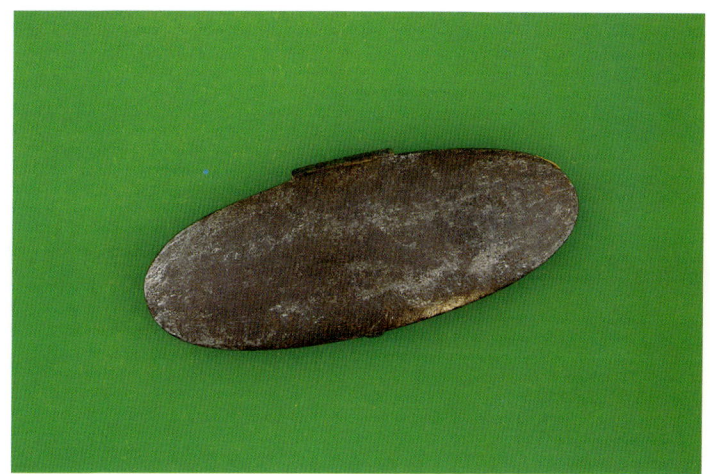

Figure 620. Clamshell steel spectacle case circa 1750.

Figure 621. Flip-top case with extensions under lid for a friction catch and to stabilize the top.

SPECTACLE CASES

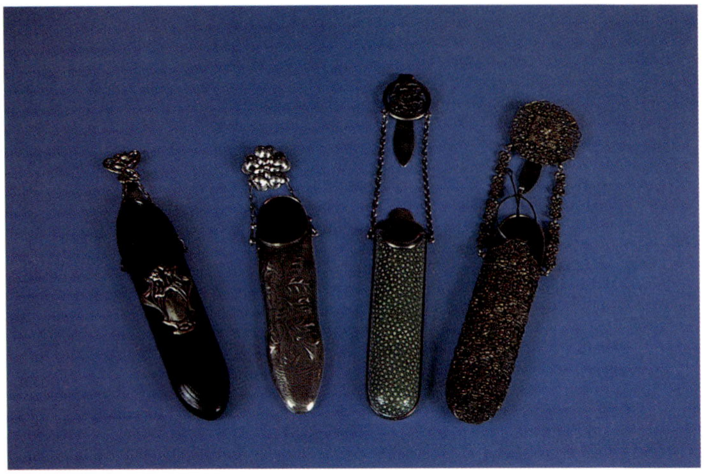

Figure 622. English chatelaine cases.

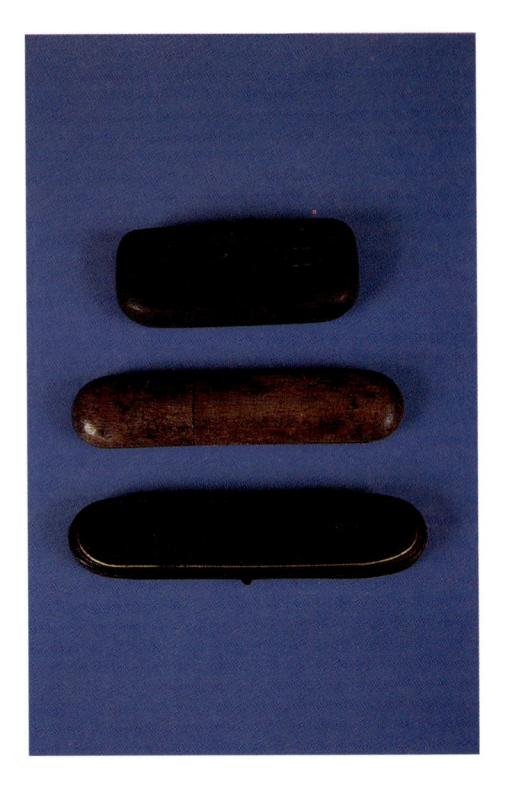

Figure 623. Slip-top and flip-top cases.

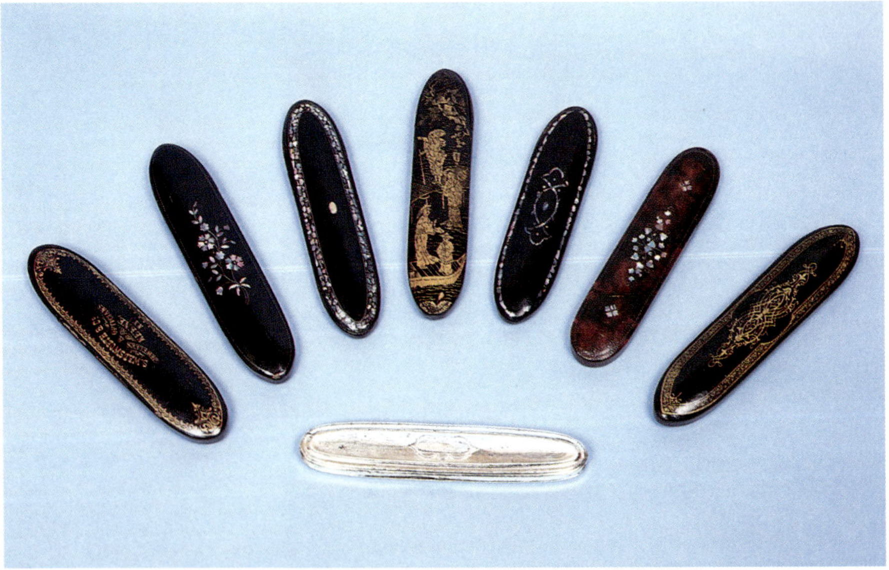

Figure 624. Lacquer, papier mache, tortoiseshell, and metal cases. Note the chinoiserie on the center case.

322   CHAPTER 31

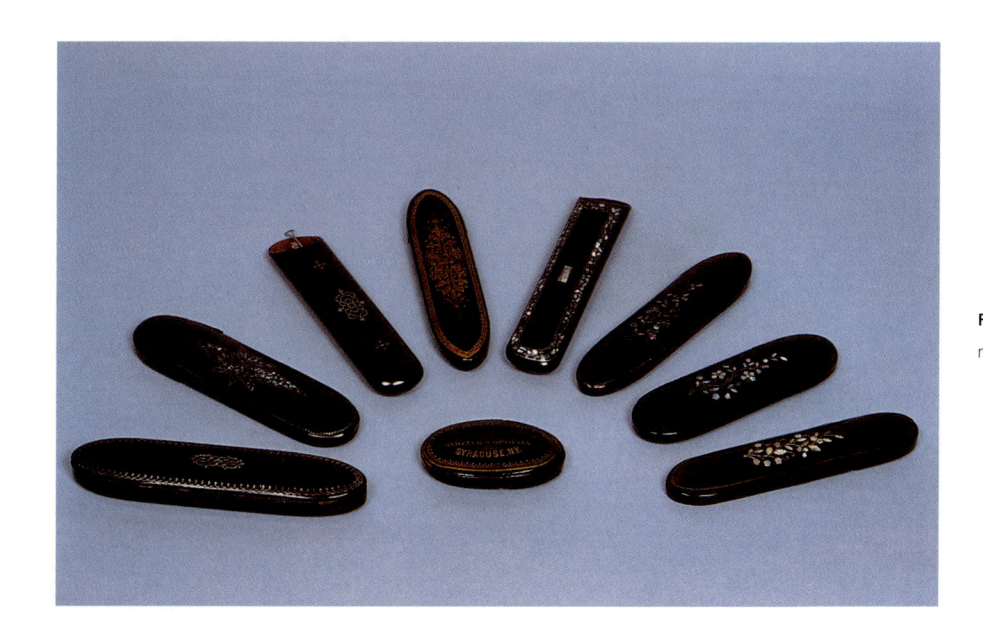

Figure 625. Lacquer and papier mache cases.

The 1800s

The early 1800s ushered in the first of the chatelaine design cases, mostly for women (Figure 622). (Chapter 32 is devoted to these cases.)

Spectacle frames were generally lighter in weight and had shorter temples than those in the previous century. They could fit into smaller cases. Extension and pivot (turn-pin) temples aided this size reduction. Wooden cases were made of thinner material, and many were of the frog-mouth opening or the slip-top design (Figure 623). Also of this design, as well as the clamshell, were those made of lacquer and papier mache (Figures 624 & 625). Some were inlaid with abalone, mother-of-pearl, silver wire, and silver flat designs. Others had transfer (decalcomania) for decoration (Figure 626). Commercial varieties plugged resorts (for tourists) or optical outlets (Figure 627).

Frames for wig glasses were usually made of tortoiseshell with short, straight temples. Many were housed in small, flat cases of silver (Figure 628), tortoiseshell (Figure 629), or shagreen (Figure 630, center). Most had flip-tops and were adorned with silver bands, hinges, and cartouches. The author has a beautifully engraved silver case from Belgium that is of the clamshell design (Figure 631, center). Tortoiseshell cases can also be found with the depressed areas festooned with gold and silver scrolls and designs. (More information on these cases can be found in Chapter 12.)

Another spectacular case comes from Italy and is made of ivory, with three inset miniatures on the top (Figure 632). Note the fine detail (Figure 633).

In the middle of the nineteenth century in America, pressed-steel cases covered with tin were produced (Figures 634, 635, & 636). They were plain at first but were later decorated by embossing. Some were made long to house longer temples, and others were shorter for folded or telescoped temples. They were used almost 50 years.

Many cases of hard leather were used in the United States (Figure 637). Some had open tops, while others had foldover

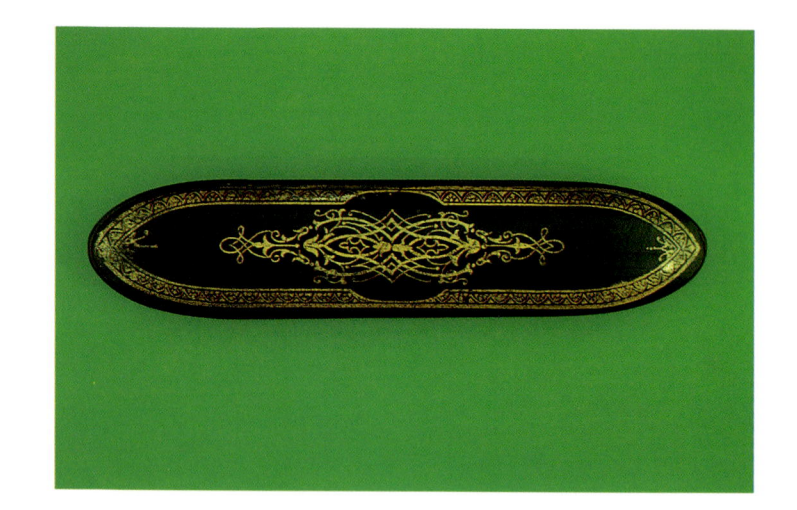

Figure 626. Lacquer spectacles case decorated with transfer.

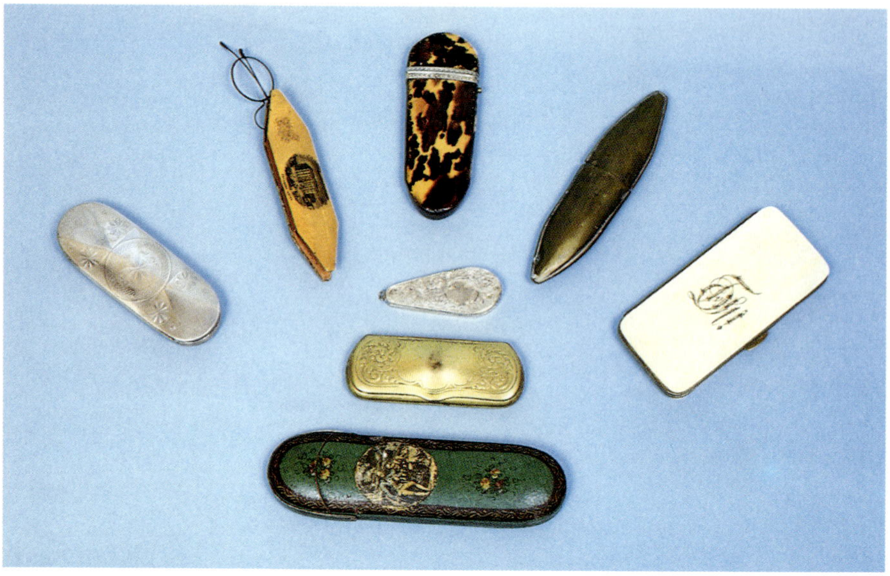

Figure 627. Various cases; one with protruding spectacle promotes a tourist attraction.

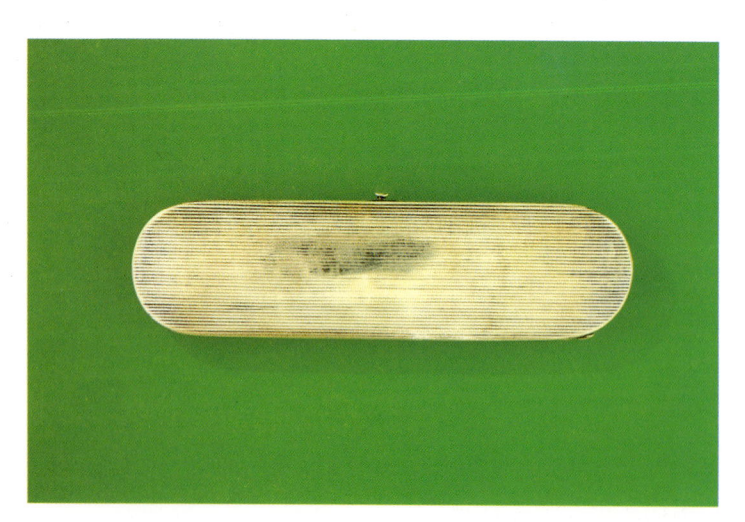

Figure 628. Silver case.

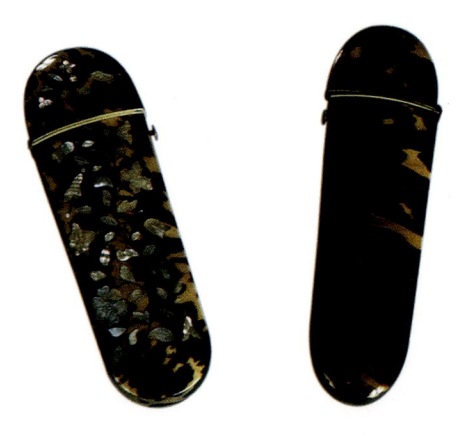

Figure 629. Tortoiseshell wig glass cases.

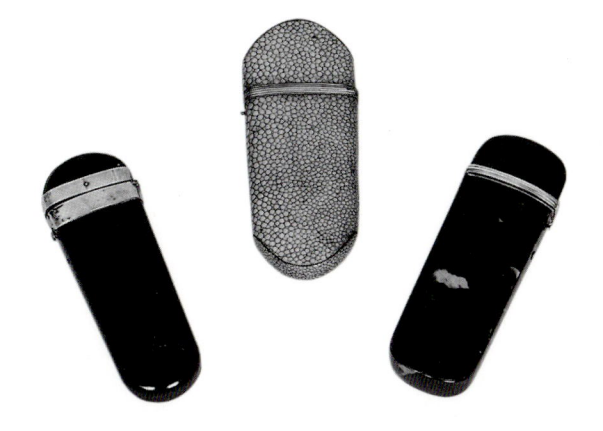

Figure 630. Shagreen wig glass case (center).

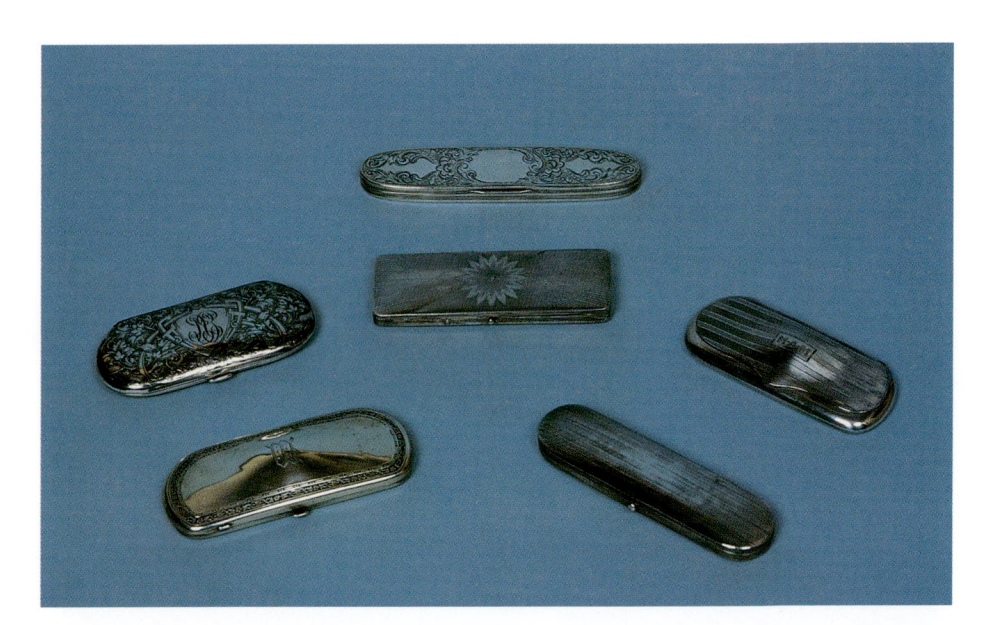

Figure 631. Silver spectacles cases.

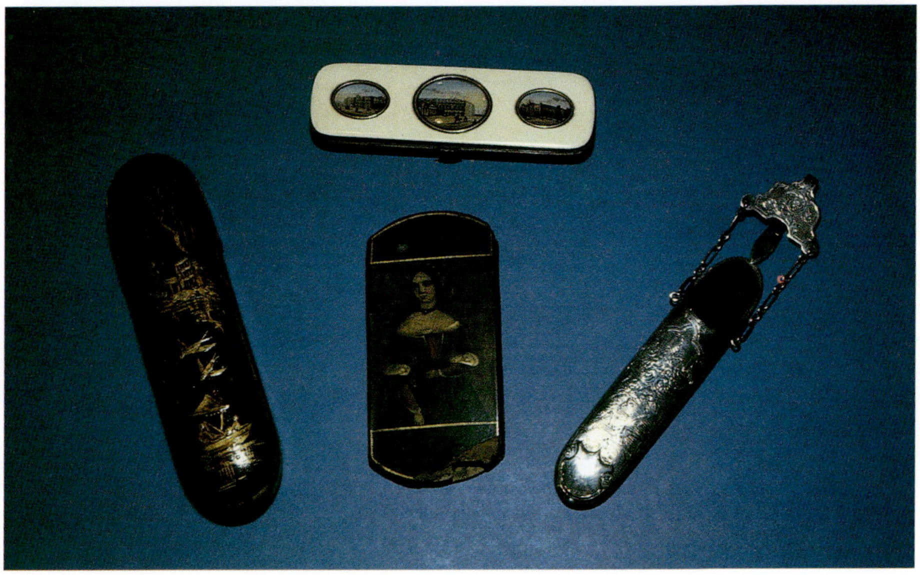

Figure 632. Lacquer, chinoiserie, spectacles/cigar case, silver chatelaine—ivory (Italian) case above.

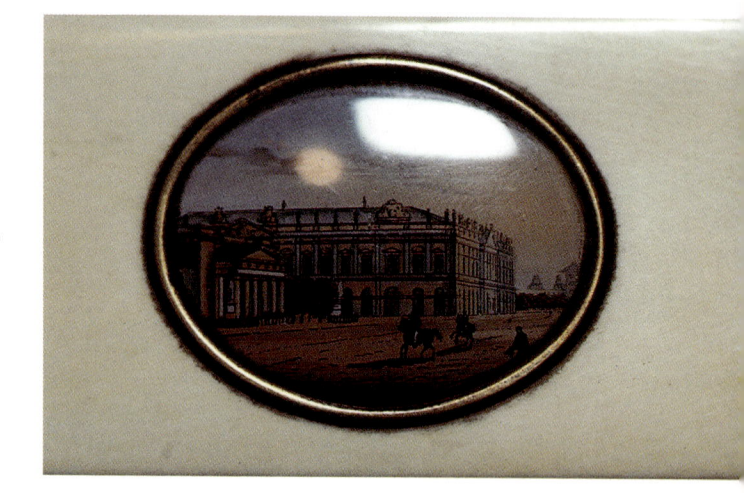

Figure 633. Detail of miniature on ivory case in Figure 632.

Figure 634. Tin-coated steel American cases.

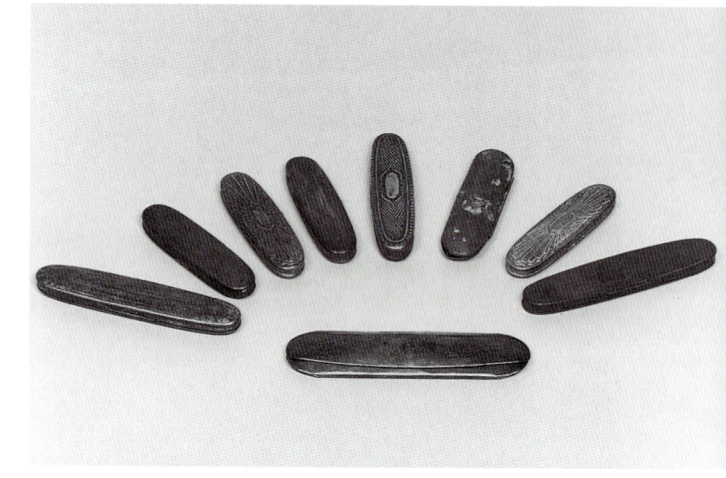

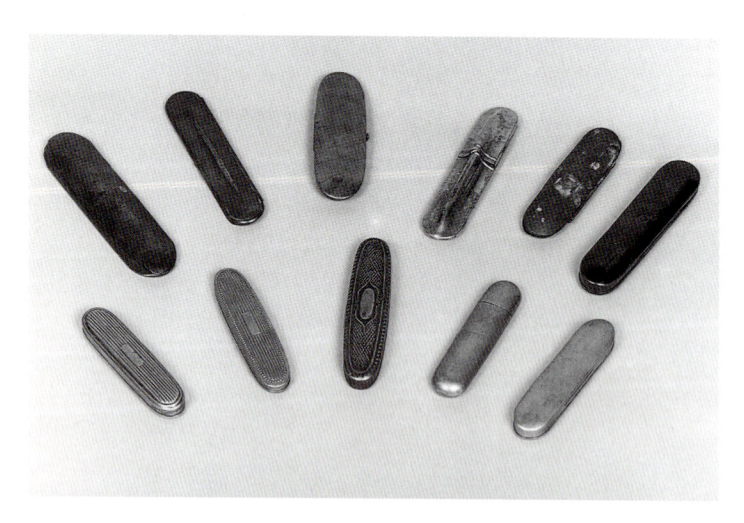

Figure 635. Tin-coated steel American cases.

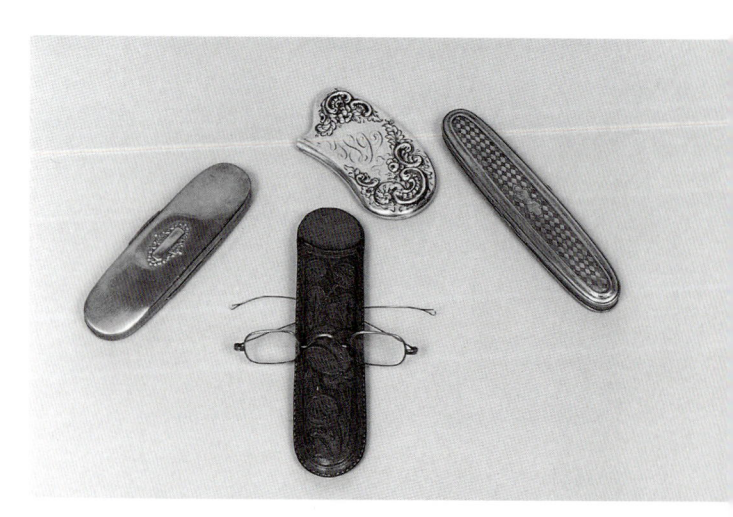

Figure 636. Tin-coated steel American cases.

326 CHAPTER 31

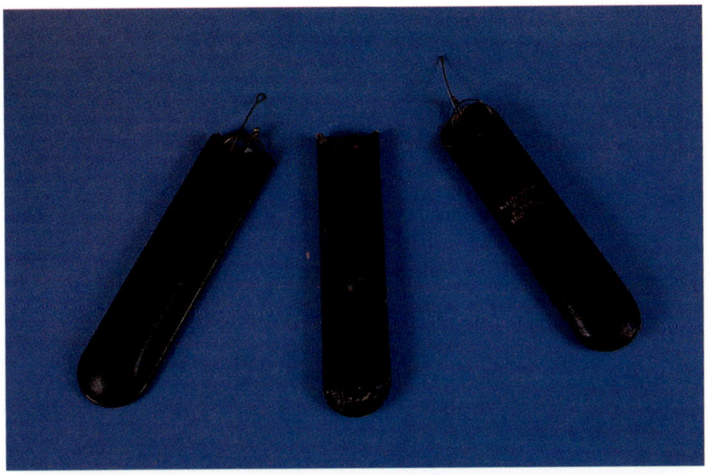

Figure 637. Hard leather American spectacles cases.

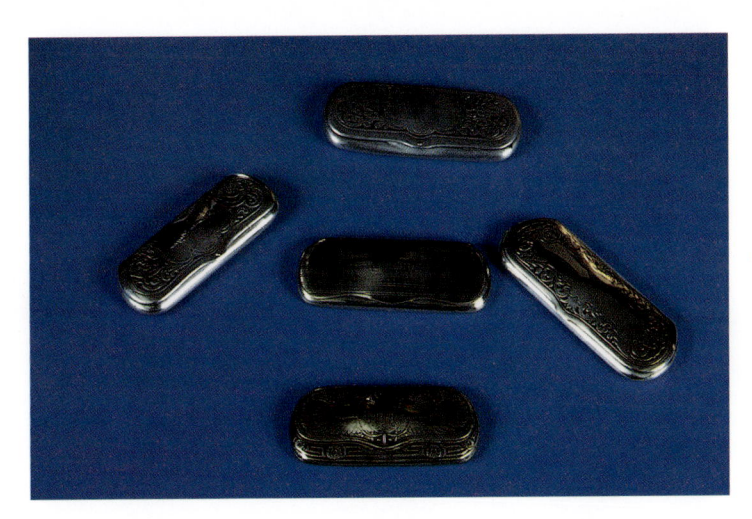

Figure 638. Aluminum cases (3 above) and silver (2 below).

tops secured by snaps or tabs recessed into the front of the cases. Quite a few sported the optical source of the glasses.

Pince-nez glasses used in the late 1800s were housed either in leather slip-in cases with tops secured by snaps or in leather-covered steel cases with clamshell openings and spring closures. Small pince-nez could be accommodated in small cases, while others simply hung from a chain, spring-mounted in a reel. Both of these types were pinned to the clothing. (More detail on pince-nez can be found in Chapter 20. Monocle cases are also described in Chapter 19.)

Toward the end of the century, the use of aluminum to fashion practical items was discovered. Aluminum opera glasses and eyeglass cases were highly prized as new and desirable items. Embossed aluminum clamshell-opening cases that closed with a spring, some of which were enameled, were very popular (Figure 638). Most all of these cases were lined with flannel or velveteen. Although the fad for the new aluminum cases faded, the cases still held a basic percentage of case manufacture.

Evening Cases

For evening wear, wooden cases were covered by extremely thin (1-millimeter) sheets of mother-of-pearl, abalone, or sea snail into various shapes and glued to the case in attractive

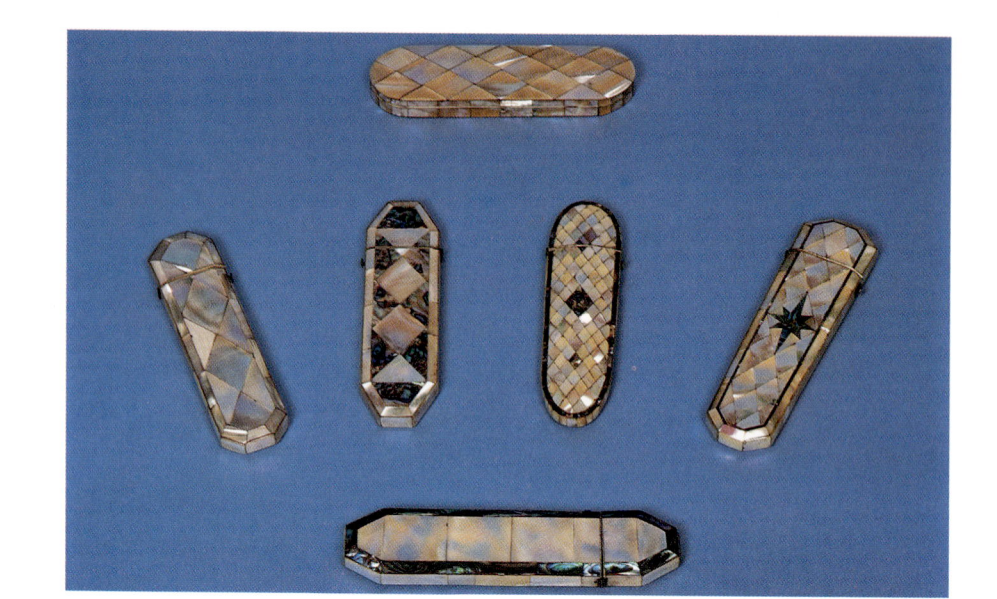

Figure 639. Evening use spectacles cases circa 1880.

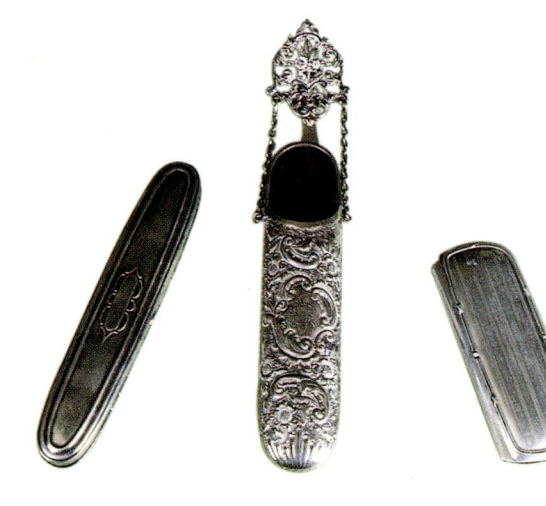

Figure 641. Silver spectacles cases.

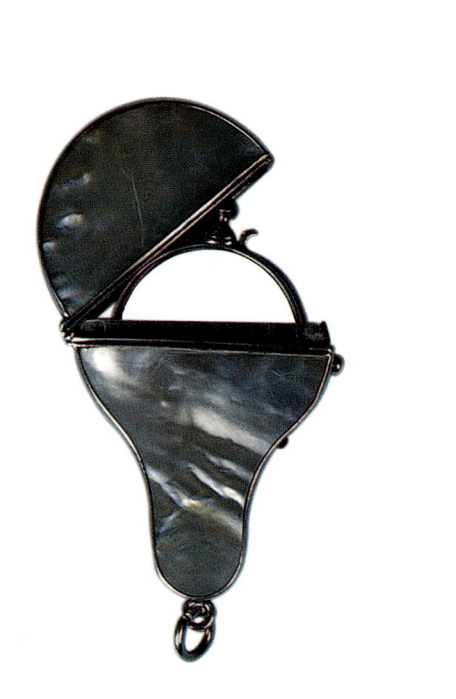

Figure 640. Evening use folding eyeglass case circa 1800.

328 CHAPTER 31

designs. These cases were made in England and contained dainty gold spectacles, usually with octagonal ribbon eye wires and extendible sliding temples (Figures 639 & 640).

Silver (sterling in the United States after 1865), hallmarked in England and on the continent, was favored by the hierarchy of elegance in the latter half of the nineteenth century (Figure 638). Some cases were chatelaines (Figure 641), but many were of the clamshell variety. Most of these were highly engraved. Sometimes the owners' initials or name or a legend of an occasion was engraved centrally (see Figure 639). Some tortoiseshell cases with silver cartouches were so engraved.

Chinese Eyeglass Cases

Chapter 8 covers the fascinating subject of Chinese eyeglass cases (Figure 642).

Manufacturing

Spectacles cases, although in demand, were not produced by many optical companies. Following is an article taken from the July 1989 newsletter of the Ophthalmic Antiques International Collectors' Club regarding one of the largest manufacturers of spectacle cases. The article was compiled from another article written for the centenary of James Willmott & Sons Company (1884–1984 brochure).

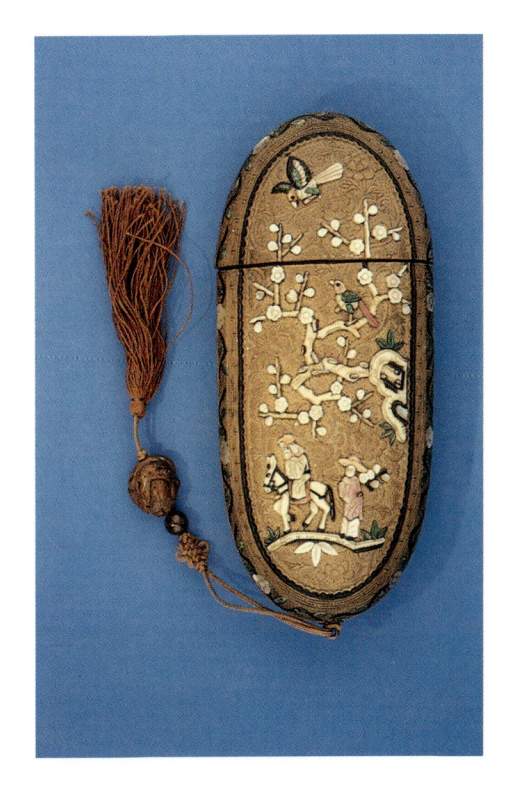

Figure 642. Chinese spectacles case.

WILLMOTTS—CASE MAKERS TO THE WORLD

In 1882 James Willmott set up a case making business in Mary Ann Street, Birmingham with a capital of £6.10 shillings. Already by 1884 the business was soundly on its feet and the name was changed to James Willmott & Sons. By 1904 the company, finding it necessary to seek larger premises, moved to Evesham, Worcester in the heart of the fruit growing Vale of Evesham. The factory in Swan Lane is on the river Avon and appears now to have its feet almost in the river.

James Willmott retired as Managing Director in 1931 and was succeeded by his son Fred but remained as Chairman until his death aged 77 in 1934. Second Chairman of Willmotts Ltd. on through the difficult years of the Second World War, was Mr. E.L. Payton. Fred Willmott retired from day-to-day work in 1939, but retained managing directorship.

The company amalgamated with the Birmingham case making firm Smyth & Co., whose proprietor E.L. Payton was also Chairman of the small but growing Austin Motor Company. Presumably it was his far sighted action in stocking up with the steel sheet required for case making. In 1940 packages of steel were everywhere, even stacked in the corridor and passages, where ever space could be found, much of which was probably used for war production.

The company was badly hit, there being little demand for jewel boxes. Their secondary production and work was undertaken for munitions. War time products included gun links for .303, .5, and 20mm ammunition. The London showrooms were closed and a general engineering firm occupied premises where Willmotts North Works now stand. Later, in 1946, their business merged with Willmotts.

The National Health Service started on July 5th, 1948,

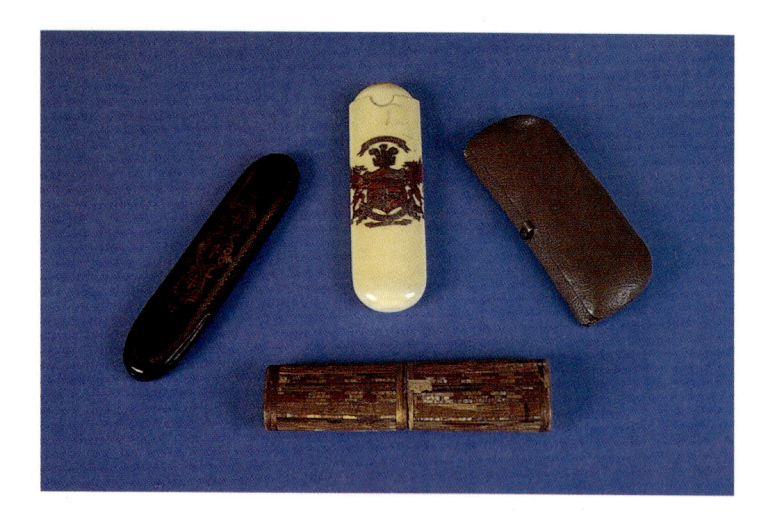

Figures 643–646. Miscellaneous spectacles cases.

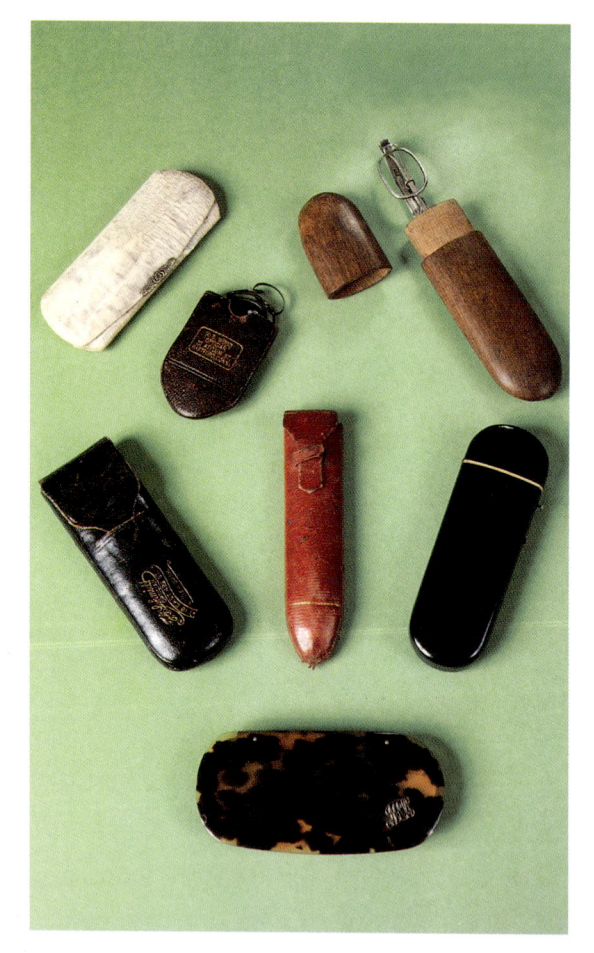

Figure 644.

and heralded a new era for Willmotts. Under this scheme most spectacles were free or with a charge of 7-½ p. if the spectacle had a pad bridge. Cases were free. Bedlam soon reigned in the optical trade and profession, and demand was beyond their comprehension. A simple order for standard plastic spectacles and simple spherical lenses took nine months from date of order to deliver, so that eight months work was constantly on the shelf. From time to time the general public would get the idea that flesh coloured plastic was in particularly short supply, and customers would call at the optician's shop and demand that their order should be changed to a different coloured plastic. The wholesaler was required to sift through months of dusty packages of unopened post in order that Madam's order could be changed from pink to blue.

The optical manufacturing trade made stupendous efforts to increase frame and lens production only to see demand drop overnight by 50% in 1951 when charges for N.H.S. spectacles were imposed.

Conclusion

Spectacles cases not only were utilitarian but were also often regarded as treasures to their owners. Since some people were recognized by their personal possessions, specialized spectacles cases were part of the genre. Petit point, knit, gold thread, embroidered, and needlepoint cases, all can be found in the history of spectacles cases. As with most items of "value," the imagination was the only boundary as to what could be used (Figures 643–646).

Notes

1. *The Ophthalmic Antiques International Collectors' Club Newsletter,* July 1989. (Compiled from an article written for the centenary of James Willmott & Sons Company, 1884–1984 brochure).

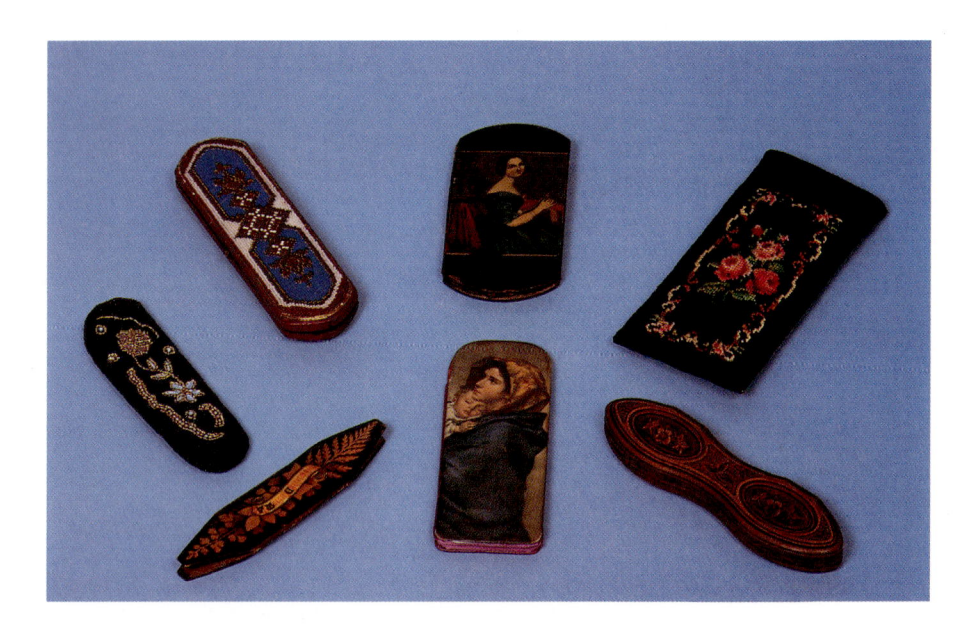

Figure 645. Spectacles cases.

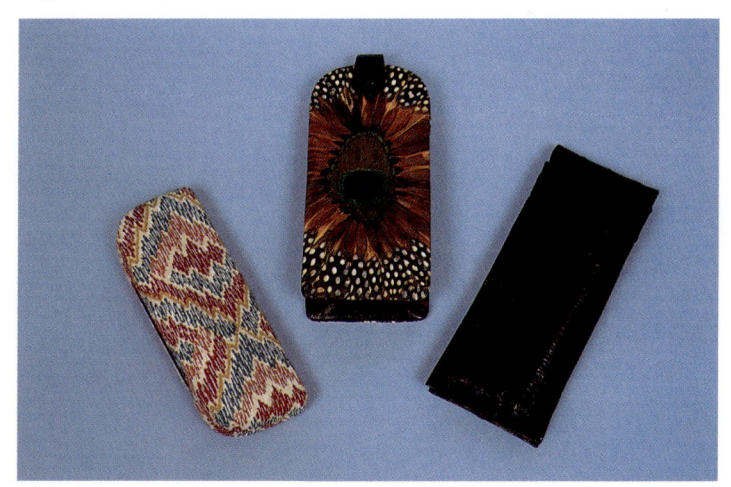

Figure 646. Spectacles cases.

Other Sources Consulted for Chapter 31

1. Elisabeth Bennion, *Antique Medical Instruments* Sotheby Parke Bernet Publishers, University of California Press: London, Berkeley, and Los Angeles, 1979), 227, 236.
2. Pieve di Cadore, *Il Museo Dell'Occhiale* (Milano: Gruppo Editoriale Fabbri, Bompiani, Sonzogno, Etas S.p.A., 1990), 99.
3. Hugh Orr, *Illustrated History of Early Antique Spectacles* (London, 1985), 11, 31, 35, 59, 60, 85.
4. W. Poulet, *Atlas on the History of Spectacles,* translated by F. C. Blodi, M.D. (Bad Godesberg, West Germany: Wayenborgh Publishers, 1978), 320.

32

The Evolution of Chatelaine Eyeglass Cases

About 1800, spectacles were beginning to be made more delicately. The more elegant eyeglasses were made of gold, silver and tortoiseshell and their protection and adornment were then considered necessary and complimentary to their style. Although some continental sweatshops turned out as many as 3,600 pairs of spectacles a week, the glasses were crudely and cheaply made and had inferiorly ground lenses.[1] However, gold and silver workers were producing frames for the upper echelons of society who certainly needed them but preferred, of course, to have them cased beautifully and to have them at hand. Thus, the chatelaine spectacles case evolved.

The History of Chatelaines

The term *chatelaine* comes from the French and means "keeper of the fort or castle," keeper of the keys, mistress of the chateau, or the castellan (the wife of the keeper). It is the combination of the French words *château* and *laine* (wool)—the latter of which was kept locked in the linen closet or armoire where there were other valuables. As a natural progression of fashion, chatelaines (Figure 647) were used since the fourteenth century for hanging articles of everyday necessity, including keys, knives, button hooks, magnifying glasses, and whistles. Some chatelaines were large and complex, and others were small, but all hung from the belt and were used mostly by women.

The Chatelaine Purse

Before the twelfth century, the chatelaine hook was used over the girdle, mostly by males with messages of state. Money and coins certainly were not in the everyday use of common people, but during the crusades, waist pouches of the king held gold coins for alms (thus the term *almoner*) (Figure 648). The chatelaine purse was used off and on as early as the fourteenth century for both daily and formal wear (Figure 649). Then it was on to the nineteenth century (Figure 650), culminating in the 1900 Gibson Girl, who also used a chatelaine purse (Figure 651).

In a French illustration of the Danse Macabre (1465), one of the participants is shown with a case hung from his belt.[2] Such shaped cases, we have found, were designed to hold folded spectacles.

Chatelaine Eyeglass Cases

Chinese spectacle wearers of the seventeenth and eighteenth centuries had problems storing and protecting their spectacles, some needing two pairs—one for near and one for distance. (Remember, they had no bifocals at that time.) Although not

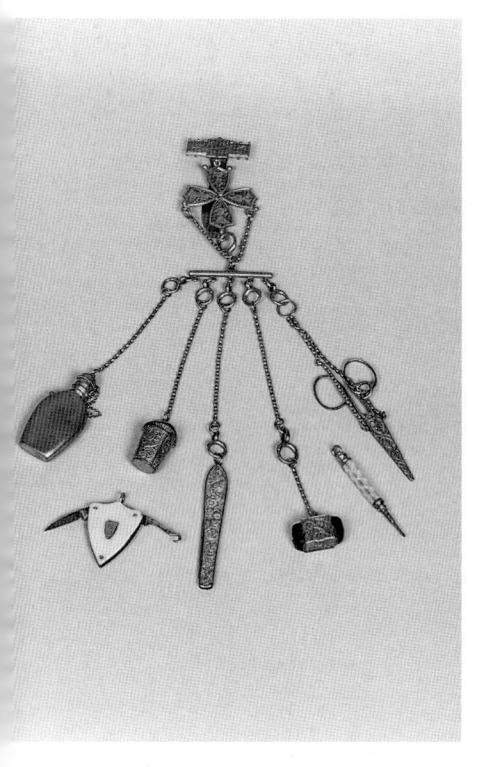

Figure 647. Complex chatelaine with extra knife and pencil.

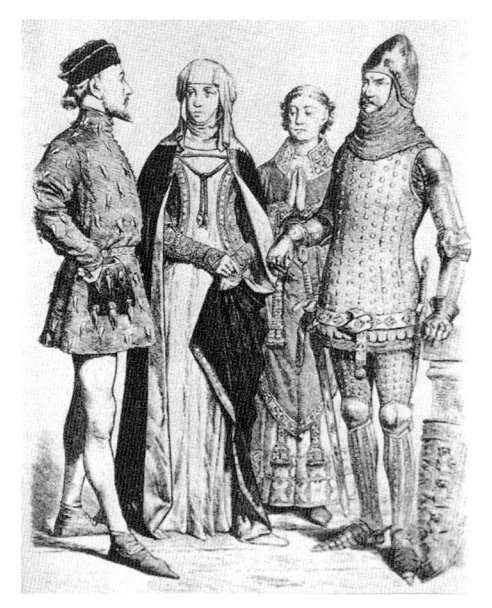

Figure 648. Pouch used for coins, fourteenth century.

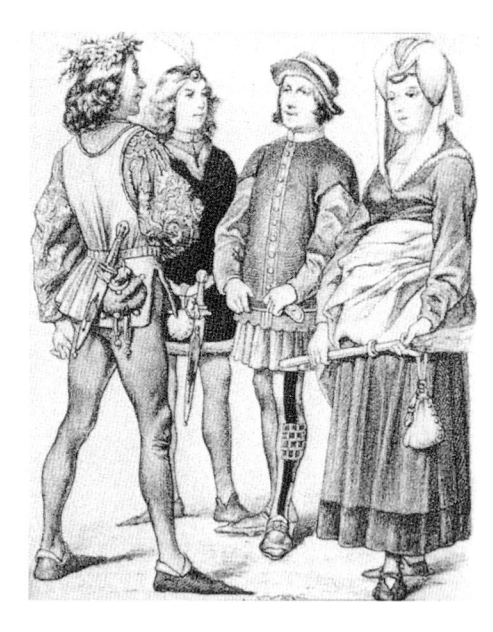

Figure 649. Fifteenth-century French use of chatelaines.

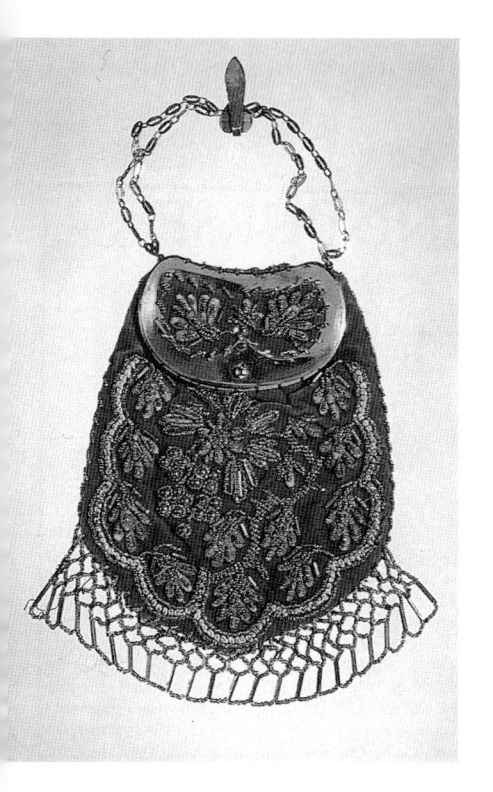

Figure 650. French chatelaine purse circa 1875.

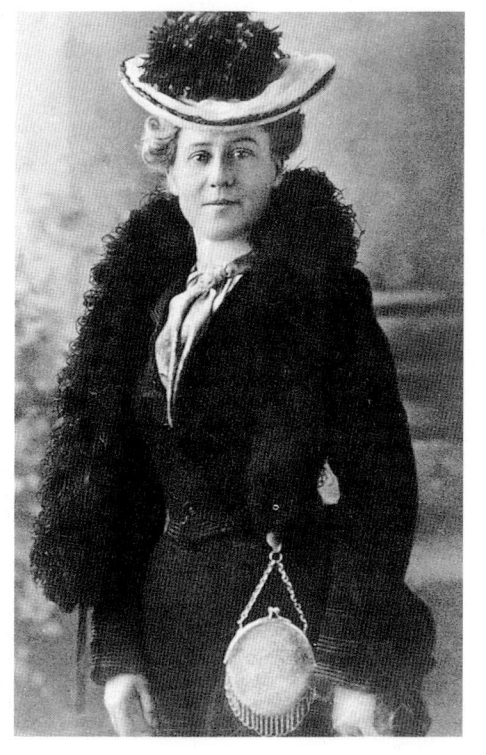

Figure 651. American woman with chatelaine purse circa 1880.

CHATELAIN EYEGLASS CASES 333

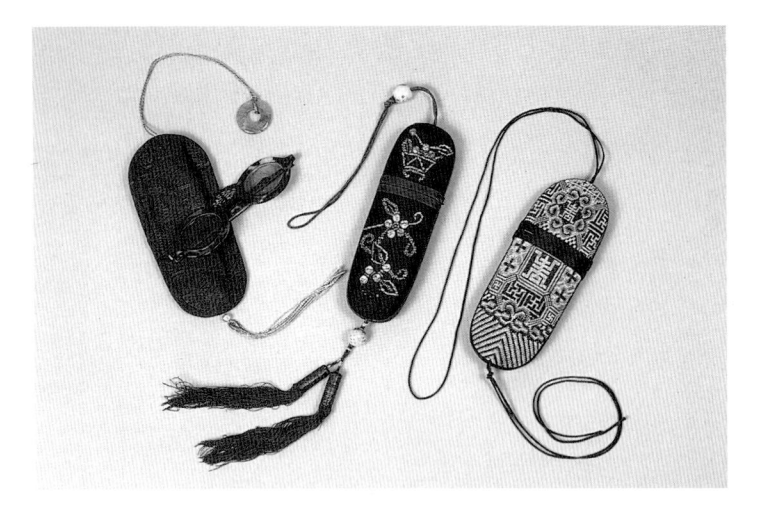

Figure 652. Chinese spectacles cases—embroidered over cardboard.

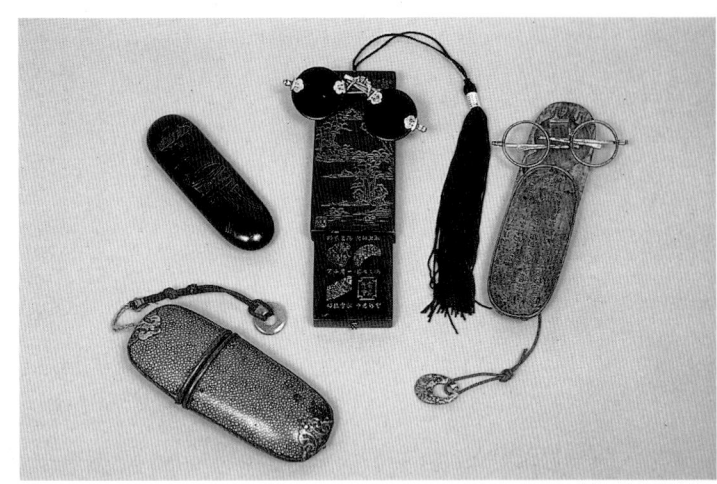

Figure 653. Above right: Chinese spectacles cases—wood, embroidered, lacquer, shagreen.

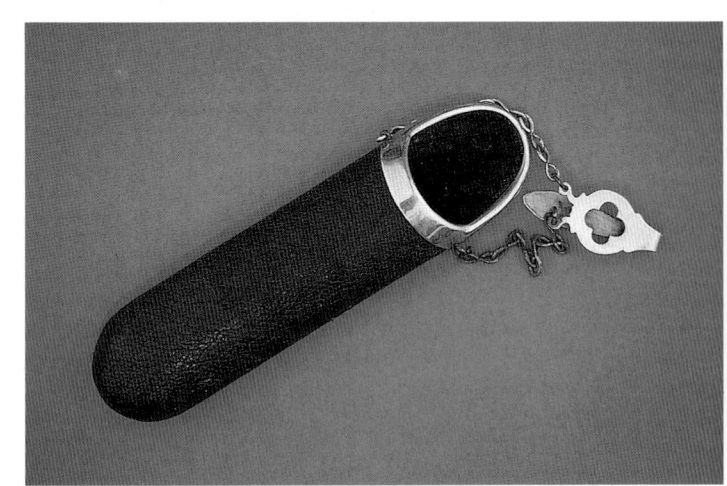

Figure 654. Leather chatelaine case.

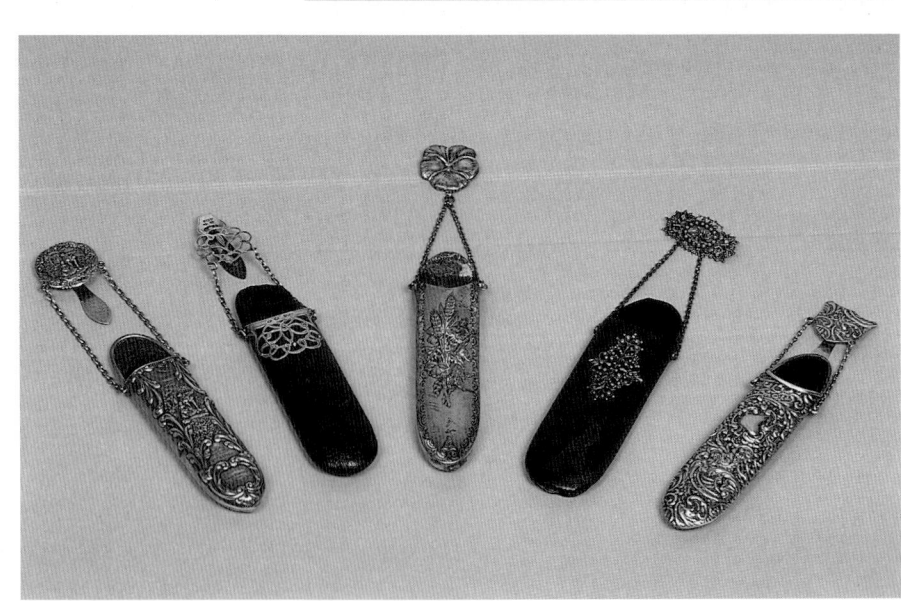

Figure 655. Chatelaine cases—silver, leather, and base metal (center).

334 CHAPTER 32

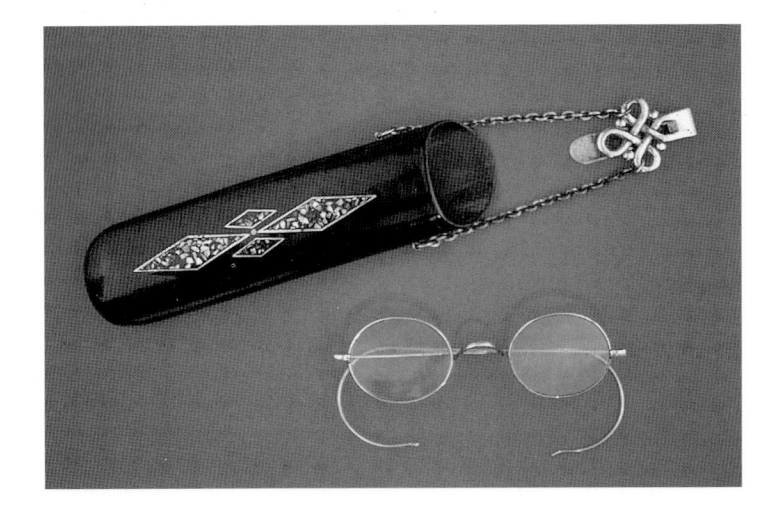

Figure 656. Lacquer chatelaine case inlaid with silver and abalone.

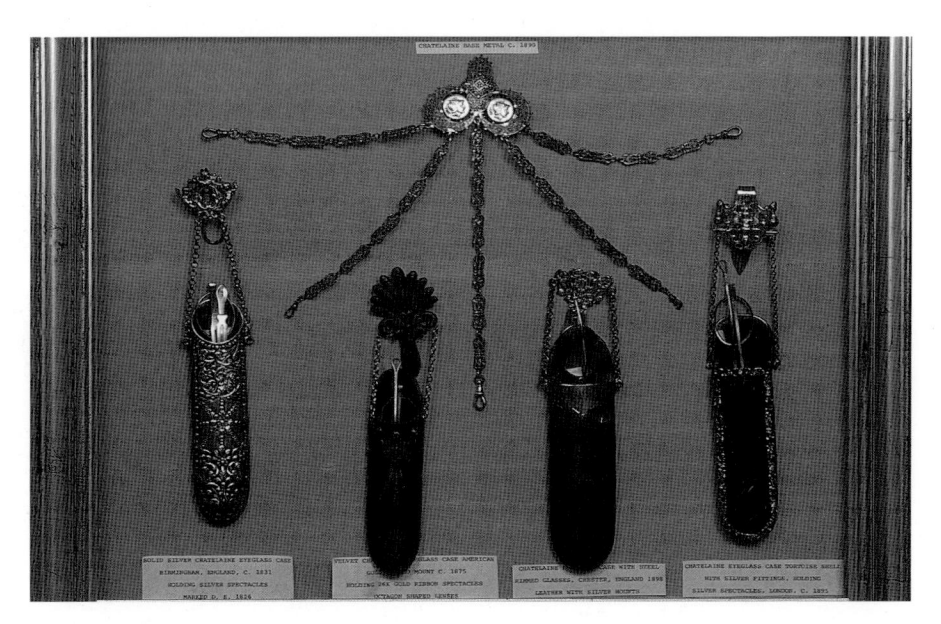

Figure 657. Silver-mounted tortoiseshell, leather, velvet and veneer, and silver chatelaine cases.

truly a chatelaine, the Chinese belt or girdle used to hang the spectacles is similar. The eyeglass cases typically had tapes attached at the top that held the case lids in place. At the same time, the tape or cord was flipped over the belt and firmly held in place by a bead, coin, or piece of jade, which could not be pulled free from the tightness of the belt (Figure 652).

The eyeglass cases were made of sharkskin-covered wood or embroidered materials over bond paper, which protected the large lenses (Figure 653). Bamboo and lacquer cases were also used to house delicate tortoiseshell or rimless frames, which were often in vogue.

Japanese spectacles cases were similarly constructed and hung over the belt and were anchored by a *netsuke*.

On the Continent and in England, chatelaine spectacles cases, made of leather (Figure 654), pressed paper, base metal (Figure 655), tortoiseshell, embossed and engraved silver, and inlaid lacquer (Figure 656), were used throughout the nineteenth century. The author has never found any cases made of gold or adorned with jewels.

In the author's personal collection (Figure 657) are English hallmarked silver cases, tortoiseshell cases bordered in silver and leather with silver throats, chains, and belt hooks. A beautiful, delicate American version (small—5 ¼" × 1 ¼" compared to the ordinary size, 6 ½" × 1 ½") is velvet, decorated with silver veneer, and contains a petite pair of 26-carat gold octagonal-shaped ribbon spectacles.

CHATELAIN EYEGLASS CASES 335

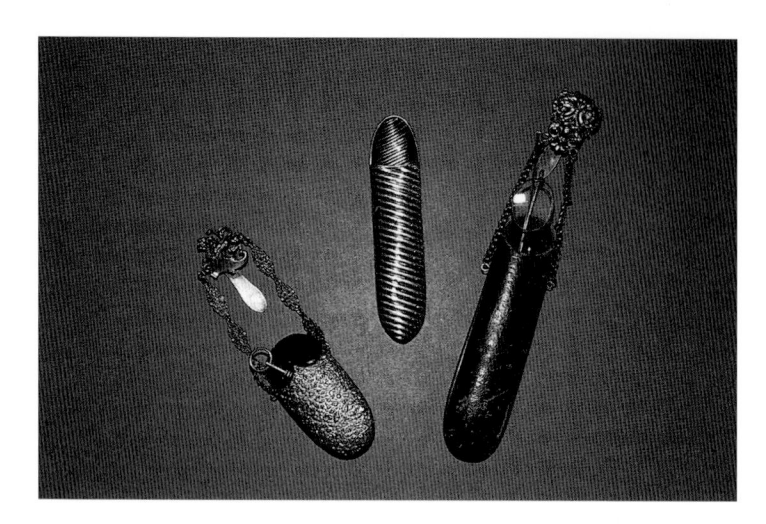

Figure 658. Small-sized chatelaine and other cases.

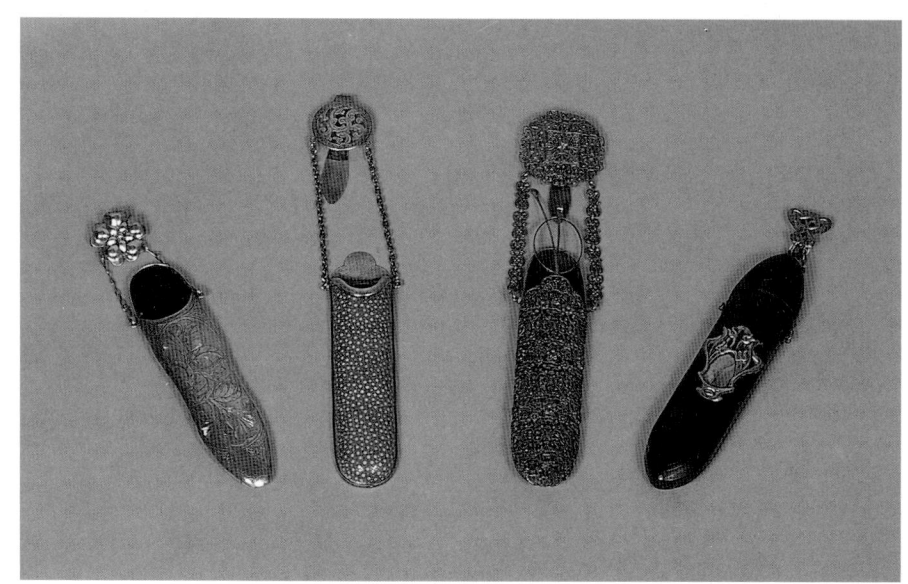

Figure 659. Engraved silver, shagreen, filigree, and frog-mouth chatelaine cases.

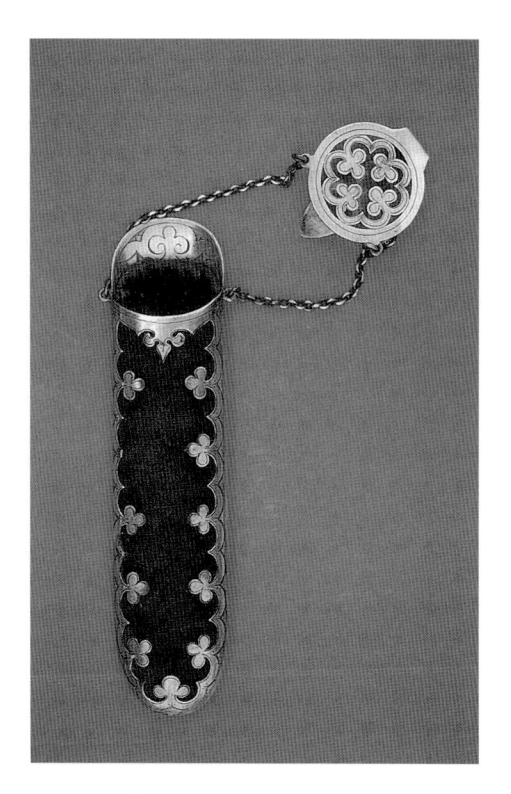

Figure 660. Velvet and steel chatelaine case.

Occasionally, we see half-sized chatelaine cases designed for folding glasses (Figure 658). Other unusual types are filigree, silver-decorated leather cases with a frog-mouth cover, and shagreen examples with silver accoutrements (Figures 659 & 660). Illustrated in author Hugh Orr's book are chatelaine eyeglass cases that Orr has collected.[3]

Conclusion

After 1900, the chatelaine fad ceased. Women held their light pince-nez with spring chains in a case pinned on their dress, attached to a hairpin, or attached to a chain held behind the ear. Thus came the end of the era of chatelaine eyeglass cases, which lasted from 1400 to 1900.

Notes

1. Hugh Orr, *Illustrated History of Early Antique Spectacles* (England: The Greenford Press, 1985), 37, 56, 63, 81.
2. Richard Corson, *Fashions in Eyeglasses* (London: Peter Owen Ltd., 1980), 25, 156.
3. Orr, op. cit.

33

Magnifying Glasses

Probably the world's original lens was a clear pebble taken from a stream bed. After being tumbled by the water, it acted as a magnifying glass. Other more sophisticated lenses made of glass or mineral followed and were used for magnifying as well as for heating purposes. (Heat was used to start fires and to melt the figures on wax writing tablets.) These lenses were finally put into frames and were later finished with handles so that they could be used more easily.

Lenses

Early magnifying lenses were not of a glass quality high in clarity and color (Figure 661). To avoid distortion, grinding was even all the way out to the edges. This is difficult to accomplish, especially in larger lenses, as spherical and chromatic aberrations must be avoided. Unfortunately, these errors are not addressed in some of the modern molded plastic lenses.

Lens strength determines the amount of magnification with these simple lenses, unlike with a telescopic device or other compound lens system. Ordinarily, a two- to ten-diopter lens is used, as it gives the most practical magnification to focal length ratio. When stronger lenses are used (10 to 20 diopters), the focal length is impractically short.

The diameter of magnifying lenses is also of interest (Figures 662 & 663). While large lenses of six inches or so are occasionally useful, those with a diameter of 1 ½ to 2 inches are the most practical. Reasons for this are the normal viewing area desired, the lighter weight of the lens, and the smaller space needed for occupancy on a desk (Figure 664). Smaller size lenses are also used for pocket magnifiers (Figure 665). These are sometimes found with protective outside cases that might hold several lenses of varying strengths.

Rims

Rims afford support as well as a guard (Figure 662) to protect the glass from excessive scratches from the desktop, etc. The most common rim is made of metal, but earlier rims were made of wood, horn, and shell. Some glasses have no frames at all and are exposed to excessive breakage.

Covers

A practical way to protect the glass of pocket magnifiers is with a cover that folds over the lens (Figure 666). Many designs are available. Mostly, the lenses in their rims simply rotated in and out of their protective cases and were held in by friction or gravity. Materials used for these covers varied. In Nuremberg in the 1700s, cases were carved of wood (Figure 661). Later, steel covers and alloy metals were used. Tortoiseshell and mother-of-pearl graced the covers of magnifying glasses for those who could afford these niceties (Figure 667). For the

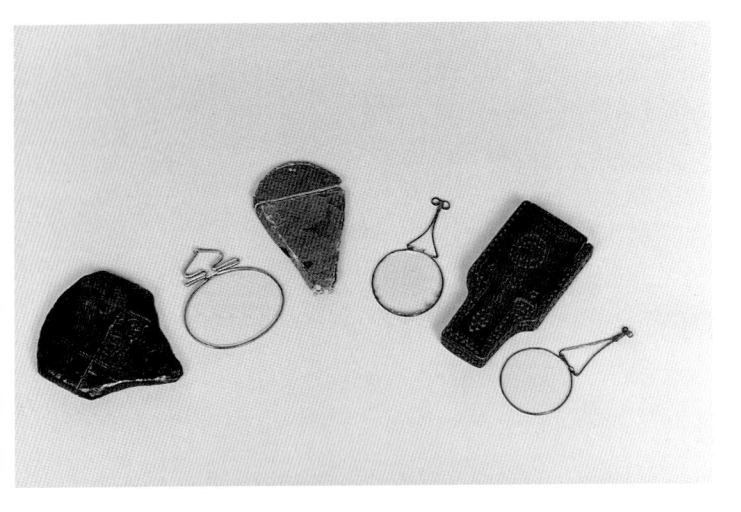

Figure 661. Various Nuremberg type of magnifiers and cases.

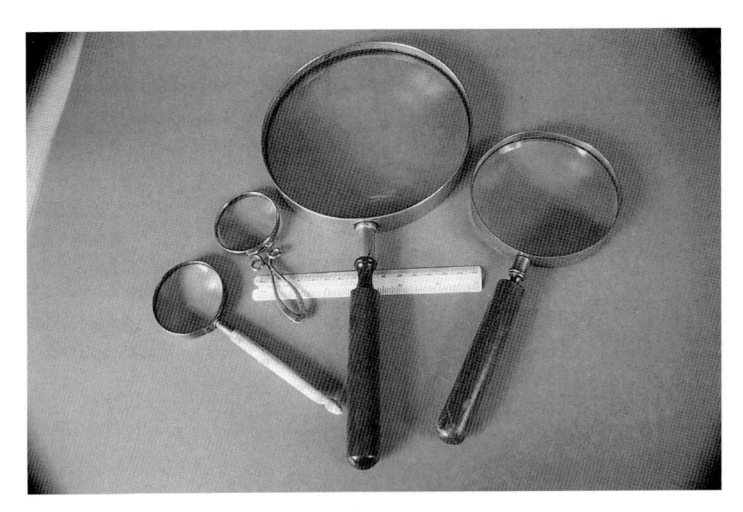

Figure 662. Various sizes of hand magnifiers.

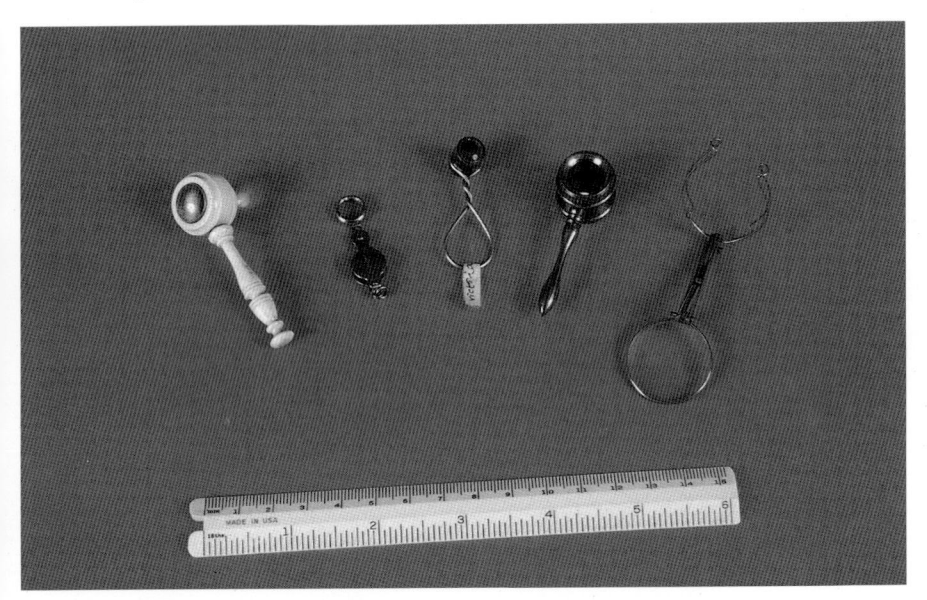

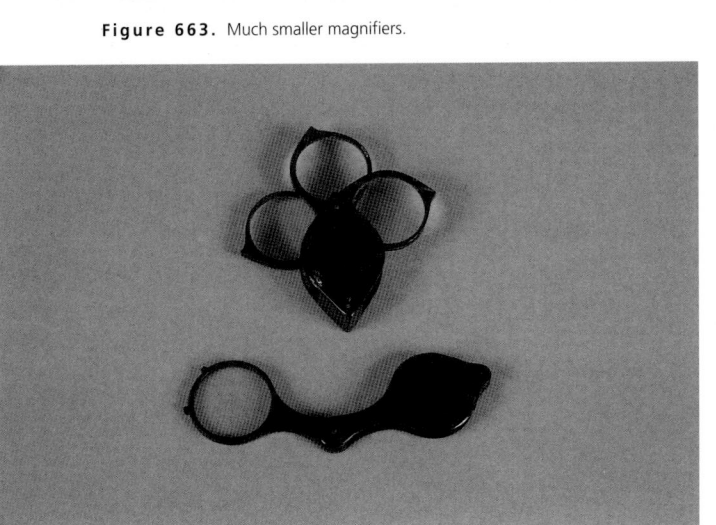

Figure 663. Much smaller magnifiers.

Figure 664. Combination letter opener and magnifying glass.

Figure 665. Tortoiseshell cased and rimmed pocket magnifiers.

MAGNIFYING GLASSES 339

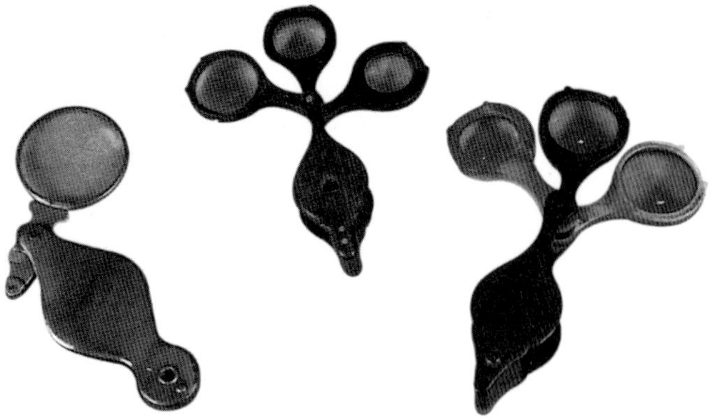

Figure 666. Horn and metal cased and rimmed pocket magnifiers—note glass cutter and breaker on metal example.

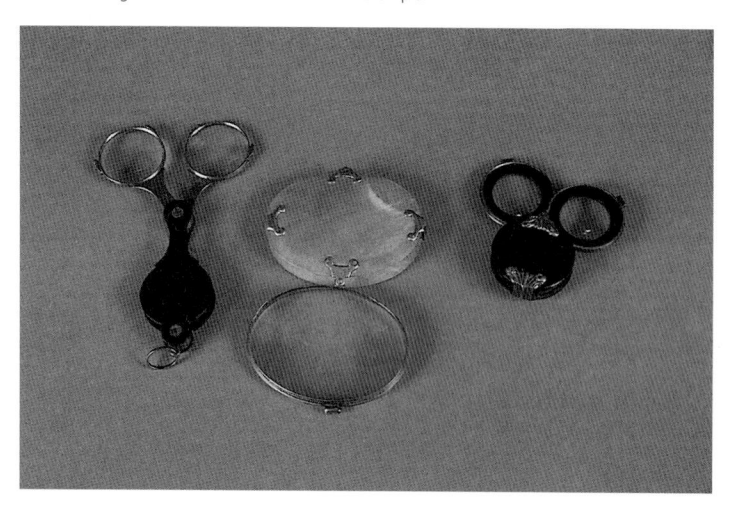

Figure 667. Magnifiers of tortoiseshell and gold, silver and mother-of-pearl, tortoiseshell and silver.

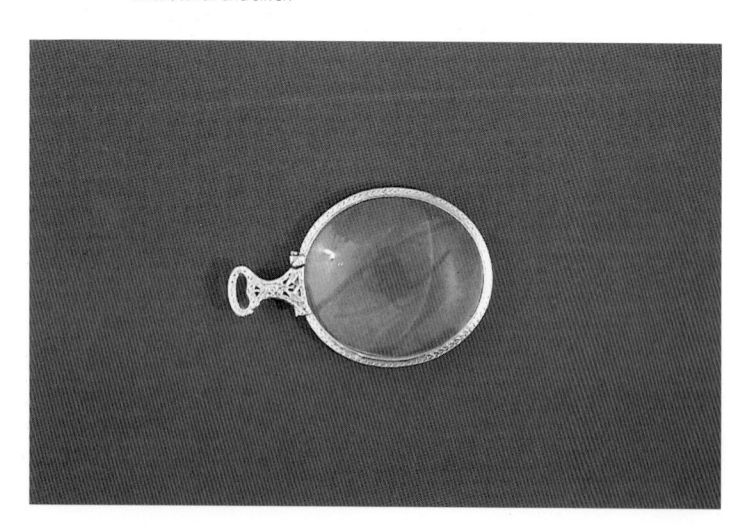

more usual varieties, gold, silver, and brass were employed, as well as hard rubber and plastic.

Another form of protection for the lenses was slip cases (Figure 661). These cases were employed with covers of leather or shagreen-covered wood or cardboard. Some had snap tabs to hold them closed.

Handles

Whereas the original handle material (wood) was continuous with that of the frame, wooden handles were also used with metal frames (Figure 662). Bone and ivory were other materials used to fashion handles (Figure 663), as was metal, as seen in older and more modern pieces.

Decoration

Some magnifying glasses were hung from a cord or chain from the neck (Figure 668), while others were merely left on the desk or vanity top. The decoration of these vision aids varied. Stones, both real and simulated, have been used to augment the decor of some women's magnifying glasses (Figure 669). Additionally, fancy metal frames have been designed as both a practical and a decorative adjunct. Not only were the cases for the well-made cased magnifiers of the late 1700s made of fine polished tortoiseshell and mother-of-pearl, but also they were banded with silver, with decorative silver supports, escutcheons, and pins.

Special Purposes

Adaptation of magnification for the use of scientists in such fields as astronomy and microbiology is well known. However adaptation of a simple lens for similar purposes may not be so widely realized. Consider the stamp collector's lens (Figures 670 & 671), the jeweler's lens (Figure 672), or the multiple lenses designed as low-vision aids (Figure 673). All of these have been gratefully used for quite some time, and surely others will appear in proper order.

Figure 668. White gold magnifier with diamonds for neckwear.

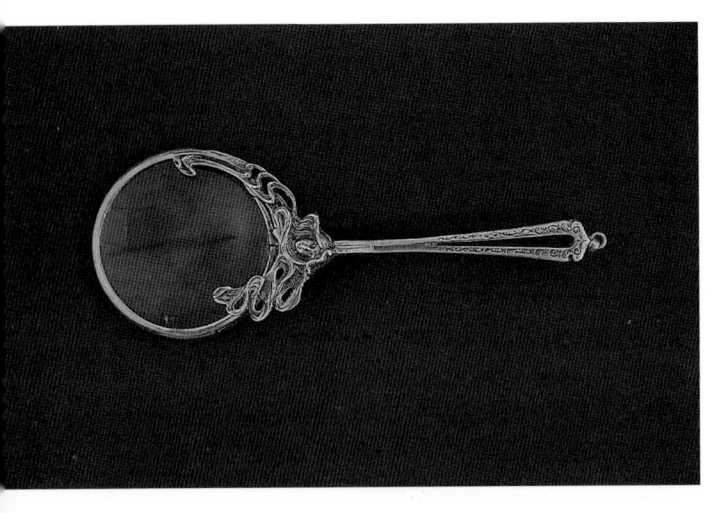

Figure 669. Woman's fancy magnifying glass.

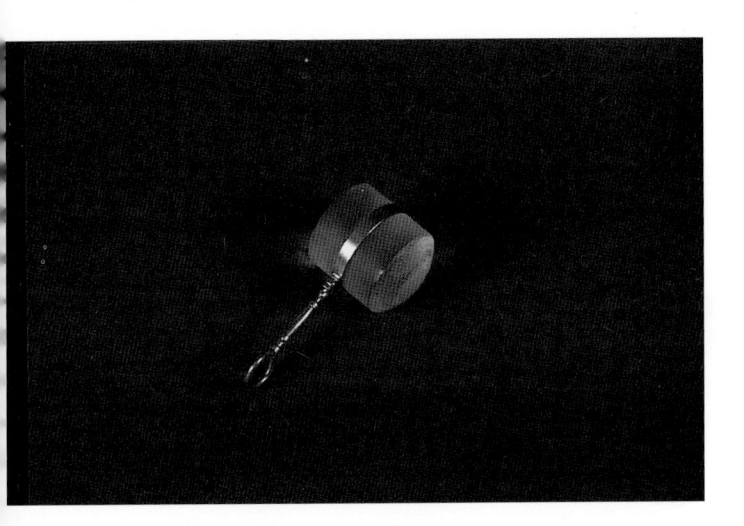

Figures 670 & 671. Stamp-viewing lenses.

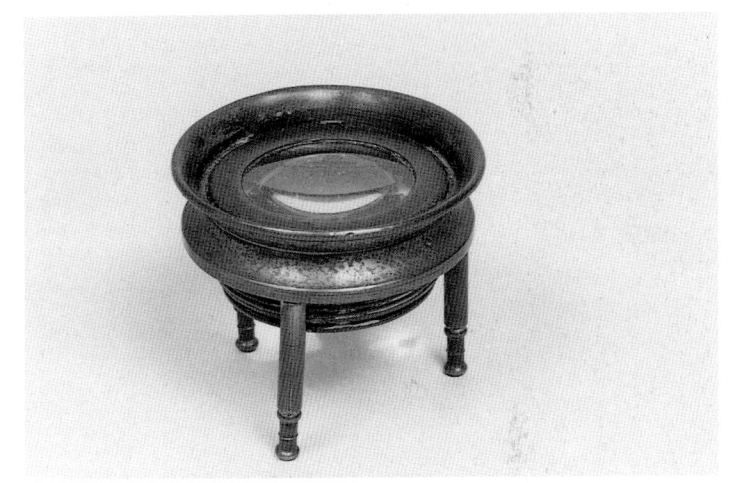

Figure 671.

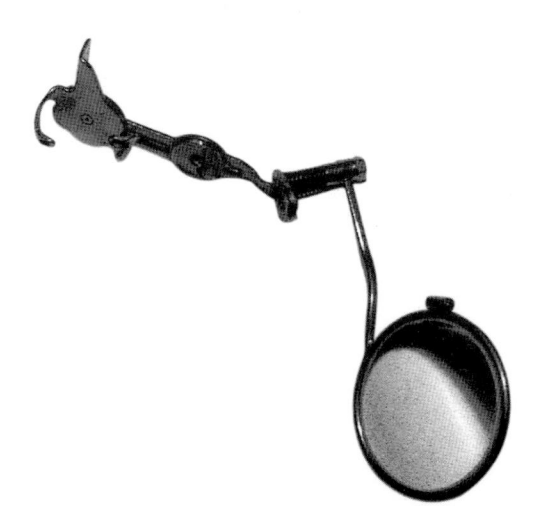

Figure 672. Jeweler's lens.

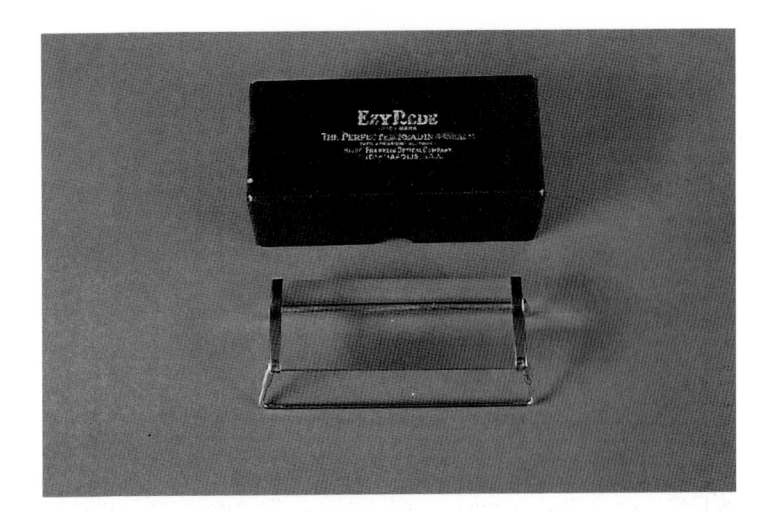

Figure 673. Low-vision aid.

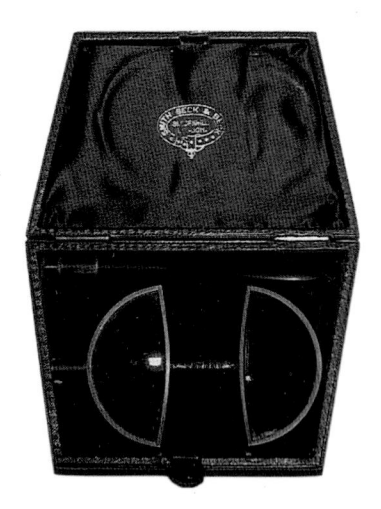

Figure 674. Binocular magnifier in case.

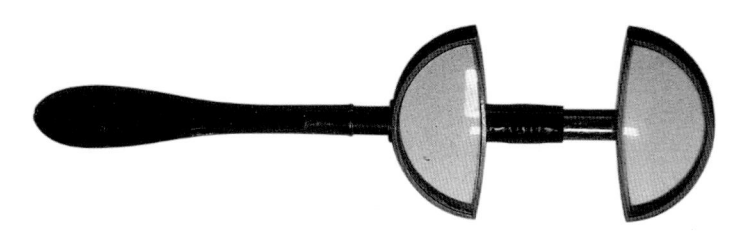

Figure 675. Binocular magnifier assembled.

Binocular Magnifiers

Another variation in handheld lenses is the binocular magnifier (Figures 674 & 675). Two lenses are connected by a small bar, and the pupillary distances are adjustable. A handle is connected to the outside of one of the lenses. Stands were available as well. Richard Beck described this arrangement of lenses in *A Treatise on the Construction, Proper Use, and Capabilities of Smith, Beck, and Beck's Achromatic Microscopes*, from which the following is an excerpt.

THE PATENT ACHROMATIC BINOCULAR MAGNIFIERS

The great advantage secured by this arrangement of lenses is the employment of both eyes when using a magnifying power which, with an ordinary lens, would confine the observer to the use of one eye only.

Under these binocular magnifiers the object retains its natural or, as it is sometimes termed, stereoscopic appearance; the light, upon which definition mainly depends, is doubled; the magnifying power is apparently much increased; and the binocular lens will, as a rule, give a better result than a single one of double the magnifying power, without bringing any strain whatever upon the eyes.

There are generally three sizes, the foci of which are 7, 5, and 3 inches, which also have another advantage, in addition to those already enumerated, in being achromatic.

Directions for Use   The lenses are plano-convex, and when in use the flat sides should always be placed next to the eyes; and the mounting is so contrived that this may be done when the magnifiers are held in either hand.

As the distances of the eyes in different persons vary considerably, these lenses have a sliding fitting, by which the proper amount of separation may be obtained; the correct distance is easily determined by experiment; but, as a general rule, if a flat object appears convex, the lenses are too near together; or when too far apart, the same surface will appear concave—the right distance being somewhere between.

It will be found by many, and especially those who have been accustomed to make constant use of a single lens, that these binocular magnifiers require at first some rather careful adjustment in holding them; for, besides the alteration of distance already described, the eyes must be directed

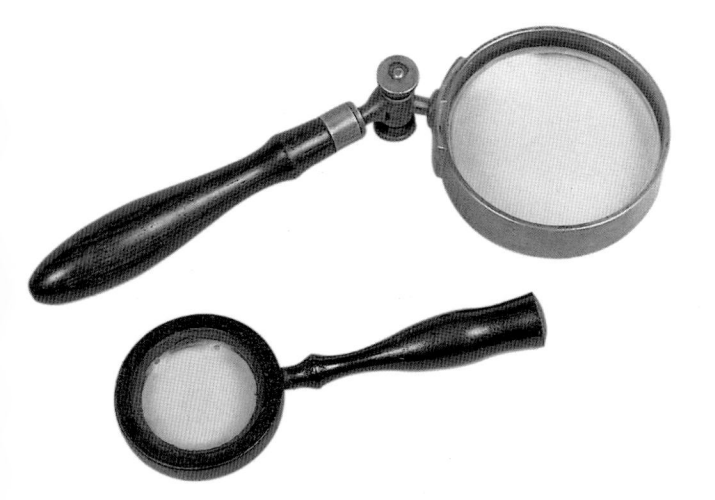

Figure 676. Above: Adjustable angle magnifier. English, circa 1900. Below: Wood magnifier, circa 1780.

vertically, upon the flat surfaces of the lenses; and each eye should see the object clearly defined. The former may be tested by slightly altering the position of the lenses, and watching whether the definition improve or otherwise; the latter by shutting each eye alternately, without moving the head or the magnifier.[1]

Conclusion

Looking back on the "dawn of lenses", and following this simple magnifier to its present sophistication, we appreciate the ability of man to adapt to its varying degrees of need and existence (Figure 676).

Notes

1. Richard Beck, *A Treatise on the Construction, Proper Use, and Capabilities of Smith, Beck, and Beck's Achromatic Microscopes.* (London: John Van Voorst, Paternoster Row Pub., circa 1865).

34

Votive Offerings

Votive offerings, also known as ex votos or (in the case of eyes) St. Lucy medals, date from before the coming of Christ. They can still be purchased today.

Found mostly in southern Europe (Italy, Greece, Spain, Portugal), these religious icons were made in the shape of the organ to be cured. Eye conditions (Figure 677), heart disease, paralysis, and many other afflictions are addressed by these offerings which are called upon by faithful believers for healing. These figures were usually pressed into a flat piece of metal (tin, brass, silver, or gold) and attached to the doorposts of the individual's home, to a wall inside a church, or near a shrine of an appropriate saint. Many people know of the shrine at Lourdes (France) or the shrine of St. Ann de Beaupre (north of Quebec City, Canada), as well as others in various parts of the world. However, Catholicism is not alone in using shrines as exhibits to the power of faith. Eastern countries and religions participate in like activities.

When an individual was cured of an illness and wished to use the ex voto as an expression of gratitude, the metal was embossed with the letters PGR (*per grazia ricevuta*)—meaning "for a grace received," or VFG (*voto fatto grazie*)—meaning "thanks for a vow realized."

One can imagine the style of these artifacts being examples of the usual decoration of the country (Figure 678). Italian types are very flamboyant, with long rococo blandishments around the oval edges. German and Flemish are usually more reserved, the former usually being oval, and the latter mostly rectangular. All of these, however, are very interesting and constitute a minicollection of their own.

Today, we do not find ex votos exhibited, as those that were fancy and expensive have largely been stolen. Since those recently produced are available, a collector who spots one in an antiques shop should be wary of the age, condition, and price.

In recent years, the author purchased a flat silver medal representing eyes, about an inch long and in the shape of a number eight on its side. A small ring was attached so that it could be hung around the neck, on a bracelet, or on an appropriate nail (Figure 678, below).

St. Lucia

Another form of votive offering is the St. Lucy medal. St. Lucia is the principal Catholic representative of the patron saint of eyes. Others have been so considered because of their pictorial representation of ocular-associated symbols. St. Lucia, however, at least in the United States, is considered the primary saint for the guardianship of vision (Figure 679). Following are three versions of her legend.

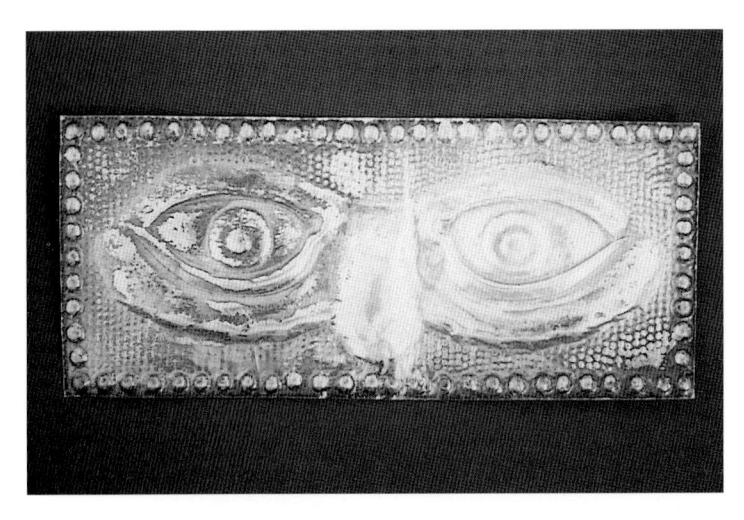

Figure 677. Silver ex voto of eyes.

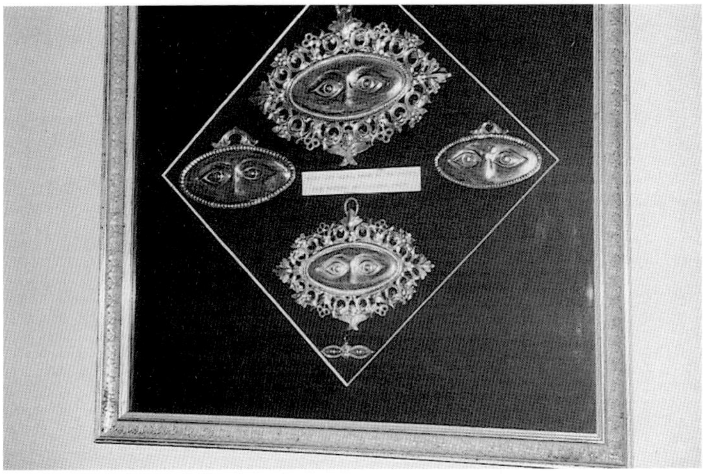

Figure 678. Frame holding a variety of ex votos; note small medal below.

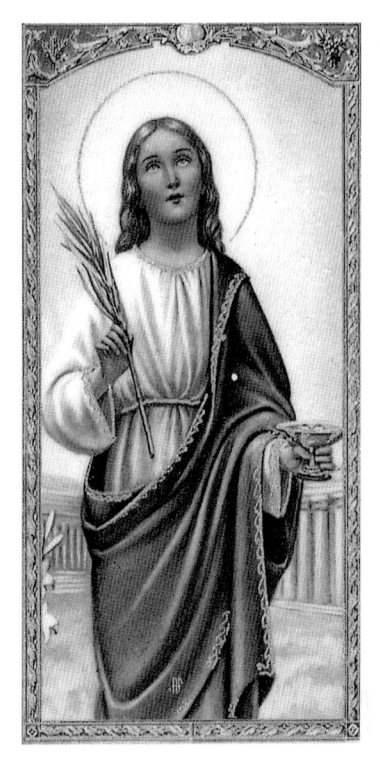

Figure 679. Artist's rendering of St. Lucy.

As found in *The Dioptic Review*.

St. Lucia, patron saint of the labouring poor and guardian against all diseases of the eye, lived in the fourth century A.D. Some early painters sought to express her name, Lucia, light, by depicting her with an eye or eyes on a plate in her hand. This gave rise to an explanatory legend. It was said that her lover had so greatly admired her beautiful eyes that she felt it was a sin. The legend continues, "considering these things and calling to mind the words of Christ, 'If thine eye offend thee, pluck it out and cast it from thee,' and fearing lest her eyes should be the cause of damnation to the young man, she called for a knife and took out her eyes and sent them to her lover in a dish with these words: 'Here hast thou what thou so much desired.' Whereat the young man being utterly astonished and full of grief and remorse became also a convert to Christ. God would not suffer that the blessed Lucia, having given proof of her courage and piety, should remain blind, for one day, as she knelt in prayer, her eyes were restored to her more beautiful than before. And this is the reason that St. Lucia is invoked against blindness and all diseases of the eyes, and that in art she is represented bearing her eyes in a dish."[1]

As found in an article from the *Benedictine Convent of Perpetual Adoration*:

> St. Lucy, whose beautiful name signifies light, was one of the great martyr-virgins of the early Church. Born of a noble and wealthy family in Syracuse, Sicily, towards the end of the third century, she early dedicated her virginity to God. A young nobleman, to whom Lucy's mother had promised her hand, accused her of being a Christian when she distributed all her wealth to the poor. Being brought to the governor, and refusing to sacrifice to the pagan idols, she was miraculously protected, first when attempts were made to violate her chastity, and later to burn her. She was at length put to death by sword. . . . Legend says her eyes were gouged out in her martyrdom and later miraculously restored, more beautiful than before. She has long been invoked as a patroness by those suffering from eye trouble. Her feast is kept on December 13th.[2]

As found in the July 1994 *Newsletter* of The Ophthalmic Antiques International Collectors' Club:

> Saint Lucia was a Sicilian, born of noble and wealthy parents in Syracuse and brought up in the faith of Christ. She lost her father in infancy, and was still young when she offered her virginity to God. This vow, however, she kept a secret, and her mother, Eutychia, pressed her to marry a suitor who was a pagan. Eutychia was persuaded by her daughter to go to Catania and offer up prayers to God at the tomb of St. Agatha for relief of a hemorrhage from which she suffered. Lucia accompanied her, and their prayers were answered. Then the saint disclosed her desire of devoting herself to God and bestowing her fortune on the poor, and Eutychia in her gratitude left her at liberty to pursue her inclinations. Her suitor accused her before the prefect of the town, Paschasius, as a Christian, the persecution of Diocletian then being at its height. When Lucia remained resolute, Paschasius commanded her to be exposed to prostitution in a brothel; but God rendered her immovable, so that the guards were not able to carry her thither. Then an attempt was made to burn her, but although oil and resin were poured on the fire of execution, she remained unscathed and even when a poniard or sword was buried in her neck (another source suggests her heart although her emblem usually shows her holding two eyes on a plate and often with a sword through her neck), she lived long enough to receive Holy Communion for the last time, at the age of twenty.
>
> Her usual emblem, her eyes, (possibly on account of her name, which is supposed to be suggestive of "light" or "lucidity") were reputed to have been torn out in various ways, but always miraculously restored. As a result she was often invoked during the middle ages by those who suffered from eye trouble.[3]

This author's personal example of St. Lucia is in the form of a wooden carving, 11 inches in height, with beautiful coloring (Figure 680). The carving is finished with a halo of light beams of metal (aluminum), which attaches to the head with a post that occupies a small recess. St. Lucia stands with her left hand holding the plate with two eyes. Her right hand has a recess, which no doubt formerly held an object (? knife), unfortunately now lost. Compare this with the description from *The Dioptic Review*.

St. Odilia

Sharing the same feast day with St. Lucy (December 13) is St. Odilia, who also is considered by some to be the patron saint of vision. Following is an account of her legend as found in the October 1994 newsletter of The Ophthalmic Antiques International Collectors' Club:

> Saint Odilia, the patron saint of Alsace and Strasbourg, was according to legend the daughter of Adalric, Duke of Alsace. She was born blind and for this reason was hated by her father and left to die. Her faithful nurse fled with her to the convent of Baumeles-Dames, near Besancon, where she was baptized by Saint Erhard, then Bishop of Bavaria, and immediately gained her sight.
>
> Subsequently she was reconciled with her father, and later founded the convents of Hohenburg (modern Odilienburg/Mont Sainte-Odile), and Niedermunster, in the Vosges Mountains, under the Benedictine rule.
>
> In recent times, an abbey has been founded by a new Benedictine congregation at Sankt Ottilien, between Munich and Augsburg.

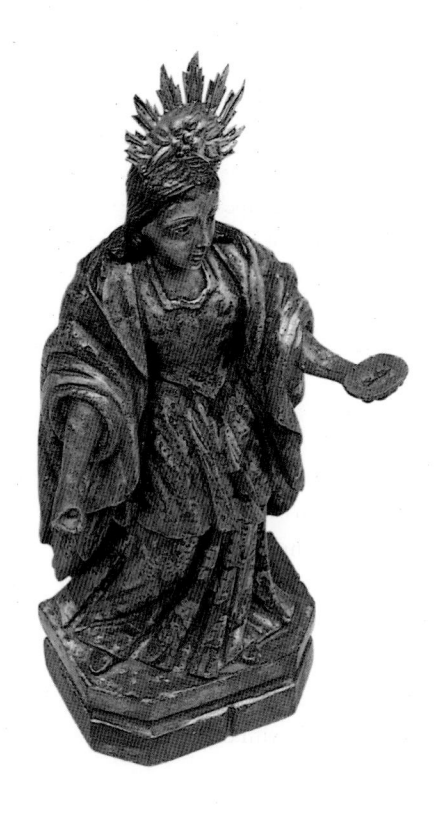

Figure 680. Wooden carving of St. Lucy—Brazilian.

Bogus prophecies attributed to her were circulating in France during World War II, whilst one of the many commemoration medals struck bears on its face a representation of Saint Odile.

She also gave her name to the Guild of St. Odilia (Consulting Opticians) early this century.

She shares the same feast day, 13th December, as Saint Lucy, while her shrine at Odilienburg became a celebrated place of pilgrimage, which is still resorted to by those afflicted with blindness or eye disease.[4]

St. Herve (6th Century)

Popular in Brittany, St. Herve was born blind, deserted by his father, and given to a holy man by his mother at age seven. He worked in a monastery and was credited with several miracles. He founded a monastry in Lanhouarneau.[5]

St. Raphael, Archangel

Saint Raphael, one of the seven Archangels, was sent by God to minister to old Tobit, who was blind. His feast day is September 29.

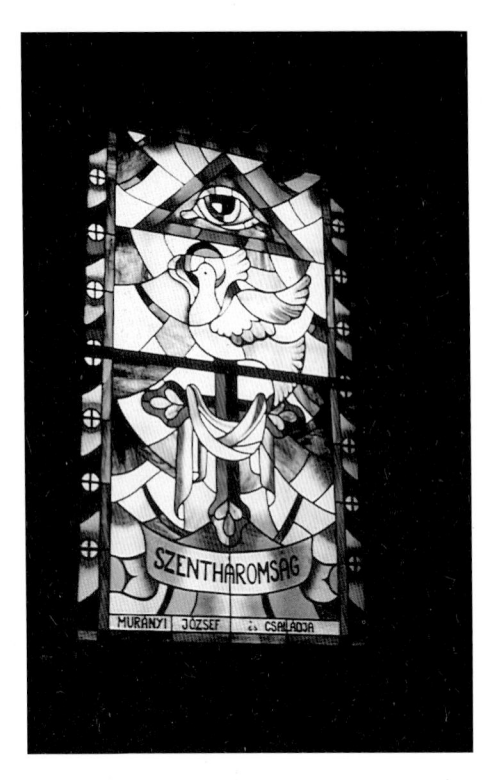

Figure 681. Picture of a modern stained glass window in a Polish church; note the eye above, which represents the all-seeing eye of the Lord.

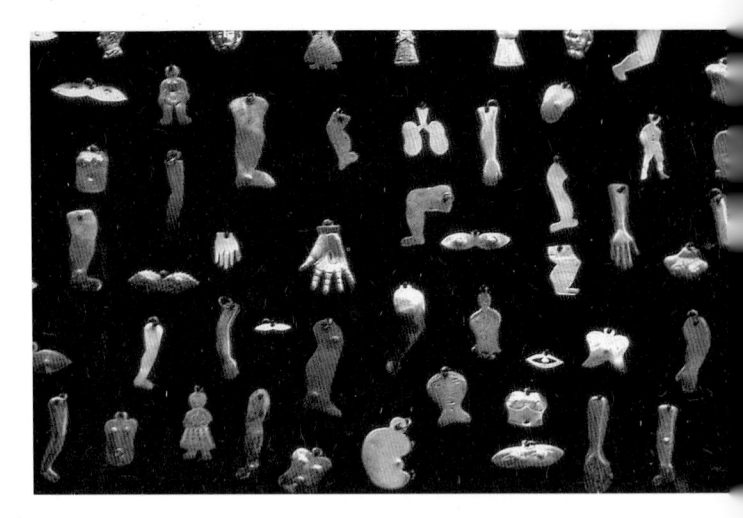

Figure 682. Votive offerings at the Cristo Chapel in San Juan, Puerto Rico.

St. Walburga

Though no information regarding his sainthood is readily available, St. Walburga is also named as an optical patron saint.

St. Audomarus

Another optical patron saint, St. Audomarus died circa 669 in Omar, France. His feast day is September 9.

Conclusion

It is interesting to note the number of articles beautifully crafted by artisans over a period of hundreds or thousands of years, not for personal adornment but as offerings to "higher beings." The advantage of these spiritual offerings was that they not only gave emotional relief to the individual and melded their relationship with the church but also gave purpose to the family in helping their afflicted kin (Figures 681 & 682).

Notes

1. *The Dioptic Review*, April 1931.
2. *Benedictine Convent of Perpetual Adoration*, article S43.
3. *The Ophthalmic Antiques International Collectors' Club Newsletter*, July 1994.
4. John Dixon Salt, "Optical Patron Saints," *The Ophthalmic Antiques International Collectors' Club Newsletter*, October 1994.
5. Ibid.

Other Sources Consulted for Chapter 34

1. *Bulter's Lives of Saints*, Vol. II.
2. V. Tabacchi et al, *Il Museo dell'occhiale* (at Pieve di Cadore, Belluno) (Milan: Del Gruppo Editoriale Fabbri, 1990), 197.
3. Ibid.
4. Delaney and Tobin, *Dictionary of Catholic Biography*
5. Andrew Ferry, "Vignette," *Argus* (San Francisco, 1990).
6. La Lente, *Collection of Fritz Rathschuller*, (Genova: Edizioni Culturali Internazionali Genova, 1988), 180–185.
7. Pierre Marley, *Spectacles and Spyglasses* (Paris: Hoebeke,, 1988).

35

Miniatures

As with many articles of manufacture, miniatures have been made of spectacles. They have been designed for a variety of purposes (Figure 683).

Guild Applicants' Miniatures

The collector will occasionally come across a very detailed miniature—one made as an exactly scaled replica of a normal-size spectacle or pince-nez. These were made by journeymen applicants to the spectacle makers guild and were part of the admission examination. The author has in his collection a fine miniature of a 1935-era rimless spectacle (Figure 683, left, second from below).

Jewelry

Other miniatures were designed into jewelry articles, some with utilitarian purposes and some simply for adornment (Figure 684). Women who use glasses for close work and who frequently put them aside are prone to use decorative pins in the shape of spectacles to hang their regular-size vision aids from their clothing (Figure 685). Occasionally, the pins are made of base metal with colored glass and sometimes are even embellished with marcasite. Other optically shaped jewelry articles found are tie tacks (Figure 686) and tie clasps (or bars) for men and metal plaques depicting vision aids of various kinds (Figure 687). Women sometimes use these as charms hanging from a neck chain or bracelet. Gold charms in the shape of spectacles (Figures 688 & 689), pince-nez, opera glasses, and even spectacles inside a case have been designed (Figure 690). Some are available in other metals such as silver. Mostly, these are well-made and indicate the optical bent of the wearer.

Stanhopes

These miniature glass cylinders, high convex on one end and with a small (2 × 2 millimeters) picture on the flat far end, are set in many forms for adornment, advertisement, and fun. One type is that of ophthalmic miniatures. Illustrated are binoculars in metal, ivory, and plastic, and a monocular, furnished with a bail to fasten to a cord or chain (Figures 691, 692 & 693).

The Evil Eye

Many variations of the Mediterranean "evil eye" are available—mostly made of glass (Figure 694). Usually, the eye is white with a blue iris and a large black central pupil. Some are hardly a centimeter in diameter, while others are several centimeters across. Bails for attachment of these to bracelets, key rings, etc., are provided. Small plastic spectacles without lenses have also been attached to key rings for adornment as well as for advertising (Figure 683, below, left).

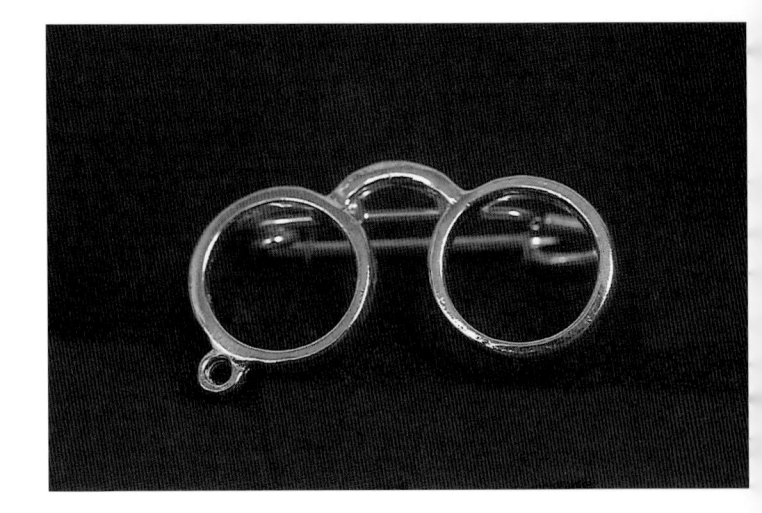

Figure 684. Gold miniature spectacle pin.

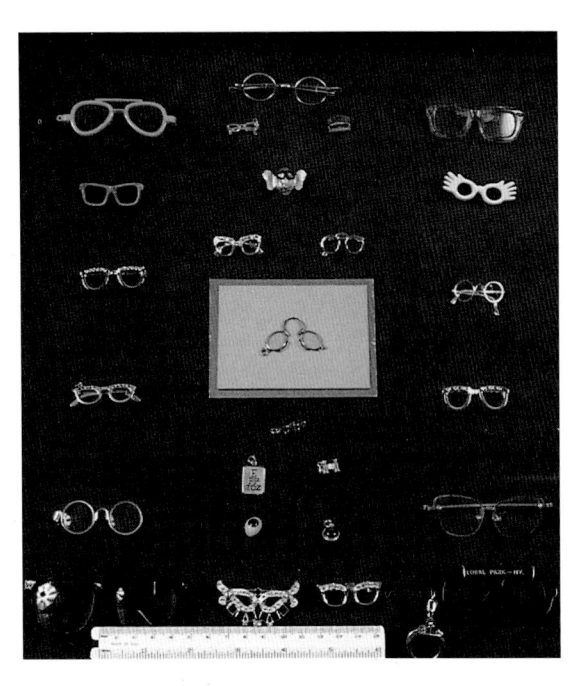

Figure 683. Collection of ophthalmic miniatures.

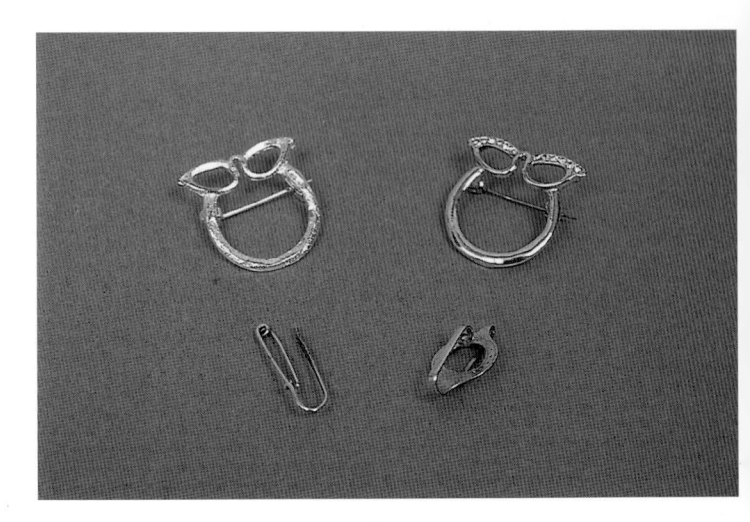

Figure 685. Group of pins for women to hang spectacles. Modern above; circa 1890 below.

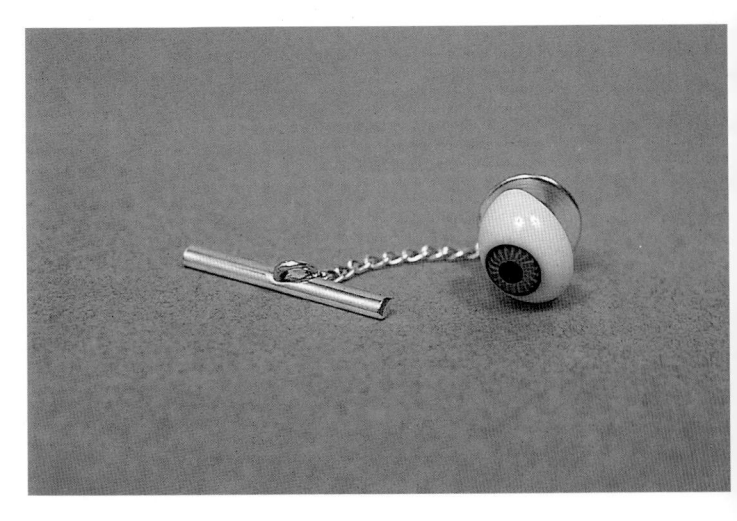

Figure 686. Man's tie tack of a porcelain miniature eye.

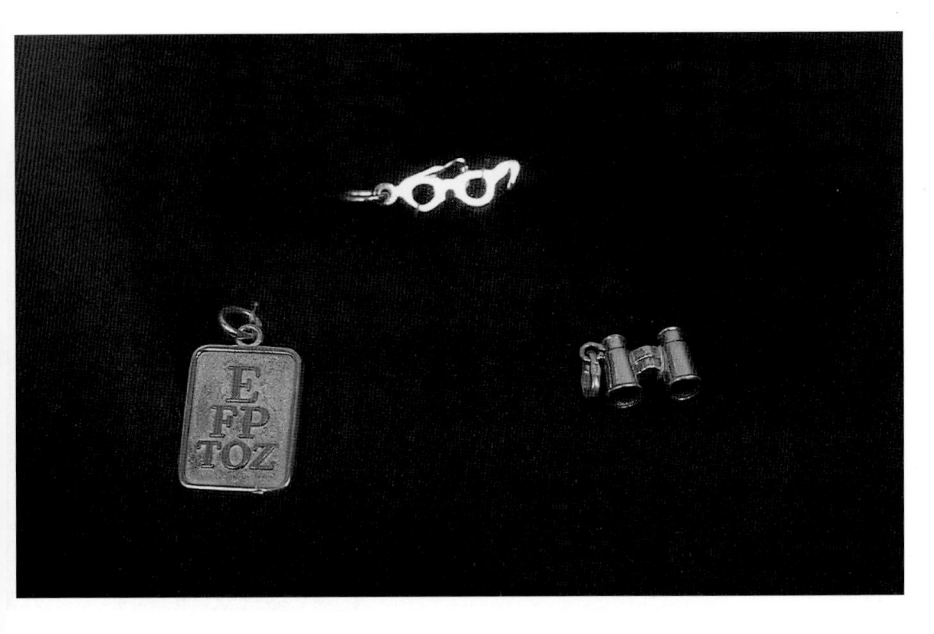

Figure 687. Spectacles, opera glasses, and eye chart in gold charms.

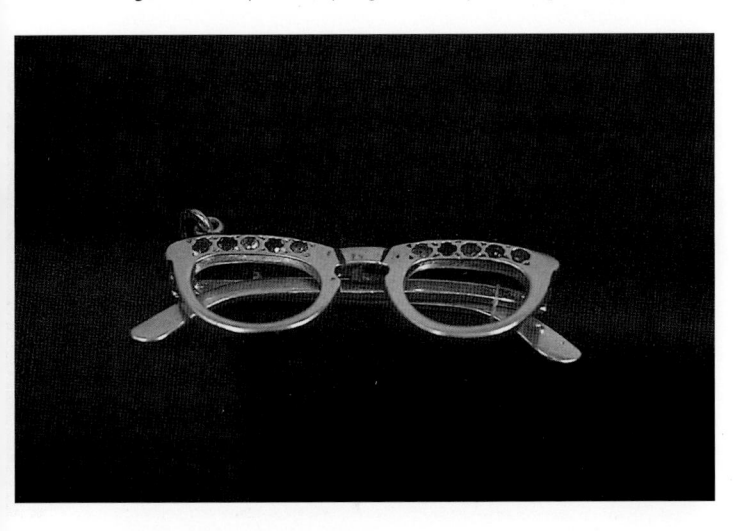

Figure 688. Miniature spectacles used as a charm.

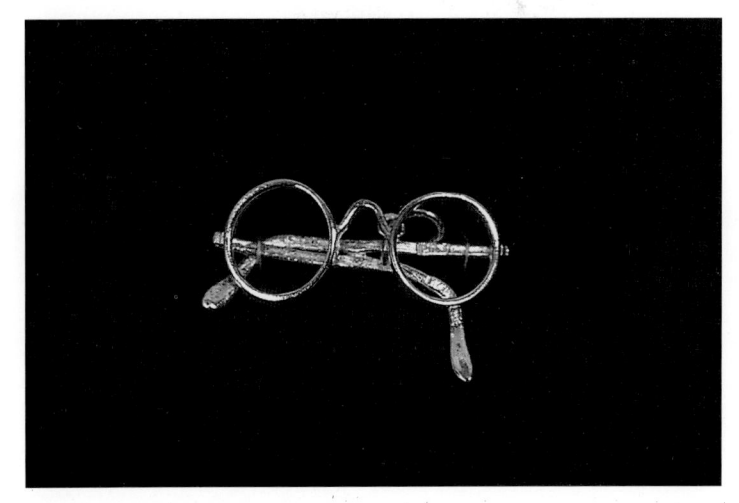

Figure 689. Miniature spectacles used as a charm.

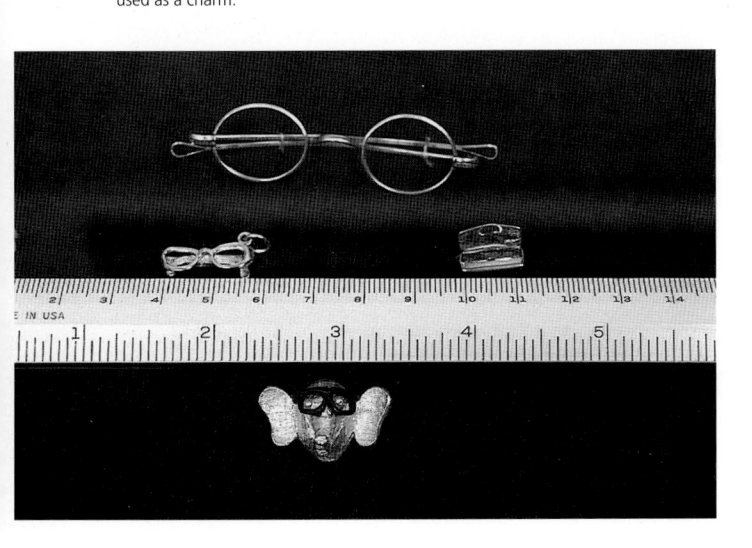

Figure 690. Additional gold charms.

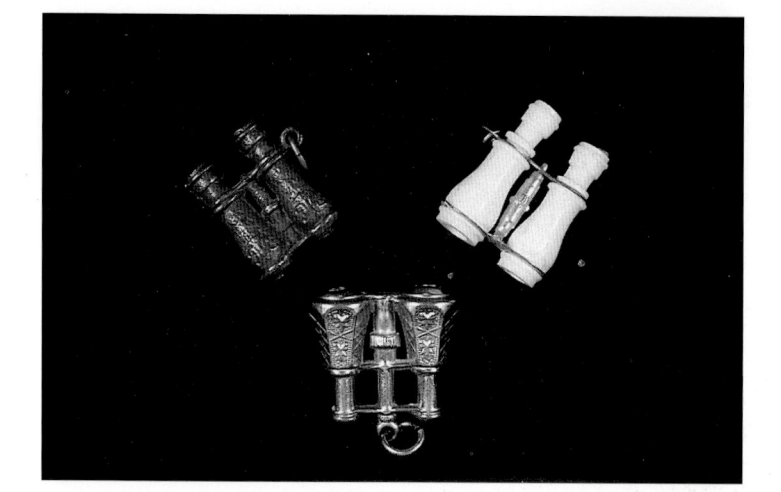

Figure 691. Two cast metal and one plastic binocular Stanhopes, courtesy John Tull, M.D.

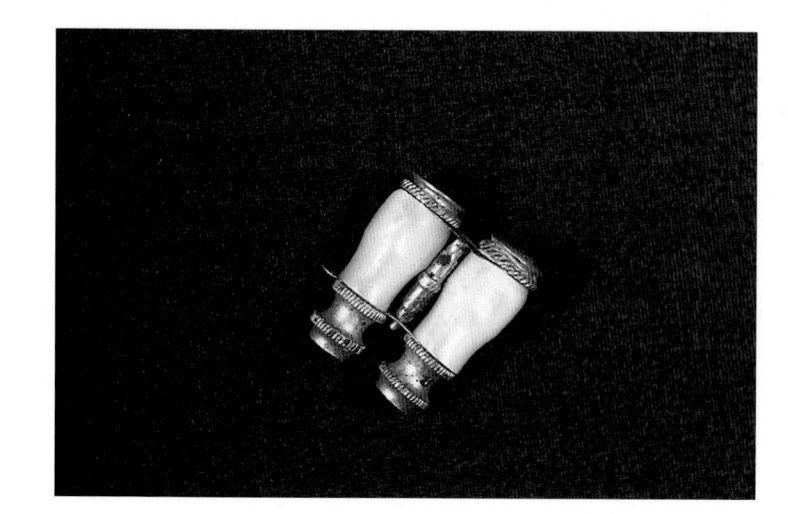

Figure 692. Fully detailed gold and ivory binocular Stanhope, courtesy John Tull, M.D.

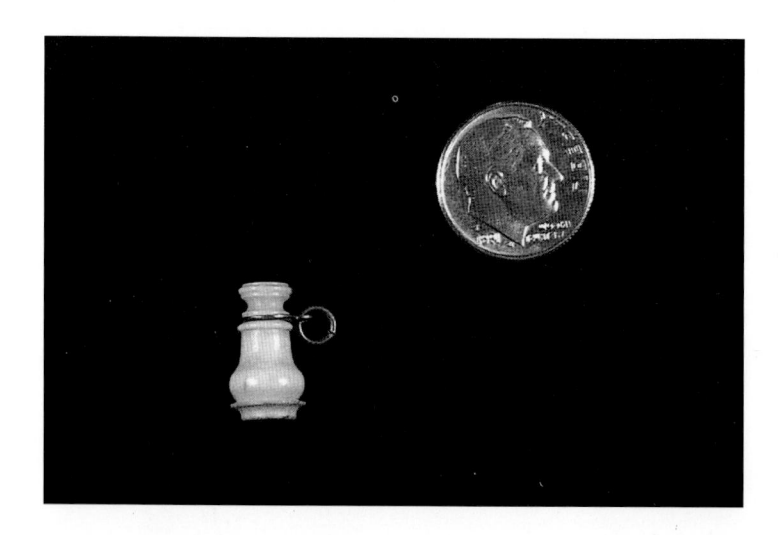

Figure 693. Ivory monocular with Stanhope, courtesy John Tull, M.D.

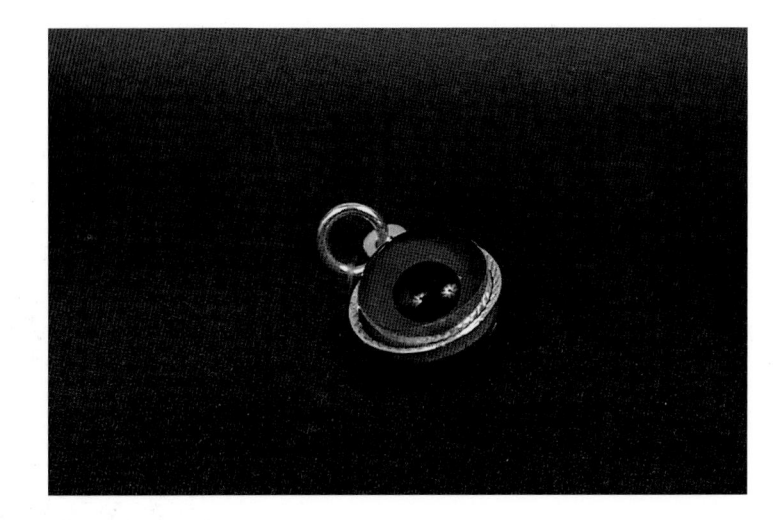

Figure 694. One type of "evil eye"—glass set in bezel with bail.

Variations

Miniature spectacles have also been made for rather unusual purposes. One such is to adorn dolls of various sizes and ages. The author has in his collection two bisque dolls, each only four inches tall and fitted with wire spectacles (Figure 695). Also, small spectacles have actually been designed for animals—much, surely, to their disgust, but to the delight of their indulged owners!

Conclusion

We see that miniatures were designed for many uses, from decoration to advertisement. Miniatures make up an interesting collection in their own right.

Sources Consulted for Chapter 35

1. J. Wm. Rosenthal, personal collection.

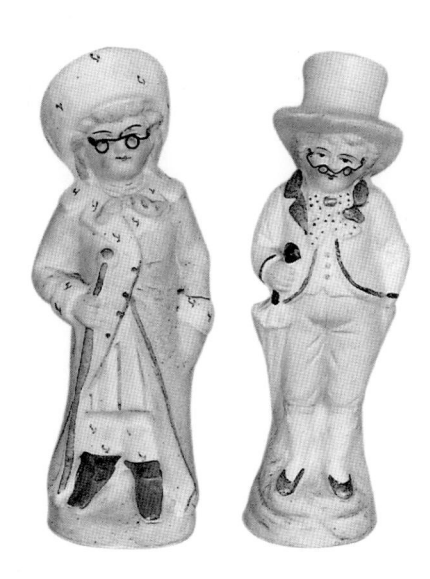

Figure 695. Four-inch tall bisque dolls, each fitted with wire spectacles.

36

Catalogs

Originating as broadsides, fliers, or posters, catalog advertisements were used by such luminaries as Benjamin Martin, Wollaston, and McAllister (Figure 696). In later years, as opticians became organized businesses with partners and workers, catalogs were printed as pamphlets. As whole optical companies or large distributors developed, illustrated catalogs were produced in book form (Figure 697).

Whereas catalogs do not usually pontificate optical theory, they do show the end result and practical application of advancement in ophthalmic learning and practice. Impractical inventions did not last from one catalog to the next. Demand took care of that.

Not only do catalogs allow us to establish when types of vision aids became available, but they also picture variations and styles of vision aids. These line drawings or prints many times solve an "unknown" that we uncover as a purchase. They also provide the original name, material, and price of many objects (Figure 698). Later catalogs (circa 1900 and following) were so large and expensive to publish that the company did not date them so that it could use them over a longer period of time. Such a tactic was expedient at the time but does not help the poor historian reading 50 to 100 years after publication.

As some of these catalogs are old, rare, and desired, their price rivals that of many academic tomes. They are therefore gratefully reserved in a separate section of any museum's library. They are, and should be, appreciated and cared for, not because of their commercial value or previous purpose but because their content opens a window to optical availability of the times covered.

Catalogs of Collections

Aside from commercial catalogs, there are those issued by museums, libraries, and owners of large ophthalmic collections. Such lists are surely a service to those of us who collect, who seek historical truths, and who need certain facts to help in these endeavors. We, in turn, use these facts to educate ourselves and others and broaden our knowledge.

Paralleling the publication of catalogs are books describing the manufacturing methods and optical theory of their time. Perhaps the first was *Uso de los Antoios* by Daca de Valdes (Figure 699). One book was published in Dresden in 1741 (Figure 700). Others, such as the *Le Lunetier-Opticien* (Figure 701) and *L'Art de L'Opticien* (Figure 702), were more of the how-to variety. They expounded the technical knowledge needed to produce spectacles, assured respect in the community, and enhanced the business of their authors.

The author's personal library's listing of catalogs follows and shows what can be collected at the present time.

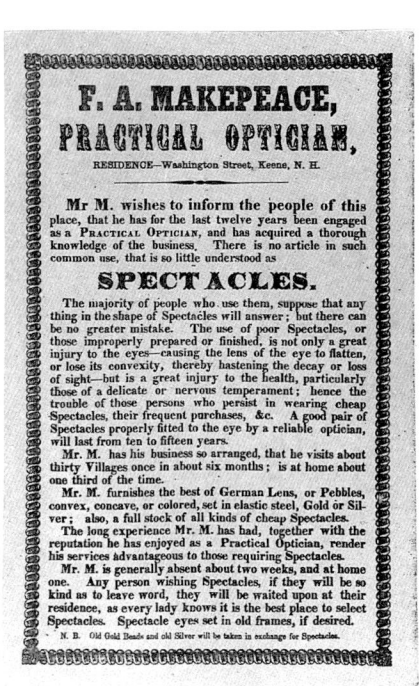

Figure 696. Flyer for F.A. Makepeace.

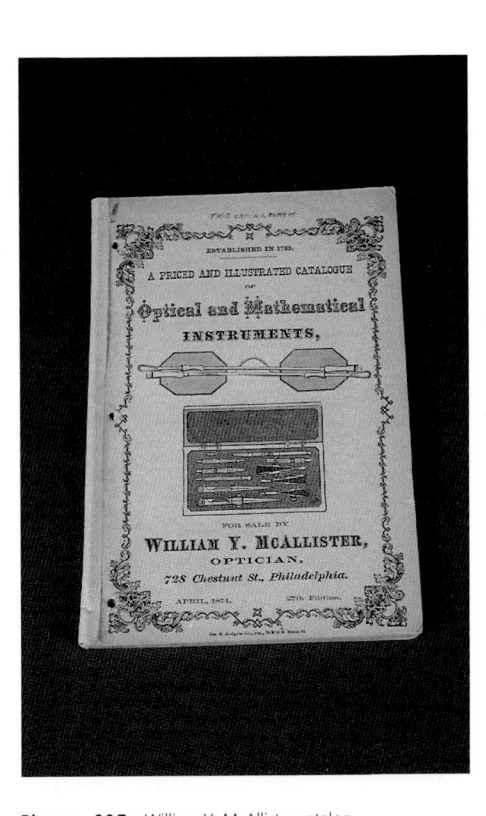

Figure 697. William Y. McAllister catalog, April 1891.

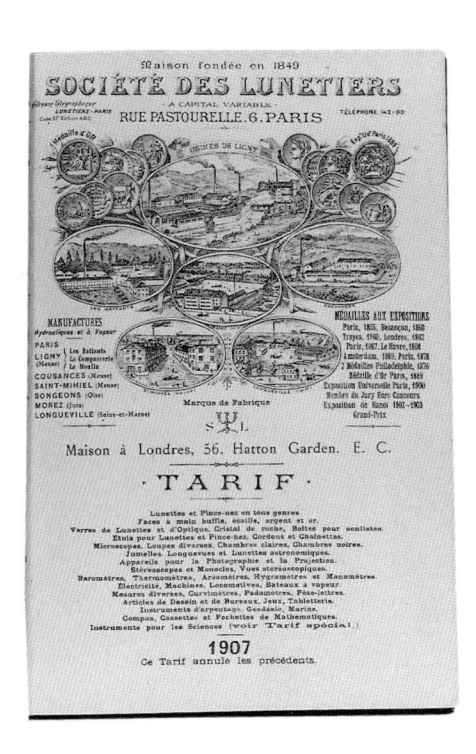

Figure 698. Catalog for the Société des Lunetiers.

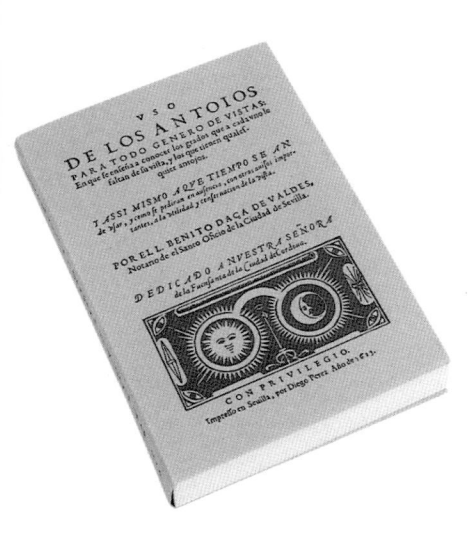

Figure 699. Daca de Valdes, *Uso de los Antoios* (Spain).

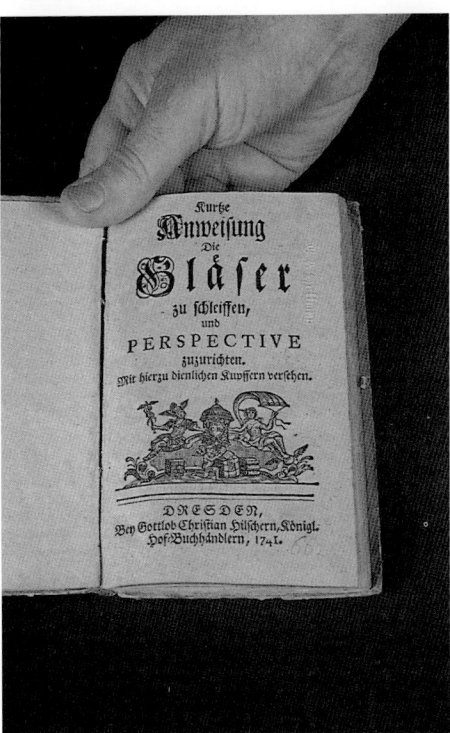

Figure 700. Dresden 1741.

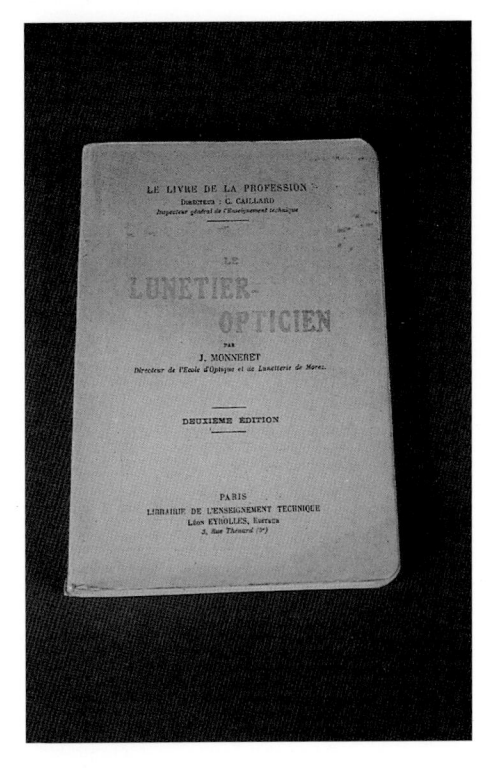

Figure 701. *Le Lunetier-Opticien*.

CATALOGS 355

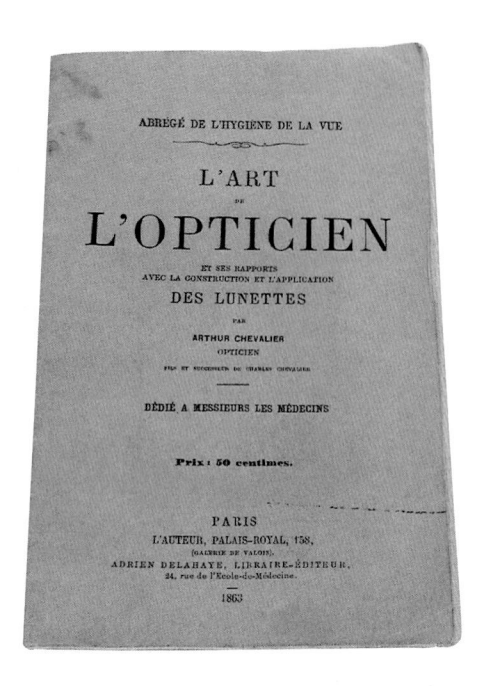

Figure 702. L' Art de l' Opticien, 1863.

List of Catalogs in Author's Collection

American Optical Company Catalog (Southbridge, MA, 1924).

American Optical Company Catalog, *Gold Spectacles*, August 1935.

American Optical Company Catalog, *Gold Filled Spectacles*, November 1935.

American Optical Company Catalog, *Zylonite Spectacles*, August 1935.

American Optical Company Catalog, *Wellsworth Eye Protectors and Sun Glasses* (Southbridge, MA, 1927).

American Optical Company Catalog, *Wellsworth Frames, Mountings, and Lenses* (Southbridge, MA, 1927).

American Optical Company Catalog, *Wellsworth Pair and Prescription Price List* (Southbridge, MA, 1928).

American Optical Company Catalog *Wellsworth Prescription Catalogue* (Southbridge, MA, 1923).

American Optical Company Catalog *Wellsworth Specialties* (Southbridge, MA, 1925).

Anglo-American Optical Company Catalog (London, circa 1900).

The Antiquarian Scientist, Catalog Twenty. .(Dracut, MA: R. V. Giordano.).

The Antique Trader (Dubuque, Iowa. May, 1972).

J. and W. E. Archbull Catalogue and Price List (London, 1884).

Bausch and Lomb Optical Company *Ophthalmic Lens* (Rochester, N.Y. 1935).

Bernard Becker, M.D., *Collection in Ophthalmology* (St. Louis, 1979).

B. C. Boekhandel and B. M. Israel, *Source Material for the History of Medicine* Catalog #100 Amsterdam.

Alain Brieux, Catalog (Paris, 1983).

British Optical Association. Museum and Library Catalog (London, 1932).

Chicago Optical Supply Company Catalog (Chicago, 1930[?]).

Christie's South Kensington, *An Important Collection of Fans* (London, June 1991).

Codman & Shurteff, *Eye Instruments* (Boston, 1960).

Geo. Elliot, & Company *Our Eyes, Spectacles* (New York, 1889).

Gemmary (Redondo Beach, CA, 1994).

Geneva Optical Company Catalog (27th Edition) (Chicago, August 1922).

J. A. Hill, Bookseller (New York, 1988).

John Howell (San Francisco, CA, 1973).

In the Eye of the Beholder University of Iowa Medical Museum (Iowa City, Iowa, 1991).

B. M. Israel, Boekhandel and Antiquariat, *Source Material for the History of Ophthalmology* (Amsterdam, The Netherlands, 1988).

B. Kahn, & Son, *Illustrated Catalogue of Spectacles* (New York, 1892).

Katalog-Einer Bilderaustellung zur Geschichte der Brille, Drs. Greeff, Hallauer, Lundsgaard, Pflugk, Reiss, Simon, und Weve (Amsterdam, 1929).

Keeler Ophthalmic Equipment (London, 1990).

Lago. Paris, Inc. (1987).

La Lente. Fritz Rathschuler ECIG (Genova, 1988).

Leon Nicole. Catalog #14 (Lyon, France).

Martayan Lan. Catalog Nine (New York).

Benjamin Martin, *New Elements of Optics—A Catalogue of W. & S. Jones* (London, 1759).

McAllister & Brothers. Catalog (Philadelphia, 1855).

W. Y. McAllister, *Optical and Mathematical Instruments* (Philadelphia, 1871).

Merry Optical Company Catalog (Kansas City, MO, 1910[?]).

E. B. Meyrowitz, *Ophthalmic Apparatus* Sixth Catalog (New York).

Musée de la Lunetterie (Morez, France, 1988).

Museo dell' Occhiale (Verona: Pieve di Codore, 1991).

National Library of Medicine, National Institute of Health (Bethesda, MD, 1987).

New Era Optical Company (Chicago, 1939).

New Orleans Optical Company Catalog (New Orleans, 1920).

Nitsche & Gunther. Hauptkatalog (Rothenow, Deutchland, 1987).

Jeremy Norman, *Medicine and the Life Sciences.* Catalog 27. (San Francisco, 1993).

Occhiali Italiani. Alberone, Francesco, F. Bassoli (Milan, 1986).

Optico Utrecht (Netherlands, 1939).

Optisches Museum, *Die Brille* (Oberkochen, 1988).

Alex Peck, *Antique Scientifica* (Charleston, IL, 1992).

Nigel Phillips, Catalog Eight, *Medicine* (London, 1989).

The Printer's Devil, Ophthalmic List (Decatur, GA, 1992).

James W. Queen, and Company, *Optical Instruments* (New York, 1872).

Riggs Optical Company, *Ophthalmic Instruments and Equipment* (1925?).

B & L Rootenberg, Fine Books. Catalog Six, 1990.

Scientia. *Historic Medicine.* Catalog #14 (Arlington, MA, 1990).

Scientific Instrument Society Bulletin (London, 1990).

Smithsonian Institution Press (Washington, D.C., March 1983)

Société des Lunetiers (Paris, 1901).

Sotheby's (New York, 1986).

Tesseract, Catalog #48 (Hastings-on-Hudson, 1995).

Librairie Thomas-Scheler, *Livres Anciens d'Ophthalmologie* (Paris, 1983).

George Tiemann & Company (New York, 1877).

Trevor Philip & Son, Ltd. Catalog #2 (London, 1984).

Trotting Hill Park Antiquarian Booksellers. Catalog Six (Springfield, MA, 1991).

Laronde Philippe Voir & Cie (Paris, 1937).

Von Augen. Museum für Kunstund Gewefe (Hamburg, 1986).

W. H. Walmsley Company, *Illustrated Catalogue of Spectacles, Eyeglasses, etc.* (Philadelphia, 1884).

John Weiss & Son, *Catalogue of Ophthalmic Instruments and Apparatus* (London, 1929).

Wessex (Portsmouth, U.K., 1995).

W. B. White, Illustrated Catalog (Quincy, MA, 1890) (cases).

37

Spectacles in Art, Pictures, and Prints

We depend on ancient illustrations of spectacles to show us their form and use when first designed. Such pictures in successive years help chronicle their development. Later, commercial catalogs not only portray the example of spectacle use in everyday life but also give specifics on their construction. The modest offering of illustrations in this chapter exemplifies what can be found in modern times.

Figure 703 shows the use of wood block prints of riveted spectacles in fifteenth-century books. This print (circa 1493) is frequently found in ophthalmic history books. However, it is not generally realized that it was used as a "filler" by printers of that era and could appear in any portion of a page found useful. Also illustrated here is a caricature by James Gilsey (1757–1815)—"Old Pushpin," (Figure 704) and several Vanity Fair prints of the 1800s (Figures 709–714).

Whereas men have used spectacles as props to embellish the aura of their professionalism in paintings and photographs, it is astonishing to see women posed for eternity with such accoutrements. The author's collection, however, contains such art in oils and Daguerreotypes (Figure 705).

Museum displays of fifteenth-, sixteenth-, and seventeenth-century art span the entire globe. It is difficult, therefore, to make a comprehensive examination without completing an extensive pilgrimage. W. Poulet has dedicated a volume of his monumental work on the history of ophthalmology to the finding of spectacles in ancient art and illustrations in his book *Art & Spectacles*.[1] Additionally, listed in Appendix 5 (courtesy Greeff et. al.) are many instances where spectacles were found in illustrations throughout history.[2] The listings should help to crystallize the location of any type of spectacle a researcher may desire to observe. The author's holdings (depicted in Figures 703–739) modestly supplement the referred-to list.

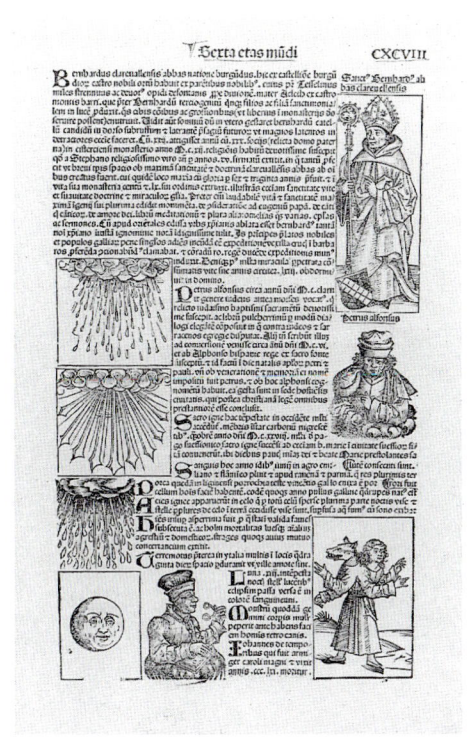

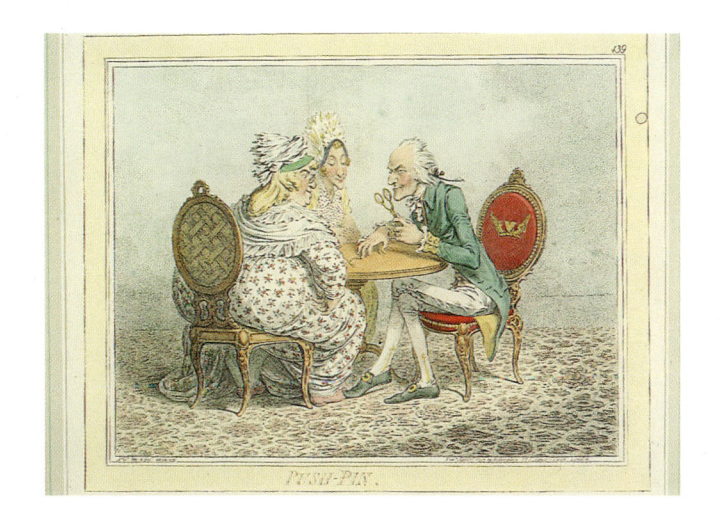

Figure 704. Print of "Old Push Pin" and his friends, circa 1797. He is using scissors glasses.

Figure 703. Wood block print from a page in a book showing "space fillers"—including one of a man holding riveted spectacles.

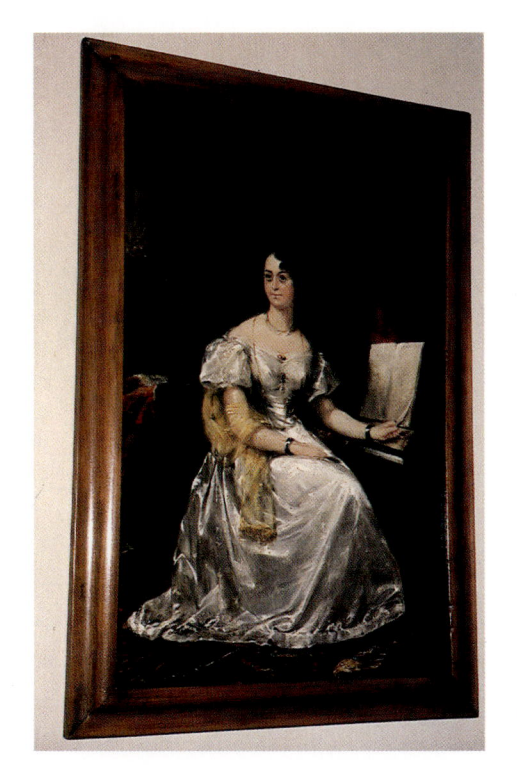

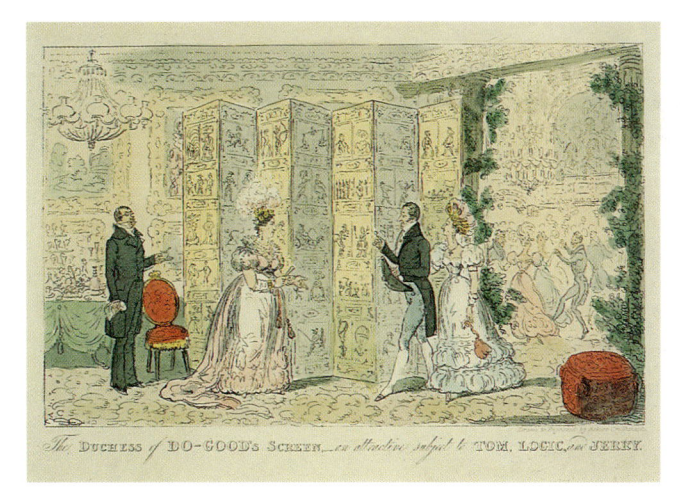

Figure 706. *Duchess of Do Good's Scream,* circa 1800.

Figure 705. Oil on board, *Lady at the Piano,* circa 1840.

SPECTACLES IN ART 359

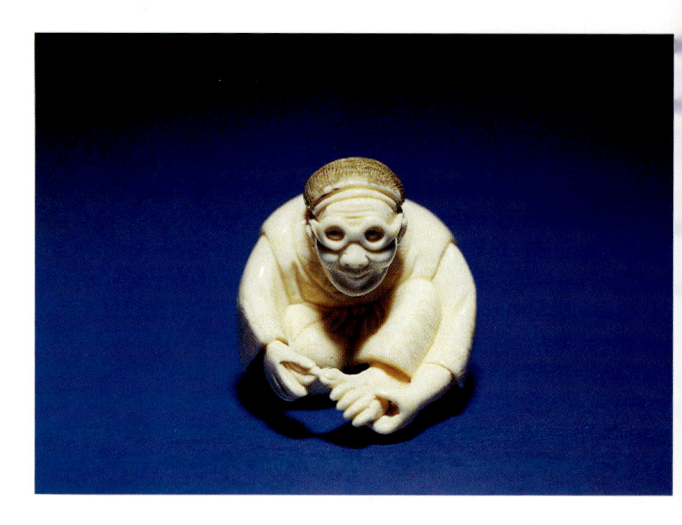

Figure 708. The most frequent netsuke with glasses is a man cutting his toenails.

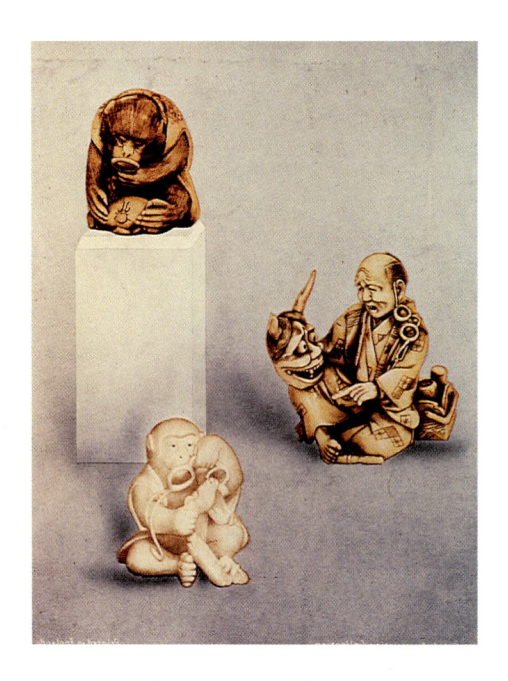

Figure 707. Netsukes wearing glasses. The author has about six of these.

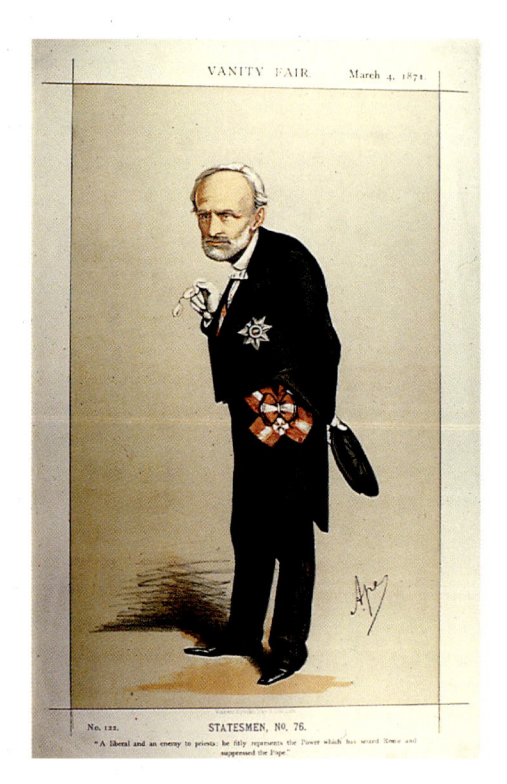

Figure 709. Vanity Fair caricature.

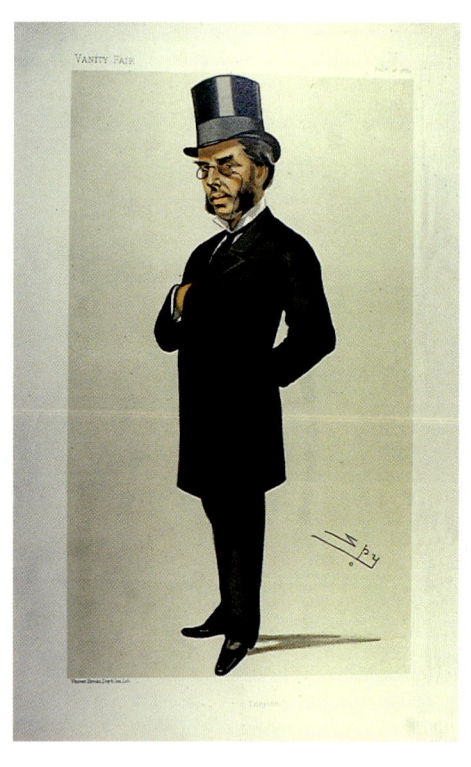

Figure 710. Vanity Fair caricature.

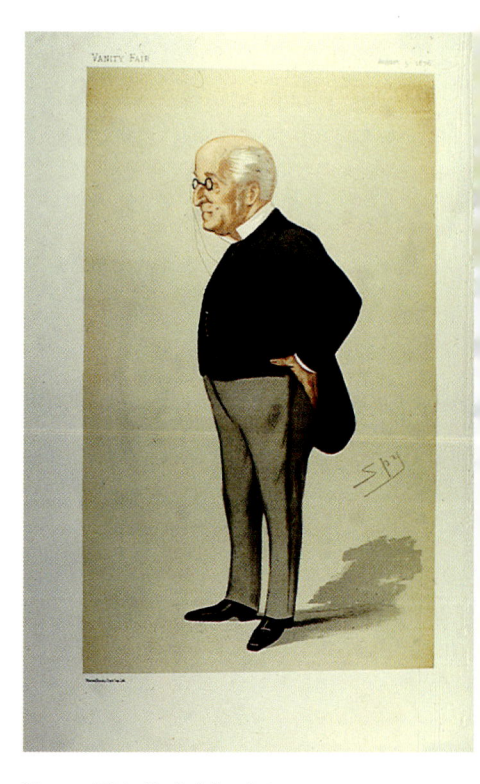

Figure 711. Vanity Fair caricature.

360   CHAPTER 37

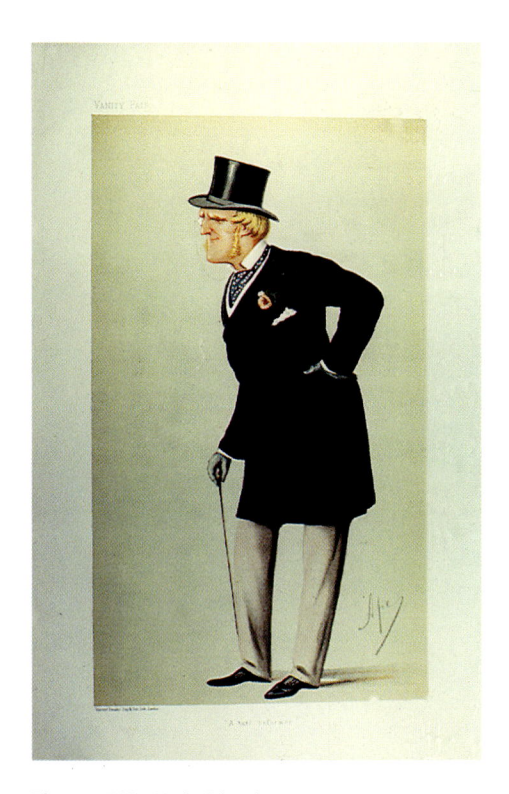

Figure 712. Vanity Fair caricature.

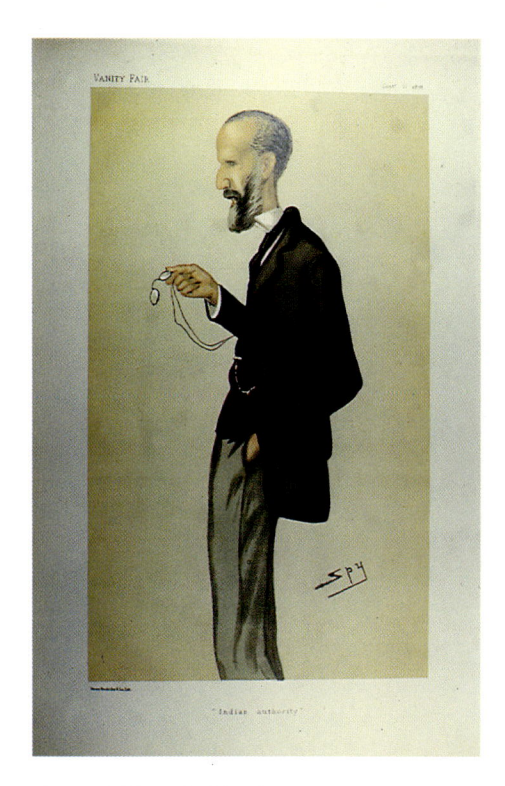

Figure 713. Vanity Fair caricature.

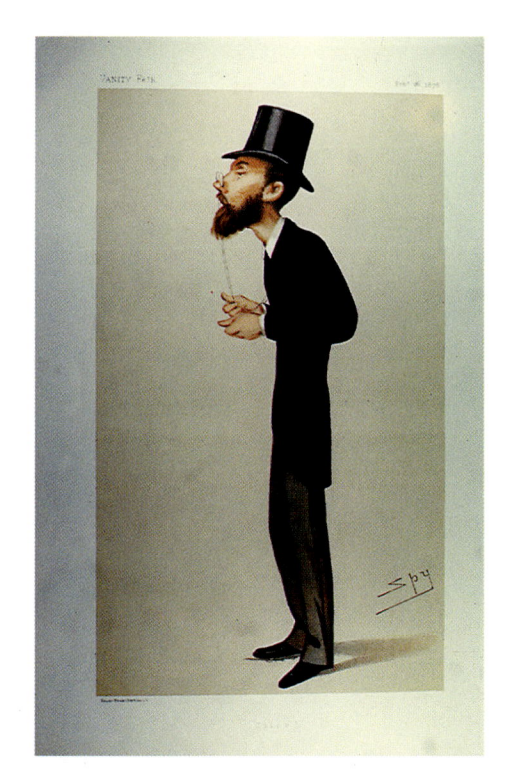

Figure 714. Vanity Fair caricature.

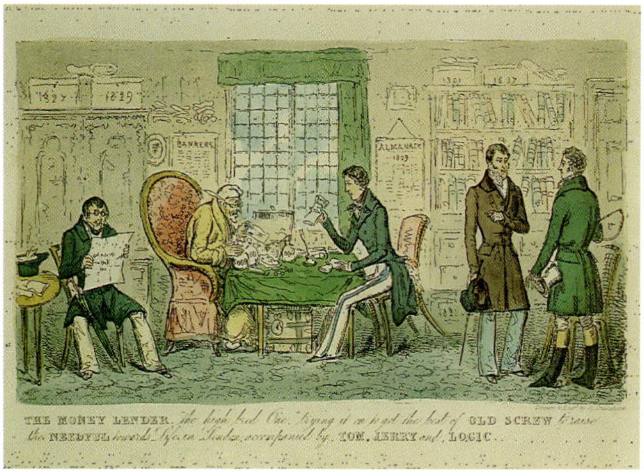

Figure 715. *The Money Lender*, circa 1800—colored print.

SPECTACLES IN ART 361

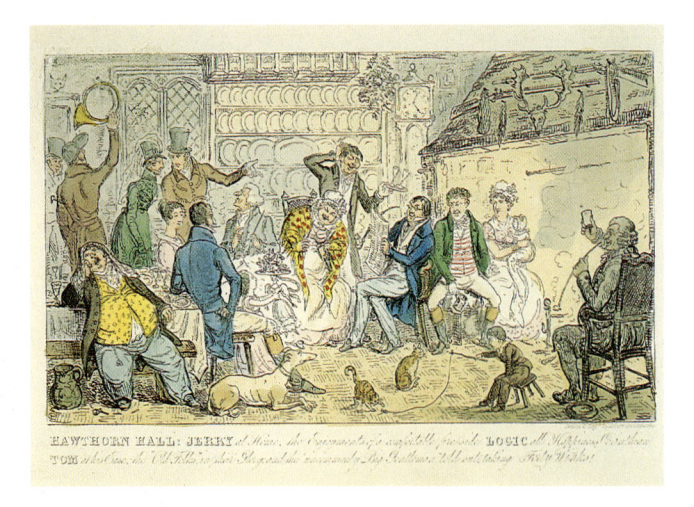

Figure 716. *Hawthorn Hall and Jerry*, circa 1880—colored print.

Figure 717. *Der Brillenmacher* (*The Spectacle Maker*), circa 1568.

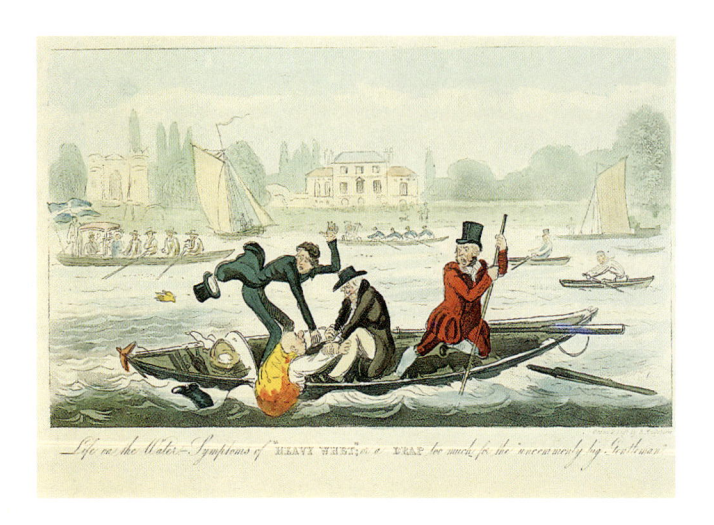

Figure 718. *Life on the Water*, circa 1825—colored print.

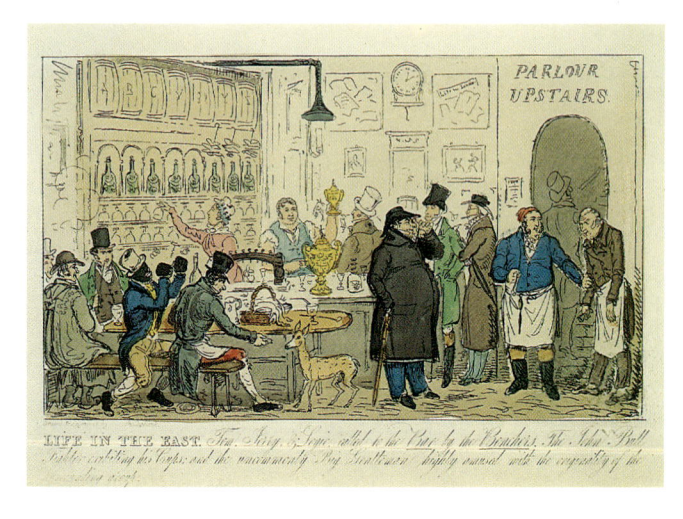

Figure 719. *Life in the East* circa 1880—colored print.

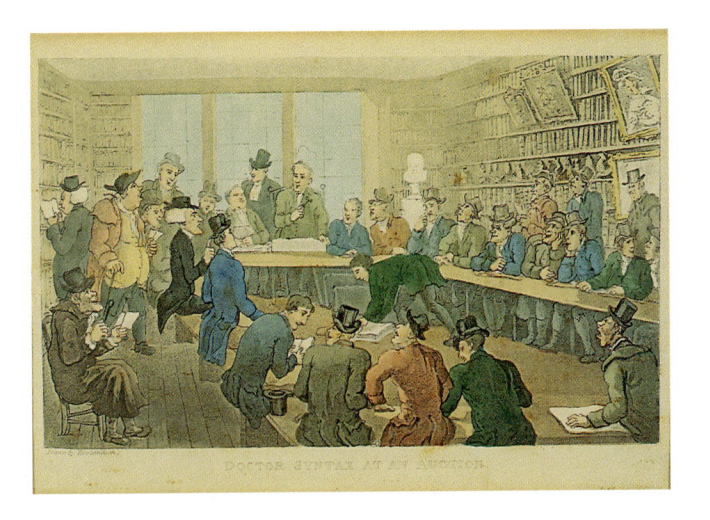

Figure 720. *Dr. Syntax at the Auction*, circa 1790—colored print.

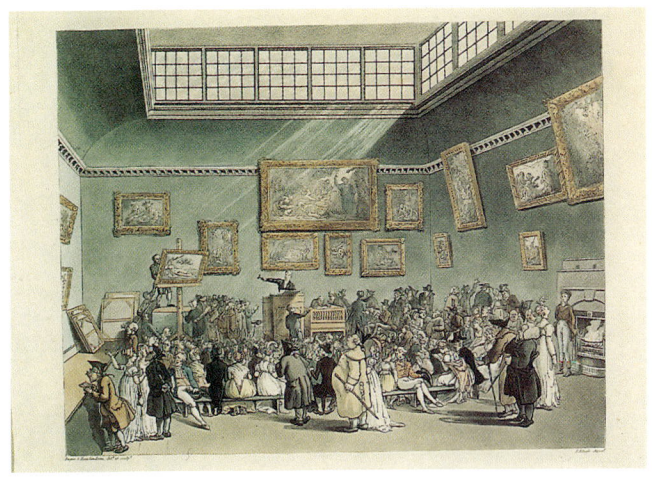

Figure 721. *Christie's Auction Room*, 1808—colored print.

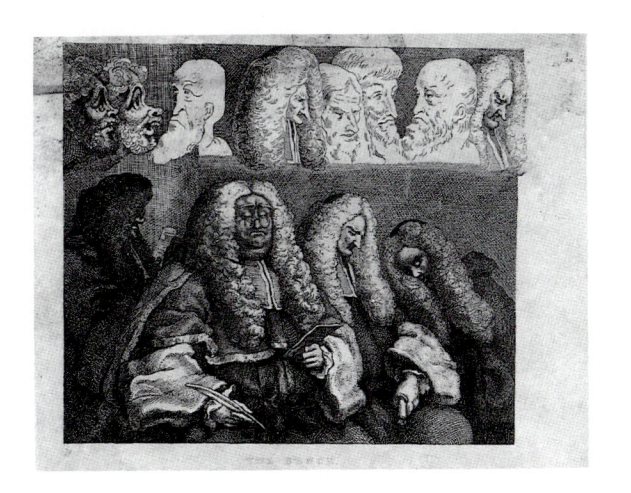

Figure 722. *At Court*—print, 1780.

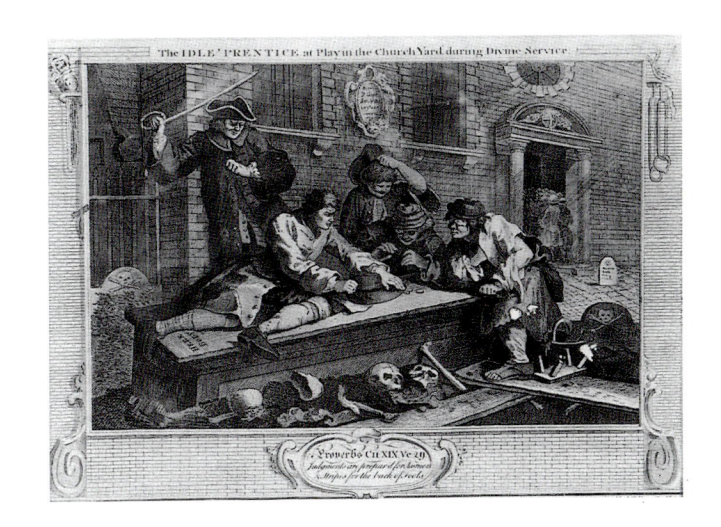

Figure 723. *The Idle Prentice*—print by Hogarth (1697–1764).

SPECTACLES IN ART

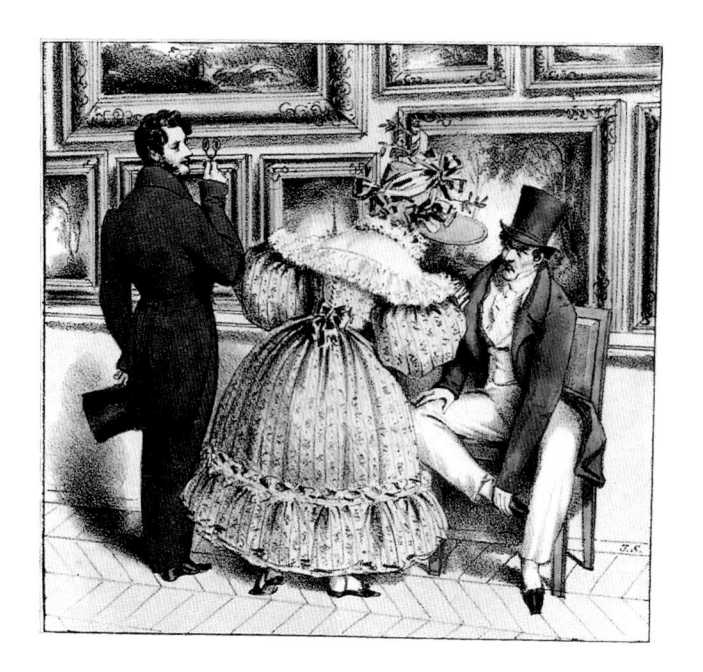

Figure 724. *At the Gallery*—print, 1800.

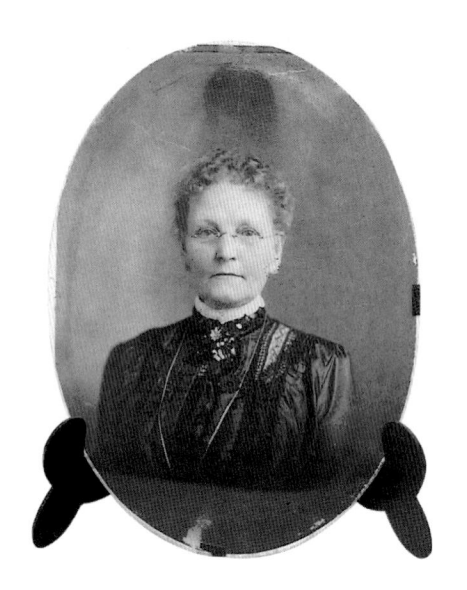

Figure 725. Photograph of a woman (on glass).

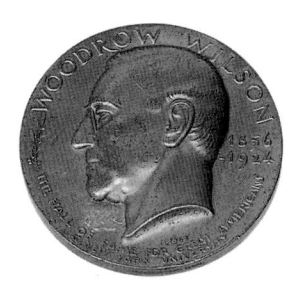

Figure 726. Medal honoring President Woodrow Wilson.

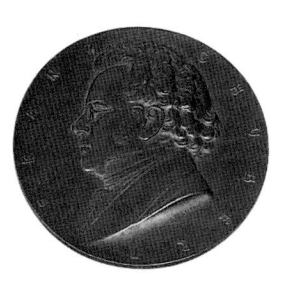

Figure 727. Medal honoring Franz Schubert.

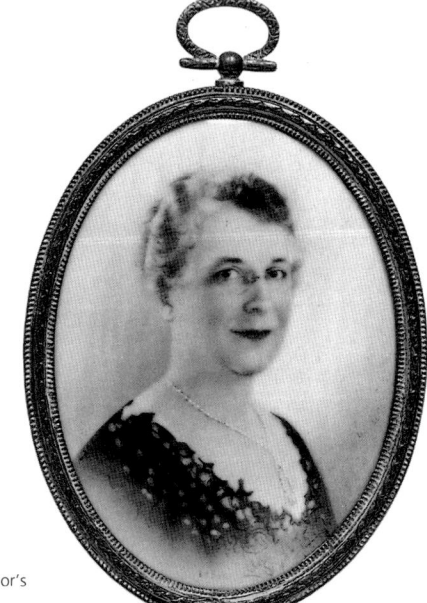

Figure 728. Enamel on ivory of author's grandmother, Bertha Rosenthal, circa 1932.

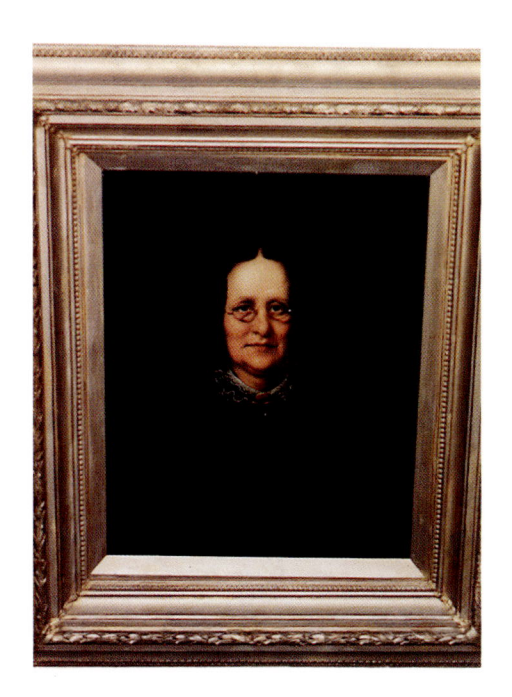

Figure 729. Oil on canvas of a woman, circa 1840.

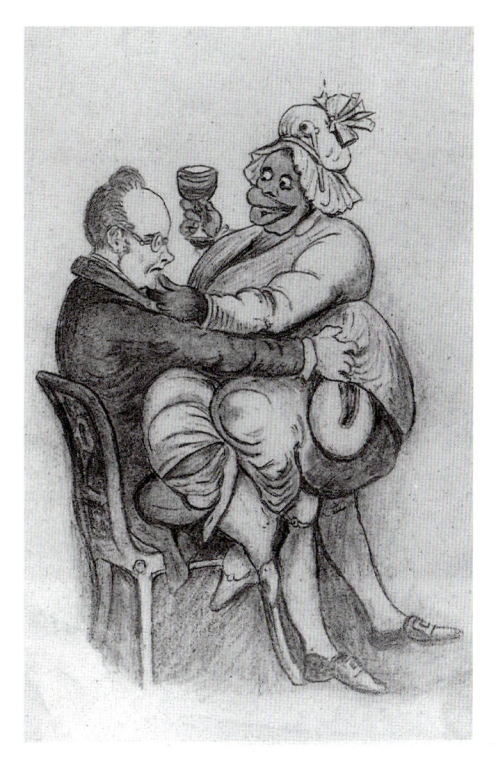

Figure 730. Rollicking pencil sketch circa 1720.

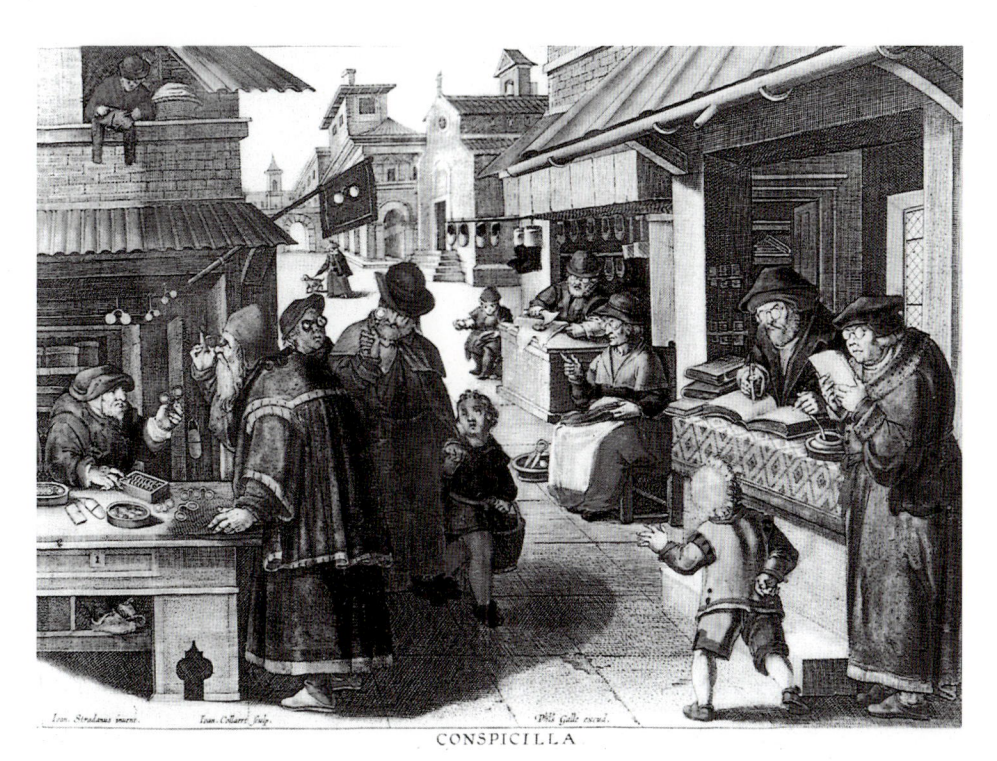

Figure 731. *Conspicilla*, circa 1650, courtesy Dr. Gilbert Blass Cohen.

SPECTACLES IN ART 365

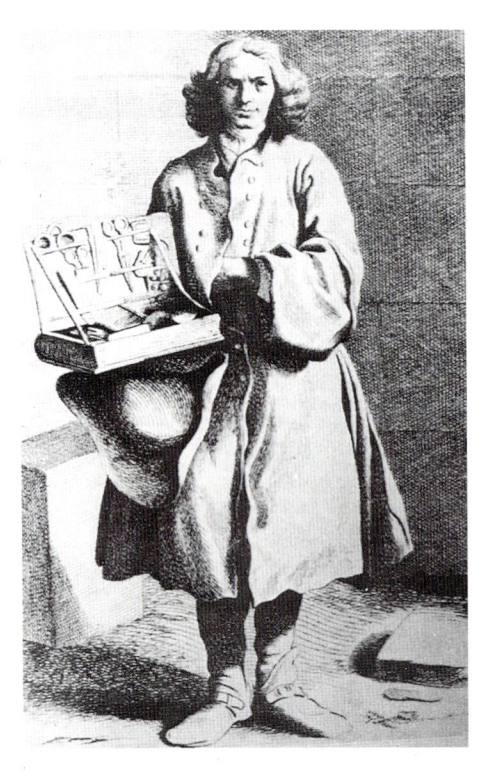

Figure 732. Print—*The Street Peddler*, 1750—note spectacles.

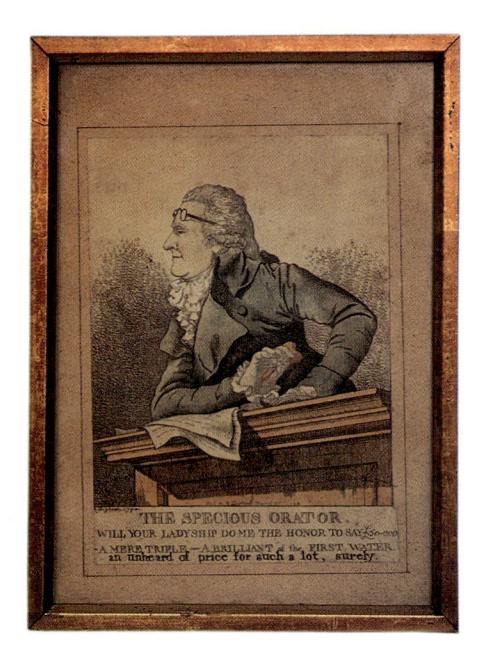

Figure 733. Print—*The Specious Orator*.

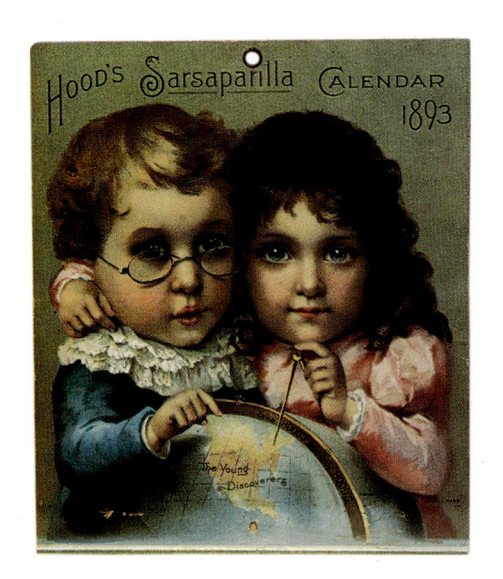

Figure 734. American advertising card, 1893.

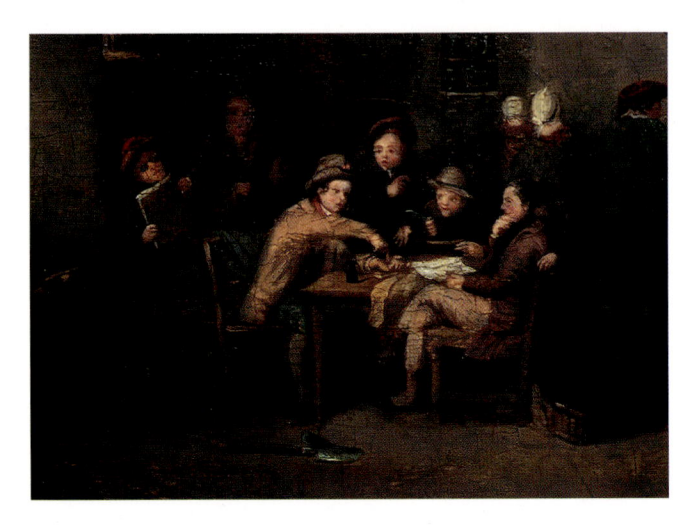

Figure 735. Tavern scene, oil on canvas, English, circa 1750.

366 CHAPTER 37

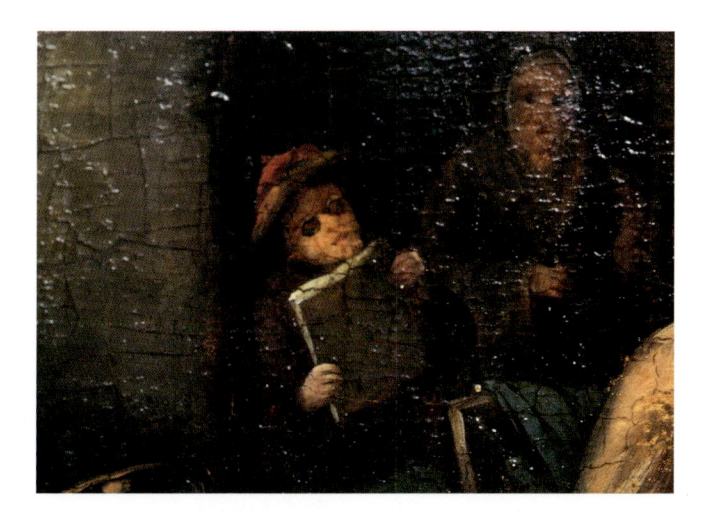

Figure 736. Detail of Figure 735.

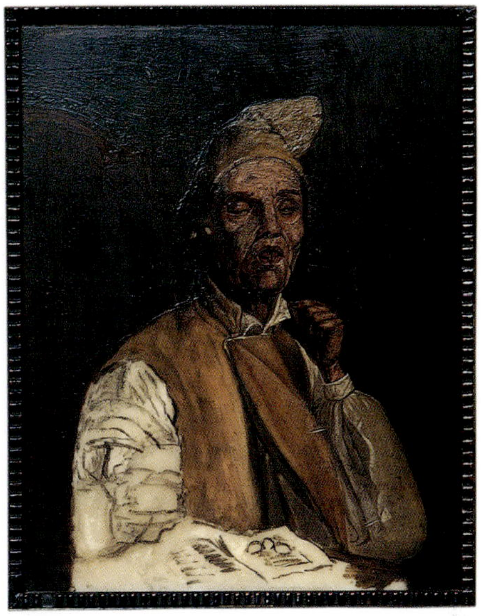

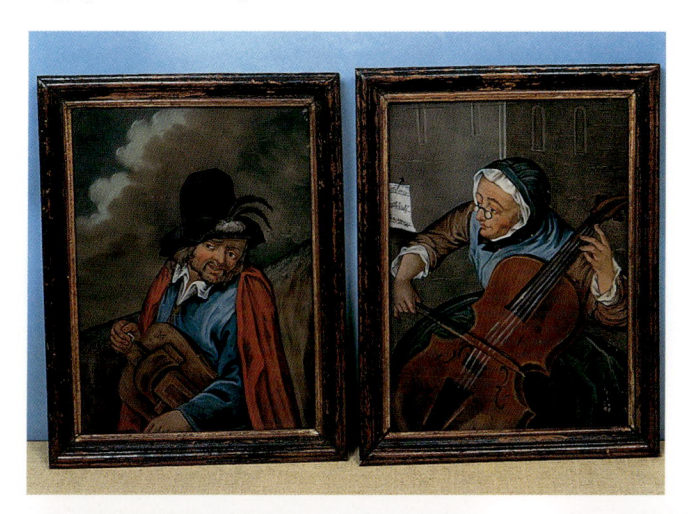

Figure 737. Man, oil on marble, Dutch, circa 1600.

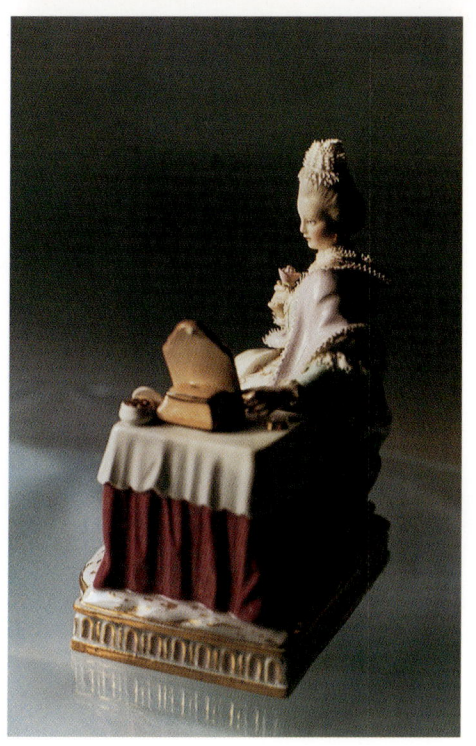

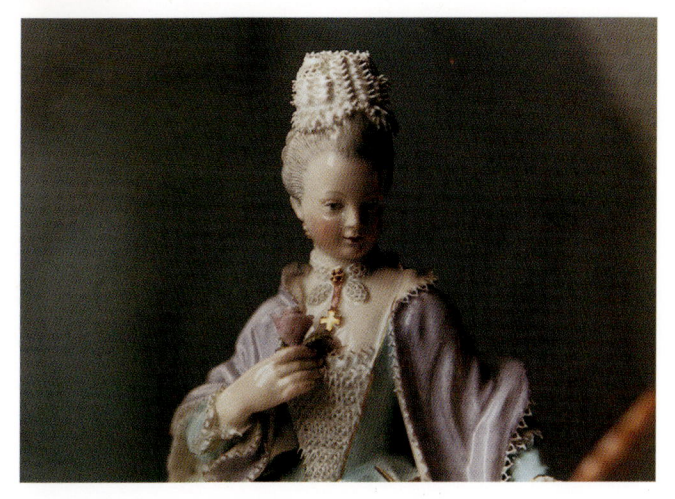

Figure 738. Pair of paintings on glass, circa 1600.

Figure 739. Meissen figure of "Sight," circa 1850.

SPECTACLES IN ART **367**

Notes

1. W. Poulet, *Art & Spectacles*, Vol. 2 (Berlin: Wayenborgh Pub., Berlin, 1935).
2. Prof. Dr. Greeff (Berlin), Prof. Dr. O. Hallauer (Basel), Prof. Dr. Lundsgaard (Copenhagen), Prof. Dr. v. Pflugk (Dresden), Dr. W. Reiss Dozent (Lwów [Lemberg]), Dr. Simon. (Barcelona), Prof. Dr. Weve (Utrecht), *Katalog Einer Bilderausstellung Zur Geschichte Der Brille* (Amsterdam, 1929).

38

The Development of Contact Lenses

Edward J. Fisher, M.A., D.Sc., F.A.A.O.

Eliminating the Corneal Power

Leonardo da Vinci is frequently regarded as the first actual investigator who conceived the idea of neutralizing corneal refractive power by immersing the eye in water.[1] In two places in his notebooks, he makes reference to the immersion of the eye into a bowl of water to demonstrate the manner by which the visual sense receives upright images. The notebooks contain some marginal notations with appropriate sketches that illustrate the principle. One sketch diagrams a glass bowl filled with water. A head is drawn, immersed in the water, with eyes wide open. The sketch is intended to demonstrate the principle of eliminating the refractive power of the cornea. Apparently, the device was proposed to further investigations of the optical and perceptual properties of the sense of vision, particularly image formation. Accompanying notations indicate a date about 1508, but it is not certain how far Leonardo proceeded with this experiment.

Enoch has pointed out that in 1837, René Descartes, the French philosopher and mathematician, described an apparatus to investigate the effect of altering the magnification of the retinal image.[2] The apparatus consisted of three telescoping interlocking cylindrical tubes. Each section was slightly conical in shape, while the whole contained water. The smaller end consisted of a plano meniscus glass lens having the same curvature as that of the cornea. The accompanying sketch shows this lens placed against the cornea. The end remote from the eye also had a meniscus curvature described as similar to that of the cornea but of greater diameter. It had parallel faces and thus was of plano power.

Optical considerations would require alteration in curvature from the corneal radius. This device, called later by Lohnstein a hydrodiascope, was designed to replace the refracting power of the cornea and produce a controlled and adjustable magnification of the retinal image. The telescoping cylinder could be adjusted in length over a range of several centimeters. It could hardly be considered as anything but a very distant antecedent of present-day contact lenses.

The Hydrodiascope

Lohnstein of Berlin in 1896 and Giegrist of Switzerland in 1897 utilized the hydrodiascope to neutralize ametropia. A small chamber filled with saline was held against the lids with adhesive tape. The forward window was fitted with a space to receive various lenses for distant or near vision. Although it could be worn longer than some early contact lenses, its cosmetic appearance and lack of field were two of its primary disadvantages.

Duke-Elder reports that in 1685, Phillipe de la Hire had diagramed a slightly different device to replace corneal refractive power by indicating a concave glass lens directly on the cornea.[3] De la Hire's sketches show a lens with a curvature on one surface approximating that of the cornea, while various concave and convex curvatures are illustrated on the distal portion. This was similar in principle to Herschel's apparatus but was made of solid material, thus reducing the tube length considerably to only a few millimeters. It is pointed out by Heitz that de la Hire was simply illustrating his theories on the nature of myopia.[4] There is no indication that de la Hire actually used such a lens.

In 1801, Thomas Young, in his experiments relating to accommodation, continued the idea of corneal neutralization. He describes his experiment as follows:

> From a small botanical microscope I take a double convex lens having a radius and focal length of 0.8 inch which is fastened in a socket one fifth of an inch deep; securing its edges with wax, I drop into it a little moderately cold water till it is three-fourths full, and then apply it to my eye, so that the cornea projects into the socket and is everywhere in contact with the water.[5]

The device neutralized the optical power of the corneal curvature, in which Young was interested for his research on astigmatism.

While these different devices were significant for their time and represented advances in the scientific investigation of vision, none of them would qualify in even a remote sense as a contact lens. They were designed to examine the nature of the retinal image, to investigate the optical elements of the eye, or to consider the effect of magnification. None of the accounts indicate any attempt to provide refractive correction of ametropia, or even to alleviate the problem of keratoconus. The reports do not suggest in any way that the devices might serve as models for contact lenses.

Bennett reports[6] concerning the work of Sir John F. W. Herschel, the Astronomer Royal, who suggested the possibility of a contact lens in 1827 and again in 1845. Herschel's article in the *Encyclopedia Metripolitania*[7] has a footnote speculating that it might be possible to improve vision in an eye having a highly irregular cornea by placing on it, at least temporarily, an appropriately ground lens and filling the small space between lens and cornea with some type of gel. Herschel suggests that such a lens might be made of an appropriate transparent material and placed on the eye with a suitable viscous substance between eye and lens. Thus, any corneal irregularity could be neutralized. No record exists reporting that any attempt was made to use such an arrangement at the time, but certainly the general principle of the contact lens had been enunciated.

The First Clinical Use of Contact Lenses

The idea of a contact lens as proposed by Herschel could not be applied clinically until the development of topical anesthetics. Although such anesthetics had been mentioned initially as early as 1860, it was not until Karl Koller reported their surgical use in 1884 that they came into general medical use. Commencing only three years after this, in 1887, the first significant clinical trials of contact lenses were reported independently by three different clinicians. Each was investigating one of three quite different applications of contact lenses to ocular problems: (1) the protection of the eye, utilized by E.T. Saemisch; (2) correction of corneal astigmatism and other irregularities, investigated by Adolph Eugene Fick; and (3) provision of ocular refractive correction, which was attempted by August Muller, who was interested in the replacement of his regular spectacles to correct his high myopia.

The first of these contact lens investigators is mentioned by several authorities, notably F. A. and A. C. Muller,[8] Duke-Elder,[9] Obrig,[10] Jenkins,[11] and Pascal.[12] All report that in 1887, Professor E.T. Saemisch of Bonn utilized the first true contact lens as a protective device. Saemisch had been consulted by a patient who required removal of the upper lid of his only useful eye as a result of a malignancy. Recognizing that the resultant, continuous exposure to the atmosphere could result in severe corneal ulceration and scarring, he requested Friedrich A. Muller and Son, noted glass blowers and artificial-eye makers of Weisbaden, to produce a transparent protective glass shell to protect the patient's eye from exposure to air. The front portion of a "reform" artificial eye was utilized, without the customary pupil and iris painting. It was suitably modified for size with appropriately smoothed edges. This lens was worn by the patient at intermittent intervals every day to avoid corneal ulceration. It is reported that this patient retained useful vision in his only eye until his death in 1908. A patient with a similar condition was fitted by Dr. Saemisch in the following year.

The second pioneer clinician who made several even more significant contributions to contact lens development was Adolph Eugene Fick of Zurich. When the sum total of his several researches is considered, certainly he should qualify as the true "father of contact lenses." An account of his research first appeared in 1888.[13] A summary of his work has been provided by Tony Sabell.[14] Fick worked with rabbits in his early experiments, fitting them with glass lenses blown over plaster-of-paris molds obtained from the rabbit eyes. Fick defines the lenses he devised in his paper as follows: "The contact lens consists of a very thin, small glass bowl, bounded by concentric and parallel sphere segments...." Both surfaces seem to have been completely spherical, with a single posterior surface curvature similar to the rabbit cornea. The lens was placed on the rabbit eye with a liquid between it and the cornea. Fick reports that the solution was inserted after the lens was placed on the cornea by levering the top edge away from the sclera with a muscle hook and dropping in a suitable amount of the liquid. Fick observed that a cloud seemed to develop behind the contact lens after varying periods of wear. Following further investigation, he reported that the clouding actually took place in the epithelium of the rabbit cornea after six to eight hours of contact lens wear. He noted that gradual adaptation to contact lenses over a prolonged period of time seemed to postpone the onset of the haziness. He investigated several different buffer solutions before finally recommending a 2-percent solution of grape sugar, which he claimed gave best results.

Fick extended his work to humans by taking impressions of cadaver eyes. Again, molds were made using plaster of paris, although today this would not be regarded as the ideal material because of its rather coarse texture. These molds readily showed the increased prominence of the cornea. Following this, he had his lenses modified to have two radii on the posterior surface—a shorter one in the central optical portion. While his first lenses were made of blown glass and tried on his own eyes, he later had Professor Ernst Abbe of Zeiss Optical Works in Jena grind lenses for him. Obrig indicates that reports were made that the early Zeiss lenses were actually blown lenses that had been reworked on the anterior surface by grinding.[15] Fick prescribed radii of 8 millimeters and 15 millimeters respectively for the corneal and scleral portions of the posterior surfaces of his lenses, with a scleral band width of 3 millimeters. The anterior surface paralleled the posterior, so that the lenses had no refractive power. However, when placed on the cornea, the liquid lens would provide concave or convex power depending on whether the corneal radius was shorter or longer than the radius of the optical portion of the contact lens.

As a pioneer in contact lens research and development, Fick deserves primary recognition on many counts—the first use of the term *contact lenses* (*contactbrillen*), the first suggestion of taking impressions of the human eye (albeit they were of cadaver eyes), observation of corneal clouding (sometimes referred to as Fick's phenomenon), experimentation with different contact lens solutions, and use of both blown and ground glass contact lenses. It was reported later by Friedrich Muller of Weisbaden (who made the lenses) that Fick fitted a large number of keratoconus patients. Contact lenses are regarded as an ideal corrective device for early stages of this condition, even today.

August Muller, a medical student from Gladbach, was a third pioneer in contact lens research. His dissertation on the subject gained him his medical degree from the University of Kiel. Muller was seeking a way to correct his own myopic refractive error of −14.00 diopters by using contact lenses, which obviously would have a better appearance than his rather thick spectacles. Muller's contact lenses were made by Otto Himmler, a Berlin optician. Muller succeeded in wearing the lenses he designed but could not tolerate them longer than one half hour at a time, despite several different trials.[16] He used cocaine as a topical anesthetic at first. Rather than improve the situation, cocaine may have contributed to some of his problems, since it tends to soften the corneal epithelium. There is no record of any attention he might have given to the relationship between the diameter of the optical portion of the contact lens and the corneal diameter of his own eye. If the diameter of the optical portion of the lens differed from the corneal diameter, this might also have been a source of difficulty, as suggested by Obrig.

Eugen Kalt of Paris was working in the area of contact lenses about the same time.[17] He designed and fitted at least one contact lens in 1888. Accounts seem to indicate that this may have been strictly a single-curve corneal type of lens. The lens was used for a patient with keratoconus, but precise information is lacking. The claim was made that contact lenses made to fit in this way would exert pressure on the apex of the cone to prevent further progression of the keratoconus. All of these early lenses were made from either ground or blown glass. Several types of available glass were used, but the principal type was that used for making artificial eyes. Apart from the difficulty of working with such very thin pieces of glass subject to breakage, body acids attack this type of glass, gradually causing the surfaces to become pitted, roughened, or corroded. This caused the lenses to become extremely uncomfortable, so that replacement was required annually or sometimes more frequently. In one instance encountered in 1940, the daughter of an engineer acquaintance of the author required lens replacement every six months until finally her father made a duplicate set of lenses from inert plastic (Plexiglas). The inconvenience of fitting—time and expense—the difficulty of replacement, and the limitation on wearing time caused many patients to discontinue the use of early contact lenses.

Ground Glass Lenses

In the first quarter of this century, the clinical choice in contact lens fitting was either blown glass or ground glass lenses. The primary source of blown lenses for clinicians was the Muller Company in Weisbaden, Germany. The scleral portion of these lenses was often made from mild white glass, which tended to hide any injection of the sclera produced by irritation. The optical portion was clear glass. No sources of blown glass lenses seem to have been developed in North America.

The Zeiss Company undertook grinding glass lenses despite the difficulty imposed by the extreme thinness required. Some of the early lenses may actually have been blown, with the outer surface ground. Zeiss continued to experiment and made ground glass contact lenses for a number of clinicians. Eventually, a standard trial set was developed with more or less standard diameters. The lenses had varying radii of curvature for both the corneal and the scleral (haptic) portions.

Obrig gives a good account of the development and fitting properties of Zeiss contact lenses and points out some of the problems encountered.[18] Because of the relative ease of reasonably exact replacement and the wider availability, these Zeiss lenses were the usual lenses of choice during the first two decades of the twentieth century, particularly in North America. On the other hand, the claim was made that blown glass lenses were more comfortable because of the smoothness of the surfaces and edges. However, the difficulties imposed by the lengthy process of fitting, replacement considerations, and limited availability were detractions from the wide use of blown glass lenses.

Molded Glass Lenses

A significant improvement in precise fitting methods began when, in 1930, Josef Dallos of Budapest did research on a procedure for taking impressions of the living eye. This resulted from a fortunate combination of suitable topical anesthetics, molding shells, improvements in technique, and several advances in glass processing.

After many trials, the anesthetic used was 1-percent pontocaine; the impression material, Poller's Negacoll (described later). Molding shells were small plastic hemispheres with stubby handles attached. The total technique involved methods of coordinating all the steps associated with procuring the ocular impressions and integrating this procedure with the manufacturing process and final adjustment of the finished lens as it was fitted to the living eye.

The proper strength of pontocaine, a cocaine derivative, provided fast-acting, short-term anesthesia of some 15 to 30 minutes, with no evident side effects on ocular tissues. It did not alter the corneal surface and had no apparent aftereffects or complications. Stronger concentrations and some other agents, such as cocaine, tended to soften the corneal epithelium and thus could affect the accuracy of the impression.

Poller's Negacoll was a substance developed in the late 1920s for dentists to use in taking oral impressions in the preparation of dentures and dental prostheses. It was a waxlike substance that liquefied when heated above 100 degrees Fahrenheit and solidified gradually as it cooled to near body temperature. As it solidified, it retained the shape assumed when in the liquid state. As a solid mold, it had a hard, smooth surface, giving an accurate negative impression of the body part being molded. The texture was excellent for ocular use and produced a smooth detailed impression of the anterior surface of the eye.

The molding shells used were small portions of a hollow sphere similar to a contact lens, with a short handle attached to the center of the convex outer surface to facilitate handling. The function was to first provide an easy method of placing the liquefied molding material on the outer surface of the eye and then to provide a rigid backing so that the solidified impression material could be removed from the eye in one piece and still retain its shape. To anchor the molding material to the shell, several small holes were drilled in the periphery, and the small handle was frequently hollow. The liquefied Negacoll would flow through the openings and anchor the impression material to the shell. These shells were available in various dimensions to accommodate different globe sizes, having a radius of some 12 millimeters and horizontal and vertical diameters of approximately 20 to 26 millimeters. Generally, three sizes were available to be used on various sized eyes, as required. Experiment dictated the size and placement of the peripheral holes drilled in the spherical surface of the shell to provide the optimum anchorage for the solidified molding compound. Suitable markings were placed on the convex surface of the molding shell so that proper orientation could be ensured for placement on the eye. Also, appropriate markings could be placed on the positive dental stone cast to indicate the horizontal meridian.

Briefly, the method used by Dallos was to heat the Negacoll in an aluminum double boiler to the melting point. The substance was then allowed to cool slowly to about 99 degrees Fahrenheit, just above body temperature. The patient was supine and the eye anesthetized. The molding compound was then placed in an appropriately sized molding shell, and the shell placed under the lids on the anterior segment of the globe. To hasten the setting of the Negacoll, cold water might then be poured over the external surface of the lids, or an ice pack might be applied. The negative impression of the eye would solidify, ready for removal inside four or five minutes. The shell and its attached impression were then removed from the eye with the assistance of a muscle hook to break any slight adhesion or suction. A dental stone or plaster-of-paris positive was made from the Negacoll impression. A pair of steel dies was made to match the plaster cast. Glass was molded over the anterior surface of the metal cast to produce an initial contact lens. Powers were ground on the front surface, and the lens outline was shaped to fit appropriately within the fornices. Initially, several molds might be made, with the eye fixed in various directions of gaze. Then, a composite was made to include the various sections. As the technique improved, good results were usually obtained with only one impression.

This was, of course, a very time-consuming process. Because one was working with extremely thin glass, there were often many breakages and thus the need for repeat moldings. When the lens was first applied to the patient's eye, the inside surface of the haptic portion might require modification in successive fitting sessions. This was accomplished by careful use of dental burrs on the posterior surface to improve the fitting properties. After a large number of patients had been fitted, a basic series of molds resulted. For some succeeding patients, one of the earlier molds might be selected and modified as required.

Dallos continued his work in Budapest but in 1937 moved to London, where he became associated with T. H. Hamblin in the establishment of a contact lens clinic.[19] His technical associate, George Nissel, also accompanied him to London. Eventually, Nissel opened his own laboratory there to produce contact lenses for other clinicians. In due course, Nissel was succeeded by his son.

Molded Plastic Contact Lenses

It has been noted that several steps had taken place in the development of contact lenses from the first suggestion of Herschel. There was the initial development of applying a lens to the eye, followed by the taking of molds of the cadaver eye. Trial sets were produced. This in turn was succeeded by the use of topical anesthetics, materials to take impressions of the living eye, and the adaptation of glass technology to produce suitable custom-made lenses for many different types of patients.

Theodore Obrig reports that about 1920 he started fitting Zeiss lenses in New York, using trial lens methods. He found long delays in obtaining specific lenses, amounting in some cases to a year or more. Often lenses were returned to Germany for power and fit alteration. Dissatisfied with the delays and difficulties, he started working on the development of his own contact lenses. He researched methods of taking impressions of the eye and in the early 1930s came into contact with Josef Dallos.

Plastics

The popular use of contact lenses was stimulated significantly in 1934 by another major milestone in their development. Clear plastic materials began to appear on the market under the trade names of Lucite and Plexiglas. These materials had many applications as a replacement for glass where transparency was required with a considerable increase in strength and safety. The fact that the index of refraction was lower than glass resulted in reduced surface reflections as well as increased transparency.

Obrig began to use these materials for his molded lenses, settling in particular on the plastic known as polymethyl methacrylate (PMMA). Plastic had many advantages in that it was easily formed and was apparently inert to body acids. However, such materials presented some problems to the contact lens laboratory. A major difficulty encountered was the need to grind accurate power on the optical portion of the contact lens. The grinding operation generated sufficient heat to warp and even melt the plastic. After much experimentation, a satisfactory method of producing good surfaces with correct power was achieved, and Obrig's laboratory in New York became the first North American laboratory to produce modern plastic molded scleral contact lenses.

This new development resulted in considerable growth in the demand for contact lenses. Many people hesitated to use glass in direct contact with the eye. There was always concern that the glass might break and cause serious injury. In addition, there was the problem of glass corrosion, which necessitated frequent replacement. Plastic was recognized as being much less subject to breakage, and it proved to be inert to body fluids. The application of this material to contact lenses increased public interest. Very few people appreciated the need to wear glasses, and contact lenses were a cosmetically attractive alternative.

Phillip Salvatori became associated with the Obrig laboratory about 1932. He made a study of the methods of taking ocular impressions and developed several improvements in molding procedures. In the mid-1930s, a new dental molding compound made from algae was developed. This material required no heating, as with Negacoll, but solidified instead by chemical action. It was also cleaner and easier to use. However, the types available were flavored with peppermint, which was satisfactory for dental purposes but reacted poorly on the eye. Salvatori, working with manufacturers of this material, succeeded in developing a derivative material that did not irritate ocular tissues. This new material was patented and marketed under the name Moldite.[20] When mixed in proper proportions with distilled water at room temperature, this material hardened to about the consistency of a poached egg within three to four minutes of mixing. The procedure for using this material was similar to that with Negacoll, but no heating was required. (The entire procedure has been described in a book by Anderson.[21])

The relationship between the posterior surface of the lens and the eye was assessed by the aid of a slit lamp biomicroscope. This instrument permitted estimates of the clearance of the lens from the cornea and its relationship particularly in the limbus area. Sometimes a few drops of fluorescein were placed on the eye to observe areas where the scleral portion allowed passage of tears under the lens. This was also used to determine where the lens might be pressing on ocular tissue. In the course of using fluorescein, Obrig observed that the use of blue, short-wavelength radiation produced brilliant fluorescence and enhanced the observation. In addition to the blue filter on the slit lamp, the use of any ultraviolet light source, such as the Hague cataract lamp or the Burton lamp, enhanced the fluorescence.[22] This discovery was another important contribution to the fitting procedures in contact lens work and has become standard practice with PMMA or gas permeable lens fitting for both scleral and rigid corneal contact lenses.

It was recognized very early in scleral contact lens fitting that impressions were made with the eye in a stationary primary position of fixation. On the other hand, the living eye, with its constant movement, may change its surface shape slightly, particularly in the area of the extrinsic muscle insertions. Consequently, methods were developed for making adjustments in the fitting properties of the lens when the eyes made extreme rotations. The philosophy behind this was that the lens should move with the eye but should never touch the corneal surface. Also, there should be no occlusion of scleral blood vessels. Clinicians thus utilized appropriate adjusting equipment on the posterior scleral portion of the lenses to alter and improve the fitting properties. A small dental motor with mandrels, burrs, and polishing discs, together with suitable abrasives, served the purpose.

Using the molding method and any subsequent minor adjustments required, the clinician could feel reasonably confident that the lens actually fit the more or less regular scleral surface. The comfort of these lenses was very good, and the plastic contact lens shield provided some assurance of safety. But the major problem of solution filtration into the anterior layers of the epithelium by osmosis limited wearing times in most patients. Vision gradually became hazy, with an annoying colored halo surrounding light sources. Some patients chose to wear one lens and, when clouding occurred, remove that lens and wear the other one. Other patients persevered and were able to attain wearing times of eight to ten hours. However, the majority of wearers were limited to only four or five consecutive hours of wear.

While Obrig was the initial and principal supplier of molded contact lenses in North America, other smaller laboratories soon began to produce lenses. One example in Canada was the Dominion Contact Lens Laboratory, started by Dr. J. E. Archer in 1942. This laboratory continued to produce molded lenses and in 1952 began experimenting with corneal contact lenses.

Plastic Contact Lens Trial Case Methods   William Feinbloom of New York began research in contact lenses about 1934. By 1937, he had developed a system of fitting contact lenses by trial case methods.[23] Feinbloom made impressions of some 250 eyes and started comparing them by means of a projection comparator. He traced the shadow thrown on the screen by each of his positive molds and began to analyze the results. He found that he could classify the scleral pattern and reduce the number of different scleral fittings required to approximately 65. In other words, with some 65 appropriate contact lenses, each with a differently shaped scleral contour, all 250 eyes could be fitted satisfactorily, with only the need to alter the refractive prescription requirements.

Having found that fitting could be accomplished by trial case methods, Feinbloom designed an all-encompassing trial lens set in 1939. Because he, too, found difficulty in grinding the refractive power on plastic material, he proceeded to develop a lens with a plastic scleral, or haptic, portion combined with a glass optical portion. The two sections were joined together by a form of vulcanizing. The plastic haptic portion was made of white translucent material, since the junction line between the glass and the plastic was quite conspicuous if made from clear plastic. This served not only to reduce the visibility of the junction line but also to conceal any injection of the sclera that might occur with continued wear. In some lenses, the vulcanizing process placed undue stress on the glass optical portion, and eventually concentric cracks appeared near the junction line.

The trial case consisted of lenses with spherical and toric haptic portions. The radius of curvature in both horizontal and vertical meridians varied from 12.4 to 14.6 millimeters in 0.2-millimeter intervals. This method of fitting was used widely by clinicians. It had the advantage of relative simplicity compared to the molding method and did not require the use of topical anesthetics. The main disadvantage was the subjective nature of selecting the proper lens by trial and error. One could seldom feel confident that the best fit had been found. Some clinicians were of the opinion that a better fitting contact lens would be obtained by the impression method as outlined previously. The trial-and-error method of fitting consumed more time and did not seem to instill as much confidence in the patient.

A few years later, in 1945, Feinbloom changed his fitting sets from spherical or toric haptic surfaces and developed the Feincone lens.[24] In this design, the haptic portion was in a conelike shape for 3 to 4 millimeters from the optic-haptic junction. There were three different angles of cone, plus a small spherical scleral tab at the temporal side. The cone shape fit on any spherical or toric sclera, providing contact at some point a few millimeters from the limbus. Such a geometric configuration required new trial lens sets as well as new methods of making adjustments. A special pliers was provided which, when warmed, could alter the cone angle. Eventually, Feinbloom turned his attention to designing and producing low-vision devices and withdrew from the contact lens field.[25]

Many other investigators began to produce preformed contact lens trial sets in the early 1940s. Solon Braff in California and Norman Bier in England, among others, developed methods of fitting scleral contact lenses from standard

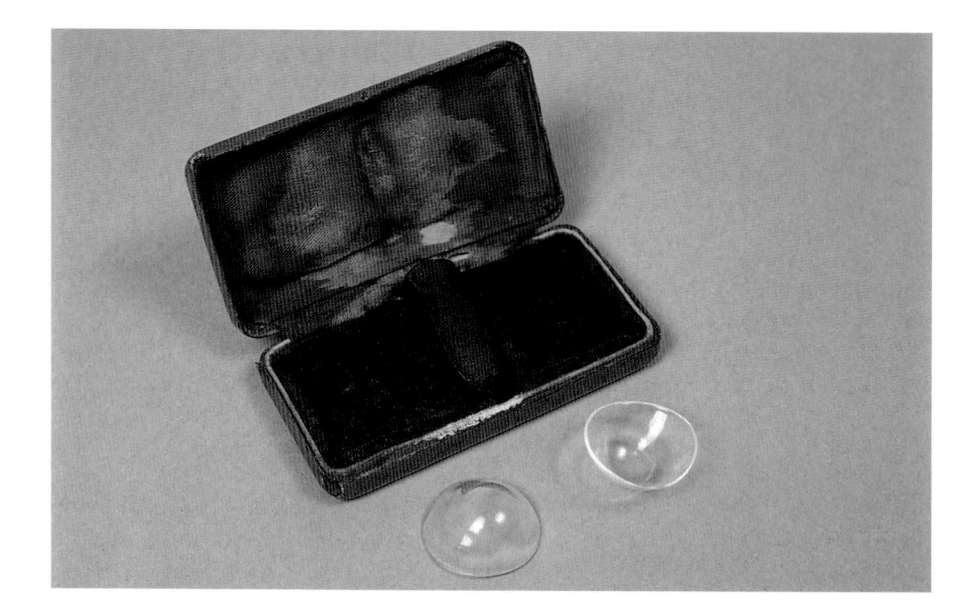

Figure 740. Hard plastic scleral lenses, circa 1953.

trial sets. Contact lens practitioners in the decades of the 1930s and 1940s continued to use both trial case and molding methods.

When a clinician acquired some skill, it was possible to provide a satisfactory physical fit in a contact lens using either the molding or the trial case method. However, patients still could achieve only limited wearing times because of corneal clouding. The solutions enclosed between the contact lens and the cornea produced a reduction in vision that had been reported much earlier by Fick. There was a marked increase in clouding and reduction in acuity after periods of wear, varying between four and eight hours. Colored halos developed around light sources. The period of clear vision varied with the wearer and also with the number of days or weeks that the patient had worn the lenses. With steady persistence, it was possible to gradually increase wearing time, but there was always some limit to the number of hours of wear. Tolerance decreased abruptly if contact lens wear was interrupted for even a few days. In addition to many other factors, the general health of the patient seemed to affect the length of wear.

Different solutions were investigated, but sooner or later the fluid infiltrated into the epithelial layer of the cornea, and vision was affected. Experiments were conducted to reduce or eliminate this, using a large number of different solutions in varying strengths. One pharmaceutical supplier[26] developed a testing kit so that patients could use a different solution every week and record results. The solution that gave best results was prescribed and was even adjusted for pH value in an attempt to improve the results. It was difficult, however, to determine whether the patient's tolerance was increasing simply from continuous wear or because of the particular testing solution. Additionally, many patients were not interested in such a tedious process extending over a period of months. As a result, rates of complete contact lens success were low, save for those who achieved great improvements in vision, as in keratoconus.

Under the assumption that continuously changing fluid under the lens would be the ideal answer to the clouding difficulty, several attempts were made to improve tear circulation under the lens. Constantly providing fresh fluid might eliminate the haziness of vision and provide extended wearing times. Some clinicians placed minute channels on the inside surface of the lens to facilitate tear circulation. Often these channels were ineffective because they became blocked as a result of conjunctival edema. Other clinicians drilled one or more tiny fenestrations (minute holes) in the corneal portion of the lens to encourage tear flow beneath the lens. Obrig designed the Lacrilens with a 3-millimeter opening below the lower lid and a shallow channel on the inner surface from this opening into the corneal portion. While these methods undoubtedly aided in some cases, they were not all universally successful. The various patents and ideas brought a rash of publicity and great promises and led to increased use of contact lenses. Ultimately, however, it was recognized that none of these methods was the final answer. The next step, about 1945, was to fit lenses in such a way that artificial solutions were not required.

Norman Bier of London had been using fluidless contact lenses as early as 1943.[27] In some of his lenses, he drilled minute holes into the optical portion. In 1950, Mueller-Welt developed a fluidless type of contact lens that utilized lacrimal fluid to fill the interspace between the lens and the cornea.[28] The Mueller-Welt lenses came to North America in 1953 through an office in Chicago (Figure 740). The optical portion of these lenses very closely paralleled the cornea with practically zero clearance. The scleral portion fitted somewhat loosely at the periphery. The space between cornea and lens quickly filled with tears through capillary action, since the gap between lens and cornea was often less than 0.5 millimeters. At times, a rather large, shallow air bubble formed under the lens near the top of the corneal portion. Both the Norman Bier and the Mueller-Welt lens types were somewhat more difficult to fit, but many patients found them very useful and could wear them for much longer periods.

Corneal Lenses

Graham describes the early development of the corneal contact lens.[29] In 1945, Kevin Tuohy left his position with the Montreal branch of Obrig Laboratories and went to Los Angeles, where he joined with Solon Braff in Solex Laboratories. He introduced and patented the first corneal contact lenses in North America (pat. 2,510,438). Vague rumors had reached America that German pilots were wearing some type of small, thin corneal lenses near the end of the Second World War, but nothing definite could be determined. Working independently, Tuohy found that small lenses, approximately the diameter of the cornea, could be worn comfortably for several hours at a time. In general, these lenses were slightly flatter in curvature than the flattest meridian of the cornea by as much as 0.5 millimeters of radius. They were 10.5 millimeters in diameter and had a single posterior surface curve and smoothly rounded edges. By present day standards, they were quite thick, running to 0.5 millimeters.

At that time, the idea of a lens in direct contact with the cornea was an innovative approach. Former thinking advocated absolutely no contact between cornea and lens, while the Tuohy lens rested on the cornea apex all the time. The Tuohy lens represented a considerable advance over haptic lenses and marked another turning point in contact lens development.

In 1951, Frank Dickinson of England, Willie Sohnges of Munich, and John Neill of Philadelphia jointly announced a microlens that was 9.5 millimeters in diameter and less than half the thickness of the Tuohy lens.[30] The relationship between the radius of the posterior lens surface and that of the cornea varied with steepness of corneal curvature, amount of corneal astigmatism, and refractive error. The radius of the posterior lens surface for a spherical cornea would be approximately 0.25 millimeters longer than the radius of the cornea—and the diameter was approximately 9.5 millimeters or less. The central thickness of these lenses was only 0.2 millimeters. The specifications suggest that the lens rested directly on the apex of the cornea and might touch lightly at the periphery because of corneal flattening. Other clinicians added a secondary peripheral bevel of varying radii and widths.

These microcorneal lenses were a significant improvement over previous scleral lens types. They proved to give superior results in comfort, wearing time, and appearance. The news media reported on these lenses with much eagerness, and almost overnight, a significant new industry developed. Enthusiasm for this new type of contact lens soon spread literally around the world. The phenomenal demand resulted in the opening of a large number of contact lens laboratories in the 1950–1970 decades. Most notable were those in Australia, Canada, Germany, South Africa, Japan, the United Kingdom, and the United States.

Foremost among the American contact lens laboratories was the one started by Newton Wesley and his partner, George Jessen. The Wesley-Jessen Laboratory, headquartered in Chicago, offered instructional classes for hundreds of ophthalmologists, optometrists, opticians, and technicians. It grew rapidly and did much to promote the use of contact lenses throughout the decades from 1950 to 1980. A great many smaller companies also established laboratories in the contact lens field.

Many clinicians conducted their own practical research, and indeed several developments occurred simultaneously from different investigators. Often, private practitioners set up their own laboratories to produce contact lenses for their patients. All that was required to produce excellent lenses was an adapted jeweler's lathe, some polishing laps, and some small, inexpensive pieces of equipment. These items, coupled with a small amount of practice, enabled the contact lens fitter to produce very good lenses in a very short time.

None of the major optical suppliers entered the field in those early years because mass production did not seem feasible. Contact lenses were individually designed and produced. Also, there were so many claims and counterclaims that no definite pattern had emerged for the design of the "ideal" contact lens.

A large amount of research was done on this new modality that could replace spectacles, and countless papers appeared in professional journals. The literature on contact lens-related research expanded exponentially. Several new journals devoted solely to contact lens material made an appearance. Contact lens societies were formed at both local and national levels. Many congresses were devoted exclusively to research reports and practical aspects of contact lens fitting. Research centered around all facets of corneal physiology, lens design, and fitting procedures.

The relationship of the posterior lens surface to the cornea was investigated. Results varied between precise matching of the posterior lens curvature to the flatter corneal meridian and lenses with radii both slightly shorter and slightly longer than this. The precise relationship often was influenced by the presence or absence of second or third peripheral posterior curvatures on the contact lens, their relationship to the main curvature, and lens diameter. Lens thickness was researched, and again many differences were reported, but the median seemed to be between 0.15 and 0.2 millimeters. Lens diameters were studied, and many different dimensions were reported. Chamfers were sometimes placed at the edge of the posterior surface to aid lacrimal fluid circulation under the lens. In one type, the chamfers had a spiral shape. Another type had four slightly rounded elevations on the inside surface to allow lacrimal fluid circulation under the lens. Some investigators advocated the placement of minute perforations at various points in the lens.[31] Much duplication of methodology with very minute variations in results was reported. Presumably, all clinicians found a measure of success with their particular variation, so one can only assume that the human cornea is extremely tolerant to corneal contact lenses!

Considerable research was also expended on the wetting, cleaning, soaking, and sterilizing solutions required. Untold numbers of accessories were developed to insert and remove lenses, store them, and sterilize them. A large number of pharmaceutical and related companies were involved at first, but later the Food and Drug Administration in the United States established rigid standards of investigation before any new contact lens or related product could be introduced. Even storage cases came under close scrutiny, with many types being developed. Many smaller laboratories could not afford the high cost of research prescribed by the rigid protocol and discontinued production.

Hydrophilic Lenses

Each stage in the development of haptic lenses, from initial trial-and-error methods to development of molding procedures, change of material from glass to plastic, improvement in molding materials, fenestration to improve fluid exchange, and development of fluidless lenses, marked enormous strides in contact lens technology. A distinct change of direction came when corneal contact lenses and then microcorneal lenses came into the picture with their many variations. An impressive increase occurred in the number of successful wearers. Considerable progress had been made in the correction of refractive errors. Surely, the ultimate goal in contact lens fitting had been reached by the 1960s, but further developments and improvements were yet to come.

Near the end of the first century of contact lens use, an impressive and perhaps even greater stimulus to contact lens wear occurred with the development of several new plastic materials. The first indication that new materials were being developed came in vague rumors around 1960. Scientists working at the Institute of Macro-molecular Chemistry in Prague developed a new type of plastic material in 1959.[32] This plastic had proven useful for orbital implants, replacement of damaged ears and chins, lining dentures, and other prosthetic purposes. It was found that the material was highly compatible with human tissue. Professor Wichterle, Dr. Lim, and Dr. Driefus worked together with this material and finally recognized that it could also be very advantageous for the manufacture of contact lenses.[33]

The new plastic material seemed to have high oxygen transmission and high fluid permeability when compared with the methyl methacrylate type of plastic used in contact lenses. Its extreme flexibility would allow it to conform closely to the corneal contour. The edges could be made extremely thin, reducing lid sensation. Since the first introduction of this hydrophilic plastic, many variations have been developed for contact lens work. The present-day story remains to be written, but a great many varieties of this type of material have become available around the world. The plastic first used was known as PHEMA (polyhydroxy ethyl methacrylate). Several types of silicone plastics have also been produced.

Two methods of manufacture have been developed to produce contact lenses using these materials. In one method, the material is cast into small buttonlike configurations, similar to those made from PMMA material. These are then lathe cut to specific curvatures, observing some essential differences from the more conventional material. The second method involves spinning a drop or two of the liquid material on a concave-topped spindle. The rate of spin and time involved must be carefully controlled to obtain the desired lens power. Today, both of these methods are used, sometimes in conjunction. The front or back surface can be obtained by spinning, while the other surface can be lathe cut. Methods have been developed to produce toric and hyperbolic lens surfaces that provide correction for residual astigmatism.

The patents for the original PHEMA material, as well as for other Wichterle patents, were acquired in 1965 by the National Patent Development Corporation of New York. Dr. Robert Morrison, an optometrist of Harrisburg, played a prominent role in the initial stages.[34]

A Buffalo optometrist, Dr. Allen Isen, and a biochemical engineer at the University of Waterloo, Dr. K. F. O'Driscoll, also became interested in the material.[35] They developed a further variation of the material. Isen not only practiced optometry but also operated the Buffalo-based Frontier Contact Lens Laboratory. Because production of the new lenses in the United States was banned at first, Dr. Isen started a manufacturing facility in Toronto under the name of Griffin Laboratories. At the time, Canadian government rules were somewhat less strict. The material Isen developed was used to produce lathe-cut contact lenses. After several months, satisfactory clinical trials were conducted under controlled situations, and the lenses came into use.[36]

In 1971, Bausch and Lomb Optical Company of Rochester obtained a license to use the Wichterle material and developed and marketed spin-cast lenses under the name Soflens. Undoubtedly, this trade name contributed to the growing demand for the new flexible lenses.

Problems with the new material were not all resolved initially. Before long, it became apparent that considerable care needed to be taken with sterilization procedures. In some cases, use of the lenses showed the development of slight blemishes that appeared to lie within the material of the lens. Investigation showed that some of these inclusions were caused by bacteria, others by metal salts.[37] Special procedures were developed to ensure satisfactory sterilization, but perhaps patient compliance was, and sometimes still is, debatable.[38] Chemical, heat, and radiation methods have been used to ensure appropriate sterilization. The U.S. Food and Drug Administration declared the lenses to be a medical device and required the adherence to a prescribed investigation protocol before approval would be forthcoming.

Soon afterwards, a number of other large companies began to work with flexible, hydrophilic lenses. Polymers were developed with very high water content and marketed by international companies. A few of them are Ciba Vision, a subsidiary of the Ciba-Geigy chemistry group; Hoya, an established Japanese producer of ophthalmic lenses; Hydron, one of the direct descendents of the Wichterle product;

Polymer Technology Corporation, developer of the Boston lenses (discussed later); and recently, Johnson and Johnson, pharmaceutical manufacturers.

The most recent development has been a group of FDA-approved lenses that laboratories claim can be worn for indefinite extended periods of time. At first these lenses were used for overnight wear or, at most, for a few days at a time. Improvements and continued investigation gradually brought about increases in comfort, safety, and length of wear. Today the claim is made that some extended-wear lenses can be worn continuously for a month or more at a time. However, there are many precautions that must be observed. The author recommends extreme precaution and professional supervision in the use of extended-wear lenses of all types. Many complications can arise that could have serious consequences on ocular health.

Still other manufacturers are producing disposable contact lenses that can be worn for a week and then discarded, a new lens being provided to replace the first. This removes most problems caused by inadequate sterilization procedures and ensures a fresh lens every week. The lenses are supplied in packages of six or more lenses at a very reasonable cost. Again, extreme caution and frequent examination are advised. Still other manufacturers have produced flexible lenses having a firm plastic center in an attempt to address certain problems of fluctuating vision that sometimes occur with flexible lenses immediately after the wearer blinks.

Gas Permeable

A result of some of the research activity involving hydrophilic plastics for contact lens use has been the introduction of fluoro-polymer plastics. One type developed from the initial PMMA plastics resulted in a material having considerably increased gas permeability. It was claimed that this gas permeability increased the transmission of oxygen through the lens, improving the maintenance of corneal transparency. The first lens made from the gas permeable material used a hard silicone polymer and was known as the Boston lens. Since the oxygen reaching the cornea is greater than that from the former PMMA materials, gas permeable lenses often provided improved wearing times. These lenses are claimed to have some advantage over flexible lenses in that sharper retinal images are produced, and thus superior acuity may be obtained. With some fittings of the flexible lenses, the flexure may bend the lens when the patient blinks, and the acuity may not return to normal immediately. The gas permeable lenses tend to overcome this difficulty. Also, they are longer lasting than flexible lenses, generally speaking. Many subsequent refinements have been made in the original Boston lens material, and other types of gas permeable materials have been developed.

Bifocals and Multifocals

The popularity of contact lenses among young people increased dramatically after 1955. Some 15 years later, many of these same patients had reached the presbyopic age and wished to continue wearing contact lenses and still retain "youthful" vision. Research in bifocal contact lenses began in earnest.

William Feinbloom had patented bifocal contact lenses of the haptic type in 1936. However, these had not proven very practical. With the obvious success of corneal and microcorneal contact lenses, attention turned to developing a similar type of bifocal contact lens. There were many alternatives for the presbyopic contact lens wearer, one of which was to wear contact lenses for distance and slip on a pair of spectacles having appropriate convex power for reading. But few presbyopic contact lens wearers were completely satisfied with this method. Spectacles had been eliminated for distance, why not for near vision as well?

For a time, some clinicians advocated the use of a procedure termed *monovision*. The dominant eye was provided with a contact lens that corrected distant vision. The nondominant eye was fitted with a contact lens that overcorrected the convex lens power, adapting the eye and lens system for near point work. For distance, this eye was rather myopic. Surprisingly, many patients found that this type of correction functioned quite satisfactorily. However, many clinicians were unhappy with the method, concerned that it interfered with optimum visual acuity for either distance or near point, and reduced normal stereopsis. Nevertheless, the use of this technique did satisfy many patients and is still used at times.[39]

Another suggested solution to the problem of presbyopia was the proposal by Newton Wesley in 1967 that some form of aperture lens could be used and thus produce a pinhole effect. Indeed, a pinhole lens was introduced, but shortly afterwards, stenopaic slit contact lenses were found more practical. These lenses restricted the light admitted to the eye to the central portion of the lens. Since peripheral rays were eliminated, a certain improvement was noted in central visual acuity for all distances. This is comparable to the use of a small aperture in a camera to increase the depth of focus.

Increasing attention turned to solving the problem created by presbyopia for contact lens wearers. Two types of bifocal contact lens were developed almost from the initial consideration of the problem. They consisted of the so-called simultaneous vision type of lens and several forms of the alternating vision type of bifocal. The former is a lens having a small area about 2 millimeters in diameter placed near the center of the pupil. This was designed to produce a focus in front of the retina, while the concentric remainder of the lens produced a focus on the retina. By simply shifting the fixation point to a reading distance, the central bundle of rays falls on the retina. The peripheral zone produces a focus behind the retina. In addition, the reflex pupil constriction, when changing fixation from far to near, helps to eliminate some of the peripheral rays. Both foci are present at all times, and simply changing the fixation point produces a sharp image on the fovea, surrounded by a more blurred image. There may be a slight haziness of vision from the overlapping rays on the retina, but for some patients, the procedure gives satisfactory results. John DeCarle of London introduced such a contact lens in 1970.[40] This method has been continued and improved to the present with the introduction of diffraction grating curves on the lens surface.

The alternating vision type of bifocal contact lens has proven to be somewhat more satisfactory for a larger number of patients. In this type, a distinct area in the lens is adapted for near vision, similar to the segment area of a bifocal spectacle lens. In the bifocal lens, there are two types. In one, the reading power is annular, surrounding the distance portion in the periphery of the lens. The lens is fitted so that the lower lid catches on the lens edge when the patient looks down, and the reading area is moved slightly upward to cover most of the pupil.

Another type has a miniature bifocal reading segment in the lower portion similar to that found in regular bifocal spectacles. The near point segment may be round, flat top, or crescent shaped. One problem in fitting this type of bifocal contact lens concerned the control of the orientation of the lens so that the segment would always remain in the lower portion of the lens. This was resolved in one of three ways, sometimes used in combination. The clinician could incorporate a small amount of base down prism in each lens. The increased weight of the prism base tended to orient the lens on the eye so that the segment was always located in the lower part. The increased thickness of the prism base also allowed the lower lid to catch on the lower edge of the lens. This served to elevate it slightly on the cornea as the gaze was lowered so that the pupil was partially covered by the segment area. Another design procedure involved a flattened area placed on the periphery of the lens parallel to the lower lid. This was known as truncation and assisted in the orientation of the lens, pushing it over the pupil as the gaze was directed downwards. A third method was to implant a small piece of heavy metal within the lens near the lower edge. The added weight kept the bifocal in the lower portion. Sometimes these methods were combined to maintain the segment area in a suitable position and ensure its proper movement over the pupil when required. A final lens for any particular patient might include any combination of prism, truncation, or metal implant.

Developers of flexible contact lenses also have produced bifocal forms using hyperbolic and diffractive surfaces. While the success rate is increasing, many patients do not achieve the desired results. The lenses are best used for very early presbyopic patients who require relatively low additional power.

Conclusion

Contact lenses have been developed through many stages since the early blown glass lens used by Dr. Saemisch in 1887. Hundreds of researchers and clinicians have contributed seemingly slight modifications and improvements, but the sum total of these developments has ended in very satisfactory results. Thousands of people are fitted every year and wear their lenses safely with much satisfaction. Still the research continues, and new developments are proclaimed regularly. Some day the "perfect" contact lens will be announced—only to be replaced by an even better one!

Notes

1. H. W. Hofstetter and R. Graham, "Leonardo and Contact Lenses," *Am. J. Optom.* 30, no. 1(1953):41–44.
2. J. Enoch, "Descartes Contact Lens," *Am. J. Optom.* 33(1956):77–85.
3. S. Duke-Elder, *System of Ophthalmology*. Vol. 5(London: Henry Kimpton, 1970), 173.
4. R. F. Heitz, *History of Contact Lenses*, 1984. (*Contact Lenses: The CLAO guide to Basic Sciences and Clinical Practice*, ed. O. H. Dabezies.)
5. T. Young, "On the Mechanism of the Eye," *Phil. Trans. R. Soc.* 16(1801):23–88. Cited by M. B. Alpern, *Am. J. Optom.* 25(1948):198.
6. A. G. Bennett, "Contact Lenses:Origin," *Optician* 141, no. 3663 (1961):644.
7. J. F. W. Herschel, *Encyclopedia Metripolitania* (1845) 4.396–404 (cited in J. Stone, and A. J. Phillips, *Contact Lenses*, 1980).
8. F. A. Muller A. C. and Muller, *The Artificial Eye* (1910) (cited by J. DeCarle, "Who Fitted the First Contact Lens?" *Optician* (supp.) (1988):4.
9. S. Duke-Elder, op.cit. p. 128.
10. T. Obrig, *Contact Lenses* (New York: Obrig Laboratories, 1942).
11. L. Jenkins, "The Development of the Modern Contact Lens," *Optician* 141, no. 3660 (1961):541–547.
12. J. Pascal, "The Origins and Development of Contact Lenses," *Opt. J. and Rev. Opt.* 78, no. 2 (1941):57–61.
13. A. E. Fick, "A Contact Lens," *Arch. Ophth.* 17(188):215–226. English translation of "Eine Contactbrille," *Archiv f. Augenheilkunde* 18: 279–289.
14. T. Sabell, "The Early Years," Optician (supp.) (1988): 6–21
15. T. Obrig, op. cit. p.128.
16. T. Obrig, op. cit. pp.129–30.
17. R. F. Heitz, op. cit. pp. 1–6.
18. T. Obrig, op. cit. pp. 137–139
19. "Hamblin-Dallos Contact Lens," *Optician* 143(1938).
20. T. E. Obrig, . "A New Ophthalmic Impression Material,". *Arch. Ophthal. N.Y.* 30(1943):626–630.
21. A. M. Anderson, *Technique of Fitting Contact Lenses* (McGill Lithograph, 1944).
22. T. E. Obrig, "A Cobalt Blue Filter for Observation of the Fit of Contact Lenses," *Arch. Ophthal. N.Y.* 20(1938):657–658.
23. W. Feinbloom, "A Plastic Contact Lens," *Am. J.* Optom. 14(1947):41–49.
24. W. Feinbloom, "The Tangent Cone Contact Lens Series," *Optom. Weekly* 36(1945):1159–1161.
25. "A Salute to the 'Father' of Low Vision—W. Feinbloom," *Rev. Optom.*128, no. 4 (1991):10.
26. Barnes Hind Pharmaceuticals, California.
27. N. Bier, *Contact Lens Routine and Practice* (London: Butterworth's, C.V. Mosby, 1953).
28. A. Mueller-Welt, "The Mueller-Welt Fluidless Contact Lens," *Optom. Weekly* 41(1950):831–834.
29. R. Graham, Evolution of Corneal Contact Lenses. *Am. J. Optom.* 36(1959):55–59.
30. F. Dickinson, "A Report on a New Contact Lens," *Optician* 118(1949):141.
31. D. R. Korb, *Clinical Observations on Current Microscopic Corneal lens Perforations* (author's publication 1950c).
32. O. Wichterle and D. Lim, "Hydrophilic Gels for Biological Use," *Nature* 185(1960):117.
33. E. J. Fisher, "Hydrophilic Contact Lenses," *Can. J. Optom.* 29, no. 4(1968):139–144.
34. K. F. O'Driscoll, "Polymeric Aspects of Soft Contact Lenses," in A. R. Gasset, and H. E. Kaufman, *Soft Contact Lenses* (St. Louis: Mosby, 1972).
35. R. J. Morrison, "Hydrophilic Contact Lenses," *J. Am. Optom. Ass.* 37,no. 3(1966):211–218.
36. H. D. E. Inns, "The Griffin Lens," *Am. J. Optom.*(1973):977–983.
37. T. Grosvenor, A. M. Charles, and M. Callender, "Soft Contact Lens Bacteriological Study," *Can. J. Optom.* 34, no. 1 (1972):11–18.
38. A.M. Charles, M. Callender, and T. Grosvenor, "Efficacy of Chemical Ascepticizing System for Soft Contact Lenses," *Am. J. Optom.* 50(1973):777–781.

39. W. E. Fleischman, "The Single Vision Reading Contact Lens," *Am. J. Optom. Arch. Am. Acad. Opt.* 45, no. 6 (1968):408–409.
40. J. DeCarle, "Bifocal Lenses," in J. Stone, J.and A. J. Phillips, *Contact Lenses*, 3d ed.(London/Toronto: Butterworth's, 1989), 595–624.

39

Modern Frames

In the first 10 to 15 years of the twentieth century, we find at first a slow evolution from the styles of the last century. Then came acceptance of sensible improvement for another decade followed by just a few frame and lens changes until World War II. Of course, after World War II, exotic styles flourished. We calmed down a bit in 1970 and 1980, espousing light, comfortable frames and visually improved lens styles and materials.

1900–1915

Frame materials used were mostly gold, gold-filled, silver, and various platings and alloys (Figure 741). Some rimless models were available as well as "round eyes" (35 millimeters) (Figures 742 & 743). Sizes of oval rims expanded from 35–38 millimeters horizontally to 40–42 millimeters. Dark Crooke's sunglasses were used. The temple eye wire gave way to the more comfortable cable temple. The crescent-shaped strap bridge gradually changed to nose pads and a saddle variety. Pince-nez lasted until the 1930s (Figure 743).

Whereas lenses were generally larger, meniscus lenses were universal, and toric lenses were commonly being used. Hang-on, hook-on, or "grab front" additions were available for near vision purposes (Figure 744). The pince-nez style mountings were popular, with the Shuron and Fits-U type predominating. Cement bifocals grudgingly gave way to the latest in kryptoks, but the former lasted past 1940 (see Chapter 21 on bifocals).

American Optical Company moved the hinge from the center of the lens to the top of the frame. This style was designed by Dr. Tillyer, an employee of American Optical Company.

1920–1930

The Hollywood, California, actor Harold Lloyd popularized the use of plastics for spectacle frames so that by the end of the decade, this material was accepted by male and female wearers alike (Figure 745). Plastics were also used as frame parts, with metal as supportive members. Eye wires and nose pads were made of plastic rather than natural materials such as baleen, cork, and tortoiseshell (Figure 746).

Lens sizes increased to 45 millimeters horizontally with round eyes. Rimless models were still available. For presbyopes, ultex bifocals and trifocals were available. Spatula temples appeared.

1930–1940

Rimless frames utilizing one or two screws gave blessed relief to those who had sore noses from heavy glasses (Figure 747). Most of these were made of white gold or gold-filled metal. No natural materials were used after this period. Few other changes occurred because of the World War II war effort.

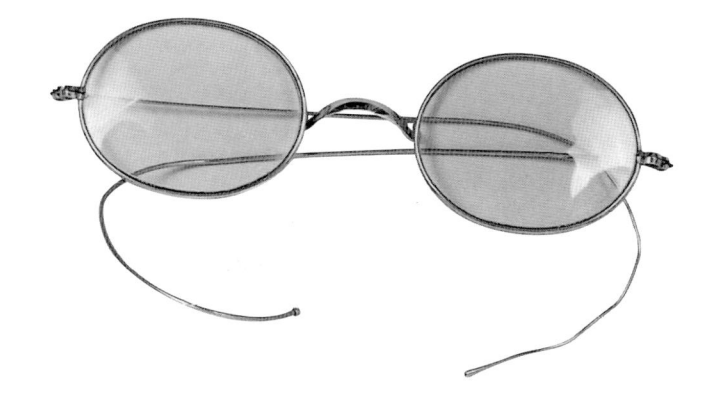

Figure 741. American spectacles circa 1910.

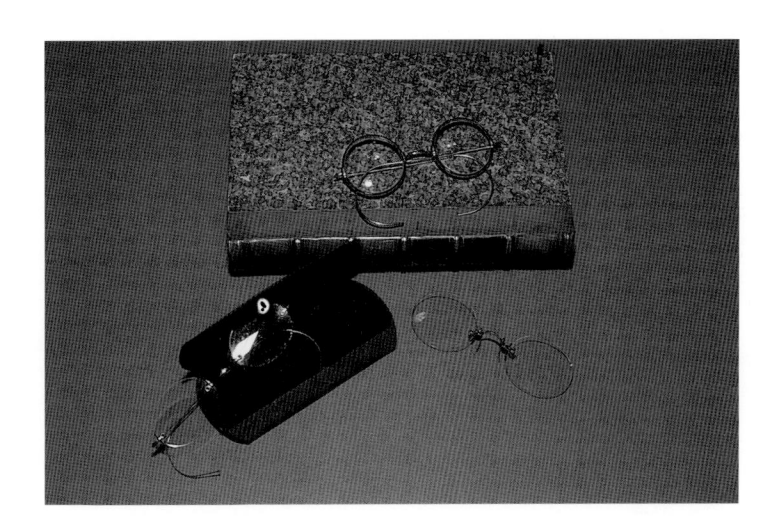

Figure 743. "Round eyes" circa 1915.

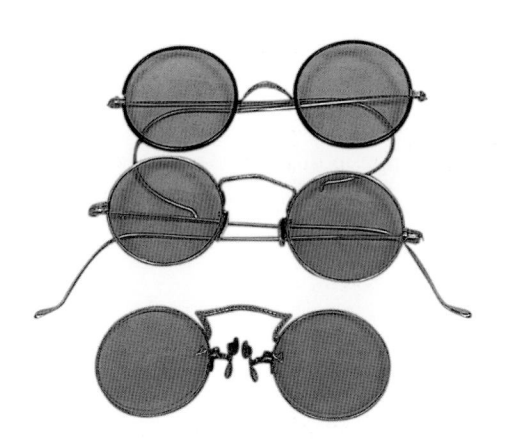

Figure 742. Spectacles of 1915.

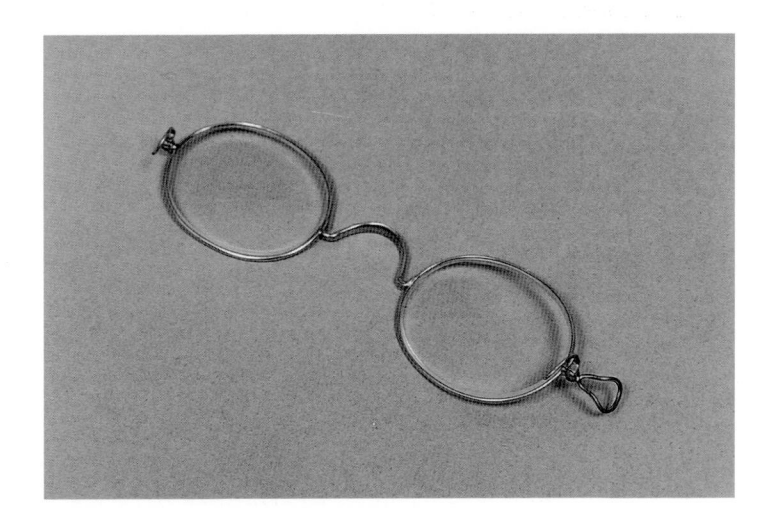

Figure 744. Hang-on near addition, American.

MODERN FRAMES **385**

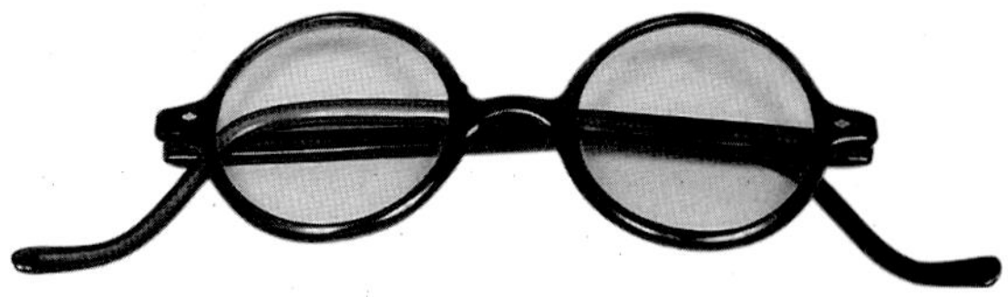

Figure 745. Harold Lloyd type of frame.

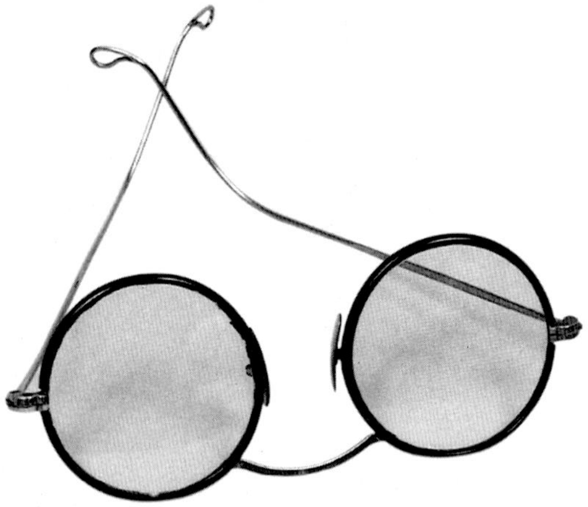

Figure 746. English frames circa 1925.

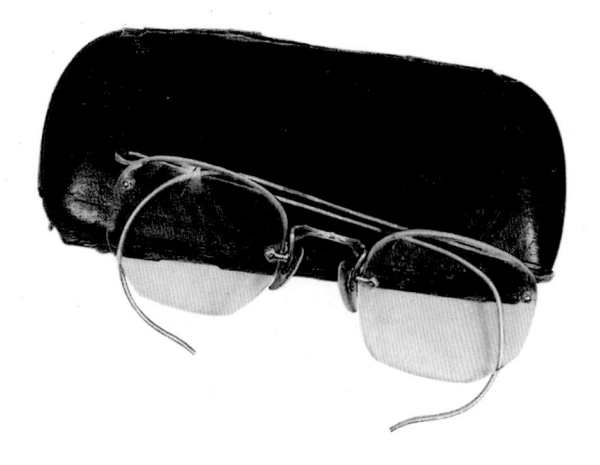

Figure 747. American rimless spectacles circa 1935.

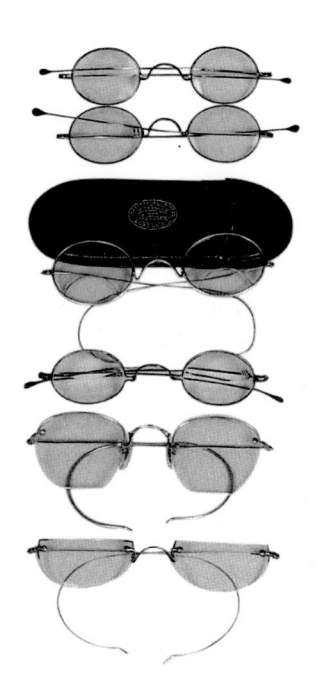

Figure 748. Progression of lens changes 1910–1930.

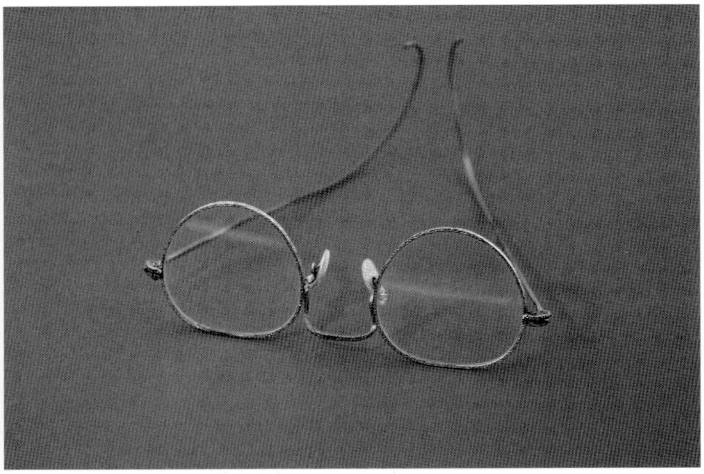

Figure 749. Gold-filled American spectacles circa 1940.

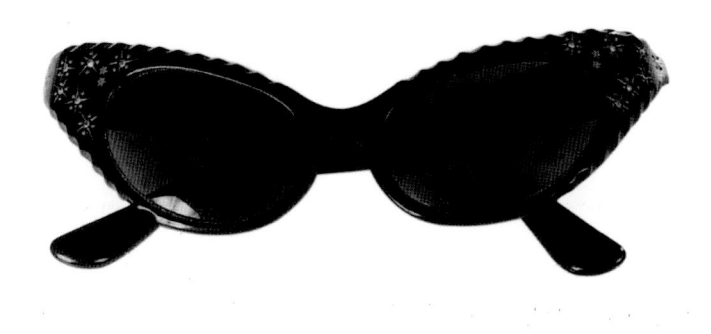

Figure 750. Typical American sunglasses circa 1950.

White metal frames were produced to fit under gas masks. Factories were happy just to obtain optical glass and enough materials to make utilitarian frames. After 1945, it took a few years to train personnel and obtain machinery and materials (Figures 748 & 749).

1950–1970

Plastics were so easy to use that most frames were made of those materials with wild colors and designs. Sunglasses were used many times day and night (Figure 750). Public figures used them as a disguise, and entertainers used them as protection from blinding spotlights. Frames were huge for both regular and sunglasses (Figures 751 & 752).

Those individuals who had cataracts removed did not yet have the benefit of intraocular lenses. They therefore had to use large plus (8 to 20) lenses to see. Plastic lenses and aspheric grinds reduced the weight for the patient in this period. Color in the lenses helped with glare.

1970–Present

Frames have come down to a sensible size and are much lighter in construction. Metals are used more and are treated with anodizing and other decorative methods. Frame materials are not only attractive and decorative but also sophisticated enough so that innovative curves and thin lines of enameling are in vogue. Semirimless lenses and lenses held in by plastic monofilament lines in the lower half give a light, airy feeling

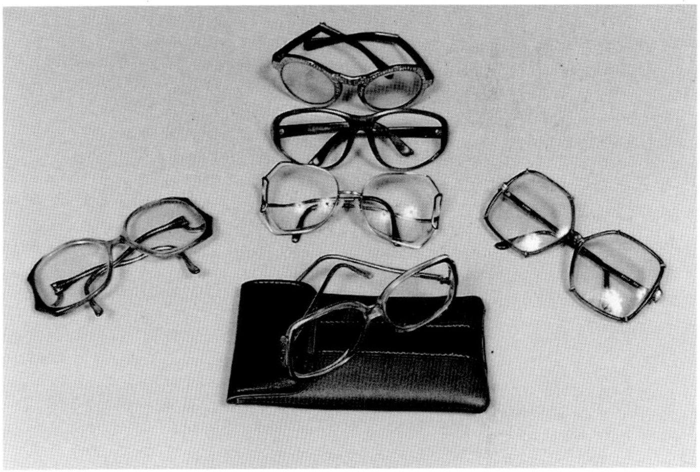

Figure 751. Large lenses and frames.

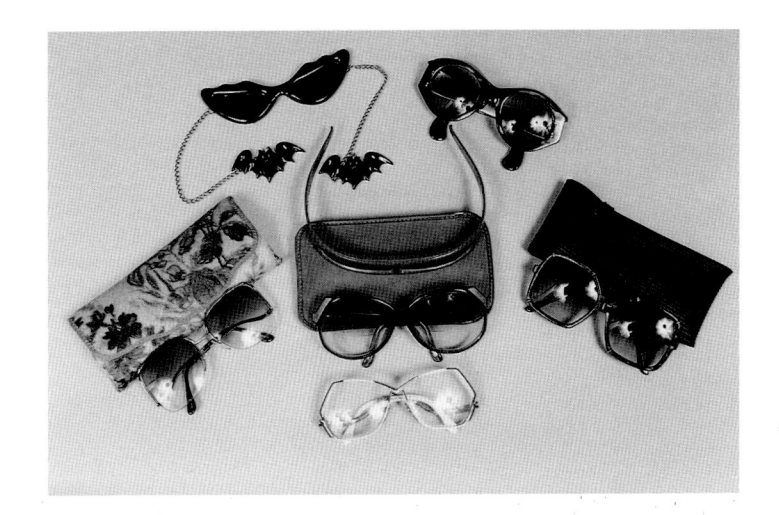

Figure 752. Other American spectacles and sunglasses.

MODERN FRAMES 387

and remove weight from frame and lenses. Frame materials such as nylon and metal alloys add durability and beauty to frames.

Lenses made of various plastics such as polycarbonate are used to bring light weight and durability to lenses. Whereas plastic lenses scratch more easily than glass, coatings applied make this less likely to occur. Other coatings to decrease glare, light, and ultraviolet are used to advantage as well.

Conclusion

Spectacles in the twentieth century showed a more rapid evolvement in materials, styles, shapes, sizes, and decoration than the previous 50 years. This chapter merely touches the tops of the waves of change. Other publications chronicle this optical, social, manufacturing, and business evolution in a more detailed manner. And so it should be.[1]

Sources Consulted for Chapter 39

1. Joseph Bruneni, *Looking Back* (Optical Laboratories Association: California, 1995).
2. Casey A. Woods, *Encyclopedia of Ophthalmology* (Chicago, 1915).

Appendix 1

Landmarks in Optical History*

3300 B.C.
: Glass beads and ornaments of this period have been found in Egyptian tombs of the pharaohs of the Fifth and Sixth Dynasties.

2000 B.C.
: Paintings on the walls of Egyptian tombs at Thebes show glassblowing. Vases of transparent glass of this period are still in existence.

1500 B.C.
: Moses mentions mirrors in the Bible, the book of Exodus. Job also mentions mirrors.

About 720 B.C.
: An Assyrian lens-shaped crystal dating from this period was dug up at the Palace of Sargon at Nimrud, and is now in the British Museum. As it contains striae and has irregular facets, it was probably only an ornamental boss and not a lens, as was first thought.

424 B.C.
: Aristophanes, Greek playwright and a contemporary of Plato and Socrates, mentions burning glasses in his *Comedy of the Clouds*, Act II. He mentions "that fine transparent stone with which fires are kindled, by which placing myself in the sun I will though at a distance melt all the writing on the summons" (referring to the waxen tablets at that time used for writing).

350 B.C.
: Aristotle, Greek philosopher, pupil of Plato, and tutor of Alexander the Great, opposes the prevalent theories that light was a material emission from a source. In a haphazard manner, he anticipates the wave theory of light when he says that light is caused by the action of the intervening medium and that "vision is the result of some impression made upon the faculty of sense." From his time, there was no real progress in the physical theory of light transmission until the time of Huygens.

About 350 B.C.
: Aristotle explains the rainbow as being caused by the reflection of the sun's rays from raindrops, pointing out that the spray from an oar will form a rainbow visible to an oarsman with his back to the sun. He also mentions eye defects of myopia and presbyopia but suggests no cure.

About 250 B.C.
: Ptolemy, Egyptian astronomer and geographer, draws up tables of refraction and reflection; he finds the index of refraction of water to be 1.33 but fails to discover the law. He also evolves the Ptolemain theory of astronomy, i.e., that the sun, planets, and fixed stars all revolve about the earth. This theory lasted 1500

---

* Also refer to Appendix 8, p. 489.

years, until overthrown by Copernicus (A.D. 1473–1543), who proved the earth's rotation around the sun.

About A.D. 50
Cleomedes, Greek philosopher in Egypt, observes bent image of straight stick in water. He also explains atmospheric refraction as the reason for our seeing the sun after it has passed below the horizon.

About A.D. 60
Pliny, Roman historian, tells about Nero viewing the gladiatorial combat through an emerald. "These are mostly concave to draw sight, but in relief form they give again images the same as mirrors when held up perpendicularly."

About A.D. 70
Seneca, Roman philosopher, states that letters, though small and distant, are seen enlarged and more distinct through a glass, water-filled globe but only concludes that all objects are larger when seen through water.

About A.D. 80
Plutarch, Roman writer, mentions myopia, the ocular defect.

About A.D. 450
Actius, Greek physician, states that myopia is incurable.

A.D. 1025
Alhazen, Arabian astronomer at Cairo, writes his famous treatise on optics, the first scientific one ever written. This, translated into Latin in 1572, was recognized for 500 years as the chief authority in Europe. He also
 —Founded the mathematical theory of optics.
 —Explained how, with two eyes, we see but one image.
 —Showed how objects are visible by a cone of rays coming from the object to the eye.
 —Explained optical deceptions, such as the apparent increase in size of moon or sun when near the horizon.

A.D. 1250
Actuarius, Greek physician, states that "myopia is an infirmity of sight for which art can do nothing."

A.D. 1250
Vitellio, Polish scientist, writes treatise in optics founded on Alhazen's, explains twinkling of stars as being caused by motion of air, compiles more accurate tables of angles of incidence and refraction of light at surface of water and glass.

A.D. 1266
Roger Bacon writes his three treatises: the *Opus Major*, *Opus Minor* and *Opus Tertius*, in which he describes the means of obtaining enlarged objects and correcting weak eyes or those of aged persons. He also describes the telescopic effect of such lenses, magic lantern, gunpowder—see 1610, Galileo.

A.D. 1280
Heinrich Frauenlob, German poet, writes a poem showing how writing can be made legible to the eyes of old persons by means of mirrors, presumably concave.

A.D. 1285
Giordano di Rivalto, an ancient Florentine document of 1305, says spectacles were invented in 1285.

A.D. 1299
Ancient Florentine manuscript by one Pissazzo tells about spectacles lately invented being an aid to vision of old men.

A.D. 1313
A manuscript from the monastery of St. Catherine of Pisa on giving a death, year of 1313, says: "Brother Alexander della Spina, a modest and good man, understood and could make all things producible which he saw or of which he heard. He made spectacles which had previously been made by no one."

1313–1320
A portrait of Pope Leo X with a reading glass is painted by Raphael and is now in the Uffizi Gallery at Florence, Italy.

1317
A tombstone in the church of Santa Maria Maggiore, Florence, Italy, states: "Here lies Salvino d'Armato degli, Armati of Florence, inventor of spectacles. God pardon him for his sins. Anno D. 1317." This is untrue.

1352	A portrait by Thomas of Modena shows a priest holding a single reading glass before the eye—a sort of a monocular lorgnette.
1352	A portrait by Thomas of Modena shows a bishop reading by means of two lenses connected by a rivet, allowing them to be folded one over the other.
1380	Chaucer mentions spectacles in *The Canterbury Tales*.
About 1410	A portrait by Jan van Eyck show spectacles joined by a bridge.
1420	Gold frames and beryl or crystal lenses come into use, followed by frames of horn and leather.
1440	The invention of printing comes about.
About 1450	Nicolaus of Cusa (d. 1464) describes concave lenses as then being known. Exact date of introduction is not known.
About 1450	Spectacles with a rigid bridge are used.
1474	Benvenute Grassi writes the first book on ophthalmology that is printed.
1480	A Fresco in a church of Ognissanti, Florence, Italy, by Ghirlandajo, a Florentine painter, shows St. Jerome with spectacles.
1483	Nuremberg has master spectacle makers.
1495	"Youthful glasses," i.e., concave for myopia, are mentioned as supplied to a monastery. Nuremberg establishes spectacle ordinances. A helmet made for Henry VIII has lenses riveted into eyeholes.
1560	Ravenscroft puts flint (lead) into glass to make it clear.
1560	Spectacles for "weak sight of old age" and for "near sight of youth" are manufactured extensively, on a fairly large scale, and graded according to age. Sales are made through traveling peddlers of novelties.
1581	A Spanish portrait by Rouyer shows a Paduan professor wearing spectacles held in place by cords running back over the ears.
1589	J.B. Porta, inventor of the camera obscura, shows that lenses were then being ground in Venice in plano concave, plano convex, double concave, and double convex forms.
1596	A portrait of a cardinal by El Greco, a Spanish painter, also shows use of cord temples over the ears.
About 1600	Regensburg frames show the use of spring bridges to grip the nose. Also, strap spectacles are similar in appearance and use to modern leather goggles.
1604	Kepler, the famous astronomer, explains the action of ophthalmic lenses as placing the image onto the retina, which serves as a receiving screen.
1609	Jans and Hans Lippershey, spectacle makers of Middleburg, Holland, invent the "astronomic" telescope, i.e., having convex objective and convex eyepiece and giving an inverted image. These lenses were of rock crystal.
1610	Galileo invents the terrestrial telescope whereby "many noblemen and senators mounted the steps of the highest church towers at Venice to watch the ships, which were visible through my glass two hours before they were seen entering the harbor." This has a convex objective with concave eyepiece and gives an erect image.
1610	By this telescope, Galileo reveals the satellites of Jupiter and breaks the dawn of modern astronomy.
1610	The much-disputed invention of the compound microscope by Galileo comes about. (?) Dallinger, in "The Microscope and Its Revelations," gives evidence at length and concludes that "Galileo in 1610 was the inventor of the compound microscope; it was subsequently invented or introduced and zealously adopted in Holland; and when Dutch invention penetrated into Italy in 1624 Galileo attempted a reclamation of his invention but as these were not warmly seconded and responded to abroad he allowed the whole thing to pass." It is highly probable that Galileo's microscope was his terrestrial telescope adapted to near focusing, while that of Drebbel the Dutchman was an adapted astronomic telescope.
1611	Kepler introduces meniscus lenses and first publishes the correct rules for finding the focal lengths of lenses.
1611	A. M. de Dominis, Archbishop of Spalatro, shows sketches of lenses correctly placed before the eye—plano convex with convex outward and plano con-

cave with concave inward. He also correctly explains the action of a rainbow and illustrates it by a glass globe filled with water.

1618 Sirturus of Milan, in a textbook on optics, advocates grading of spectacle lenses according to their radii of curvature instead of according to the age of the persons they best fitted—the system then in use. He also complains of the low quality of Roman and Venetian spectacles lenses, saying that the glass was poor and full, the grinding forms unequal and inaccurate. He describes grinding methods then in use at Regensburg, Germany.

1621 Drebbel, a Dutch mathematician to court of James I, invents a compound microscope that probably had a convex objective and convex eyepiece.

1621 Snell, professor of mathematics at Leyden, discovers the law of refraction, later (1637) put in trigonometric form by Descartes.

1622 Richard Bannister writes the first English book on ophthalmology.

1623 Daza de Valdez, a Spanish priest, writes a book on spectacles. He describes cases of anisometropia, i.e., with one lens convex and the other concave (more exactly—this type is called "antimetropia"). Also he describes lenses bevel-edged to fit in frames and tells how tests for glasses were made at an optician's establishment.

1629 Worshipful Company of Spectacle Makers is incorporated in England. This is today the foremost such association abroad.

1637 Descartes independently discovers Snell's law of refraction and puts it in its present trigonometric form. In French books, the law is called "Descartes' Law."

About 1650
The use of spectacles with a split bridge begins

1662 The Royal Society is chartered by James I of England.

1664 The Royal Society (England), on March 6 hears its first paper on "An Improvement in Optick Glasses . . . to work great optick glasses with a turne tool without any mould and to show without rainbow colors," by a Signor Campani of Rome.

1665 Grimaldi publishes his discovery of diffraction, i.e., the slight bending of light rays on passing by a straight edge or through a relatively small aperture.

1666 Sir Isaac Newton's famous prism experiment shows decomposition of white light into colors by one prism and recomposition of these colors back into white light by another.

1666 First Optical Patent, No. 149 English, is awarded to Francis Smethwick on a more perfect form of lens. From his description, this appears to be a crossed cylinder.

1667 Telescopic spectacles for the very nearsighted are described by a Jesuit priest, Fr. Eshinardi.

1675 Romer, Danish astronomer, discovers that light travels with a measurable velocity. He finds it to be 192,000 miles per second by observation on the satellites of Jupiter. This is doubted everywhere until Bradley's different method indicates similar results (see 1728).

1678 Huygens enunciates his wave theory of light but fails to explain many important phenomena. Hence, his theory is untenable until the time of Thomas Young (1807) and Fresnel.

About 1690
Oxford type spring glasses are introduced at Regensburg. Chinese at this time were using shell-framed glasses with temples. Test glasses in belts displaced the old "trying on" method of spectacle fitting.

1704 Sir Isaac Newton announces his corpuscular theory of light, the prevailing one until Young and Fresnel's experiments on the wave theory. Today, neither theory adequately fits all the phenomena with which we are acquainted, and scientists within the past ten years predict that the next theory will probably be a combination of the two theories.

1727 Edward Scarlett invents temples—London.*

1728 Bradley, English astronomer, confirms Romer's estimate of the speed of light by a different method through the discovery of astronomic aberration of light.

---

* Note Scarlotti p. 419.

392 APPENDIX I

1747　Daviel's does the first planned intracapsular cataract extraction.

1758　Dollond, English optician, invents the achromatic lens.

1783　The first spectacle patent is issued to one Addison Smith, English, for achromatic lenses in spectacles.

1784　Benjamin Franklin invents the first bifocals.

1801　Thomas Young, English scientist, discoveres and measures his own corneal astigmatism and writes an epoch-making treatise on physiologic optics, which is far ahead of its time.

1804　Wollaston gains the English patent on meniscus lenses, the first wide-angle ophthalmic lenses.

1810　Sir David Brewster suggests trifocals.

About 1815

Thomas Young discovers interference of light waves, and founds modern theory of color vision.

1815　Frauenhofer locates over 600 lines in the solar spectrum.

1820　Nickel plating of instruments is started.

1827　George Airy, director of Greenwich Observatory, corrects his own ocular astigmatism by a pair of spherocylindrical lenses.

1837　The "solid up-curve" bifocal is patented by Schnaitmann of Philadelphia.

1840　Gauss publishes his general theory of refraction through centered spherical surfaces by use of principal points and planes. In 1845, Listing discoveres two additional nodal points.

1850　Helmholtz invents the ophthalmoscope.

1851　Helmholtz invents the ophthalmometer for refraction.

1854　Helmholtz invents the plane parallel plate ophthalmoscope.

1860　Wollaston invents the periscopic lens.

1864　Donders publishes *Refraction and Accommodation.*

1865　William Bowman invents retinoscopy and cycloplegics.

1866　Nagel advocates the metric system of designating the powers of lenses to displace the old inch system. The term *diopter* is proposed by Monoyer of France.

1871　Cuignet invents the retinoscope.

1873　Abbé announces his theory of the microscope.

1882　The Javal-Schiotz ophthalmometer is invented.

1885　The first toric lenses are ground in America.

1886　Jena glass is put on the market.

1888　Morck patents the cement bifocal.

1889　Morck patents the perfection bifocal.

1890　Prentice's paper "Ophthalmic Prisms" originates the prism diopter.

1895　Prentice's paper "Why Strong Contra-generic Lenses Fail to Neutralize" results in sweeping changes of trial set lenses.

1899　Borsch patents the original cemented Kryptok.

1906　Stainless steel is developed.

1900–1923

The rise of modern ophthalmic optics comes, during which Tscherning of France calculated the first anastigmatic lenses, Von Rohr of Germany calculates Punktal lenses and originates vertex refraction, Gullstrand of Sweden invents aspheric anastigmatic cataract lenses, known as Katral lenses, Borsch of America invents Kryptok fused bifocals, and Connor of America invents Ultex one-piece bifocals.

[The other discoveries and inventions of this half century are as yet too recent to be properly classified according to their significance or importance.]

OPTICAL LANDMARKS　393

Appendix 2

English Translation of D. M. Manni's Book about Salvino Armati

Italian translated by Richard Cardoni

Latin, French and Greek translated by Dr. Martha Beveridge

We note that in 1271, Marco Polo, on his first voyage to China, observed spectacles being worn. These were, however, being used for other than optical purposes. Even before this, lenses were described by Alhazen, and an emerald was used by Nero.

Without a doubt, the definitive, recognized, authoritative, researched, and basic publication on this subject is that of Edward Rosen. In 1956, Rosen wrote a two-part article entitled "The Invention of Eyeglasses," in the *Journal of the History of Medicine and Allied Sciences*. This article exhaustively approached the subject from many reasonable angles—national, religious, industrial, scientific, and psychological. Rosen conclusively ascertained that the true inventor is unknown and selfishly tried to hide his invention for personal gain. Or was it forbidden by the doges of Venice for him to share his invention?

In either case, this intention was thwarted by Friar Allessandro della Spina, who saw the first eyeglasses, reproduced them, and introduced them to the public.

One of the hurdles in determining this truth was a book written by Domenico Maria Manni in Florence in 1738. Manni salutes Salvino Armati as the inventor. Rosen unveils this as a fabrication in his article.

A full translation of Manni's book follows in an effort to:
a. Bring to the English-speaking public a direct translation of Manni from the ancient Italian, Latin, and Greek.
b. Indicate some of the problems Rosen solved in his monumental work.
c. Allow interested parties their own opportunity to judge this material.
d. Show that even Manni made typographical, reference, and translation errors.

The author managed to have Mr. Richard Cardoni of Loflin, Pennsylvania, translate the old Italian and Dr. Martha Beveridge of New Orleans to translate the ancient Latin, French, and Greek passages. This effort was truly a labor of love and a difficult feat well done.

Following is the complete work of Manni for your review.

Sources Consulted for Appendix 2

Cashell, G.T.W. "A Short History of Spectacles," *Proceedings of the Royal Society of Medicine* 64(Oct. 1971):1063.

Kuisle, Anita. *Brillen*. Deutches Museum, 1986.

Maggeridge, J.F.C. "The Discovery of Spectacles," *RSA*: 4, 1982.

Poggendorf. *Geschichte des Physik*, p. 99.

Rosen, Edward. "The Invention of Eyeglasses," *Journal of the History of Medicine and Allied Sciences* 11(1956):13–46, 183–218.

Young, John M. *The History of Eyewear*. American Optical Company Museum, 1985.

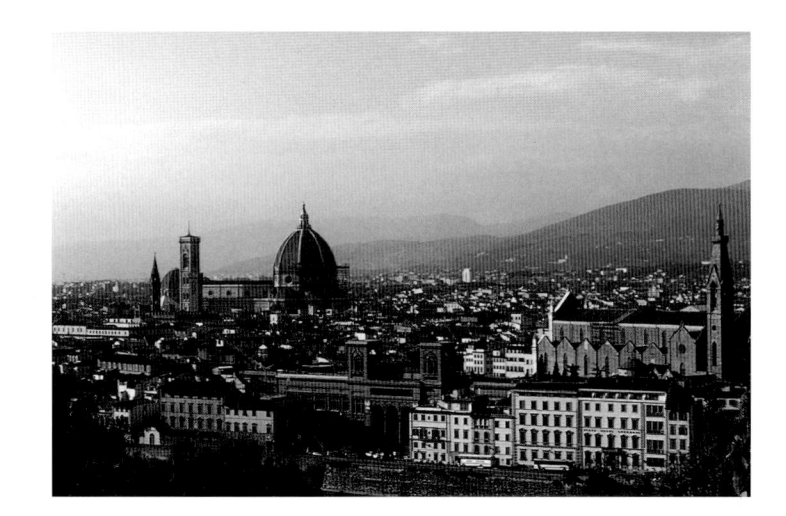

Figure 753. Florence 1994. (Rosenthal)

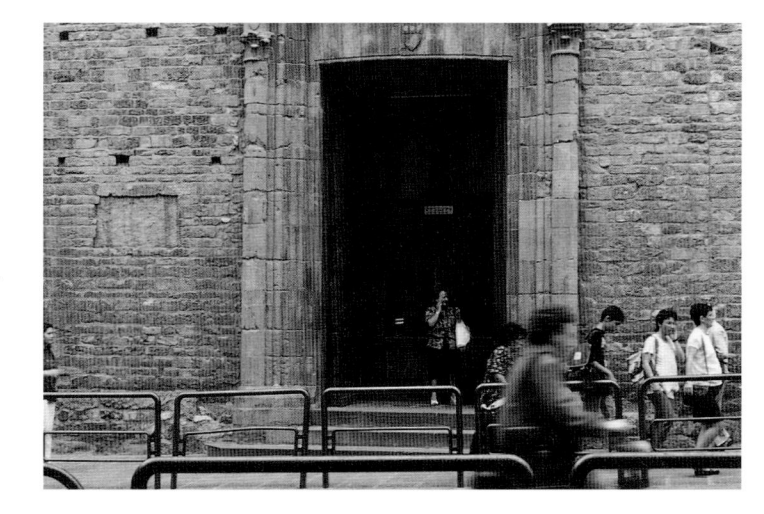

Figure 754. Main entrance of the Santa Maria Majore Church. Florence 1994. (Rosenthal)

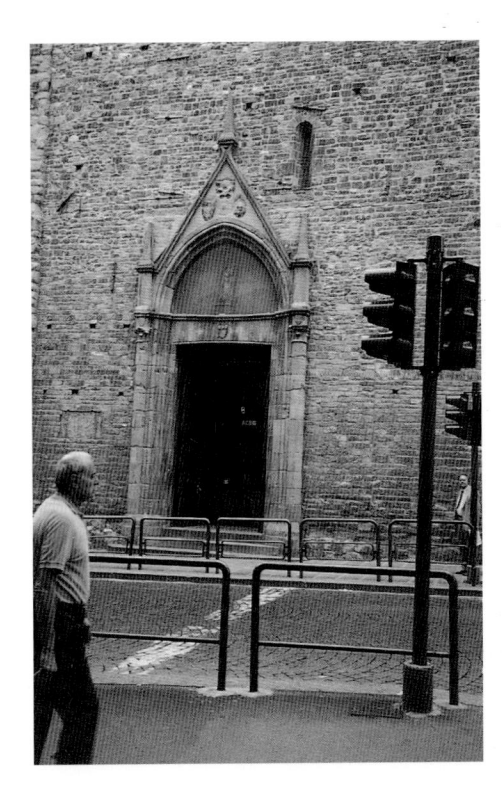

Figure 755. Side entrance of the Santa Maria Majore Church. Florence 1994. (Rosenthal)

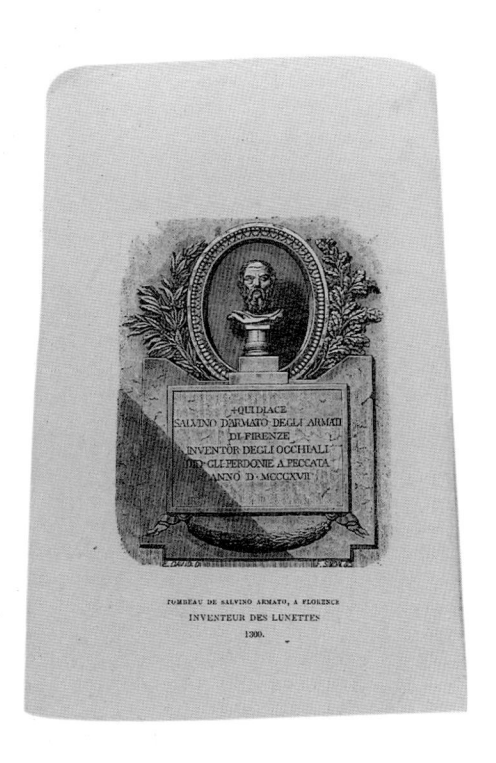

Figure 756. From Arthur Chamblin, *L' Art de l'opticien* (1863).

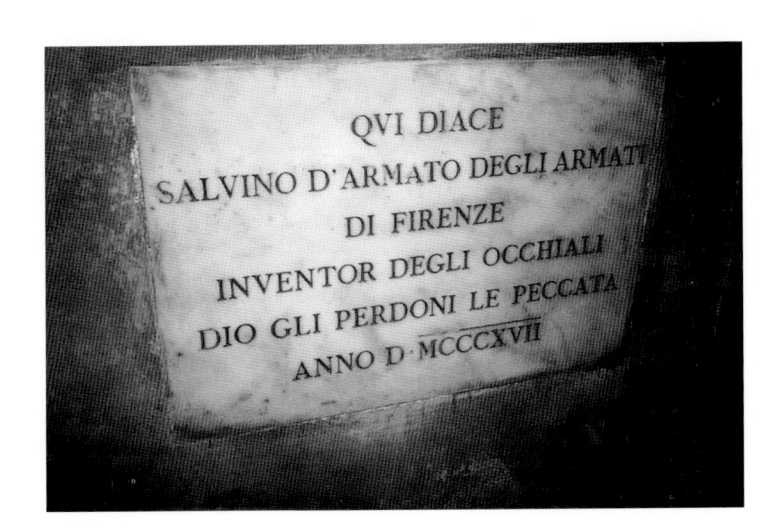

Figure 757. Plaque honoring Salvino d'Armato, Santa Maria Majore Church. Florence 1994. (Rosenthal)

About Eyeglasses for the Nose
Invented by Salvino Armati
Florentine Gentleman

Historical Treatise

by

Domenico Maria Manni

Florentine Academy

In Florence—1738
at the Printery of Anton Maria Albizzini
with Permit of the Superiors

To the Illustrious Sir
Andrea Da Verrazzano
Nobleman (Cavalier) of the order of Saint Stefano

If your most respectable person vs. Ilustrissima might be so pleased with the little work that I am devoting to you how ardent is the desire that I maintain to show by means of my homage.

About Eyeglasses on the Nose
First Part

Prologue

The propensity of man to search into the truth of all things is such that in spite of the hatred of whom now and then finds it (truth) throws things away, he who doesn't make a noble search by himself, for who seems to be born from Aristotle, deceives himself. You could also add the internal effort with which he feels pleasantly induced to search for the truth, enjoying in spite of anything, as Tullis said, to publish. With all this though many difficulties appear against the person who searches for the truth, the old people say it and the new philosophers, that the major part of their living was that they were employed in exploring and searching and usually in vain; Man, is for the most part, subjected to restricting the apparent appearances of things when the substance seems to be grasped: and they find more false things, and there are many more than the truth, which is the only thing, alone, transitory and hidden.

But since it was the disposition of Heaven that the world be subjected to the arguments of men it might not be too serious (heavy) to see hear the discussion of the present question if in as much as the unskillful hand of the writer can render (translate) the same devious reasoning; it will seem alright to me (if) the one that I did is joined to that one if for the benefit of time things become revealed I will know how to remove those false (things) that truth has hidden. I am not even one to believe to be in a hurry to find what others many seasons before, much more knowledgeable than I because of their serious maturity and expertise; didn't find; that is to say that give what might be the subject of my reasoning a meticulous search if the ancients might have had use of that very useful instrument called Eyeglasses worn on the nose. (1) (on) the truth, on which every intellect rests. I would believe frankly to be able to publish it not caring in any way what men might know or say about it. But then (since) as the poet says "What I do, I see, and the truth that is misunderstood doesn't deceive me." It is necessary for me to confess because I am doubly afraid to bring the same thing to light; first because for as much as I have forced myself to manage well the present argument, however I could still believe in not having succeeded in a great deed; Secondly because if it happens this way I won't even get my principal end of unloading on the World universally my observance towards You Illustrious Gentleman, while this same badly conducted work of my natural talent, will not have as an adventure the defected course among learned men.

Another work is due you (all) that you have inherited by blood those rare learned selections from which your relatives were all beautifully adorned (complimented) clearly no less for their prowess than for their knowledge (two) virtues emulated in them and in you along with compassion. Whereas the great actions of two of them are known among the others of your lineage (family) with the name of Lodovico: that one of them extremely brave in the military regarded in particular high esteem by Philip IV king of Spain, was general of the galleys of the Religion of St. Stefano and Governor of the City and Port of Livorno, where he left along with various others indelible monuments of virtue in the Church of Saint John: The other Monsignor Suddecano of our Metropolitan, and Spedalingo of St. Mary of the Innocents who together with Cavalier Ulisse his brother was both (together) founder and bestower (dowry) of one of the most illustrious exemplary colleges of Holy Mary that there are in Florence. The great Diovanni da Verrazzano is very famous throughout the universe as discoverer of the new hidden region named New France about which I have spoken much elsewhere and not that (only) me, many bright writers make an honorable mention of it. Nor do you have it here from us of whom the prudence of the now Senator Filippo your father might not be evident and that you don't admire highly the sublime talents of the intellect of Senator Neri, your beloved brother, who form the accredited Depositary Care of the City and form the state of Siena, with sadness of those people and with supreme applause not only from ours, but from everyone he was now promoted form the wisdom of the Royal Sovereign to the Care (Charge) of his General Depositary (Treasury).

Whoever has all these things present and in sight as I have them; whoever knows your house has become the abode of Men of Letters and of those disposed to fine arts, that they find refuge there and welcome reception and favor; (he) who knows about studies, that you have always done in every manner of erudition, regarding principally history, sees very well the truth about which I'm saying and as long as I am here every shadow of adulation will by long, particularly where I omit in silence, so as not to put your modesty, all your talents and your most beautiful prerogatives on trial. Nor did I indicate nevertheless, as it is said, by the way (in secret) Giuseppe Manni my father when he also was given the honor of adorning *with your name V. S. Illustrissima* a pamphlet, inedited up to now, by the celebrated Cardinal Giovanni Batista De Luca: which makes me blush in the face in considering the inestimable diversity of the authors that come (are) dedicated to you.

But as he is certain, that not every error that is committed is for every pernicious mind: That's my way of seeing it, because the method of operation that I now have, this advantage may not be to prosecute (pursue) because the present little work in the name of V.S. Illustrissima will be had in some time in whatever considerations, in a way, I point out, of those descriptions (made), by an unhappy paintbrush, which are surprising when decorated by a vague pleasing design, or else at least they entertain the eye of the least intelligent. This I feel is my expectation (confidence) while with deep honor I confirm (ratify) to V.S. Illustrissima the dedication and my unchangeable (immutable) respect. How much we see to be already passed in uninterrupted continuity, any book has had the custom of publishing this new material. As much as or maybe more than is necessary at this time, although the argument (plot) about which it revolves, seems like one that at first sight might be a trifling (unimportant) even though it isn't.

In the moment when it is brought to its most tender effect that I nurture for the glory of my country, I prepared 8 years to put together the beautiful and useful findings of the Florentines that afterwards in the printings from Ferrara came to light. The inventions of the eyeglasses seemed worthy of special mention not only for their marvelous usefulness that it cause, (but) even more because it restores and it repairs the bas reputation (voice) of the Florentines already from olden times of whom (says) the Divine Poet: (Dante) In the world the blind are called bad (old) reputation. This attribute is truly given to us by some people (populations) of Italy. For this reason Adriano Polity Senese in his *Tuscan Dictionary* to (about) the v. Bescio wrote that ours (our people) used to say (Bescio) and they used to call ours blind (*ciechi*). Landino, then, about the mentioned verse by Dante noted in this way: Because the Florentines were called (*ciechi*) I can't find anything authentic in any writing nor even useful, because these people are sharp and ingenious if it's not this, what Boccaccio still writes: The Pisano already went to the acquired Balearic Island of Mallorca with their big fleet that their city almost remained unguarded. Because the Florentines were their friends in those times they entreatied them and asked them to guard Pisa until they returned because they feared an outburst from the Lucchesi (Lucca) who were preparing an army against them and it would be an ignominious thing to leave their enterprise behind. Therefore, faithfully and with diligence it was guarded by us. The Pisano returned victorious and for the conquered island they reported rich booty: and in those two noble remains, which are the very ornate doors of a Temple and two columns of crystals. They wanted to donate one of these two things to the Florentines and to give them the captures (things) and estimating that they would select the columns, stirred by envy, they obfuscated them with fire and broke them and later they covered (dressed) them with pink cloth. The Florentines not aware of such a fraud took them away nor were they aware of the defect until they were on their way back to Florence that they discovered it. So the Florentines were called blind for such inadvertence and the Pisans, for having deceived their friends who with such faith had guarded their city, were called traitors. *It was cited before in various origins by Vilani in Chapter I of the second book of his history, talking about Totila*: He ordered that Florence be attacked and the longer you are there is in vain because seeing that he couldn't have it (Florence) because it was well fortified by a wall and moats and towers and very good people; He got the idea to conquer it by flattery and deceit in this way, because the Florentines were constantly at war with the city of Pistoia. Totile stayed in the city to guard it and ordered telling the Florentines that he wanted to be their friend and in their (favor) he would destroy the City of Pistoia showing their great love and promising to give them freedom with many liberal conditions: (terms) The Florentines, badly advised, (that's why in the proverbs they were called blind) believed their false flattery and vain promises, opened the doors, and he went in and his people and he lodged in the Campidoglio. *Another occasion is cited by Francesco Da Buti Pisano who about the long alle-*

gations by Dante leaves this written: It's an old reputation (fame) more so antique, in the world they are called blind (destitute) more so blind (*ciechi*, ignorant) and this is because they were little aware of their facts. On the other hand, the honorable Egidio Menagio writes differently saying: the Florentines are smarter, more ingenious and witty than any people of Italy, to this the proverb testifies: He who deals with a Tuscan must not be short-sighted. However the reason for this attribute of theirs is not too well known. The assertion of that writer makes an impression on me, as a foreigner, passionate estimator (judge) of things but more than that I value the writing of another stranger, a man of state as of doctrine, I mean Filippo Maria Visconti Duca de Milano, who I having heard, personally was renovating near us the old spot (mark) on Bracciolini Hill, wrote that, according to a certain impudent and shameless appelation that tramples on what has been ordained, the citizens of Florence are said by some to be blind, and that, as far as the worthiest and best men are concerned, this infamy of a falsely ascribed name is rightly demolished by nothing better than by our dignity. For who could be found so unaware of everything that he would think them (i.e., the Florentines) blind, when he gazes at the beauty and adornment of that City, but would not rather feel himself captivated not only with his eyes, but with his intellect. Indeed we, who are drawn to judge by no affection, no ill will nor malevolence, are so far from thinking them blind that we confess rather that they are at times most wise and keen-sighted. It is certain that the perspicacity of the ingeniousness of the Florentines is asserted by many. Even the Doctor Arciprete Baruffaldi wrote about it:

   It was a worthy thought of eternal memory
   Illustrious thought
   That of an ingenious person
   Extreme Florentine wittiness and ingeniousness

It is worthy of the Florentines to be industrious, witty, and smart, etc. And to this wittiness of much ingeniousness the nature of the air in Tuscany is very young, by itself very subtle. With all this yet, we have to be called (named) blind (*ciechi*) and the truest occasion for assigning it (the name) comes from the above mentioned Menagio when he says: It could also be that the Florentines are called blind because truly many of them suffer from "sight problems" for reason of their climate which is too subtle especially in the winter. And if that is the case everyone sees well they have repaired advantageously the harm done, with the present invention, which were those already found by me about inventions, which in order to be more brief, and to the best order of that book, it suits me to leave it behind; and as many as there were before, about which it seemed to me to pick out the most necessary part, and taking opportunity I'll throw out the rest (remaining). One of those arguments, however, that a variety of documents of congruence of authority, of offerings was certainly this matter about the invention of eyeglasses. In a manner that I was able to make a copious serving (reading) of these same writings from the advanced relics to Chapter 25 about my commentary on the Florentine inventors by saying it this way, in two Academic Reasonings that I extend (extensively) to recite, if the opportunity presents itself, in one of our meetings, in which, as a reward, I enjoy the honor of having written (them). If it wasn't that I read them before because adhering to a gentle friendship request by P.D. Angiolo Calogiera Camaldolense, very noteworthy in letters, also in doctrines and erudition for the beautiful collection that he orders published in Pamphlets that I had sent to Venice the same discourses they came out to the public in Volume IV from this collection. It's not long that it came to my notice (news) and from me going along studiously in search and with more zeal maybe than before, as with him, who was looking to give another system to these discoveries, it came to me then, the fact to reduce them in the present way.

   I can't deny that with this new publication, the approval of the learned would serve me as a stimulus, that the mentioned discoveries excused (had pity on). So if an act is of genuine reverence, on mentioning Plinio, confessing an indication from where our advancement was born, I say here how Sig. Dott. Giovannandrea Barotti my friend in the scholarly annotations to the very agreeable work that despite the humbleness of the title, the ingenuity of the learned subjects stands out, that recently they have put to verse and published with grandiousity, therefore in telling Bertoldo etc., he wrote concisely: the Eyeglasses are thus a modern invention, and from the 13th century as Manni shows in the *Discourses* (*Reasonings*) inferred (deduced) in the 4th Volume of the *Opuscoli* that P. Calogiera is compiling and in his Commentary on the Florentine inventors Chapter 25. Lately I have still had the heart to continue the enterprise of having read as the very clear author of *Literary Observations* that could serve as a continuation of the literary Journals of Italy in this way goes the Article V excusing my labor. It seems to have something to do with the *Mathematical Material Treatise* of Mr. Domenico Manni in the 4th Volume (of the *Opiscoli*) dealing with the invention of the eyeglasses, as much as it seems, that this made way for that one about telescopes (spyglass) to which is owed many beautiful discoveries in the sky, and to that one about the microscope to which is owed many beautiful observations of natural things. It first shows how the ancients didn't have such an instrument, and afterwards how the first inventor of it (them) was not Brother Alexander Spina Pisano, but it definitely was Salvino of the Florentine Armati Family in the end of the 13th century.

Everything is revealed then up to here, that was preceded (said before); if that is the way you could say it, the present impression, that has gone along with it must be kept near. The reader although will observe in its place what was my opinion about looking glasses (mirrors) that the ancients were able to have had, not dismissed, by my advice from any glass that might be compared to the lens. After this was written this way and even printed in this manner, Dr. Anton Francesco Gori public professor of history of the University of this country (region), whose name itself is enough to praise him, having questioned Francesco de Ficorini, a famous antique dealer in Rome, at my request, has responded to it this way on the 12th of April, the current month. I am glad to hear from your grace that a friend of yours is going to do a dissertation on the (nose) eyeglasses that I esteem as a very worthy work. I (in my opinion) have never had in so many years any indication that these were used (as a custom) neither by the Greeks, nor the Latins. I know well that I've seen little figures engraved in gems so tiny that it is impossible for them to be engraved only with the eye and without a lens. For that reason they must have had a lens. Besides, as much as, you read Archimedes, I have never had any proof. Considering that for thirty years I have been an excavator (digger) of sacred relics outside the wall of the St. Lawrence Catacombs with a candle (probe) and on the first level of the order, that there are also two levels above them, full of nicks and deductions that I copied. I myself found a lens in the wall sealed with plaster or fine lime, and this lens was just abut the size of a coin and it marvelously made things larger. So that Mr. Ficorini who afterwards continues to say that having shown it to a friend of his, indicates little with his great displeasure. He was bewildered.

And here, since incidentally one speaks (discovers) about Archimedes, I confess, that I would have voluntarily said some more about him in Chapter 8 of Part I, referring to that (matter) that the learned Count Gio: Maria Mazzucchelli in his scholarly work about Historical News, Critiques of Life, Inventions and writings of Archimedes Siracusano. If first I could have seen it. (under my eye)

It remains finally, that I made the reader arrive (get to) some errors in printing (that) happened, and they are: on page 7 I Surgendosi, should be Scorgendosi, perceiving on page 29 in the margin LXXXIII should be LXXXXIII on page 51.V.9. and says who wants to read about those prodigious ways of Andrea Avellion and of finally on page 74 change it (lo) to I read (leggi).

Index of Chapters
First Part

Introduction
Page 1

I. About the words: Ocular, Oculare, Ocularium that were found to mean eyeglasses.
II. The word Specillum is examined, improperly attributed to the eyeglasses.
III. About the words: Perspicillum, Perspicilium, Conspicillum, Conspicilium
IV. About the words: Specularius, Conspicillarius, Faber Ocularious, Oculariarius, and others
V. A place in Divine scripture is explained, (which) was from a bad intention (misunderstanding)
VI. A doubt of Egidio Menagio becomes clear
VII. The kinds of glass that were available to the ancients.
VIII. Other looking glasses (mirrors) that the ancients had.
IX. About a glass, that was used instead of eyeglasses in the past.
X. An impropriety concerning eyeglasses is proven in some pictures.
XI. A popular error about an old mosaic is removed.
XII. Indications that the ancients didn't have eyeglasses.
XIII. Authors who sustain that eyeglasses were a new invention.
XIV. Other authors who affirm that such inventions were modern.

Second Part
Prologue 43

I. About various types of nose eyeglasses.
II. About the material and form (shape) of the eyeglasses.
III. About the various shapes of the eyeglasses.
IV. (Those) who had spoken about our invention, with foundation.
V. Letter about the invention of eyeglasses written from Francesco Redi to Paolo Falconieri.
VI. How Redi didn't otherwise attribute the first invention of the eyeglasses to Alessandro Spina, as soon as some (others) appear.
VII. About the real (true) and first inventor of eyeglasses.
VIII. Other testimony (proof) of this invention.
IX. Some information about the person and the family of the inventor is given.
X. How the Florentines were determined (could be sincere) to make the memory of this discovery eternal.
XI. Writers who record the new discovery of the invention.
XII. Other writers who mention this invention.
XIII. How in Florence, more than anywhere else, the industry of eyeglasses was advertised.

Certified by me below (underwriter) Chancellor of the Sacred Florentine Academy, as in the watchful Row of Memories and Registry of this Academy which is kept in the Chancellery of the same (academy), besides the other writings of the present year, the following testimonial letters are found originally in the text, that is near (here).

We, below, Censors (critics) in the current year of the Sacred Florentine Academy on commission of Mr. Consolo of the same (academy) and by order of the dispositions of the Chapters and Statutes of that (academy) we have seen and reviewed (considered) well the present book entitled: *Historical Treatise about Eyeglasses on the Nose*, composed by Demenico Maria Manni Florentine, and one of our Academicians, and we believe (choose) to be able to give license to that author to be named in the publication of the worthy Florentine Academy work. And to certify its truth we make the following affirmation (attest) on this May 19, 1738.

Filippo Gondi Canomico (Florentine) Censor
Francesco Maria Gabburri Censor.

The above mentioned account, etc., concedes to the author of the present work to be able to be named in the publication as one of the Florentine Academy, which he is (already)
Date this May 21, 1738.
Cammillo Piombanti Cancelliere
Francesco Antonio Feroni Consolo.

Part I. Chapter I.
About the words Ocular, Oculare, Ocularium, found to mean Eyeglasses.

Chapter I

None too soon I prepare myself for the proposed research that the most solemn lexicographers, vocabularists and Grammarians of centuries before this, have challenged me with beforehand, with several credible names and qualified to signify such an instrument (research). And indeed if the name, which seems to be Nonio, that's how it was said (*a noscendo*) it can't be disjoined from the matter which is spoken about nor the matter of the name itself because it is becoming knowledge in such a way that given the fact it is found in old times or else in modern times the name of whatever: it comes as an infallible consequence to have had the same thing. Although there are many terms that come to be used for our Eyeglasses that you couldn't put any more of them to use for whatever reason for a more necessary instrument.

It is true therefore to start with the terms Ocular, Oculare, and Ocularium, where according to some people our Tuscan Eyeglasses had its birth, we are sure, if among the writers of the Latin language who were flourishing at the time, the terms might have never been used. As for what I remember, one of the first who put to use such words in this sense was eventually F. Bartolomeo Da S. Concordio Domenicano. Those about whom at length

Those about which I might have spoken another time at length, like the authors of the teaching of the ancients, and which using the Chronicle that he wrote from the Celebrated Convent of S. Caterina of Pisa, pleased them (the ancients), discussing accidentally the same invention of Eyeglasses.

Bernardo Gordonio follows immediately, one of those first professors of medicine that they were made clear in Mompelieri in the University, there it was straight from Niccolo IV in a work observed by me that he wrote in the year 1305 about which elsewhere we will do a long discussion.

The third (person) to use this term in such a sense was the celebrated Francesco Petrarca; those to tell the truth who let the Latin dialect stand in which he conducted with admirable cleverness his poem about Africa, whence (i.e., for which) there was a noteworthy laurel tree on the Capitolium as a reward for him. He therefore, as the two writers indicated above, not being famous, at least not in the 14th century, they couldn't make use of other words than those that were used as the custom of that time. Petrarch, however, in speaking about the remedies for each kind of fortune (good and bad), it pleased him to explain his feelings thus by saying: He restores a weak sight by glasses (ocularibus) and when, in a letter, he discusses the origin, life, frequency and result of his studies, he thus likewise left written that he had to seek help and refuge in eyeglasses (Ocularium).

However, the very bright Tommaso Reinesio in the learned annotations in his inscriptions (records) affirms frankly by the names Ocular, Oculare and Ocularium is indicated nothing other than the following: the part in the iron helmet which is opposite the eyes, through which things happening can be seen, although the whole face is covered.

What I took our Tuscans to mean (customarily) helmet visor and I took the Latins to mean Visorium, and really as for the word Ocularium, no one less than Carlo d'Aquino adheres such a meaning to it in his scholarly military lexicon, from the one that the learned Carlo Du Fresne makes in the useful work of the glossary, because if L'Aquino explains Ocularium as the opening (foramen) of the helmet, the other man defines it as the crack in the helmet, through which one sees. Al though it quite seems that L'Aquino took it from Du Fresne. Therefore in one not so old word a great fact, which if this, the examples are clearly in this time (sense) of history a little after 1200 although they report, in agreement, a killing done by way of a sword passed into the brain through the top of the helmet. Rigordo Medico, a notable historian, is the first who wrote the life of Philip II. King of France, called Augusto, of which he was still Chaplain recording in it around the year 1215, such a fact by saying he was killed by a knife wound received in the head through the Ocularium (i.e., opening) of his helmet. Matteo Parigino uses the same term in the year 1217 (referring jointly to the mentioned Du-Fresne) thus discussing (how) a certain one of the Royal Princes rushed in and, piercing his head through the Ocularium of his helmet, drove out his brain through the middle of the helmet's windows, to which is given the name Ocularia (plural), through which the pupil of the eye admits light. Finally

Guglielmo Britone, Latin poet barbarian who put the life of Rigordo in verse.

But as for the word Oculare, Du Fresne's feeling is not too different which is reinforced with the authority of the examples, he writes Oculare, the skin which is near the eyes.

Similar case comes to mind now in consideration of a stanza of a major Tuscan Poet, in which treating the problem, the souls of those translators are suffering in hell, who were living in the semblance of charitable (benevolent) people, they had much convenience in deceiving others, the Poet wrote (about them) Italics

Therefore it appears in which form the visor might have been in those times. Since the poet affirms that the cold (frozen) tears used to fill up under those eyebrows all the hollow of the eyes: or as the commentators explain the entire socket of the eye, (which) visors of crystal (glass), the intelligence of who confess and the commentary of that same century, made by Francesco Da Buti, Public Reader of Dante in Florence and still the model of those miserable people, that is seen in the beautiful example of it in the Academy of the Crusca, where they were (put) secretly in a pool of ice (glass), with only their face out (of the ice), (face) turned toward above, it seems precisely that they had Eyeglasses (Took place in Dante's writings—Ed.) submerging in the void of both the eyes two small plates of plate glass (ice) and they put the nose in the middle, perhaps these thinqs were for vision. (visor)

The name Specillum is examined, which is improperly attributed to the eyeglasses.

But turning what was some digression it was certainly curious for me to see something of the word Specillum, the mistake taken for ours by another prudent writer Cristofano Landini, when in translating the Natural Story of Caio Plinio from the Latin into the Florentine language joined to that passage in Chapter 53 of Book VII by the same author, which says: Gaius Julius Medicus, while he was anointing (his eye), drawing a probe (Specillum) across it. I turn into Tuscan: C. Julio Medico, while he anoints (engraves) he wants to put on his Eyeglasses, with that which follows. I am mistaken, about which they didn't stumble between the translators of Plinio, nor Lodonico Domenichi nor even Antonio Brucioli and Celio Rodigino had it well in consideration according to my estimation writing; "Finally in this part I should like those who are learned men to be advised that, in respect to that passage of Pliny concerning sudden deaths (which comes) from Book Seven (particularly the words "Gaius Julius Medicus, while he was anointing [his eye], drawing a probe across it"), there are those who relate (this word specillum) to Conspicilia, which, when placed on the nose, miraculously help vision. But this (argument) is easily beaten down by Varro, in whom we read as follows: Hence, specillum, with which we anoint the eyes with which we see (specimus).

Therefore in order to make the truth right Landino wasn't the only one to give the word Specillum a false bizarre meaning becasue other writers did the same thing as he did (his example). Gio: Batista Porta gave it worth in the 17th Book of Natural Magic (witchcraft) entitling an added chapter *De Specillum*. Much more, nevertheless, Ambrogio Calepino made it famous in the Dictionary, Filippo Venuti also in his collection of history and poetry scraps and even Giuseppe Laurenzi in the anniversary Amaltea and not least Maurio Nizolio in the Treasure of the Latin language, where each one of them give to this word Specillo the meaning of eyeglasses, the first, for example, saying "Certain people also give the name Specilla (plural) to those little glass circles, which old men bring up to their eyes so that they can see more clearly." The second one defining it as Eyeglasses and the other two almost with the same words calling it "the glass, which we bring up to the eyes, so that we can look at something more easily."

But why digress in talking about them, because others used the same words that they used without having examined the real meaning of it. It seems to be more useful to see the real genuine value of these words, because it is that one that I see to denote then, that among the surgeons is used to see (recognize) the wounds and similar things for these actions they order (say) Speculare—as of the Specillo, besides Cornelio Celso making it a word, it is assigned from (by) Marco Tullio because of being an inventor and doctor. And without this meaning (the word) Specillum comes to be used to mean a roll of cotton (lint) of linen thread cloth to anoint (soothe) the eyes, which is the stated feeling of Varrone. Then the Nizolio in the treasure mentioned discourses of that one that he says in the Ciceronian Dictionary it is alright to excuse it just so in this last one he hits the mark. Therefore the very bright Jacopo

Facciolati wisely removed the false meaning of this word, keeping the true one, the legitimate one, in amending what the dictionary of Ambrogio Calepino did as a good deed through which this came justly to amount to great worth.

But not Chapter III satisfied however by this we pass on to others to consider how Perspicillum and Perspicilium are upheld, because these, for what I hear (feel) about them, they were words used to mean eyeglasses, but at first they weren't seen in print until the 15th century; Although then until our days the writers used them, especially those writers of medicine. The first word is certianly valued in the place indicated above and the other one I can't find even the oldest mention of it in the life of F. Francesco Piso, in a place, where they were talking about eyeglasses and in the Vissio which treats *Math Science*, I point out where that writer praising the invention of eyeglasses says clearly that the ancients had not even a notion of these.

Much less it seems then to maintain the name *Conspicillum* (wrongly written by Garzoni *Conspecillum*) to mean eyeglasses used recently if not still by resemblance, seeing it used by Filippo Iacopo Sacsio Tedesco, since he is discussing various kinds of Microscopes. It is certain, that if Guido Pancirolo, a man of many selected letters, (in his work) On New Discoveries, and Salmuth in the notes about the same work wanted to persuade everyone to use this word to mean eyeglasses, expect a false definition because Nizzolio first with his memorandum adds (gives) to the mistake, already enlarged by who heard it through hearsay because the same word was used by Plautus in that visionary verse "Bring glass, it is necessary to take advantage of (this) place from which to look" if Pancirolo, and Salmuth, as I was saying will take a factual term for the eyeglasses Vossio will respond that they (i.e., Pancirolo and Salmuth) are deceived in many ways, adding, "First I deny that these were (words) of Plautus; I also deny that they are read in any ancient author." I then, could say that for the care done in Plautus, no less in MSS. than in the best editions in the back of the guide by Filippo Pareo diligent illustrator of that Comic Writer looking for it even in Frammenti and in Lessico Plautino I haven't been able to find it there. It is not a marvel either that he didn't see it in all Plauto Vopisco Fortunato Plempio as he affirms Girolamo Mercuriale didn't see it who saw it cited by others, he was among two who believed it might have been there and he left it written: It might not be therefore that you marvel because of many things believed and what is more many writers not unknown registered to see (verify) me, or since they are not sure don't admit, or s absolutely false with frank refused, which I now owe to Plautus' lesson because the establishing of a certainty from one lesson that is not done, who might have read it in Plautus nor in some Comedy the foundation of an important thing is too ridiculous. I am reminded that a valuable annotator of Marco Tullio says the following concerning the above: In the writings of ancient authors, either taking something away rashly or adding something (rashly) has always earned the indignation of all learned men, nor should it be tolerated. Therefore, when I see those emendators asking questions like the following: "What if you were to read it like this? What if like this?" And again: "Could it happen to be possible that this is correct? Is it possible that this is (correct)?" And when I see them asking more things like this one after the other, I am sometimes inclined to laugh. In our case then by testimony of Guisto Lissio whoever knows that in Plautus many things were made said capriciously due to the unskillfulness of the translators which also influenced the works of many other authors. Similarly in the Latin Dictionary of Dante you can read conspicillo, conspicillonis, Plautus who keeps espion(?) before the esteemed Sig. Abate Facciolati could respond, as few have done before, in his learned corrections, "Neither Plautus nor any Latin author has this word, as far as I indeed know." Through which things you see well how much we owe this Latin Comic Writer returned in his genuine Lesson (form) to Pareo who protests: "Having obtained the oldest and best manuscript Codices from the famous Chief Library of the Palatine, when, with truly unutterable labor, I seriously compared this untouched author with the same (writers) once more, I restored innumerable passages to their pure antiquity by right of postliminium[1] so to speak: I wiped away the remaining blots, by which it happened to have been defiled, with the genuineness of the old parchments. Indeed in this hard work of mine, I relied on

---

[1] the right to return home and resume one's former rank and privileges.

the greatest faith and feeling of respect, and I took great pains that to this author nothing was added which I did not deem right and most obviously true from the sacred consensus of sacred antiquity." Pareo then says here that Plautus was by chance defiled with blots. The corruption comes to my memory, because in a similar fictious verse the grammarians inform (recognize); because it should be iambic trimeter verse or sex verse that is not seen, they write: Bring glass, it is necessary to take advantage of (this) place from which to look.

The verse limps in that Conspicillo. That fact however was known by those few, that would be supported by Plautus. They allowed themselves to write Conspicilio which was an honest expedient means, and they weren't noticed about which responds Cristiano Becmanno (1) that Conspicilium isn't said right, it should always be said Conspicillum, the origin and the analogy attests to it. Indeed, they say, just as Baculus is formed into Bacillus, Furcula into Furcilla, so also, according to Varro (in) Book V of his *Latin Language*. Speculum is formed into Specillum, and later into Conspicillum.

Gerardo Vossio says a lot about it in the Etymology, disapproving of what Adriano Giunio let run in the edition that he did of Nonio Marcello, the word Conspicilium, he should have put in that word instead of Conspicillum in his Nomenclator; where there it was born, it is for his imitation and by the one of Celio Rodigino the second editors of the Crusca Vocabulary, Francesco Eschinardi and others used the word Conspicilium to denote eyeglasses.

But let's put Conspicilium as the true word. Therefore does it follow, if the vocabularists define it: (that) from which you may be able to see. So along with others Eilardo Lubino in his interpretation of the Latin words least used, citing the authors, who before him treated this material skillfully.

The same reason militated by Perspicillum because it is a modern word is not admitted for the most part in the Latin dictionaries.

Gio. Iacopo Hofmanno uses it in his universal Lexicon praising the invention as modern and making it a word from the passage of Plautus.

But to what end do we dispute this blessed Plautine Verse, almost from goat's wool, investigating so studiously what could have been without joining to find what the truth really was. The Grammarians who want to say that with or without the finished Verse they will never lose since that was never read. This exists you well know and the fact comes from Plauto. This then, is stated from the Cistellaria and not from the Mostellaria. As Hofmanno writes from a lack of memory: As I was returning home, he pursued me secretly with close watching (Conspicillum) all the way to the door. In which place then the word Conspicillum is intended to mean our (word) eyeylasses in the Mercuriale has only one meaning that Mr. Facciolati assigns to it, therefore to say that by judgement of Vossio of Hofmanno and others among which are very considerable and the opinion of old Nonius Marcellus: Conspicillum is a place from which someone can see; just as Nonius Marcellus interprets, who brings up (the following) from Plautus' *Medicus*:

"I was keeping watch on a lookout, I was guarding the cloak" where you would not be able to take it otherwise than in that passage of his play *Cistellaria*.

Salmuth writes about this unique definition equally in the annotations to the Pancirolo, which seems, that it finishes (answers) the present question, after having related (referred) the first verse, that undoubtedly is not Plauto's nor can it be of any other old (writers), let it be understood that about this word that almost nowhere is mention made (of it) in the classical writers.

None of those words to mean eyeglasses existed in old times. They were seen to be used before, much less I am of the opinion that the same ones express a desire (as someone could suspect) for that name (appellation) that in an inscription in the Doniane you can read namely Auxiliary Instrument as much as Petrarch used the same terms for eyeglasses saying help for the eyes (*ocularium auxillum*): much more than Dr. Anton Francesco Gori in the scholarly annotations of this work, he suspects, rather, that this meant the staff (walking cane) used as an aid to age or to make traveling (walking) more comfortable.

The words Specularius, Conspicillarius, Faber Ocularius, Oculariarius, and others.

Chapter 4

Up to now the eyeglasses have certainly supplied a delicate subject to discuss and hear about. More than anything the most tiresome is the speech of the Grammarian who are wandering around. Because they (those) who thought such a usage was old supported themselves with the authority of the words which were modern or had little proper use really were intended wrongly, they have nothing to do with our argument. We could say something more about Celio Rodigino, who affirms that there are those who, being makers of Conspiciliorum, are thought to be called rightly Specularios. He keeps adding that the same word used in ancient times is from the Jurist Ulipiano in agreement with them that glass is used for windows. We could say a lot about Fabiano Giustiniano who in giving advice in his catalog of writers, that whatever material (subject) they treated, they used the word Conspicillarius to denote eyeglass maker. Although these, like him, often in modern times such a term came to be used, which did not exist (before).

Allow me truly to consider some kinds (of words) after so many artisans in our country and others and in the lengthy catalogs we read we do not find mention ever of the Eyeglass maker.

And also they had glass-maker—mirror maker and so on, that you can read enumerated in the books of our Arts. That's what the makers of eyeglasses were called by us around 1400. He makes eyeglasses and no other thing indicates to me that the skill didn't exist much before, in a way that there wasn't even the word in the anthology, I will say that the other words formed by us, like Eyeglassmaker as was said later, which, if the fear of not being overly tedious didn't prohibit me I would like to exemplify the work of the artisan who stains glass for the windows of the churches using the expression he makes glass around the mid-14th century.

In such a way scholarly people would take (i.e., interpret) Faber Ocularius and Oculariarius[2] when the smart compilers of the third edition of the Crusca didn't show any doubt that the Faber Ocularious really denoted Eyeglassmaker because after they ordered that equivalent and the old note books (which are nowadays purged) the notebook makers kept putting and later adding Faber Conspicillarum—Ocularius—which is found in old editions. It is really wisely doubted that the compilers made any better observations in their fourth edition—they threw away freely the word Faber Ocularius. So then you could suspect Mr. Facciolati, mentioned before, when defining the Ocularius of the latins which was founded on the words of the Reinesio, who had said that Faber Ocularius was one who prepares glasses serving more easily either for protecting the eyes against injuries of the air or for representing and grasping objects in a larger form. Thus he writes: The craftsman, who makes glasses for protecting the eyes or for representing objects in a larger form. This word is read in (the work called) *Inscriptione apud Reinesium Class. XI. num. 66*, but the word does not seem really ancient, because there is no agreement in ancient authors about this instrument for the eyes.

In this place, first, the opportunity to talk about it is less, I remember to indicate in following Faber Conspicillarum used in the past vocabulary of the Crusca, as you also find the word Conspicallator used in a modern sense for eyeglassmaker, by Fabiano Giustianano in the above mentioned book.

But turning to the objective, it is certain to have been used in the old times for making crystals and glass like gems and the nobles put eyes in statues especially when they represented some Deity. For which I don't see, nor does Cesare Calderino see it, how you could doubt that from the name of an artisan Oculario or Oculariaro might be designated as an artisan who in old times flourished and who didn't go back to the times of Jesus Christ, but until the 13th century was in existence. We have much proof of such a custom but similar to any other the author is irrefutable, which was of the notable people of our country, Senator Filippo Buonarroti who in page 12 of his scholarly work on the Observations about the Medals in the Carpegna Museum, says this about the old artifacts. Nowhere did they use more skill or diligence in making eyes for the statues either from glass or crystals or precious stones: A certain man named Rapilio in an inscription was attributed to him in praise for having used this craft (skill). (The inscription refers to a man named Rapilius who placed eyes in statues.—Ed.)

Whereas you can see much evidence of these eyes hollowed out and deteriorated as appear in a bronze mask of Jupiter and on another of a Bacchus priestess or aquatic Nymph and particularly on a certain strange God from Egypt sculpted in a green serpentine stone with small spots. Plinio mentions a lion of marble that had emerald eyes and maybe those on Minerva in Vulcan's temple in Athens, which are described by

---

[2] Both these Latin terms were used by some to refer to the maker of eyeglasses.

Pausanias as the color of the sea, they were of Aquamarine, that is a kind of beryl of the ancients. In the life of S. Silvestro four silver statues of angels donated to the Constantin Basilica with precious stones of Alabanda[3] in their eyes. In our Museum there are many small bronze statues with silver eyes. Among the others there are a horse of great design—a dog, a Mercury shepherd with a ram on his shoulder and a Genius with a Patera.

In a small gallery in our country, observed by me many times, there was an ordinary serpent with silver eyes. Felice Ciatti in the historical memoirs of the city of Perugia the one that he calls Etruscan Perugia, and before he wrote it there, he wrote it in a pamphlet, that was printed under the seal of that city in 1631 with the title *Historical Paradox*, on the statue of bronze already in the Territory of Perugia rediscovered and then put in the Gallery of the Grand Duke of Tuscany, you (he) observes that the statue had eyes of gems. About which the renowned Signore Dottora Anton Francesco Gori elsewhere notes that in this type of art it is permitted to suspect that the Etruscans surpassed the Greeks and Latins, who pursued this custom thereafter and he confirms the same in his Etruscan museum where he reports there are some Etruscans with silver eyes. And to add to that which is well seen by all others, in the pulpit in the San Miniato of Monte Church there are some lads (rascals) with eyes made from other material which the lads are not made of. And in a portico of the interior courtyard of S. Maria Del Fiore you could distinguish a big image of Virgin Mary sculpted in marble already having two glass eyes, but one was lost because of its antiquity. On the street outside the S. Miniato door which leads to the Giullari floor, not too far from the same door you find a certain tabernacle, inside of which is a messenger of white marble that has black marble eyes or metal incased like mosaic.

This was an Epigram by Lucilio that is translated in the Latin anthology: Demostratus, before you anoint the sacred eye, poor fellow, say: Dion is so cautious. Not only did he blind the Olympic god, but in this way also the statue, which he had, lost its eyes through his doing.

Giovanni Saresberiense learned of a citing by Cecilio Balbo that is not far from our argument. It says this: For who of the Gods would forgive the person by whom he knows he has been tricked? Who would not rush against the man who tears out the golden eyes of Jupiter or, having removed the silver and stones, strives to disfigure his clothing? Who, with rash claws digs out the hard eye from Mar's head?

I am indebted to Doctor Anton Francesco Gori, Prof. of History for this learning and for others. He is the illustratr of old memoirs of our country and others. He, therefore, puts the citing of Cecilio Balbo, where the Greek, Roman and Latin inscriptions are illustrated next to the grave stone erected in memory of Rapilio who used to furnish skillfully, statues with eyes so that this comes to be one of the many rare monuments possessed by Carlo Tommass Strozzi, Cavalier of great intelligence and benefactor of Fine Arts in his villa Montui. There are others in Rome, by our mentioned illustrator made with the same marble about which he stated, as I see by Facciolati, Reinesio, Dausquio, and Grutero, the last of which is given entirely in this way: To the spirits of the departed. Gaius Licinius L.L. Patroclus, a maker of glass eyes, has made (this monument) for his beloved brother, Lucius Licinius Statorianus, son of Lucius.

Because in Aldo Manuzio's Orthography, it differs than in the one L. Licinius wrote in the third verse, another similar marble is mentioned a lot in the inscriptions of Marquardo Gudio which is found in the Cardinal Carpegna Museum. A lot is stated about the Oculario (i.e., maker of eyes for statues).[4] But it is certain that however a person might want Faber Ocularius and Oculariarius, they cannot be any different from (saying) this: They made eyes. Oculos Conficiebant.

So they also had another use of the same eyes made from gems, or of shiny material, and they had to be consecrated with some ceremony and dedicated to the Gods of the Gentiles in the temples as Clemente Alessandri refers. Where eventually we frequently put as a donation an offering of two silver eyes on our altars as a sign of heavenly thanks for our power of vision, and especially from which century is taken the images of S. Lucia. It is my opinion it is from that time that they started to depict the same images of the saint with a vase in the form of a cup, having on it two eyes, instead of the old vase of fire as her descriptions wanted to depict of her at first.

---

[3] A wealthy city in the interior of Caria in Asia.

A place in Divine Scripture that was understood in bad terms, is explained.
Chapter 5

It is not, to pass on to something else, who might suppose because in that passage of Ecclesiastes when the guards of the house will be frightened and very strong men will bend and the grinders of grain, small in number, will be idle and those looking through windows (Foramina) will grow dark, there you understand the design (purpose) of eyeglasses, the style, that supposedly came from Geiero in his commentary on the preachings of Salomon, so you understand the same from P. Agostino Calmet on the same Ecclesiastes where he with the learned words and understood the same passage with his prudent opinion, and he disapproves together putting in his opinion the feeling (opinion) of Geiero. He said that the eyes of old men are dull and sluggish. Concerning the pupil of the eye he also explains the word Foramina (openings or windows), whether these windows are the eyelids,[5] or whether they are the circle of the skull itself, where the eyes are buried. Geierus (incorrectly) thinks that they are the Conspicilia of old men, just as in the time of Salomon the use of Conspiciliorum was prevalent (to mean eyeglasses).

Nor is Calmet's opinion different than Giovanni Lorino's saying: Openings or windows, i.e., Foramina (Symmachus refers to acts of seeing "in the eyes" one eye or more eyes as they say in Greek; Chald. say through the window-bars of your head, or—in Greek—through the eyes) and it's the same for Hesychius, that is θυρις[6], or window; Although additionally, as the former author teaches, it may be said—in Greek—"the eye of the ears," i.e., the opening of the ears, or the passageway through which the voice penetrates. Nevertheless he indicates a word pertaining to seeing, (saying) that the discussion is about the sense of sight, although it is allowed sometimes that (a word concerning) sight is transferred to the other senses. The Italians commonly say in their homes, palaces, or temples the word "eye", or rather "eyes" in place of windows, or for an opening or openings, especially round ones through which light is admitted.

Finally Iacopo Tirino on the same passage from Ecclesiastes: Those looking through windows. The pupils, which look out through the cornea, a covering furnished with windows; or more simply, the soul looking out through the eyes, will grow dim, from the absence of those spirits, which, being bright and clear, leave a person in darkness and overwhelmed without light when they are not present, as Hippocrates said. Valesius adds that for old men, partly because of dryness, partly because of an accumulation of excretions, the fluids of the eyes thicken and grow hard and that the membranes become hard and wrinkled; and also that the optic nerves and passageways are stopped up or closed for many. I am quitting in order to avoid an excessive diffusion of referring the current opinion of even more commentators who go about interpreting this passage (extended to mean only Geiero's eyeglasses) and contemporaries of these, and older, among which Ugone Grozio: He explains "And those looking through windows (foramina) will grow dark" as follows: Obviously in the phrase "those looking through windows" (fenestras). He also explains this in Greek[7] he understands "eyes", for which the eyelids which intervene are—as it were—windows and I refrain from putting in consideration to the readers who have knowledge of eyeglasses you can never understand these however full of holes and open they are (not).

A doubt of Egidio Menagio becomes clear.
Chapter 6

Because of some real appearance fallen suspect to Egidio Menagio scholarly French gentleman, really in the middle of the 12th century there might have been eyeglasses or not. I see it as my obligation to refute a similar appearance that was there. He says in this way: "Around the year 1150 the eyeglasses were in use, as it appears in those verses of Procoprodomo in

---

[4] The 2nd inscription was put up by the heir for an Ocularius named Gaius Venuleius Aristocles who lived 38 yrs., 7 mos. and 2 days; his wife Marcia Venuleia, 29 yrs., 4 mos. and 8 days.

[5] The word palpebrae can also mean "eyes" in Ecclesiastical Latin.

[6] Manni writes θopις, but the word θυρις means window.—Ed.

[7] Manni writes οιπακυπλουτες but οιπακυπτουτες means "those looking through windows."—Ed.

his political verses against Alegumeno a book written in pen from the library of King Christianissimo; In which place was suggested to me by Mr. Du-Cange.

Procoprodomo is talking here about the doctors of the emperor Manuele Comneno, who he's making fun of: they came (the doctors) they saw immediately they took his pulse and with a glass they looked at his excrement with a glass therefore an eyeglass. But maybe this glass was put on the excrement so as not to smell its bad odor.

It is certain that if Menagio wasn't undeceived here, as he did, I guess little honor would have been brought to him for establishing the oldness of the eyeglasses in documents more bold than ambiguous, sophisticated which is the maximum by Geiro referred to above. A glass (pane) however was that put upon a garbage container to impede seeing inside because it kept a stinking vapor (inside). As to what we know, even today in some places this custom still lasts. If likewise a kind of lens might not have been used from a short distance (up close), which I doubt, because they could have been supplied to man since ancient times, as we see it.

The kinds of glass that was [sic] available to the ancients.
Chapter 7

It wouldn't be outside of reason to support the fact that the ancients could have made use of a glass to make objects bigger (magnifier). Since omitting that fact that some refer to by saying that Tolomeo already used a crystal (glass) to (look) at ships a hundred miles distant, a fable that is useless, because Count Antonio Manzini sets himself to deny it since it is proven by everyone who has little knowledge it still seems that the astronomers to look up into the Heavens made use of some instrument, that took the place in a way, of our lens. It seems that they might have had need sometimes of the Divine Law especially in order to use it the right way during the circumcision of infants. Besides all this there was the Idolatry with the diviners (witch doctors) and an old rite concerning the observers of animals' bowels which Dionisio, and more clearly Tertulliano. The crowd creates for itself the lots of the gods, auguries, the illustrious names of the planets, creations of their beginnings, and afterwards it (the crowd) sees and awaits for future events by means of inspecting the entrails of animals, from which they discerned some good observation or a sad omen. Since Plinio the younger, without delay he makes the sacrifice, he declares that the entrails agree with the meanings of the stars. In these functions the old superstitious customs observed it seems they made use often of a glass to make objects bigger, which, as we indicated, it could have been made in the shape of any big lens, which maybe was lost, they had recourse subsequently to some (balls, Bowels) about which we will make special mention in its own place.

Other mirrors (glasses) that the ancients had.
Chapter 8

Meanwhile therefore it is allowable to keep imagining (mentioning) like this similar glasses, in as much as we know for sure, because for many years there were many uses made of crystals. You had mirrors first made from silver or tin, later in glass, in which men didn't look (use) as much as at first with the simple use of water where Lucretius says: Finally whatever images appear to us in mirrors, in water[8] and in every shining surface.

Afterwards came mirrors that they frequently represented in bas-relief, afterwards grown in splendor and exceeding luxury out of necessity, not of decoration mainly (about) near the feminine sex; where among astronomers the mirror is given to Venus as her particular emblem, therefore the glasses in the shape of a sphere distributed on the walls of the rooms and in baths to bring light and to protect from the cold; Even Seneca (said) they didn't only put them in rooms they put the same plates of glass (crystal) in graves maybe to reflect the darkness of them, when maybe some kind of light might open them (get in), where eventually some appearance of light had origin in them. They had glasses on the windows of various kinds according to the styles of the centuries, mainly in a round shape presented in our times; As for at first they made use of some thin panes of transparent marble because glass wasn't invented yet. These windows used were Specularia: where Marziale (Martial) Glass casements facing the south winds of winter let in pure suns and a day without sediment.

And Pliny the Younger. The dining halls become an excellent place of refuge against the weather: for they are protected by windows and much more by the overhanging eaves of the roof.

They had some mirrors in the service of the acts of war to damage the enemy with them, mainly to see where they should hit the marks with the bows (and arrows) they had a parabolic mirror or burning mirror that grouped the rays on one point and succeeded in setting fire. And this is quite famous because Archimedes used it to set fire to Marcello's boats that were attacking Syracuse, and later Proclo imitated this in Constantinople in reference to Zonara. Aristophanes tells a debtor that he wants to burn the bills with such a mirror when the creditor shows them to him. Eustasio took then a certain Artemio who had a bad problem with his neighbors and to get rid of them it is said that with such a mirror he set fire to their house a few times, so that they thought that this was some kind of a disgrace sent from the heavens and they went away to find another place to live.

A glass, that the ancients used instead of eyeglasses. Chapter 9

The ancients made use however of some balls of glass instead of our eyeglasses. They still weren't the ones about which an inscription referred to by Grutero says this. Ursus Togatus who first (made) glass balls, but certainly the others about which Francesco Petrarca (Petrarch) affirms. It (the glass) restores a weak sight; in this matter you have thought more keenly than your ancestors, who made use of small glass vessels full of water (as Seneca recalls), almost a delightful game of nature. Concerning the remedies for each kind of fortune, that which opens the passage upon understanding what these glass balls might have been call to mind Lucio Anneo Seneca in his time who was flourishing under the empire of Nero while he comments on the Natural Questions added to Chapter 6 in the first book: The letters, although tiny and obscure, are seen larger and clearer by means of a glass ball filled with water. However such an instrument as eyeglasses is seen to have been (come) from the ancients.

Because the glass with water makes you see the objects better (bigger) in a way that Morale continues to say: It will become clear, if you fill a cup with water and throw a ring into it, although the ring is lying on the very bottom, its face is rendered larger on the surface of the water. Whatever is seen through liquid is truly much larger. Many of the goldsmiths are trying a similar experiment even today and with them when they have to apply the exercise of cutting small lines, particularly while they are working at night, they put between the design to be worked on and the light of a full bottle of clean water.

These are the mirrors that the ancients made use of. Of eyeglasses, not yet, since we don't see any sign that they still might have been found (invented) in olden times.

An impropriety about eyeglasses is proven in some pictures. Chapter 10

You must give a good amount of reflection to some painters who in representing ancient history the modern instrument of eyeglasses intruded (in their paintings). One of these was the famous Lodovico Cigoli who in painting a beautiful table for the San. Francesco de Frato Church in which he had to depict the Circumcision of our Redeemer we do not remember how to say the inscription that is there, which is believable because up to now there existed on the floor of the Saint Mary Maggiore Church in Florence where he had the comfort of practicing painting as well as architectural works that he conducted in that church, He made old Simon appear on that Table with (nose) eyeglasses on in order to show (supply) the defect of his old age in perceiving the holy part, that he had to engrave. If not rather to show in his was with some evidence of that fabulous thing. The scholarly Ignazio Giacinto Amat de Graveson says about Simione to prove it: There are some who think that that old saint was deprived of his eyes, and that from the mere touching of the boy Jesus he recovered his sight; but since that relies on no authority of scripture or of the old writers, it ought by rights to be attributed to other more recent stories which the Greeks force (upon us). That however he showed not to admit since the eyeglasses for the blind (weren't produced) to wear. Really therefore Cigoli didn't even examine this painting to (see) if it might be Salomon or even Saint Joseph or others who were surrounding the Child Jesus, if they were priests or laity and if in the temple or in another place the sacred circumcision took place, about which there might be some controversy among the writers, where you could also believe, according to my advice, that even though he's a learned man, simply made a mistake about these eyeglasses on the face of Simeone with intolerable anachronism.

---

[8] Manni writes *qua* instead of *aqua* which Lucretius writes.—Ed.

In the same way you can see that Paolo Veronese put in his Painting in the drawing room of the auditorium of the Royal Palace of Versailles where Jesus Christ with the disciples in Emaus some of which have the crown around their waist. Similarly the Red Florentine Painter, painting for Saint Lorenzo of our country the Spoliation of Virgin Mary represented (painted) a Dominican Brother in the history (painting). It isn't worth saying, and the people who study it try to defend it: who could know that in olden times if any person might have dressed in the habit of a Dominican. Not seeing the (history) painting that this representation was an impropriety. The painter of course is worthy of being excused of this deed, whose hand often cannot obey the corrupt intellect that guides it. In the case of our Cigoli it is worthy to give him some compassion since the discovery of eyeglasses was already anticipated by Domenico del Grillandaio in that painting that came from his brush that you perceive on the side wall on the left hand side of the All saints Church in Florence in which San Girolamo is shown staring with some books in front of him in the act of reading and with a pair of glasses hanging from his reading desk. Father Francesco Albertini in his Memorial of the Florentine painting attributes this work to Sandro Botticelli.

But as he sees it shown like this, a blunder often repeated is reason for many others (to happen) so it proves even more that it gives to it an erudition not entirely despicable which I briefly indicate (beckon). In the city of Venice in 1660, there was an old sign on an eyeglass maker's shop. The venerable Doctor S. Girolamo's with these words on it: San Girolamo inventor of eyeglasses. What foundation this fabulous memoir might have, I don't know.

It is enough for me to know that in the work and in the life of this saint you don't find even the least sign or any other things that maybe he dreamed it up, they were attributed to him. I heard say that he was explaining the Divine Scripture, these words (are) in the papal see, When he wanted to express the irresolution of S. Girolamo on the interpretation of a difficult passage: Here S. Girolamo rubs (strike) eyeglasses in order to say that he was irresolute and he was taking time to respond. Of the remaining one doesn't want to make marvel out of similar errors about which and especially about another picture of S. Girolamo we read thus in the second volume of the work entitled. (*Essay on Popular Errors*—Ed.)

We must not omit here the painting of St. Jerome which (the painter) has depicted in his cell with a clock next to him. Although the intention was pure and although it is very likely that this saint took into careful consideration his time, one must not give place to a belief that he calculated in this way. The ancients make no mention of clocks; Panicirolle observes that they are among modern inventions, etc., but St. Jerome lived under Theodosius I in the 4th Century.

Finally in Rafaello Borgnini we see many problems concerning the anachronisms and the disagreements in the truth of history introduced by the painters or by those who ordered the paintings.

A popular error about an old mosaic is taken away. Chapter 11

I can't do any less (more) here to indicate, that after having made sure about how many times there were many basis on the origin of eyeglasses I happened to hear rumors about the Mosaic in the Tribunal of S. Miniato at Monte, Church that is always closed nowadays, there was a lion as a symbol of the evangelist Saint Mark (very improper thing) with eyeglasses on the nose. For which recourse to history was made first, about the Basilica that they mention, and the Chronicle of S. Miniato was under his eye, where it seemed, that if you had to talk about this mosaic one didn't even know how to find it; I saw that Ildebrando Vescovo of Florence, seeing the Basilica of S. Miniato conducted on bad terms in the year 1013 was almost rebuilt and the ornaments of mosaics and marble were made beautiful. And doubting that this Mosaic indicated by the Admirer could have been the one of the Tribunal where in 1013 it wasn't possible to have the eyeglasses since they weren't painted. I observed that Ferdinando Leopoldo del Migliore not too distant from that time used to write of it like this. That Mosaic picture was made about 1100.

Finally reminding about what Giulio Cesare Scaligero (Scaliger) left written that the true understandlng or knowledge of such things is in the things themselves. I went up there and I had to get a ladder, and who might have helped in approaching the Mosaic with my eye I not only perceived that there weren't eyeglasses, because for such things people are commonly baptized, there certainly was a dark stain under both eyebrows, but what maybe is more, I saw that under the Mosaic on a stripe of the trimming was the record of the year of this work MCCXCVII (1297) by which you could correct Migliore in the place indicated above.

Indication that the ancients might not have had eyeglasses. Chapter 12

All the things mentioned made me clearly see that the ancients had not had the use of eyeglasses to which you could add the consideration that after various kinds of instruments that the old times had in use, their memory was never clouded in any way about any relic that they might have found at one time or another. It is all incredible because in discovering so many gems, cameos, medals, coins, rings, symbols, presents, idols, and what do I know (else), there was never any chance over so many long centuries of finding a glass that might show that it was an eyeglass, since other kinds of glasses were found by the thousands, and many kinds of colors, painted and carved. More so, Great Marvel (Francesco Redi used to say) it would be, presupposed, that the Greek comics, and the Latins might have had knowledge of eyeglasses if they never took the occasion in naming them or in joking about them through their announcers, when, to tell the truth, in modern times the examples are frequent in the Morganas of Pulci and in the Rhymes of Burchiello and in the Rhymes and in the prose of Alessandro Allegri also, in many pleasant Tuscan Comedies and poetry. It would be a marvel (as Redi continues) if the diligent Plinio in the chapter about the inventors of things didn't make any mention of it. In another not even Authors of Medicine said a word about eyeglasses as Mercuriale observes: Let me with confidence assert that to the ancient doctors a glass instrument, suitable for weak eyes, was unknown. The Arab, Greek and Latin doctors advised thousands of remedies for vision but not yet eyeglasses. There wasn't a statue or a picture in ancient times that showed eyeglasses.

Equally an indication that seems to me to be of some importance is that of not seeinq on the ecclesiastical ceremonies of any antiquity waiting for Mass, nor any order, nor decree nor rubric that conforms in any way to the eyeglasses that were frequently used to read and examine with exactness which was owed to that holy sacrifice. As many other things are found to be spoken about. The only mention that you read about it (for that which I might not know of) is in Bartolomeo Gavanto Modern Author who in this way reasons about it saying: Those who use eyeglasses (Perspicilla,[9] pl.) are accustomed to putting them down first in this place. However, let them indeed put them down on the altar, but never on the body.

Count Carlo Antonio Manzini in his eyeglass to Eye Dioptrics practices writes this in the beautiful beginning of his work.

"For how much diligence I might have used in searching for the first inventor of eyeglasses that are worn on the nose, that I simply call them. It was not possible for me to discover a trace. I searched all the Cornucopia of Sipontino Pontefice, all Polidoro Virgilio, Garzoni, Isidore, and other authors that come into the memory of the inventions, and of the facts of famous men of centuries gone by and it wasn't possible to have any account of it." And a little later, art is very modern however it doesn't have any mother who needs it. The first centuries saw the world created by men of robust condition who tired the centuries themselves struggling with them not one by one but one man would surmount seven of them and eight and more than centuries as you read in Iared that he lived 962 years, and his grandson Methusela who was 7 years older; where I don't argue about it because they were not in need of eyeglasses, like those, to which in any thing weren't lacking the nature to render them healthy and perfect. To which argument I do not feel like subscribing as to the universal sturdiness of vision. This certainly pleases me here to indicate in favor of the truth because not all the nations prove about eyeglasses the same great need that some (nations) have of them.

But turning now, Baldassar Bonifazio advances even further, saying that he would bet any beautiful thing that the ancients didn't have eyeglasses, with the following words: Although in truth, from that passage of Plautus (which says) "Bring a glass, it is necessary to take advantage of (this) place from which to look", many believe that those little glass circles which we bring up to the eyes and fit to the nose were even familiar to and used by the ancients, I, on the other hand, would contend on any terms one cares to wager that although the ancients were perhaps much wiser than we are, they lacked our eyeglasses.

---

[9] Earlier Manni disputes the use of this term to mean eyeglasses; the author he is quoting, however apparently uses it in this way.—Ed.

Authors who sustain that eyeglasses are a new invention. Chapter 13

If however all the things divised were gathered to demonstrate that the discovery of eyeglasses might not be too old, it will rest quite clearly to see that the famous Francesco Redi was of the sentiment that the invention of the same eyeglasses might be new in respect to the ancient Hebrews, Greeks, Latins and Arabs. Adding also that such is still the feeling of Pietro Borello, of Monsignor Pompeo Sarnelli in his letters on the Ecclesiastes and of Abbot Giacinto Gimma in the Idea of Italian Literature. This like the opinion of a great deal of other writers who in old times had treated (wrote about) such an instrument factually uniform among themselves, that is, one could refer to it for the common satisfaction of the others. The illustrator of the above mentioned work of Pancirolo which is worth saying the Salmut where he discourses about eyeglasses: Moreover, Pancirolus relegated this chapter to this back part (of the work), because, since no mention of eyeglasses is made practically anywhere among the ancient writers, it seemed (to him) that they could properly be considered among those things which had been discovered recently.

We saw however Mercuriale who constantly says: Let me with confidence assert that to the ancient doctors a glass instrument, suitable for weak eyes, was unknown, and others confirm the same thing saying in Latin language that the instrument of eyeglasses was infallibly unknown to the ancients.

Giusto Lissio, saying in great confidence to his friend Carlo Clusio, he tells him in faith, that not yet being 20 years old has begun already to see little (bad) and if it weren't for eyeglasses he wouldn't be able to even read nor write, adding what is important: (I thought I was) rather undeserving (of such a situation), even more so because I do not read that the ancients used this kind of aid to ease their predicament.

Giovanni Gerardo Vossio treating *De Scientiis Mathematics* as above I indicated said absolutely about the eyeglasses that the ancients had not even an idea about these.

Gio. Iacopo Hofmanno referred another time as follows: People who are aged and myopic indeed owe a great deal to (the science of) Optics, because they see both more sharply and at a greater distance by means of glasses (Perspicilla, pl.) which are adapted to the sight of each (condition) and of which there was no inkling among the ancients.

P.D. Secondo Lancellotti Olivetano in order to prove his subject in the *Nowadays* certainly had necessity of some authority, or proof, that this use was close to the ancient people in some way however it was an obligation for truth to confess: "The ancients, as a consequence, didn' t have the use of eyeglasses made of glass as they are used today to help the weak and thin human vision.

Finally Doctor Gio. Andrea Barotti Ferrarese in his scholarly notes about the pleasant modern work of Pertoldo, Bertolino, and Cacasenno composed in eight rhyme (stanzas) about clear subjects and with magnificent printing in 4 Bologna 1735—goes on to say: The eyeglasses are a very modern invention from the 13th century.

Other authors who affirm such an invention to be modern. Chapter 14

It is not denied here by my advive, the bringing of two passages by Florentine writers one from the middle of the 16th century the other from the end of the 17th. The first one of these was Senator Giulio de Nobili well deserving of the good Arts which he loved greatly, as with him, whom he induced with his requests the Famous Pietro Angelio de Barga to translate into Tuscal the Four part of Tolomeo the original in the own hand of the Translator gotten (possessed) by me. This Senator however, although abandoned by them who speak about the writers of our country and by anybody from common poetry and about the subjects that grew from that he has spoken, Berneschi composed two chapters the first in praise of near sightedness the second in praise of eyeglasses, addressing the two of them to Cavalier Lelio Bonsi his friend, manuscript taken by the learned Doctor Antommaria Biscioni, in the second of which pretending, as a poet, that the eyeglasses were an old invention, and fabulous, he comes to refer playfully the opinion that was going around (although to his advantage he puts it in just) that the invention of eyeglasses was modern, with the following extremely joking verses:

Some ignorant person I see here is self-concerted and he says the invention is modern too much perfume and too much flattery and maybe it could be some novice the author who writes in jargon to you he will show well that he deserves eternal fame but not to others now, because I am not going to have it except to give a copy or a remark keeping the good always for ourselves the clear story for us denotes the origin of eyeglasses to be divine and in use even in the most remote age who uses it a lot and who less than miserly with great art hangs them on the brow who wants them on their nose night and morning but blessed is Giuliar of the Ricci (rich) who has two on his nose, on his chest and one in his pocket changing their use to his whim and the ancient opinion of Mercuriale was precisely revalidated of late because it affirms in his lessons as a certain thing that the ancients did not have knowledge of our instrument. Of late, he said, since the year 1537 he dedicated his Gymnastic Art to Maximilian the second emperor in 1583 was declared Palatine Count and golden horseman.

The other writer finally is our Filippo Baldinucci in his vocabulary of Design affirms a useful artifact is that which was not known in antiquity is renewed and rediscovered again.

You see more writers yet who deny that eyeglasses are an instrument of ancient times. With these however two pens go in company which before being finally named as far as making major proof they should get it from us: so much more, in our city, for this well deserved instrument, they stopped a long time: and these are Beato F. Giordano da Rivalto mentioned by us other times and F. Bartolomeo da S. Concordio both of the Order of Preachers: The last of which speaking a little after 1300 about our such instrument, he said New Invention. And the first one demonstrating already in those years in which he preached, to be a discovered fact, he added that it was New Art that never was (before) which testimonies as they are rendered entirely convinced that this invention was modern so they obliged of them to investigate the inventor another time.

Eyeglasses worn on the nose
Second Part
Prologue

It was a great providence from heaven, to say the truth, that through the means of a glass the most noble and necessary sentiment to man which is potent vision could in any way in spite of the years (age) supply and restore, saving the advanced in age a premature death. Therefore, to a great cause the eyeglasses (as of Giovanni Ferro in the theater of business, and of Picinelli speaking of the enterprise made a profit) they were taken away separately and begun (made) by some cautious men, attributing to them as a joke (device) when they said "far" or "at a distance" (Procul) and "evidently" or "clearly" (perspicue) and "more through you" (Per vos magis).

Which the only benefit leaning aside you still have them, they offered something more, the eye glasses on the nose conciliates reverence and respect because the person who wears them is seen to be in a pitiful costume (state) where Michelangelo Buonarroti at the fair (says)

He knows how important it is to him
Gout in his feet, and a gray beard on his chin
and a pair of glasses on his nose
to the man, who agitates (is sad), makes proof (that he is) of himself

About various kinds of eyeglasses on the nose.
Chapter 1

There are certainly various kinds of eyeglasses, some being concave, others flat, some convex whose use is as was noted to make things bigger and clear up the object and to bring it closer. I am not talking about the Microscope or the Telescope or the Helioscope or the Polemoscope nor of that mirror with which at night, not otherwise, that with the light of a lamp you could recognize an army in the distance. And much less than those eyeglasses that are worked into facets multiplying the objects weirdly. Our reasoning will only follow those which produce (as an old writer of the Family Government said) in giving value to reading and writing to the poor old people and

by which as says Batista Porta, they are able, though weak in vision, to read very small characters, the ancients when their sight is lessened (these are words of Antommaria Salvini). (They made their readers read scrambled sayings.) And about that we have testimony in Cicero, in Cornelio Nipote and in Suetonio. Giusto Lissio wrote about it: Unless glass aids were to come to my relief, I would hardly (be able to) read or write. The benefit of these eyeglasses however was known and praised by many, among which is the Salmut about the Pancirolo and Giovanni Imperiali in the Beridhe Notti and by many others who in order to avoid lengthiness abandoned it being content in only indication the French for the appearance of small moons (glasses) they are called Lunette and the Spaniards—Antoio almost Antoculus (glasses) as Egidio Menagio wants.

About the material and the shape of eyeglasses.
Chapter 2

The material used is important in the shape of this considerable instrument, I am not one who is far from believing the fact that the material was derived from the visors of military helmets having two small plates in place of the eyes, sunk for the most part, but maybe still again of glass. These were in use in every century, as faithfully the ancients made bronze sculptures and the statues of every subject, especially those of Pallade. A well certified document is also supplied Monsignor Rafaello Fabretti about the Traiana Column where on the images of the Batone Gladiator and in such a shape (form) the visor of the helmet is precisely made, that you see there hanging on the trunk of a tree. Another one had an older origin which was that visor of an Etruscan hero demonstrated on Table III. in the Etruscan Museum of Anton Francesco Gori mentioned before and other Etruscan visors you could see scattered on that work. And to descent to the low centuries, this is how the visors are on some seals reported in that beautiful work of Johannes Michael Heineccius "Concerning Ancient Seals of the Germans and Other Nations" where similar visors are seen among the others on a seal of (that) distinguished gentleman Wilhelm of Ysenberch and on another of Master Ulrich of Hainovve with similar plates bored, corresponding to the places of the eyes and therefore already indicated as Orbiculi by Ammiano Marcellino. The visors went into disuse in the later centuries, they were still in use in the times mentioned above, and even with an uninterrupted continuation (of use) in the middle (centuries). They were used without doubt in the same time in which the eyeglasses were established to be discovered that is to say a little before 1300 reading that in the year 1289 the helmet of the great warrior Vescone Guglielmo d'Arezzo was brought to Florence in triumph, remained extinct (dead) in fragments, given by us under Campaldino to the Aretini. And that they might put crystals in the visors you could suppose for the reason of stopping the passage of dust in battle and in part you could infer from the words of the divine poet in the year 1300 who writes like this in the 23rd *Canto of Hell*.

And yes like a visor of glass to which then the commentator Francesco Da Buti in the same century in which Dante lived, he wanted to apply the figure of these visors as we indicated above.

In others the name Ocularium is seen because for the authors a little previous to 1200 it is defined "opening of the helmet" (foramen galeae) and indeed "crack of the helmet" (rima galeae).

"But now let's look at the material better, the description of Baldinucci is just: This instrument is composed of two crystals, or glasses joined with a wire of brass, silver or other metal or encased in enclosures of bone or of leather: you hold them on your nose in front of your eyes, thus the visual ray which is between the objects and the eyes passes through them" And a little later: "They make eyeglasses in diverse manufacturing ways, proportioned to different uses, which we make use of them. And firstly if you take care of yourself they help the short vision or the weakness. they are to see far away and also nearby. For nearsightedness and the effect of seeing far away they make eyeglasses scooped or concave which show the objects close reduced to less than their natural state. For the other they make eyeglasses convex, also said lenses, which make the objects appear although far bigger than what they are; and in proportion of the greater or lesser sphere to which the center responds, according to how they are worked (made) they receive the virtue of enlarging or making smaller than their natural state, the objects. Some though are called eyeglasses of first others of second vision, they make the convex and the concave from crystal or glass non colored but very clean (neat) and without stain. They make eyeglasses to comfort the vision, so that the vision isn't scattered or fatigued from the whiteness of the paper you are studying; and these are made from flat colored glass, more or less dull, others are used for traveling so that the vision or the eye doesn't get the reflection of the sun, nor receive damage from the dust, and for this effect certain bands of leather are joined to them, attaching the temples and to the head they stop at the ears.[10]

And here after having said something on the effects of this instrument, I like to report then what is read in the physical pastimes (amusements) of Aristo, Eudolfo and P. Regnault. The eyeglasses of convex glass (it says there) from the perpendicular they make things farther and this distancing brings them nearer and they unite at a point in a common focus. Therefore with these eyeglasses objects get bigger because they are seen under a large angle and the image of the object as we already said, corresponds to this angle. These eyeglasses are good for the old people from which crystal they are cut they can't soften nor become thick from any strain from the eye by which having the focus beyond the retina they don't join the rays in the same way as the one like a pencil (might make) they meet at the same retina, so these eyeglasses procure their union on the retina.

Tommasco Garzoni da Bagnacavallo in his universal place left such a thing written about the manipulation of eyeglasses: In France they make them perfect and even in Venice, rendering them and account in this way: Murano, pleasant and sweet place near Venice is better than any place in the world for its glass and crystals, partly because of the salty water that is very appropriate for this sort of work and partly for the abundance of the wood from the forest that makes beautiful and clear flames. And because in other places they don't make salt from soda (Dali) as they do in Murano, so for this reason they make beautiful crystals.

I don't believe finally that authority might be for bringing confusion because below we will refer to making eyeglasses from beryl: since by beryl is intended certain non artificial crystal but native to this name, also put among the gems of the writers who spoke about such material and particularly of Baldinucci in his Vocabulary of the art of design from which is used to make rings of very little value.

About the various forms of eyeglasses.
Chapter 3

It would certainly seem useless for us if we wrote something about the form and shape of the eyeglasses as that one that seems notable to everyone if we didn't say something worthy of particular reflection, that is here known. In his Lecture on Death by Friar Girolamo Savonarola author as everyone knows, in 1490 you can read in this way: "Because the eyeglasses fall often, it is necessary to put a cap (bonnet) on them or some hook to attach them so they don't fall." I don't doubt that this need of Savonarola thus harshly placed under the eye, wouldn't be reduced in obscurity to the reader when he might not be mindful of that because a scholarly subject was communicating with me. Therefore to say that to be of the opinion that the first to affirm that the eyeglasses are put on the face were by means of an attachment of them to a small bonnet (cap). And one of them they covered the fore head up to the brow in 1300 according to the memoirs of the time that you could clearly comprehend. Therefore it still gives way to the intelligence that is read in a sacred history in the City of Pavia from which the author Iacopo Gualla Giureconsulto entitled *Papiae Sanctuatium* that is to say there are kept with veneration in that city Birretum and Ocularia S. Bernardini de Senis: which things although today maybe they were disjointed, they could be either connected or ready to be connected together S. Bernardino was living therefore in 1440. They used to keep these relics in the fortress of that city where they were transported to the major church in the year 1499. The reader shouldn't expect now that because of having incidentally named the eye glasses of a Saint, that I was going to speak about some others of the same kind as of those miraculous ones of Saint Filippo Neri that are kept in Rome and about others, because this doesn't belong to my scope (objective).

But in order to stay on our proposal, it is a true thing, that things go on perfecting themselves with the passage of time, The Time of Grillandaio didn't arrive yet, which means the end of the 15th century in which the eyeglasses were made to attach to the nose, as in that picture of all the saints named above appears. It still is not clear from the passage of Franco Sacchetti if from the year 1346 to 1361 in which time Tommaso Baronci a loyalist of the Prior of Liberty, many times eyeglasses were made with that new attachment, reading that Rommaso in order to recognize a joke made in that time which was about the Prior of Liberty: you took off the glasses from the side and put them on (from there) and with them you looked down (bent down) as much as you could. It is also shown that in the time of the famous Luigi Pulci dead in the end of the 15th century and even in that writing of the witty Burchiello who passed from this life in 1448 this instrument is recommended only for the nose, singing (saying in one of the Morgans):

This also seems to me the newest case
Quickly going out of the palace

---

[10] Note Scarlotti's invention of temples on eyeglasses.—(Rosenthal)

He became before the one without a nose and he goes toward Rinaldo like a crazy person he had a long beard and a shaved head Rinaldo looks at that doglike (ugly) face that doesn't look like a man nor an animal and said: Where do you attach (hang) your glasses?

And the other that is well before that time about a certain particular nose he wrote as a joke (play around) and its all aquiline (eagle like beak) and it has a pair of eyeglasses hung on real well that they never move from their support.

From which things it all seems that you could conclude that between 1440 and 1450 eventually you should change the fashion of having them on the face and their attachments and in the Preaching of Savonarola they recognize both of these ways putting the oldest one first by saying: It is necessary to put the bonnet on them or some hook to attach them. And in fact in a choral book from the Convent of Saint Marco written in Florence, and painted in miniature around the middle of the 15th century you see a miniature that shows a Friar with eyeglasses having this posterior attachment.

Those who had spoken about our invention with foundation.

Chapter 4

The first one, to tell the truth, who undertook to talk about the eyeglasses with foundation was certainly the learned Francesco Redi in his Letter that you read in Volume IV of his work in the edition of 1724 as in the one of 1731 and it is the following contents:

To Mr. Carlo Dati

I am sending to your grace the Camdeno and I render to you those graces that I know and I put (give) greater ones. etc.

About the inventor of eyeglasses on the nose, I will write the precise words of the Chronicle a manuscript in the Convent of S. Caterina in Pisa. "Brother Alexander de Spina Pisanus used to produce whatever he wished with his own hands, and, overcome with feelings of kindness and generosity, would communicate (this knowledge) to others. And so, when, at that time, a certain man had for the first time discovered glass instruments, which the common people call glasses—obviously a beautiful, useful and new invention—and (this man) did not want to communicate the actual skill of making (these glasses) to anyone, this good and clever man (Brother Alexander), once he had seen the glasses, learned (how to make them) right away, with no teacher, and he taught others who wanted to know. He sang melodiously, wrote elegantly and decorated books that had been written, which they call the red ones. There was absolutely not one of the manual skills of which he was unaware."

The author of this said Chronicle was Friar Domenico da Peccioli Pisano of the order of San Domenico.

The mentioned Friar Alessandro Spina died in the year 1313 in Pisan style and in 1312 Roman style.

This Chronicle is written in a book in pages (in-folio) but small, on ordinary paper, but thick, and in characters (letters) pretty good for those times.

In the margin of that paper, on which Friar Domenico da Peccioli mentions the death of Friar Alessandro Spina there are painted a pair of eyeglasses, but if you know (about it) it is a more modern work (fact).

If your Grace wants other news about that I would favor one verse that will be served to you with great punctuality. It is good weather these nice days and if it wasn't much of a bother to you, I beg you to advise me if you have any news of the original because the stars of Castore and of Polluce are called in our language Saint Ermo or Sant'Elmo. I am honored by your orders (demands) while with all the most reverent affects I kiss your hands.

November 8, 1673—Florence

It could well be that the passage above referred from the Chronicle of S. Caterina might be read twice because of the diversity that we perceive in it, Therefore in the annotations in the margins of this letter it says: See the letter of our author about the invention of eyeglasses addressed to Mr. Paolo Falconieri where there is reported another passage similar to this Chronicle.

Neither is it any wonder, because, the followers of similar histories used to frequently repeat what was already said by others. And in fact Friar Domenico da Peccioli Pisano wrote—reporting as much as was narrated by their first ancestors as a confession of the same, Redi in the Letter that we refer to published by itself alone the first time in the year 1678 and then with something added years afterwards.

Letter about the Invention of Eyeglasses written from Francisco Redi to Paolo Falconieri, In Florence by Francesco Onofri Stampore—Printer of the Grand Duke—1678.

Illustrious Signore

That evening, during which Mr. Carlo Dati, of celebrated memory (fame), in the palace of the prior (head of convent) Orazio Rucellai read his favorable and scholarly Tuscan tales about eyeglasses to Mr. Francesco di Andrea (priest) famous neopolitan man of letters and to many other Florentine gentlemen no less noble than virtuous, they spoke familiarly and they talked and they mentioned many things about the uncertainty of the time when (in which) that instrument was invented as being very useful for helping sight (vision) and really worthy of being named as one of the most useful discoveries of human ingenuity. I remember that then I was of the steady opinion that the invention of eyeglasses wads (all) modern and totally unknown to the ancient Hebrews, Greeks, Latins, and Arabs: and that, also, which I won't dare to affirm that it wasn't unknown to them, it then was lost for a long time, and a little before the year 1300 it was found again and re-established: and I remember also, that I promised then to give to Illustrious V.S. (title of respect) all the news which, more by luck than by study, came to me (my possession) all put together (assembled). I'm never satisfied with my many worries rather with my obligation having made daily debt after debt, I'm afraid now that it started with the rigidity of creditors to really force (squeeze) me, and the natural softness of the spirit is gone, he-she bitterly rebukes me, and I'm angry (she he) reprimands me with asperity this little gracious failure to pay. Therefore, in order not to live in such contumacy (defiance of authority) I'm now scraping up the payment in this letter writing to her, him that in the Library of the Dominican Fathers of the convent of Saint Catherine of Pisa you can find an antique Latin manuscript chronicle on parchment which contains many things that happened in that venerable convent and it begins; Here commences the Chronicle of the Convent of Saint Catherine of Pisa, O.P. Prologus, in Toga this chronicle was started by famous Friar Bartholemeo of Saint Concordio Predicator, and author of that pamphlet about the *Teachings of the Ancient People* in which, over the years, reduced to its true (real) lesson, was printed in Florence by the learned and noble Mr. Francesco Ridolfi under the name of Rifiorito Accademico Della Crusca (Florentine Academy of Letters) Friar Bartolomeo de san Concordio died in 1347 in decrepit age because he saw about 70 years in the Dominican Religion, the chronicle was continued by Friar Vgolino of master Noui Pisano of the popular family of Cavalasari, the latter died of continuous fever in Florence Visitor of Ordine and it happened to him according to Fra Domenico writing about Peccioli Pisano, that reporting as he himself affirms as much as was narrated by the first two of his ancestors, he lasted then to write up to his own death which followed in the month of December of the year 1408 as the same chronicle relates the teacher Fra Simone da Cascia a son of the convent of Saint Catherine who after him continued to compile it. In the beginning of this chronicle it states on page 16 the death of Brother Alexandro Spina Pisano which came in 1313 in Pisa with the following words: Brother Alexander de Spina, a modest and good man—whatever he saw or heard had been made, he even knew (how) to make (it). He himself made glasses, when they had been made for the first time by someone, (but that man) was unwilling to communicate (the knowledge) and he (Alexander) willingly and cordially (?) communicated it. By his ingenuity in corporal matters, this ingenious man created a dwelling place in the house of the Everlasting King.

From which you gather, that if Brother Alexander Spina wasn't the first inventor of eyeglasses, he at least was the one who by himself without any instruction finds the way to work them and at the same time in which he lived comes to light for the first time this very useful invention. In that way I point out that for a certain sameness of fortune it happens to our Galileo Galilei, who having heard of by fame, which by a certain Fiammingo that long eyeglass was invented, that in Greek vocabulary is called Telescope, he worked on a similar one of them with only a knowledge of refraction, without having ever seen it. That in the time of Brother Alexander Spina came to right the invention of the eyeglasses, I have another detail of proof because in my old books written in pen (ink) there's one entitled *Treatise of management of the family of Sandro de Pippozzo, of Sandro Florentine Citizen made in 1299*—by Vanni del Busca Florentine Citizen his son-in-law. In the introduction of such a book there makes mention of the eyeglasses as a thing discovered in those years. I find myself sad in years, that I don't have any value in reading and writing without glasses (pieces of glass) called eyeglasses, recently found to be useful for poor old people when they fail to see. Besides in the lectures of Fra Giordano da Rivalto del Testo in the pen of Filippo Pandolfini cited from our Vocabulary of the Crusca to the word Eyeglasses clearly it is said, it still isn't 20 years that the art of making eyeglasses was found, that they make you see better, that it's one of the best arts and one of the most necessary that the world could have. Fra Giordano was a man of a holy life, and great teacher of Divinity who after having lived a space of 30 years in the Religion of San Domenico in the Convent of Florence and of Pisa finally in year 1311 in the month of August he died in Piacenza, called by brother Amico Piacentino head teacher of the Dominicans to send him a Lecturer for the Paris Studio. Therefore Fra Giordano passed from this life to the other in 1311. He flourished in the time of Brother Alexander Spina discoverer of eyeglasses who died then in 1313 and lived with him in the same Convent of St. Catherine of Pisa: Therefore he was able with undoubtable certainty to affirm much about the eye glasses he said in his above mentioned lectures. So as soon as Fra Bartolomeo da San Concordio was able to write truthfully that Spina in his own ingenuity discovered the way to work the eyeglasses, and he communicated it to everyone, that he wanted to learn it because that Fra Bartolomeo was a contemporary of Spina and lived with him in the same Convent of Santa Caterina of Pisa. Therefore it is that for me to be able to ingeniously affirm that the art of making eyeglasses is a modern invention, and discovered in Tuscany in those years, that ran, to take it the longest, from 1280 up to 1311. And this space (of time) you could still shrink to an advantage, of you knew, or if you could guess in which year Fra Giordano recited his lecture that even in some written texts I have found to be written after those that he said in Florence about 1305. With the above mentioned news it will please V.S. Illustrissima to observe that from the time of Brother Alexander Spina in which are found books of the Writers many a time, and clearly named were Eyeglasses, and that before that time you don't see any memory (mention) of them, at least that I know of. Bernardo Gordonio Professor in Mompelieri, in a book entitled *Lilium Medicina*, started by him, as acknowledged, in the 1305 in the month of July in the chapter *de debilitate Visus* = *Concerning Weakness of Vision* after having instructed a certain Collirio he replies with great vivacity and a little too impudently: And it (collyrium) is of great virtue because it enables an old person to read tiny letters without glasses. A letter of this same author (Petrarch), with the title "Concerning the Origin, Life, Frequency and Result of His Studies"—Francis Petrarch (gives)

greetings to posterity. One reads concerning glasses; It had fallen to my lot as a young man (to have) a body not of great strength, but of much dexterity; I do not boast of outstanding beauty, but of what can be pleasing in one's younger years: a bright color between fair and dark, lively eyes and vision that was very keen for a long time, which unexpectedly, failed me beyond my 60th year, so that, to my indignation, I had to seek help and refuge in eyeglasses: old age invaded a body which had been extremely healthy all my life and surrounded it with the customary army of diseases. I was born to honest Florentine parents, whose origin and fortune were ordinary and—to tell the truth—verged on poverty, but they were driven out of their country, (so that I was born) in exile in Arezzo in a year of this last century, the year 1304, beginning from the time of Christ, on a Monday at dawn on the 1st of August.

Guido da Chauliac Professor also from Mompelieri in his work *Major Surgery*, composed in the year 1363 it carries in it some good medicines for weakness of the eyes and adds besides with greater sincerity than Gordonio's. If these and similar things don't help it's necessary to resort to eyeglasses. In some acts of Parliament from Paris on November 12, 1416 cited, although in another proposal from the scholarly Egidio Menagio in the book entitled *Amoenitates Juris Civilis*. Niccolo de Baye Signor de Gie makes a petition to the Parliament in which—Because furthermore I have become somewhat weakened in my vision and cannot make entries well without having glasses—Giovanfrancesco Pico in the tenth chapter of the *Life of Fra Girolamo Savonarola*.

And Fra Timoteo da Perugia in the life of Savonarola himself in Chapter 48. To search out the truth also and to put to flight jealousies or hatreds and the other wicked strivings of the mind, he very often would repeat this proposition—(namely) that it was necessary for him, who would like to see very accurately what was false, to put aside his eyeglasses* for if the glasses* are pure and clear, the aspects of things are received on the pupil as they are; but if the glasses are green, blue, purple, wax-colored or brown, the forms which are drawn from things are adulterated in a certain way, and such forms usually appear like the glasses[II] are. It happened that a good man who was making (doing) the art of eyeglasses going out of the door of the convent with his slippers in his hand, he started with good and loving words to scold the common

people this was heard by one of the Compagnacci he hit him on top of the head with a big club. I will make it too long and fastidious if I bring forth too many examples, it's enough just to indicate that they are frequent and in the Morgante (lordship) of Pulci and in the Rhymes of Burchiello, and in the Rhymes, and in the prose of Alessandro Allegri and in other pleasant poetry and Tuscan Comedies (plays): Therefore it would be a great marvel, presupposed that the Greek and Latin comic actors (writers) might have had knowledge of the Eyeglasses, if they never had taken the occasion either to name them or to joke with you about them through the mouths of their interlocutors (actors). Likewise it would be a marvel if the very diligent Plinio in the Chapter about inventors of things hadn't made any mention of them. I know well that from some modern Lexicographers are cited certain fragments from (of) Plauto; neither is it unknown to me the *Faber ocularius, and oculariarius* made of sepulchral marble the figure carved in the marble of Sulmona that I already communicated to Mr. Dati and finally how much Plinio refers to the Smeraldo (emerald) in the fifth chapter of the 27th book but these things that I hear now V.S. Illustrissima I hear it from that story (tale) of Mr. Dati, worthy of coming to light together with the others that remained manuscripts, after the death of that scholarly gentleman. And here V.S. Illustrissima I humbly kiss your hands.
Florence

How Redi did not otherwise attribute
the first invention of the eyeglasses to
Friar Alessandro Spina as it seems to some (people).

The illustrious Redi was always accustomed to writing about each one of his things (matters) with wise foresight, and he spoke so much about the present Invention, after having referred to the passages of the above mentioned Chronicle, he passes on (made) this inducement: From what is gathered, if Friar Alessandro Spina wasn't the first inventor of eye glasses he at least was of those who by themselves without any teaching at all invented the way to work (make) them and that in the same time he lived this extremely useful invention came to light for the first time.

Not appearing was the fact that Filippo Baldinucci clearly expressed the sentiment of Redi in his Vocabulary of Design published in the year 1681 left room to believe that Redi made Friar Alesandro Spina the inventor of eyeglasses by saying in this way: Doctor Francesco Redi Noble Aretino First Physician of the AA. SS. of Tuscany, celebrated writer, Poet, and Philosopher and in our century valued in Florentine eloquence in one of his scholarly letters written to the virtuous and noble Paolo Falconieri already first gentleman of the Chamber of the Serene Grand Duke proves and evidences, that this useful invention was discovered in Tuscany around the years 1280 and 1310 by Friar Alessandro Spina Pisan of the order of Preachers, etc.

It still seems that the lawyer Giacinto Gimma, a neopolitan, made a mistake when he said in the history of Italian Letters published in 1723 where he reasons about eyeglasses (1) Francesco Redi proves in the letter about the same invention written to Paolo Falconieri that they were discovered in Tuscany: showing from various manuscripts and from a predication of Friar Giordano de Rivalto that the author was Alessandro Spina from the Convent of S. Caterina in Pisa. Where he absolutely wanted the word Author to be taken for Discoveror.

There is no doubt that Gio. Cinelli writing a scholarly work about our writers, seen by me Doctor Antommaria Biscioni, urged he reasoned thus about Spina, with having gotten, as I estimate, the news from Redi himself, because Redi it appeared wrote about eyeglasses as a monk in 1678 and Cinelli lived until the year 1706. It could be then that Friar Alessandro might not have been the first discoverer of this art, but having heard about such a new thing as a man of ingenuity he began to speculate and at the risk of working, he guessed it. The Tuscans are sharp. (ingenious)

Monsieur Spon did not employ this method because in order not to alter the facts he translated by word Redi's letter in his scholarly Collection which is titled "Curious Researches of Antiquity" in the decimated differences where Menagio and Moreri attracting such learned things, propagated them.

---

[11] In this passage, *conspicillia* and *perspicillia*— two words Manni rejects as correct terms for glasses—are used.—Ed.

The real and first inventor of Eyeglasses.
Chapter 7

Although the great news that was provided by Redi doesn't seem to satisfy the eager desires of the person who is asking for the truth, however in the question of eyeglasses one does not withdraw therefore who might have been the first inventor of them; nevertheless gave material to recover what was missing while in the year 1684 Fernando Leopoldo del Migliore published his Florence illustrated, it came under everyone's eye his estimable existing document in his old Sepoltorio manuscript with the words that I transcribe in talking about the S. Maria Maggiore Church of this country.

There was another memoir that went bad in the restoration of that Church registered faithfully in our old Sepoltorio, so much nicer, when in the middle of it we came across the knowledge of the first inventor of eyeglasses having been a gentleman of this country, highly adorned in wit on every subject that demands sharpness of him: This was Sir Salvino of the Armatis, son of Armato, of noble lineage, of which they still call today the blind alley of the Armati's that narrow lane, because such is the significance (meaning) of Chiaso (blind alley) situated behind the Centaur. You also want to make note here that nowadays in fact the alley is closed to which the house of Mr. Venturi, in the back, responded to the contrary. But let's continue; You see the figure of this man, a flag was stretched in civil custom and with letters on it that said this.

Here lies Salvino D. Armato of the Armati of Florence inventor of the eyeglasses God pardon him his sin year 1317. On this important document it seems to me to see that the reader might be able to observe many more things in passing. First the beginning, a cross like that one, that reportedly doesn't come from Crescimbeni provided in the Commentaries about the history of Common Poetry of Epitaphs. (He) is referred to with such an Inscription. But this you want to judge as an error of the copyist or the printing, as such is the omission of a letter, writing the same: Savino instead of Salvino; whereas the Cross on the Epitaphs is an observation of educated persons who (guess) they might have lasted up to 1500. It could have been badly cut into the marble (the word) La Peccata (sin), which maybe said Le Peccata and so the Crescimbeni corrected it. Yet it could have been a fault of the engraver as similar mistakes, not by the pen, but of marble I have seen examples of them. But turning to Migliore these (he says) is that one not named, nor expressed in the old MS. Chronicle in the Convent of the PP. Domenicans in Pisa cited by Francesco Redi, an excellent doctor of our time is his Narrative on Eyeglasses; reading how Friar Alessandro Spina who lived in those same times and who maybe was a Florentine and not a Pisan, searched to learn the invention to make eyeglasses from one who knew it (who) didn't want to teach him and by himself he found a way to work (make) them. Up to here are the words of Migliore that treats S. Maria Maggiore. Gio. Vincenzio Fantoni one of the learned gentlemen of this country speaking about that Church does little about the vanished (stolen) death, so he left written in confirmation in the additions made by him in the abridgement of the notable things of Florence fourth edition 1733 saying: One singular memoria was already in this Church, today decayed; The monument then was made of Salvino D'Armato of the Armati in 1317 with the specific title as Inventor of Eyeglasses. And he himself possessed no different a memoir originally composed in another Sepoltuario (Sepulchre), according to what he believed a little after 1600 and it is that under a coat of arms of the Armati family, it existed there already next to the belfry it was written Seppilliorium Armatt but today it isn't there any more.

But the document of Salvino d'Armato on the Sepulchre of Migliore assures me it exists even today taken by Mr. Gio. Batista from Migliore grandson and heir of the historian. Another person who sees it contemporarily is the famous Captain Cosimo della Rena truthful writer as much as accurate, who in the introduction to his Series about the ancient Dukes and Marquesi of Tuscany, so he decided to research the occasion and treat it. "Many inventors of less useful things in the world were omitted, and again as among the others a Salvino d'Armato of the Armati who before anyone else found the use of eyeglasses, so efficient as to revive vision to man; Ferdinand Leopold del Migliore found this memory again after many years, he was an indefatigable illustrator of the memoirs of the country which he still brings with much approval to the printing." By which words you could eventually suppose that Migliore might have not yet published his work, as that one that although was under press (in the) year 1684 you still know that after the one of Rena it was finished.

"These (Rena says himself) were investigated to be the burial place of the body of said Salvino in S. Maria Maggiore of Florence died in 1317 according to his epitaph."

Other testimony about this inventor.
Chapter 8

Although there were many things so validly shown by Migliore that he might be the inventor of eyeglasses, but nevertheless I would like to confirm it along with the authority of the previous writers. Mr. Marco Antonio Mariti Florentine man of endowed with much education as the year 1730 is increasing, the Chronological ledger (torch) of P. Gio. Domenico Musanzio of the Society of Jesus with abundant entries put Armati among the illustrious men because of his discovery. Even the above praised Fantoni considered him a very brilliant man and made him a (governor) in praise.

But that, shouldn't be omitted in any way, if it is the assertion of the foreign writers, as the scholarly Archpriest Gio: Mario Crescimbeni mentioned in a place above, calling the Florentine Armati the inventor of eyeglasses: and more than wore that of Doctor Carlo Taglini Public Professor of Philosophy of the University of Pisa who is almost like a national of Friar Alessandro Spina, about the first invention he had no doubt in underwriting for our Armati in his scholarly Philosophical Letter printed in Florence in year 1728 with the printing of Giusseppe Manni my father.

Some news about the person
and the family of the inventor is given.
Chapter 9

It is true that we don't have any memory about the person of Salvino Armati outside of knowing that he was a well deserving and noble citizen of this country. From some writings of the Convent of S. Maria Novella in the handwritings of the celebrated Senator Carlo Strozzi are conserved in the famous Strozian Library you deduce that Salvino D'Armato had a brother.

He also was of the congregation of S. Maria Maggiore, named Bartolo, who passed to the other life a few years before him, he left Lapo, Salvino, and Vanni his own sons, that were seen mentioned in the years 1294 and 1295 many times in a lawsuit pending among them and Canda de Ser Aliotto di Mazzocchio, or Mazzocchino of that Salvi of the Armati his relation. Vanni then and Salvino from some memoirs provided by the kindness of Lorenzo Maria Mariani antique dealer and custodian of the secret archives of S.A. Reale of Tuscany, who died a short while ago, are found sworn into the Art of Change in 1321 and just in that year Vanni was perceived as seated as Signori (Sir) in the Priorism for the first time along with five other times so he stayed (in that organization) until the year 1341. Salvino likewise enjoyed the supreme honor of the Florentine republic 4 times from 1328 to 1337, still being alive also in 1341 and his monument, the way Stefano Rosselli says on his sepulchre and others upon referring to the tomb (grave) (that is how they call it) in S. Maria Novella among the mislaid tombs, it was in the cemetary in front of that church. Finally a daughter of that Salvino, Bartolo's son, is found in the year 1345 and 1346 to be already a widow of Baldo de Dingo de'Marignolli her husband.

Then our Salvino through authentic writings in the mentioned Royal Archives is understood to have had a son named Parente, who passed from this life in the year 1333.

Their coat of arms consisted of a red field full of white stripes on the plane (flat) and you can see it near our inscription in the Church of S. Maria Maggiore.

How the Florentines
took the eternalizing
of the memory of this discovery to heart.
Chapter 10

The inscriptions for more diverse reasons deserve from posterity all faithfulness, mainly because of their antiquity, and as a fact, according to what is credible, from the same sons of the inventor because as the Roman orator says, "it is almost a given of nature that whatever honor or glory has by chance flourished in some family, the family's descendants practically pursue this glory most eagerly, so that people's conversation may be filled with the virtue of their ancestors to keep it in the memory" and that should be eventually much more to the heart of these Armati, since it concerns not so much a very useful invention, but also some jealousy in respect to Friar Alessandro Spina who found the way to copy the same eyeglasses by himself.

Writers who make a record
of the newly discovered invention.
Chapter 11

Florentine was the invention of the eyeglasses. Florentine wasn't only the first memoir, that was left in the marble, but also, from the beginning was put in letters, 'which thefts do not injure and over which the ages have command, and these monuments alone do not know death. Because the oldest record, that was found, we have from a particular manuscript that the brilliant Francesco Redi had, work of a Florentine, of those kind that our Nation because of economics left written in pen: Although some modernly were made for the public in print, and it was entitled: *Treatise of Government of the family of Sandro de Pippozzo di Sandro Citizen of Florence* made (done) in 1299 assembled by Vanni del Busca Florentine Citizen his son-in-law. It was this Sandro, rather Alessandro, man who was a friend of literature, and intelligent; because the Archpriest Crescimbeni in the Commentaries to the History of Common Poetry, reasons (talks) about him like this: Sandro de Pippozzo di Sandro Florentine Citizen in the last stage of his old age in 1299 compiled a treatise of the Governing of the Family as Redi refers, who possessed his verses, and he says the truth; since Redi himself in his annotations to the Dithyramb (emotional writing) tells of having the Rhymes, and that in the last of his doting old age he composed a treatise of the government (conduct) of the family. This Allessandro de Pippozzo in his prologue of his work goes among others in saying and showing that these eyeglasses were found (discovered) in those years: I find myself seriously old, and I don't have any power to read and write without pieces of glass called eyeglasses just discovered to help the poor old people when they weaken in seeing .

This fragment from the prologue reported comes also in the History of the writers by Giovanni Cinelli, who adds here: this good old man lasted until after 1308. It is then true that Cinelli made a big (gross) error when he showed in that history not to believe that the invention of eyeglasses might be modern rather than not. And you see clearly the basis for his error, so that it wasn't necessary to do another examination about him; since he neither gave the reasons, that being unskillfully supported in part by a doubtful passage, the source still not discovered by him, but seen cited by others and having believed because of a truth that was shown above to be a mere mistake of Cristofano Landini in his translation of Chap. III of the VIII book of the history of Plinio.

In the years I note what the mentioned Sandro wrote, the blessed Giordano de Rivalto in one of his learned sermons in the Piazza of S. Maria Novella when he was in Florence as reader of the works, on February 23, 1305 on a Wednesday morning, thus pronounced. In finding arts (skills) you never see an end. Everyday you could find one of the arts. Does the buffoon find them all in the ballad? No he doesn't find them all because there are those in the world that he doesn't know (exist) quantities (of them) are made: Where in Paris there are great arts of engraving or cutting precious stones which is great art; and so in ths world there are many of them that you don't know about. It is still not yet 20 years (observe the time/date) that the art of making eyeglasses was found, that they make you see well, it is one of the best arts, and of the most necessary that the world had, and it is seldom that a new art that never was before is found. And the reader said: I saw with him who first found it, and made them and spoke about them. That's how it was left registered by he who from the lively voice of the Preacher, told similar sermons such as the ones that exist in the old Code of Mr. Duca Gio: Vincenzio Salviati, praised highly by the Cavalier Lionardo Salviati, and in another one of the Library of Mr. Marchesi Riccardi, which now are published with the stamp (seal) of this city. It is also notable that the compiler added there: and the Reader said: I saw with him, who first found it, and made and spoke about them. And to exemplify the last words, and together clear them, I allow myself to refer to a similar note, that I read in a little history of Florence manuscript, compiled by Agostino di Iacopo, and others by Lapini, where in the year 1518 it was left written: the way to make small balls for the crossbows was found, and the first inventor of them was a beautiful spirit named Giovanni de Mona Piera del Mucione, who to them was always called Giovanni of the Crossbows; and before this time they didn't use these said crossbows. He was a very whimsical man, and I knew him and ate with him many times.

The place exemplified then, you read in the Preaching of Beato Giordano, it remains to be seen how it becomes very credible that Beato might have seen with him, who first found it. Beato Giordano lived more years in S. Maria Novella in Florence as I have shown before in his Notices: And I note, there close by were the homes of the family of the inventor, therefore of Salvino Armati, and that to the exclusion of Allessandro Spina; because you read with him, who first found it, because you can't say that about any others except Armati; and besides this he saw and spoke about them something you can't understand about Spina, with whom besides seeing him and speaking about them, he had spoken with him earnestly, living with him in S. Caterina di Pisa and about which he couldn't abstain from naming the habit (monk) and the profession.

Also presented here is the third Memoir of the Florentine writer from those same first years, and this is of the famous Francesco Petrarca, who on the assertion of Monsignor Lodovico Becatelli Archbishop of Ragusa in his life he was past 60 years of age, therefore near the year 1365 he had to resort to the help of eyeglasses. And he says the truth; while he himself in the devised letter, which has as a title in the printings "Concerning the Origin, Life, Frequency and Result of His Studies" he went on writing like this. It had fallen to my lot as a young man (to have) a body not of great strength, but of much dexterity; I do not boast of outstanding beauty, but of what can be pleasing in one's younger years: a bright color between fair and dark, lively eyes and vision that was very keen for a long time, which unexpectedly, failed me beyond my 60th year, so that, to my indignation, I had to seek help and refuge in eyeglasses. Where it happens, that writing "Concerning the Remedies for Each Kind of Fortune" he put others in his mouth: A weak vision is rekindled by the use of glasses, with what follows, already referred to above.

Other writers, who make mention of this invention.
Chapter 12

That is how, briefly, our invention of the instrument became famous, that even the writers who were strangers to discussion began to discuss it quickly; which through a continuous series of occasions have always proceeded to do. Which (this) fights against allowing to appear (see), that the silence of the writers in every ancient period (age), gives a great sign (clue) about the lack of eyeglasses.

Bernardo Gordonio, Professor of Medicine wrote a book entitled Lilium Medicinae, whose printing came, according to P. Pellegrino Orlandi in the year 1494 in Venice, and there also in 1496 where Pascual Gallo adds to it a third printing in 1498. This was even reprinted in 1542 in Paris, and edition taken, by me, and afterwards by the celebrated Rovillio de Lione in 1574. And that, which makes our case which is that the work was composed in the year 1305 because in the prologue you read: This book has been undertaken moreover with the aid of almighty God, in the famous School of Montpelier, after the 20th year of our reading, in the year of our Lord 1305, in the month of July. This Reader of Mompelieri in the men tioned work where he speaks of the sufferings of the eyes, Part III, Chapter V "Concerning the Weakness of Vision." After having proposed various eye-waters, says about one of them: And if it is winter, it should be prepared on the ashes, where there is warmth in the manner of a nesting hen and it should be shaken and boiled in a glass vessel and dropped into the eyes; and it is of such great virtue that it makes an elderly person read very tiny letters without eyeglasses.

In a similar way Guido da Caulliac another professor of Mompelieri, who flourished upon saying (talking about) Gio: Iacopo Frisio, and about P. Orlandi from 1360 to 1365 compiled in 1363 a famous work about Surgery seen by me, Whose title "Surgery by Professor Guido of Caulliac, highly experienced in the Art of Medicine" printed, according to Pascual Gallo in the year 1499 in Venice and according to Orlandini in Venice also in 1490 and in Bergamo in 1498 besides you can also find an edition by Lione in 1537 and one made there in 1572. In this work then such writer in Treatise VI *De Decoratione* (Treatise VI Concerning Embellishment) says these words: For the same purpose are water of fennel, rue, swallowswort, euphragia, verbena and the expensive water of Master Peter Hispanus and similar things. And if these things do not help, one must come back to eyeglasses or to those made of beryls.

The famous Redi, having reported this passage of Caulliaco in Tuscany gives some indication that he didn't make use of the indicated printings, which are Latin. And since the brilliant Mr. Antonio Bastero a Barcelonian nobleman, in the first volume of his Provenzal Crusca quoting this Surgical

Work that he asks of Monsignor Guido di Cauliacco, he cites from it a text in pen numbered Cod. 4804 from the Vatican Library, this one not being in Latin, as the author wrote it, a version previously made well believed by the scholarly annotator of the lives of the Provenzal poets, published again in Venice by Lorenzo Baseggio in 1731 besides the two referred to authored by Gordonio, and by Caulliaco were first observed by the Cavalier Girolamo Mercuriale Forlivese, learned Doctor, since he in his various lessons wrote in this way: I would declare with confidence that an instrument made of glass suitable for weak eyes was not known by ancient doctors; however, it is by no means such a new invention that I would absolutely think our grandparents' parents lacked it, since it is clearly mentioned both by Gordonius, who was renowned a little less than 300 years ago, in his chapter about weakness of vision, and also by Guido Gaulliacus, who was 50 years younger than Gordonius, in that chapter about eyeglasses which old men use to see tiny letters.

In some acts of Parliament in Paris (before we leave the French authority) of November 12, 1416 cited by Egidio Menagio, he has there the passage referred to above by Redi.

Similarly Gio: Francesco Pico, in turning to the Italian writers in Chapter 10 of the Life, that he wrote about Friar Girolamo Savonarola, says in the way, that Redi himself relates.

How in Florence, for the first time and not anywhere else, they went about propagating the skill (artifice) of eyeglasses.

Chapter 13

We touched above the authorship (authority) of Tommasco Garzoni, the flourishing, that he does and did in his time with this art in Venice because of the closeness of Murano, to which the exquisiteness of glass increases its reputation; from which they also make faithfully the following verses by Batista Guarini the elder, written to Girolamo Castelli Medico di Borso Duke of Ferrara:

> Until I might tell you about the Glass Vessels of Murano,
> jewels outstanding in their skill,
> a place which, being next to the beautiful city
> of Venice,
> makes that city famous.
> Do you see how beautiful brightness shines in the glass and cold ice yields,
> and the water which runs over the pebbles
> of the flowing river?

But it is also here to remember, as before, that in the industrious city of Venice the excellence of this work was transported, but without leaving our city deprived of it, that always is conserved by the professors, here and nowhere else was it flourishing because omitting some passages of writers, who demonstrate how among us (is) the master of eyeglass making, so (thus) called, always had diverse skills explained in that document that I would like to indicate confirmation and it is an original letter from Zaccaria Barbaro from Venice dated June 26, 1476 that Dr. Anton Francesco Gori has kept (near) in which (letter) he thanks him for 12 pair of eyeglasses, that along with his order he received from Florence with it (the letter).

The end.

Appendix 3

Alphabetical List of (Mostly) United States Spectacles Makers from 1700–1850

The following list is taken from stampings on actual specimens in the author's collection. The collection contains at least one artifact (pair of spectacles) made by each of the following spectacles makers. Many are lacking city and date of manufacture. Any information the reader may have regarding additions or corrections to this list would be greatly appreciated by the author.

A

J. A.
A. L. & Co. (Noel's Patent Jan. 11, 1859)
A.L J C
AO (1869)
Ackley
E. Ackley
Henry Adams, Elmira
Henry Adams & James Peters (Philadelphia, PA)
Ammidown—precursor of American Optical Co., Southbridge, MA, 1840.

B

B & C
BH & Co. B & L (after 1851)
BSO = Bay State Opt. Co. 91885) B.S.O. Co.
E. B. (possibly Edward Bogleston) (Stockbridge, MA)
E. E. Bailey (Portland, ME, and Claremont, NH)
Ball, Black & Co.
W. Barber (Philadelphia)
Pete Bateman (Eng)
W. Beecher —Southbridge, MA
B. Benjamin
Benz
Bohli
Bolles & Day—Hartford
Borhek
Boss
H. Bowles
Brewer
Briggs
Brown & Kirby—New Haven, Conn.
Butler & McCarthy (B & McC) (Philadelphia, PA)

C

C.C. & S.
C.F.
C.R. Co.
C & R
Cadwell
N. W. Cass
Diamont Chandler N.Y.

Chandler & Darrow, N.Y.
G. E. Cobb
I (?) Colton
G. Cooper
Elias Coup (Bridgeport, CT)
Cow
Cromwell
Curtis & Stills (Woodbury, CT)

D

◆ = Diamond
H. (M & a deer)
M (M & a deer)
Darrow (see Chandler)
Diamanta
Dorner
M. Doster (Phila.)
Dwelle

E

E. Eldridge
Eltonhead (Baltimore)
Evans

F

F. & Co.
F.E.C.N.
J.C. Farr—Phila.
Firce
Fisher (Phila.)
N. & T. Foster
G. Fox
Franklin—Wash. D.C.

G

G B (& picture of a deer)
G. T.
P. Garrett
Giamanta

Good
N.C. Gray
G. Griswoll

H

⌂H⌂

H & H (Hall & Hewson) Albany
Habermeier
Hall & Hewson (Albany, circa 1850)
Hall, M.B.
Harwood Brothers
Higgins
Hillner
A. Hobron
Hoffman
E. Hughes
Hyde
B. Hyde
James Hyde (New Orleans, LA)

I

Ilikit

J

J. & H. T. (England)
J. & J. R.
J. K.
A. B. Johnson (Hill, NH)

K

T. & W. Keith (Worcester, MA)Peter Kempston (Eng.)
W. B. Kendall
J. Kent
Kern
Kiltner
King (gold) [circa 1875]
J. King
Julius King-Trial Frames (Oph.—Cleveland)
Kippen

L

L. B. & Co.
L & H
LO N.Y.
LSF & S (Noel's Pat. 1859)
Lambe
Lazarus & Morris
A. Lewis
Lloyd
Andrew J. Lloyd—Boston (optician)
W. Lock
T. Lyon & Bro.

M

Wm. Mannerbruk, Reading, PA 1820–35.
Wm. Y. McAllister (Phila.)
Merriman
P. Miller & G.U. Wright
Pardon Miller (Providence, RI)
Daniel D. Moody (Monson, MA)
M. Munroe

N

Newberry & Co. (Brooklyn, NY)
Newbury Phila.
Edwin Newbury (Brooklyn, CT)

O

Lawrence O'Dell (New York, NY
C. E. Oerte (Phila.)
Nathaniel Olmsted (Farmington and New Haven, Conn.)
J. (?) Owen (Phila.)

P

Parker (case)
A. G. Peck (Osterbrooke, OH)
Peirce Phila. & Boston c. 1810.
Peters
G. Peters (Phila.)
J. Peters (Phila.)
John Pierce (Boston, MA)
J. O. Pitkin (Hartford, CT)
O & W Pitkin c. 1820.
Platt
L. C. Porter (Hartford)
J. Price
Pugh

Q

Queen & Co. Phila.

R

Reich
F. Roberts (Philadelphia)
Robinson
C. Rumse

S

J. E. S. & Co.
S. F. & Co.
S.G. N.Y.
S.T.D.C.
J. Sargeant (Hartford, Conn.)
Scheidig
Schild
Schildknecht 1820
Schnaitman, inventor-optician
Schneider
Schneirer
Schneizer
Schreiber
Schweizer
K. Segttz
E. Shaws
Shuron after 1864
Slofman (Indistinct)
Smith, J.L.
Smith & Still
A. Solomons
Wm. P. Stanton (Providence and Nantucket, RI)
C. Staples
J. P. Steiner (Philadelphia, PA)
Stern (opt. Co.)

Stevens & Co.
Stevens & Gold
F. Stll—gold
Strauss

T
P. L. Taylor & Co. (Brooklyn, NY)

U
Geo. Unite (Birmingham, England)

V
Voelk

W
(see P. Miller & G.U. Wright)
J. Watson (Phila.)
L. Wells
Wilcox (Alvan) New Haven, CT.
Wildnecht Jos.
Willmore (Eng.)
M. Wise (New York, NY)
Wright Bros.

Appendix 4

History and Bibliography of Astigmatism Original Work by Emile Javal

Translated from the French by Linda L. McDonald

1801. The discovery of astigmatism is due to Thomas Young who measured this defect on himself. With the help of Porterfield's optometer he ascertained that, for his eye, the most remote distance from the distinctly perceived was about 7 or 10 inches so long as he placed a chart near his eye with two pierced pinholes on a straight horizontal line or a straight vertical line. He expressed the value of his defect with a spherical lens composed of:
1/7" − 1/10" = 1/23" = 1/700 mm.

He established undeniably the changes of form that the image received from a luminous point placed at a variable distance from an eye affected with astigmatism; he believed that he recognized for his eye, that the defect had its place in the crystalline lens and that its cause was situated in a position oblique to this organ.

1810. Ten years later, Gerson of Hamburg, in an inaugural dissertation, cited a letter by Fischer, his professor of mathematics; Fischer, without knowing of Young's work, had discovered astigmatism in himself, and by the measurements (of which he had not given the details) had proved that this defect often recognized for its cause an irregularity in the shape of the cornea. From there, Fischer proved that the defect existed to a variable degree in the greater part of humanity. In place of comparing the cornea to an ellipsoid, Gerson likened it to the surface of a torus, which is not simple since the torus is a surface of the fourth degree.

Yet, neither Fischer, nor Gerson thought of correcting astigmatism and in the selections of their work that I was able to obtain, they did not say that the vision of astigmats suffered keenly.

1818. Mr. Cassas, an historical painter, worked in the studio of Mr. Gros during this year. He despaired because his instructor always added horizontal strokes to his drawings: He carefully studied his visual aberrations, and in his travels asked all the opticians and physicians that he met to procure lenses for him that would enable him to see the horizontals. It was only toward 1840 or 1844 that an optician from Rome named Suscipi, cut some lenses that passibly corrected the defect. These lenses, convex spheres on the anterior surface, introduced a concave toric surface to the side of the eye. Much later Cassas, through the Parisian, Soleil, had some glasses made with cylindrical surfaces crossed at a right angle, which corrected very nicely all astigmatic problems he had.

When I saw him in 1865, Cassas had been wearing, for a long time in front of his left eye, a lens formed of a concave cylindrical surface with a horizontal axis of 8 inches from the focus and of a convex spherical surface of 36 inches; in front of the right eye he wore two crossed cylinders at 6 1/2 inches horizontally and 36 inches vertically, both of them concave. Despite my great care, I found it impossible to make a better correction. All I was able to do was to give him some lenses with double focus and to bend the correcting lens of the right eye to about ten degrees on the horizontal. I also prescribed the cylinders to his son who was a myope. His overcorrected 1/24 showed a correctable astigmatism with a concave cylinder 1/18. Note that the father and son were affected by a slight color blindness. If I have overborne a little on the case of Mr. Cassas, it is because he is not mentioned in the literature, although from what follows, one may be unable to assign him a specific date. This case is, except for that of Airy's, the first case to have been corrected usefully by lenses. Like Airy, of whom we are going to speak, Mr. Cassas gives us an example of an astigmatism, the degree of which remained stationary during a long period. The reason apparently was that his defect was congenital and varied little with age.

1827. Airy, director of the observatory at Greenwich, remarked that his left eye was not only myopic but amblyopic. With a certain concave lens he observed a star which appeared to him not round at all, but in the form of a luminous shaft. Then he observed that a cross traced on paper was not clearly visible at any distance for his left eye: in accordance with the distance from the eye where he placed it, if he bent it to 35 degrees, he soon perceived one and then the other of the appendages of the cross. In relaxing his accommodation, a luminous point, placed at 6 inches from the eye, appeared to him like a shaft forming an angle of 35 degrees with the vertical; placed at 3 1/2 inches, the delineated point followed a perpendicular line to the preceding. He then had an astigmatism of about 1/8 and a myopia of 1/6. He corrected the two defects by using a spherical cylindrical lens, made by Fuller at Ipswich. Twenty years later, when he spoke about his astigmatism in front of the 'Cambridge Philosophical Society', he evaluated it at 1/10 and attributed the difference to some error of observation between the amounts.

Airy's case is interesting because the author indicated the first use of cylindrical lenses for correcting the visual defect to which his colleague, Dr. Whewell, proposed to give the name "astigmatism".

1834. Plateau published a report on the asymmetry of the eye.

1847. Hamilton described a case of astigmatism.

1848. Godde, an astigmat himself to a high degree, in one eye at least, described five cases of students or professors from Cambridge. Only one of his own eyes presented the defect, whereas his mother was an astigmat bilaterally. Godde himself posed the fundamental question: Is astigmatism hereditary?

1849. Schnyder, a clergyman, described his own astigmatism. Stokes invented the ingenious lens called a bicylinder, which bears his name.

1852. Young had discovered astigmatism (1801); Airy had been the first to point out that this anomaly hinders vision and employed cylindrical lenses to correct it (1827); other persons cited their observations, usually made on themselves. However, in combining the subjective with the objective, all had neglected to determine whether the abnormality frequently merited being corrected in others and, since Young and Gerson, no one bothered to search for the cause of this anomaly. On July 12, 1852, the brilliant Goulier, professor from Metz, dispatched to the Academy of Sciences a sealed envelope containing a note which had been printed the last year in the report. In the contents of this note it was concluded that Mr. Goulier had been able, by use of cylindrical lenses, to clearly restore vision in a great number of people. For several years, Mr. Goulier had prescribed glasses and examined eyes, and he was preparing to put his findings in a comprehensive paper when he learned that someone had already done so. Mr. Donders, presenting a study difficult to compile for a professor of geodesy, came to reap a rich harvest from a field which Mr. Goulier had worked so hard to clear. To be sure the attainments of Knapp and Donders remained intact, but the hour had come where the discoveries of Young and Airy had spread into common practice.

I must give my thanks to Mr. Goulier for the report he had drawn up as early as 1852 and for the principal conclusions that he had hidden in the sealed envelope of which I have spoken most highly. I am going to borrow different passages from Goulier's work, some of which contain interesting facts and warrant publication here for the first time. I only heard of Goulier's work toward the first of March 1866:

"Doctor Young had pointed out, that there long had been, a certain common visual abnormality, in which rays parting from a luminous point came together in a section of the eye formed by the visual axis, converged in different points following the position of this diametrical plane. Following the steps of this learned man the focus of rays brought together in a plane, passed by the axis of both eyes, would generally be more remote than the rays brought together in a perpendicular plane.

"This remark appears to have surprised the physicians, the physiologists and even the oculists, for among the French works that we have consulted on this question, we have not found any mention of this remarkable fact, and we have even discovered, in the works of the oculist, some references to extraordinary visual phenomena which the authors found unexplainable, and of which the defect appeared to follow a flaw in conformation as pointed out by Doctor Young.

"After several years, without any knowledge of Young's prior studies, we recognized that this defect in the conformation of the eye was very common, but waited to study it, until we found a subject afflicted with it to a marked degree. In a few months we found the subject. The observations we had made on him directed us to restudy this defect with more care, and to correlate the case with the experiences on a great number of subjects. The conclusions of this research are:

"1. That this defect is almost general.

"2. That the defect exists in a great number of people to an extent that is considered more or less serious. It dulls their vision, however no one looked for a way to correct this recognized error.

"3. That one may very often remedy it, as we have already done several times by lenses of a special form, easily applied."

Mr. Goulier explained then, how he measured astigmatism: first, with the help of Young's optometer; second with the help of a screen with a hole placed near the eye which appeared oval; or third, by means of hatchings traced on paper in two rectangular directions which he placed at the 'punctum proximum' and which he sought to make one see in succession with the greatest possible clarity, with the help of suitable spherical lenses. When he employed the first or the third of these operations Mr. Goulier exercised a certain amount of precaution, overlooked by Knapp, to have the subjects keep their glasses on whether they were myopes or presbyopes.

1853. Fliedner established that in distance the greater part of people see horizontals better than verticals. Powell recognized, in himself, a difference in the distance of distinct vision for the verticals and the horizontals. Vallee established a similar difference.

1854. Hays published three cases of astigmatism and their correction by employing cylindrical lenses. Helmholtz described his 'ophthalmometer' on which the use of it is the basis for the greater part of the findings of Donders and Knapp relative to astigmatism.

1855. Wharton Jones and Wilde attributed astigmatism to a defect in the cornea.

1856. A French architect, Trelat, and in the same period, Le Verrier, the director of the Imperial Observatory, corrected their astigmatism in a way similar to Airy, with the help of cylindrical lenses that the optician Soleil provided.

1859. Knapp, equipped with the ophthalmometer of Helmholtz, his professor, sought to determine the shape of the cornea on the living. An observation of Senff (1846) made him ask himself the question whether astigmatism was not due to an irregularity in the shape of the tunic of the eye: He communicated this idea to the oculists reunited in a congress at Heidelberg in September 1859, and when he came back to this subject, in 1861, Donders was able to present the results of some measurements that he had made and in which he found himself in agreement with the oculist of Heidelberg. Since this time, Knapp published a more complete work on the same subject (1862), but he appeared to be a little concerned about prescribing glasses for these errors. In 1861, Helmholtz was again far from suspecting the frequency of pathological astigmatism, and he was very certain of the current work of his student. The work of Knapp appeared in 1862 and demonstrated that irregularities in corneal shape were ordinarily the principal cause of astigmatism. Sine (1864) asked himself if the muscles to the right of the eye were not sometimes the cause of the deformity; this idea had come to him after learning about a verified diminishing of astigmatism with a strabismus patient after an operation. I have heard Doctor Dor cite an analogous case, and I have seen astigmatism diminish in a strabismus patient, by following the treatment that I had made him follow for the cure of his deformity by means of stereoscopic exercises. Be that as it may, this question is under consideration: none of the three cases that I have come to cite were clear enough to persuade the conviction of the observer.

We must come back again to Knapp (1864) for an account on the diagnosis of irregular astigmatism, very interesting but not too practical.

The most important reason that we may have in the discovery of this author, however incontestable may be the attainments of his work, is to have brought forward the question of monochromatic aberration, in making the exact measurements of the cornea with the help of an ophthalmometer.

1862. Some days before Knapp's fine work on physiological and pathological astigmatism, Donders brought out his book, "Astigmatisme en cylindrische Glazen," which was translated the same year in German and French. It is a complete theoretical and practical treatise.

Some of Donders's students, in particular Middelburg, assisted the professor in including some new observations and, in 1864, the 'Society of Sydenham' made a translation in English, after the original manuscripts, and combined them in one fine volume, together with the research of the physiologists of Utrecht on 'the anomalies of refraction and accommodation of the eye'. "It is a work which gives honor," said Mr. Monoyer, "to the illustrious savant who is the object of a similar distinction and to the men instructed who have conceived the idea; it is above all a marked service rendered to science, and it is hopeful that French literature is not delayed in being enriched by the translation of this work."

Mr. Donders's book is going to appear shortly in German: the importance of this work and the facility of obtaining it for oneself, either in English or German, will make it unnecessary for me to present any analysis of it: it is in the hands of all the people that are interested in these things.

1862–1866.

The appearance of Knapp's and Donders's work, in 1862, had been followed by a veritable explosion of little summaries, which had not added a great deal to our understanding. To be mentioned, however, is a work by Schweigger (1863) in which excellent advice is found on the diagnostic objective of astigmatism, reproduced in part in his book on the ophthalmoscope (1864) of which there exists a poor French translation. From a practical point of view, a brochure by Knapp (1865) indicates that his specialist did not prescribe 20 pairs of glasses per year. I think that Donders and his assistance give it more detail. Now the use of exact lenses seems to me destined to spread beyond the walls of Utrecht which really did not take place yet in a serious manner.

Without naming anyone, I may frankly say that the cylindrical glasses which were often shown to me by patients, who consulted other doctors, were frequently very inexact and there is nothing surprising about it. I demonstrated some time ago (1865) how much the present methods used for the choice of glasses are defective. While considering theoretical knowledge I had also shown (1866) how without understanding preliminaries each doctor may, in putting forth a little care, choose the glasses as well as a specialist.

Appendix 5

Listing of Art and Illustrations Demonstrating the Use of Spectacles

[Author's note: the information contained in Appendix 5 is taken from the sources listed on page 463. Any spelling or grammatical errors contained in the text appear as they did in the original sources. Most of the information comes from the early part of the twentieth century, and therefore may not be valid today. However, it is hoped that the reader can use the information contained in Appendix 5 as a starting point for further research.]

Tong-Spectacles
by
H. Weve

1. A 14th. ct. choir book of the monastery St. Marco at Florence shows us some monks at choral singing.

Nail-Spectacles (Riveted Spectacles)
by
Prof. O. Hallauer

1. Tomaso da Modena. Hugo de Provins. Treviso — 1352
2. Initiale d. Bible historiaele. Nat. Libr. at Paris — 1380
3. Konrad von Soest. Panel. Niederwildungen — 1404
4. Ulrich von Richenthal. Chronicle. Prague — 1417
5. Panel in the Cathedral at Saragossa — 1441
6. Sepulchral monument of Otto III. Munster in Konstanz — 1445
7. Venetian woodcut. Circumcision. Nurmberg — 1450
8. Liber Pontific. St. Mariae. utrecht. (v. Pflugk); — abt 1450
9. Pisano Vittore. Album Valardi. Louvre, Paris; — before 1451
10. Pius Joachim. Museum in Basel — 1460
11. Hans Multscher. Death of St. Mary. Karlsruhe; — after 1460
12. Friedr. Herlin. St. Peter in spectacles. Rothenburg. — (prob.)? 1466
13. Friedr. Herlin. High priest in spectacles. (prob.)? 1466
14. Friedr. Herlin. Jesus in the temple. Nordlingen; — abt 1470
15. Copper-plate with Prophet. Univ. Libr. Munchen. (Munich) — 1461
16. Master E.S. Buchstabe. N. Kupf. St. K. Munich — 1466
17. Martin Schongauer. Death of St. Mary. K. St. K. Basel — 1469–71
18. Anonymous. Woodcut. "Pythagoras". Lubeck — 1475
19. Michael Pacher. Four Evangelists. St. Wolfgang — 1477–81
20. Niccolo Alunno. St. Hieronymus. Corsini. Rome; — abt 1480

21. Schilling Spietz. Chronicle-writer. Univ. Libr. Bern 1484
22. Gil de Silve. Self-portrait. Miraflores Burgos 1486–96
23. Glass pane with nail-spectacles, in the collection of v. Pflugk 1480–90
24. Danse macabre, from Mainz. K. St.K. Berlin 1491
25. Schedel's World-chronicle. "Rasis the Doctor 1492
26. Mns. Univ. Libr. Heidelberg. Trainband-captain 1496
27. Brunschwig. Surgery. Medical advice 1497
28. Lazarus-tapestry. Hist. Mus. at Basel; abt 1500
29. Berh. Striegel. St. Servatius. Germ. Mus. Nurmberg; abt 1500
30. Hans Holbein. Sr. Death of St. Mary. Basel Museum; abt 1510
31. Majolica by San Sebastiano. Venice 1510
32. Tyrolese painter. Patriarch. Kaiser Friedr. Mus. Berlin 1510
33. Thomas Murner. Strassburg. Guild of the knaves 1512
34. "Quartet of singers." Collection Hallauer; abt 1515
35. Woodcut representing Pope Leo X. wearing spectacles 1519
36. Hermann Thom. Ring. "Virgil." Augsburg 1530
37. Nail-spectacles. Ornament from Palace of Canossa in Verona; abt . 1570
38. Nail-spectacles from the castle of Ambras. Mus. of the Hist. of Art, Vienna, abt 1570
39. Carlo Crivelli. Berh. v. Sienna. Nail-spectacle case on girdle . 1477
39a. Nail-spectacle case, epoch Henry IV. in leather (Mc.Heymann).
39b. Nail-spectacle case of wood; carved. (Me. Heymann).
40. Later forms of nail-spectacles. Link-spectacles, besicles brisees.
40a. Link-spectacles with case belonging to them. Mus. of. Hist. of Art Vienna 1570–80
40b. Link-spectacles with case belonging to them Rosenborg, Copenhagen 1597
40c. Link-spectacles with case belonging to them (Priv. Poss. of v. Pflugk) abt. 1750–1800

Group A. Fancy-Spectacles (esp. in Spain)

1. El Greco Theostocopuli, Cardinal Nino de Guevara (1596–1598). Collection Havemeyer, New-York.
2. El Greco Theostocopuli, Cardinal Nino de Guevara, bust (1595–1598). Coll. Nemes, Buda-Pest.
3. Pacheco (Francisco), El Padre Luis del Alcacar (1599). Libro de Description de verdaderos Retratas de Illustres y Memorables Varones.
4. Pacheco (Francisco), El Frai Pedro de Valderrame (1599). Libro de Description de verdaderos Retratas de Illustres y Memorables Varones.
5. Pacheco (Francisco), Baltazar del Aliasar (1599). Libro de Description de verdaderos Retratas de Illustres y Memorables Varones. Facsimile-edition in the national picture gallery Amsterdam.
6. Verasquez, The Poet Franc. Gomez de Quevedo, about (1628).
7. Murillo, Portrait of a Spaniard (abt. 1660). Coll. Benedict Berlin.
8. P. Simon the elder after P. Ronche, Portrait of Ant. P. Alvarez. Orosio d'Avila Astorga. Vice-king of Naples (17th ct.)
9. Clement Ammon, Portrait of Hier. Capivacceus Nobus Patavinus (Medical Prof) (1652). Bibliotheca Chalcographia. Frankfort 1652.
10. Jerome David (signing himself H. David. F.), Engraving of Hier. Capivacceus (before 1670).
11. Spanish School, Portrait of the Marquess d'Altamura (16th ct.) Pinakothek at Parma.
12. B.E.Murillo, Santa Isabel de Hungria currando un tinoso (1618–82). Prado, Madrid.
13. B.E.Murillo, The foundation of Sa. Maria Maggiore. The Patrician John before the Pope. Abt. 1665. Prado, Madrid.
14. Zurbaran (Francisco), Spanish School, S. Pedro Nolasquez.
15. Jacques Callot, Les 26 Martyrs du Japon (1597). Engraving by Israel Sylvestre, edited 1621–1691.

Group B. Spectacles for Mountebanks and Quacks

1. H. Curti after C.M.H. Mitelli, The Theriac-trader (17th ct.). Reprod. in Peters: Der Arzt und die Heilkunde. id. in Bock: Die Brille und ihre Geschichte.
2. A. van der Venne, Engraving, The Seller of rat-traps (17th ct.). Atlas van Stolk, Rotterdam.

Group C. Protective Spectacles

1. Paulus Furst after J. Columbia, The Plague-doctor (1656).
2. John van der Straat (Stradanus). Engraving, Coral-Fishing (16th ct.) Collection Dr. Bierens de Haan, Amsterdam.

Group D. Spectacles as Emblems

1. Ehrhard Schoen, "Die Klage des Unschuldigen Niemand" (1500–1550). Statsbibliothek, Munchen.
2. Anonymous, "Nobody is my name" (16th ct.). Coll. Weve, Utrecht.
3. Breughel the elder, Every one looks for his profit (16th. ct.) Rijksprentenkabinet, Amsterdam.
4. Master E.S. Monk in Letter N of the Alphabet (before 1466). Rijksprentenkabinet, Amsterdam.
5. P. Breughel the younger, Tyl Uilenspiegel. Black-and-white drawing. Reprod. Cat. verz. Klinkosc. 1889.

Group E. Spectacles in Masquerades and with Jesters

1. J. de Cheyn, Masquerade group with woman in spectacles (17th ct.). Rijksprentenkabinet, Amsterdam.
2. De Wael, Masquerade group with woman in spectacles (end of the 17th ct.). Rijksprentenkabinet, Amsterdam.
3. Anonymous, Dutch School, Twelfth Night Festival. Masquerades with imitation of spectacles round the eye-sockets (17th ct.) Central Museum, Utrecht.
4. P.B., Dutch School, Copper-plate (1642). Coll. Dr. Bierens de Haan, Amsterdam.
5. Anonymous (German School), "Hans Hinderfur" Wood-cut (17th ct.). Kupferstichkabinet, Berlin.

Group F. Spectacles for Seeing Sharply at a Distance

6. Anonymous, Italian School, The miracle of Drusiana, Fresco (2nd half 14th ct.). Church of S. Augustinus st. Rimini (Described by A. Tossi).
7. Anonymous, French School, Miniature from manuscript Galeni opera varia lat. interprete Nico de Regio (Middle 15th ct.). M.S.Db. 92 of the Sachische Landesbibliothek. Described by A. von Pflugk.
8. Anonymous German, Wood-cut from "Chirurgie von Braunsweich" (1497 and 1537). Coll. Dr. De Lint, The Hague. Occurs also in Pracelsus.
9. La Hire (Laurent de), Pope Nic. V in the crypt of St. Franciscus (1st half 17th ct.). Louvre, Paris.
10. Rubens P.P., Jesus with Simon the Pharisee (1615–20). Ermitage Leningrad.
11. Octave van Veen, Jesus with Simon the Pharisee (Before 1629). l'Eglise de Bergue-Saint-Winnoc.
12. Lucas Granach the elder, The Adulterous woman (abt. 1540). Alte Pinakothek, Munchen.
13. Bonifacio Veroneses, The Adulterous woman (before 1540). "Brera" Milan.
14. Corn. de Baellieur, Antwerp, The Adulterous woman (middle 7th ct.). Gemalde-Galerie, Brunswick.
15. Frans Franken, Antwerp, Christ, 12 years old in the Temple (first half 17th ct.). Cathedral, Antwerp.
16. Jacob Jordaens, Antwerp, Christ, 12 years old in the Temple (middle 17th ct.). Alte Pinakothek, Munich.
17. Jan Steen, Leiden, Christ, 12 years old in the Temple (middle 17th ct.). Museum Bazel.

Group G. Spectacles for Myopes

1. Hier. Bosch (Dutch), Juggler on the market (Le Charlatan) (abt. 1480). Museum St. Germain en Laye.
2. Hier. Bosch (Dutch), Juggler on the market (Le Charlatan) (after 1480). Galeria Crespi Milan.
3. Rafael Santi, Portrait Leo X with concave glass 1516–1520. Palazzo Pitti Florense.
4. Anonymous (Bazel), Wood-cut Leo X in Spectacles 1519. Reprod. in Hallauer Festschrift, 50 Jahr. Bestehen der Augenkl. zu Basel 1915.
5. School of Titian, Christ and the tribute-money (2nd half SVI ct.). National Gallery, London.
6. Jan Corn. Vermeyen (N. Niederl.), The raising of Lazarus (Triptique des Micault) (1st half XVI ct.). Museum Brussels.
7. John of Calcar, Title-page of Vesalius: "De humani corporis fabrica". Wearer of Spectacles as well as myope with handle-monocle (1543). Univ. Lebr. Amsterdam.
8. Wandelaar, Copper-plate after above-mentioned wood-cut (1672). Vesalius Editions by Boerhave and Albinus.
9. Pieter Breughel the elder, The Adoration of The Mages (1564). Nat. Gallery, London.
10. Collaert after van der Straet, Street with spectacle-shop. Old man with monocle with handle (2nd half XVI ct.). Reprod. a.o. by Bock.
11. Van der Straet, Black-and-white drawing, Wearer of spectacles and figure with monocle with handle (2nd half XVI ct.). Museum Boymans, Rotterdam.

12. Hendrik Goltzius after Dirk Barentsz., Venetian evening-party. Engraving after drawing (drawing before 1560). (Reprod. in Hendrick Goltzius von Otto Hirschmann in meister der Graphik Bd. 7).
13. Cl. J. van der Heck, Otanes before King Chambyses (1620), Sted. Museum, Alkmaar.
14. Jordaens, Christ before Pilate (Middle XVII ct). Drawing Museum Boymans, Rotterdam.
15. Cornelus van Kittensteum after Dirk Hals, "The Sight" (abt 1630). Reprod. Vol. II. "Amsterdam in the XIIth ct."
16. Is. van Ostade, Man's portrait (1681). Museum Boymans, Rotterdam.
17. A. van der Venne, Fishing for Souls (1st half of the 17th ct.). Rijks-museum, Amsterdam.

The Spectacles with a Round Bridge
by
Prof. H.J.M. Weve

1. Italian Anonymous. Miracle of Drusiana. Fresco (End 14th. ct.). (Church of St. Augustin at Rimini).
2. Anonymous. Watermark, Palermo 1392, Les filigranes 1907. Repr. by C.M. Briquet.
3. Jan v. Eyck, Madonna with Saints and donor-Joris van der Paele 1436. Museum Bruges Replica: Museum Antwerp (Musee des beaux arts).
4. Flemish Anonymous, School of Prevost. Wing of a triptych. Founder with patron saints. Panel-picture (abt. 1440). Museum Bruges.
5. Anonymous, Circle of the master of Flemaille. Ecole d'Artois? St. Gregorius (abt. 1451). Private poss. in Paris (M. Martin le Roy). Repr. Henri Bouchot: "L'exposition des primitifs Francais".
6. Anonymous, French or Flemish? Tapestry: Bishop accepting gifts (15th. cent.) Repr. without further explanation in Mme. Heymann: "Lunettes et Lorgnettes de Jadis".
7. Anonymous. Gothic Tapestry (15th. ct.). Assueres et les juifs. Musee de Nancy Repr. La Prese med. Aug. 1928.
8. Anonymous Flemish, Portrait of a man (15th. ct.). Museum Straszburg.
9. Geertgen tot St. Jans. Holy Family St. Ann with spectacles. Panel-picture 1470. Rijksmuseum Amsterdam.
10. Masters of the Swabian School, Deat hof Mary from Dinkelsbuhl (abt. 1490). Germanisches Museum, Nurnberg.
11. Israel v. Meckenen, The Evangelist Mattheus (Etching) (abt. 1490). Museum Boymans, Rotterdam.
12. Cologne Master of the Holy Fmaily, Antwerp infl. Vision with founder (1492). Nat. Mus. Nurnberg.
13. Anon. painter of Frankfort, probably Antwerp artist. Death of Mary from the Dominican Church of Frankfort (1492). Hist. Mus. Frankfort.
14. Flemish Anon. Vision of St. Bernard (15th. ct.). Museum Bruges.
15. School of J. v. Oostzanen, Dispute of St. Catherine, Embroidery (1520). Rijksmuseum Amsterdam.
16. North Netherland, Anon. Portrait of Jacob van Driebergen (1512). Central Museum Utrecht.
17. Engelbrechtsen or Jacob v. Oostzanen. Spectacle-shop (painted) (beginning 16th. ct.). Private poss. (Formerly Coll. Freund, Berlin).
18. Anon. Flemish or North Netherl., Wood-cut (abt. 1510). from the book: "Der vrouwen Nature ende complexie". Libr.: Nederl. Maatschappij ter Bevordering der Geneeskunst.
19. Hieron. Bosch, Christ expels the traders from the temple (abt. 1500). Coll. Claude Philipps Londen reprod. Paul Lafond. H. Bosch 1914.
20. Quinten Metsys Portrait of Etienne Gardiner, Lord Chancellor of England (abt. 1525). Furstl. Lichtenstein-Galerie.
21. Quinten Metsys, Portrait of a man (1525). Frankfurt a.M. Stadelsches Institut.
22. Hieron. Bosch, Evangelist John on Patmos (abt. 1500). K. Friedr. Mus. Berlin.
23. Hier. Bosch, Concert (Allegory) (end 15th. ct.). Coll. Pontalba. Senlis Reprod. Paul Lafond.
24. Jan Mostaert, Haarlem, St. Hieronymus (before 1550). Coll. Hermsen: The Hague.
25. Joos van Cleve or van Beke, Antwerp, St. Hieronymus (before 1540). Formerly Coll. Rich. von Kaufmann.
26. Adr. Isenbrandt, St. Hieronymus (before 1530). Exposition de la Toison d'or 1907, Bruges, nr. 214.

27. Hemessen, St. Hieronymus, A series of pictures reprod. Hier. partly as a scholar with skull, book and spectacles, partly as penitent with stones and bare chest; they are partly ascribed to Jan Metsys, v. Reymerswall, a.o. Painters of the Antwerp School.

28. Lucas van Leyden, Picture Evangelist Marcus (before 1518). Museum Antwerp.

29. Lucas v. Leyden, Etching, Evangelist Marcus (Meister der Graphik. Vol. XIII. M.J. Friedlander).

30. Simon Bening, Bruges, Les heures de Notre Dame dites de Hennesy, St. Marcus (before 1530). Also in a livre d'heures in Munchen. Repr. in Les Heures de Notre Dame par Jos. Destree.

31. Maarten van Heemskerk (Haarlem), The Evangelist St. Lucas (1532). Frans Halsmuseum Haarlem.

32. Van der Pas after Lucas v. Leyden, St. Lucas (before 1530). Reprod. Etching. Rijksprentenkabinet, Amsterdam.

33. Joos van Cleve or van Beke, Holy Family, Joseph with spectacles (before 1540). Nat. Gallery London 2603 and Coll. Salting London.

34. Flemisch Anon., Joseph with Spectacles (beg. 16th. ct.). Kon. Museum Antwerp.

35. Flemish Anon., Joseph with Spectacles (beg. 16th. ct.). Coll. Spiridon. Reprod. Ludwig Baldass Joos van Cleve.

36. Flemish Anon., Joseph with spectacles (beg. 16th. ct.). Wallraf Mus. Cologne. (Nr. 428 Ct. 1915).

37. Van Orley, Holy Family: Joseph with spectacles (before 1540). Galerie Sigmaringen.

38. Maitre du St. Sang (Bruges), master of the chapel of the Holy Blood Holy Family: Joseph (abt. 1520). Kunsthalle Hamburg (Formerly Coll. Chillingworth ((auction Lucern 1922).

39. Abraham Benson (school of), Death of Mary (abt. 1515). Conn. with the two following pictures. (formerly Coll. Smallenburg).

40. Hugo van der Goes (attributed to), Death of Mary (abt. 1480). K. Friedr. Museum Berlin.

41. Hugo v. d. Goes (attributed to), Death of Mary (abt. 1480). Nat. Gallery London Nr. 658.

42. Swabian-Tyrolese Anonymous, Death of Mary, Altar-wing (abt. 1500). Auction Heberle, 16 Nov. 1909.

43. Joos van Beke (v. Cleve) or Master of the Death of Mary (Antwerp), Death of Mary (before 1530). Wallraf Museum Cologne.

France

44. Anonymous, Wood-cut from "Ordonnances 1510", Scholar in the Library (1510). Reprod. without further explan. by Mme Heymann.

Spain

45. Anonymous, Retable de St. Martin, Head-altar of the Church of Medina del Campo (1520). Reprod. Coll. Dr. Simon Barcelona.

46. Anonymous, Spanish or Catalan, St. Paul Altar picture (beg. 16th. ct.). Musee de Cluny, Paris (in Bourgeois and in Catalogue of the museum wrongly mentioned as French 15th. ct. Prob. the spectacles with round bridge were painted here wrongly when being renewed).

German-speaking Countries

47. Cologne Master of the St. Bartholomew Altar, St. Peter (abt. 1500). Nat. Gallery London.

48. Anonymous, wood-cut on the title-page of the "Augenspiegel" by Dr. Joh. Reuchlin (1511). Repr. in Hallauer. Memorial Vol. Bas. Augenklinik. Orig. Coll. v. Pflugk, Dresden.

49. Hans Holbein the elder, Painted table-leaf (1515). (Repr. Hallauer).

50. Hans Holbein the younger Portrait of Thomas Morus(?) (before 1543). "te vitanda" (Eobanus Hessus?)

51. Anonymous, Title-page wood-cut of "De generibus ebriosorum et ebrietate vitanda Eobanus Hessus?

52. Anonymous, Goldsmit at work, wood-cut (1523). Repr. in Hallauer.

53. Anonymous, Discussion of physicians, Painted window (1524). (National Museum Zurich). (Reprod. in Hallauer). (Poss. of Prof. B. Rhan in Zurich).

54. Edward Schoen, Wood-cut, The complaint of the innocent, No one (abt. 1530). Statsbibl. Munchen. Reprod. Geisberg: Der Deutsche Einblatt Holzschnitt. in der 1st. Halfte des 16. Jahrh. II. 31.

55. Hans Fried. v. Freiburg, Picture, Jesus 12 years old in the temple (1512). Art. Coll. Basel, also mentioned in Prausnitz p. 32.
56. Anon. wood-cut, A. Durer's influence "The book-jester" from Sebastian-Brandt's "Narrenschrift" (1494). Hallauer p. 132. (Die Brille 100 Jahre vor und 100 Jahre nach der Erfindung der Buchdruckerkunst).

Leather Spectacles
by
Prof. von Pflugk

1. Oldest pair of leather spectacles, from before 1500. Germanic Nat. Museum; Nurnberg.
2. Spectacles from the Carthusian monastery at Nurnberg. Abt. 1500. Collection v. Pflugk. Dresden.
3. Monocle. After 1500. Germ. Nat. Mus. Nurnberg.
4. Three pairs of the so-called "Pirckheimer Spectacles". Abt. 1520. Wartburg. (Thuringia).
5. Two pairs of spectacles, one of them in an iron case. Abt. 1520. Bavarian Nat. Museum. Munich.
6. Pair of spectacles from before 1547. Collection v. Pflugk. Dresden.
7. Spectacles of Gustav Adolf, from before 1632. University Art-collection. Upsala.
8. Reading couple with monocle. (Oil-painting). Abt. 1650. Coll. v. Pflugk. Dresden.
9. Leather-spectacles with steel bow. (English make?). Abt. 1750. Coll. Zeiss. Jena.
10. Leather-spectacles with steel bow. (Enbl. or Spanish make). Abt. 1750. Coll. v. Pflugk. Dresden.
11. Together with these old Chinese leather-spectacles. Coll. Hallauer. Basel. Place and time or origin unknown.

Spina-Frontalis Spectacles, Super-Orbital, Arch-, Bonnet-, and Wire Spectacles
by
Prof. Dr. H.J. M. Weve

A. Spina-Frontalis Spectacles (Stirnstangenbrille)

1. Claes Jansz. van der Heck, Picture: Otanes before King Cambyses (1620). Sted. Mus. Alkmaar.
2. Rembrandt, Woman reading, Etching (abt. 1650). National Gallery of Prints, Amsterdam.
3. Anonymous copyist of Rembrandt, Woman reading. Etching (?). Hans Singer: "Rembrandts Samtliche Radierungen".
4. Nic. Maes, Studies of a woman's head, drawing (abt. 1650). Brit. Mus. London.
5. Anonymous, Un trio convaincu. Aquarel (18th. ct. French.). Reprod. Mme. Heymann: "Lunettes et Lorgnettes de jadis."
6. Greeff, Repred. silver specimen (18th. ct.). Rijksmusssseum, Amsterdam. Reprod. Greeff Kl. Monbl. f. Aug. 1913.
7. P. Minguet, Reprod. Specimen (abt. 1763). Reprod. Von Rohr: "Geschichte der Brille.

B. Super-Orbital Arch Spectacles (Stirnreifenbrillen)

1. Dudley Adams, Reprod. in letter patent (abt. 1797). Reprod. a.o. In Von Rohr: "Geschichte der Brille."
2. Anna Dorothea Therbusch nee Lissenzka (1722–1782). Kaiser Friedrich-Museum, Berline.
3. Grenier, La loge rotie (abt. 1800). Reprod. Mme. Heymann:"Lunettes at lorgnettes de jadis."

C. Bonnet-Spectacles

1. Anonymous, Title-page Codex, Pal. Germ. 126 Drawing (1496). Heidelberger Univ. Libr. (treated by Von Pflugk).
2. Hans Holbein the elder, Martyrdom of Sta Bartolomaus. Picture (abt. 1503).
3. Hieronymus Bosch and Jerome Cock, St. Martin in a Bark Engraving (abt. 1500). Reprod. in Paul Lafond.
4. School of Durer, Christ, 12 years old in the Temple (1505). Dresden, Gemaldegallerie.

Pinching-, Clasping-, or Spring-Spectacles
by
Prof. Greeff

1. Spectacles from the work of Cornelius Meyer: Degli occhiali, anno 1689. 4. A. Cushion-spectacle.
2. Lamellar spectacles. (from the collection of Greeff).
3. Pinching spectacles with a copper plate inserted by way of link. (from the collection of Greeff).
4. Pinching spectacles from a length of leonic wire. Nurmberg. (from the collection of Greeff).
5. Bow-spectacles and pinching-spectacles. From the Regensburg guild of spectacle-makers. About 1600.

6. Pinching spectacles from the Regensburg guild of spectacles-makers.
7. Jacob Adriaensz. Backer. (1608–1651) (Amsterdam). Portrait of an old lady with a pair of pinching-spectacles in her hand. Kaiser-Friedrich-museum in Berlin.
8. J. A. Backer, Portrait of an old gentleman with Nuremberg pinching-spectacles and case belonging to them.

Cable Spectacles, Temple Spectacles, Real Spectacles
by
Prof. Greeff

1. Temple-spectacles from the collection Greeff.
2. Anton Greeff (1736–1813). The painter Chodowiecki in temple-specacles. Picture-gallery, Dresden.
3. Silver-temple-spectacles with broad plate at the end. (After E. Pergens abt. 1780–90).
4. Temple-spectacles with double joint hinges and broad plate at the end. (After E. Pergens).
5. Old English temple spectacles of 1728. The broad plates at the end are formed by spiral winding; of English model.
6. Temple-spectacles with broad plates at the end. Here after P. Minguet, abt. 1763 (v. Rohr).
7. Three old Nurmberg spectacles with gilded brass mounting. (Greeff).
8. Old ear-spectacles (Coll. Greeff).
  a. simple temples b. double temples directed inward c. double temples directed downward d. telescope spectacles.
9. J.H. Jeldershuis 62 years old with spectacles with double temples with end-plates, model according to Smith; abt. 1791. Spectacle-bridge with double hinges. (v. Rohr).
10. The first rimless spectacles, model Waldstein in Vienna.
11. The painter Chardin of Paris with spectacles with large round lenses; self-portrait. 1775.
12. A Myopic presbyope.

Scissor-Spectacles
by
Prof. von Pflugk

1. Page No. 5 of the statutes of the Regenburg Spectacle-makers. About 1550. Germanisches National Museum. Nuremberg.
2. 3. Scissor-spectacles mounted in horn with old facet lenses, abt. 1750.
4. Scissor-spectacles mounted in brass. abt. 1750.
5. Scissor-spectacles mounted in brass, gilded with beautiful lacquer painting. Abt. 1800.
6. Ordinary scissor spectacle spectacles mounted in horn. About 1800.
7. "Push Pin", caricature by James Gillray. 1797.
8. Boulevard de Gand: Caricature by Isabey. 1798.
9. Monocle abt. 1810 with silver mounting and mother-of-pearl case (Danish private property).
10. 11. 12. Eye-glasses with mountings of various metals, after 1800.
13. Eye-glasses with fixed handle and old facet glasses, abt. 1800.
14. Eye-glasses (Coll. Werner) Dresden, abt. 1840.
15. Eye-glasses, mounted with silver, coll. von Pflugk.
16. 17. 18. Eye-glasses which can be shoved into a horn case.
19. Caricature by Opitz, Leipzig. Abt. 1820.
20. "L'Original", caricature after Carle Vernet, abt. 1798.
21. Old bronze specimen with traces of the old gilding. Abt. 1790.
22. From the coll. Zeiss. Jena. Abt. 1800.
23.–28. From the Collection v. Pflugk, Dresden.

Lenses for Seeing at a Distance with Covers

30. Old glass of the period of about 1600. Germanisches National Museum, Nuremberg.
31. "Lunettes simples montees en corne ou ecaille. a. La Lunette; b. L'etui." After Diderot et D'Alembert. Encyclopedie (1761–63).
32. "... don una convessa, para los que son cortos de vista". From the winning number of the Pablo Minguet. Madrid 1763.
33. Lenses for seeing at a distance, from the property of King Frederik of Prussia (1740–1786). Hohenzollern Mus. Berlin.
34. Similar lenses from the last years of the 18th. ct. Coll. v. Pflugk.
35. English caricature by Brandin after the engraving by Grignion.

36. The optical contrast. English caricature. London 1772.
37. German foldable lenses from the middle of the 18th. ct. Nuremberg workmanship?
38. 39. German foldable lenses from abt. 1780–1800.
40. English? foldable lens of abt. 1820.
41. The monocle of the painter Anna Dorothea Therbusch from the years 1760–1765 after the self-portrait of the artist. Portrait at the Grand-Ducal Museum at Weimar.

The Monocle as a Help for Taking Aim

42. The monocle used by Frederick II of Denmark, placed on the rifle as a help for taking aim. 1585. Rosenborg Museum near Kopenhagen.
43. Lenses for the above purpose from 1500, depicted in the Statutes of the Regenburg spectacle-makers (original size of the page). Germanisches National Museum.
44. Lenses helping to take aim to be placed on the rifle, abt. 1600. From the electoral Saxon property, Dresden, Coll. v. Pflugk.

The Monocle Pinched in the Contractor of the Eye

45. French caricature by Gavarni, abt. 1821.
46. English caricature after Charles Hunt, abt. 1825.
47. 48. "Les Lunettes" and "les amateurs de tableaux". French caricature by Boilly, abt. 1821.

The Monocular Spectacles by Prof. von Pflugk

1. Cardinal Nicolas of Rouen, 1352, Treviso, St. Nicolo. To this belonging the Fresco of Tommaso di Modena and the reconstruction of v. Rohr.
2. Pope Leo X, by Raffael 519, Florence, Palazzo Pitti. Photo of original size.
3. Part of the frontispiece of Vesalius; De corporis humani fabrica. 1543. Basel.
4. Part of the wood-cut; Johannes Mandlin, 1577, Tubingen.
5. Part of the: Sale of spectacles in Italy, copper-plate by Collaert, after the drawing of John Stradanus, 1580.
6. Spectacles for presbyopics from the picture by Andries Both, before 1650, after the etch by Peter Schenk.
7. Spectacles from Cornelius Meyer Nuovi Ritrovamenti. Romae 1689–1696.
8. Etch after the drawing by Piazetta, about 1750. Copper-plate gallery, Dresden.
9. Spectacles for Myopics from the Picture "La Vue" by Gabriel Spizer, about 1750, after the contemporary etch by I.J. Haid, Augsburg.
10. Neuremberg Glass for Myopics, by "Frierich Schroder", about 1760.
11. Glass for Myopics mounted with horn from the period of about 1780.
12. 13. 14. 15. 16. 17. Glasses for Myopics to be worn round the neck, about 1800.
18. Bronze medal, referring to the death of Sir Ralph Abercrombie—28 March 1801.
19. Costume Parisien, 1810.
20. French 21, German caricature, about 1810.
22. Reading man. Picture of about 1650. Collection v. Pflugk.
23. Reading couple with monocle in leather mounting. Picture about 1650. Collection v. Pflugk; belonging to this the monocle in original size and the corresponding specimen from the Germanische National Museum at Neurenberg.
24. Reading glass, marked: "Schwartz wonhafft in Furth 1749".
25. 26. 27. The customary reading glasses of the last years of the 18th. century.
28. Reading glasses, French workmanship, about 1800.
29. Reading glass, German. workmanship of the same period.

East-Asiatic Spectacles by Prof. Greeff

1. 2. Old Indian show-spectacles with pagodas and elephants, cut of red fragrant sandalwood. (Coll. Greeff).
3. Korean, foldable string-spectacles with prop-plate on the root of the nose. With case belonging to it. (Coll. Greeff).
4. Chinese string spectacles with 2 eyes, without bridge-plate. The bridge is foldable in the middle: folding-spectacles. (Coll.Greeff)
5. Chinese spectacles with weights. These spectacles are held on to the ear by weights.

6. Japanese string-spectacles with one eye and a prop-plate. With case belonging to it. (Coll. v. Pflugk).
7. Japanese string-spectacles with 2 eyes and a prop-plate. Folding spectacles with case belonging to it. (Coll. v. Pflugk).
8. Japanese string-spectacles with long prop-plate for forehand and nose. Foldable. Case belonging to it. (Coll. v. Pflugk).
9. Japanese spectacles with temples. Case is attached to the belt with ribbons. (Coll. v. Pflugk).
10. Old-Chinese temple-spectacles. Glass planparallel of smoky topaz (tea-stone). Case made of black lacquer with gold writing. (Coll. Greeff).
11. Chinese rimless spectacles with case. (Coll. v. Pflugk).
12. Chinese rimless spectacles with case. (Coll. v. Pflugk).
13. After a drawing by the Japanese painter Hokuzai (1760–1849). A monster with 3 eyes is tried on spectacles with 3 lenses.
14–20. Seven reproductions after coloured wood-cuts but the Japanese painter K. Utamaro (1754–1806) from his series: "The education of the children through the spectacles of the parents." (After the Originals in the Coll. v. Pflugk).
21. After a coloured wood-cut by Utamaro. Man with two girls reading in a written scroll.
22. Wereschtschagin (Russian painter): Toengoezin with string-spectacles with 2 eyes and a prop-plate before the forehead.
23. Davis: A Chinaman with spectacles with weights.
24. Ferrario: Chinaman with string-spectacles.

Spectacles for Seeing at a Distance
by
Prof. H. Weve

a. Show- or fancy-spectacles (Renomierbrillen) as wore by the Spaniards.
b. Spectacles to draw the attention as worn by the quacks and mountebanks.
c. Protective spectacles mostly made of coloured glass widely spread till in the 18th. ct. so that the cases were calculated to keep two pair of spectacles. We here also mention the protective glasses used by the divers when fishing up red coral. (Pozuola 16th. ct.)
d. Not seldom spectacles were represented as the emblem of learning or of defective eyesight e.g. with priests and with the "Nemo" figure. (The devil).
e. With masquerades the spectacles served as a laughter-moving means at the same time making people unrecognizable. Also jesters often wore spectacles often even making part of their attire.
f. Spectacles serving an optical purpose but probably not serving for correction of myopes.
g. Spectacles for myopes.

Spectacles for Seeing Near at Hand
Anachronisms
by
Prof. H.J.M. Weve

The anachronisms may be divided into the following groups:
1. Prophets, Aposteles and Patriarchs
2. Death of Mary
3. Circumcision and Instruction in the Temple
4. Christ in the Temple at the Age of Twelve
5. St. Joseph and the other members of the Holy Family
6. Christ and the Tribute-Money
7. Christ and the Adulterous Woman
8. Vocation of St. Matthew
9. Healing of Tobias
10. Adoration of the Magi. (l'Adoration des Mages)
11. Descent of the Holy Ghost. (Whitsuntide)
12. Christ Chasing the Merchants from the Temple
13. Christ before Pilate and Ecce Homo
14. Other representations

Spectacles for Women
1. Apostles, Prophets and Patriarchs

1. Hermann tom Ring, "Virgilius" in nail-spectacles (abt. 1550). Gallerie Augsburg. Cf. Copy Hollander: Die Medizin in der Klass. Malerei 1923. Pict. 147. Prophet called "Virgil". Also repr. in Deutsch. Opt. Wochenschrift, Jan. 1927. Further at Prausnitz's.
2. Riberia ditto Spagnoletto, Moses und Aaron (1588–1652). Galeria Corsini at Firenze. (Florence). Copy, Kunsthist. inst. Utrecht 3183.

3. Bernard Striegel, St. Servatius (1461–1528). Swabian School. Germ. Mus. Nuremberg. No. 888. Copy Prausnitz and Greeff.
4. Master of the St. Bartholomew-alter, Cologne School, St. Peter (1490–1515). Nat. Gall. Also repr. at Prausnitz. Under influence of M. Schongauer and the Dutch masters.
5. Simon Bening, Les Heures de Notre Dame. (Hours of Our Lady) (early 16th. cent.). Dites de Hennesy originates from first-class studio at Bruges, probably of Simon Bening's. 1530. Sint Markus. In the breviary of Munich same copy by same hand.
6. Friedrich Herlin, St. Peter in spectacles (1466). Altar St. Jacobs-church at Rothenburg. Influence of Dutch masters. Pupil of Rogier van der Brugge, 1400–1480. Copy at Prausnitz.
7. Maerten van Heemskerck. Haarlem School, Pupil of v. Scorel, St. Luke painting the Virgin. (1532). Frans Hals Mus. at Haarlem.
8. Lukas van Leyden (1494–1533), The Evangelist St. Mark (1518). Copy cf. Meister der Graphik. Vol. XIII, Lukas van Leyden by M.J. Friedlander.
9. Lucas van Leyden, The Apostle Mark. Coll. Barbier. Sale Brussels Juni 1912 (sale of 4 apostles framel together. Probably this is a copy (with small variations) of a painting in the Antwerp Mus.).
10. Rembrandt, St. Peter in prison. Paris. Ch. Sedelmeyer. Copy Rembr. wiedergefundene Gemalde, 1910–20. W.R. Valentiner. 1921.
11. Spanish School? St. Paul (16th. cent.). Nat. Gallery, London.
12. Henri Goltzius, See St. Paul (16th. cent.). Engraving repr. in book Mrs. Heymann; written underneath: Henri Goltzius. This is certainly incorrect; probably engraving N. de Clerc, Delft. 1614–1625, publisher and engraver. After painting of Spanish? anonymous, now in Nat. Gall. London.
13. Anonymous, Apostle Paul in spectacles (1380). Miniature. Man. Bibl. Nat. at Paris. Repred. by Heymann (the oldest representation of spectacles but one). Lettre ornee (Historia) of the "Bible historiale". Bibliotheque Richelieu. Manuscrit francais No. 7. 1380.
14. Joh. Schensperger (1497). Liber Cronicarum, Augsburg. Aartsbissch. Museum Utrecht. Nr. 53. Jacob Julius Africanus a. others.
15. Sorobabel, Jacog (1492). Incunabulum. Schedels Weltchronik. Copy at Hallauer's. Also in Liber Cronicarum 1493, Nurnberg, as Sorobabel. Further in Nurnberg. Cron. 1495 as Jacob. (Cf. pict. 9 Bourgeois 1923).
16. Anonymous, St. James (15th. cent.). Wood-cut on ceiling of Reception-room of Academia. (R. Galeria di belle arti), in Venice.
17. Jorg Syrlin from Constanz (or Heinrich Yselin3. Bust, Evangelist St. Luke (1480). One of the 12 apostle-busts cut in oak on choir-stalls in the former Benedictine Abbey of Weingarten in Wurtemberg. Swabian School. Now in Nat. Mus. at Munich, Copy at Prausnitz's.
18.—
19. Van der Pas, Engraving of St. Luke after a drawing by Lucas van Leyden. Rijksprentenkabinet.
20. L. Geyn, Engraving St. Luke (inv. et exc.). Rijksprentenkabinet, Amsterdam.
21. Meister, E. S., St. Philip (middle 15th. cent.). Engraving (Lehrs 119).
22. Meister, E. S., St. Philip (middle 15th. cent. not later than 1467) Engraving (Lehrs 131). Copy in book on Meister E. S. in Libr. of Rijksmuseum Amsterdam.
23. Ecole d'Artois, St. Gregory in bow-spectacles (abt. 1450). Les Quatre Peres de l'Eglise. Property of M. Martin le Roy, Paris. Connected with the master of Flemalle and the artists of the Duc de Berry. (wings of a diptych). Copy Henri Bouchot. l'Exposition des primitifs francais. La peinture en France sous les Valois (1292–1500). Le miniature du Pontifical d'Etienne Loypeau presage l'auteur de ces peintures.
24. School of Aragon. Registration of St. John by his father Zachariah (end 15th. or beg. 16th. cent.). Musee d iBelle Arti de Barcelona (cliche Arzius Mas). Copy Dr. Simon: Ulleres angulares de molla.
25. Anonymous (Catalonian), The prophet David? Fragment of a pradella from the coll. of D. J. Estruch, Barcelona. Cliche Serra. Copy Dr. Simon. Les ulleres angulares clavades.
26. Anonymous, Moses in spectacles (1450). Miniature, now at Heidelberg. (Von Pflugk): Der Biblische Moses mit der Brille). Deutsch. Opt. Wochenschrift. 1920.
27. Monogramist. J.B., The Evangelist St. Matthew (1525). Engraving (Waldmann. Die Nurnberger Kleinmeister 1910).

28. School of Rafael, Baptism of St. Paul. Sacristy-church of San Pietro in Perugia. (mentioned in "De Tijd". Vol. 4. '27. Page 3. p.q.k.s.
29. Carlo Crivelli, St. Peter and St. Paul (1468–1493). Academia di belle Arti. Venice.
30. Michael Pacher, St. Luke (1481). On back of predella of altar-painting at St. Wolfgang in Salzkammergut. (Mannowski: Die Gemalde des Michael Pacher. 1910. Munich and Leipsic). Friedr. Wolff, Michael Pacher, Berlin 1909.
31. Q. Metsys (style of), St. Peter. Wallraf Mus. of the city of Cologne. Verzeichnis der Gem. des Wallraf, Richartz Mus. of the city of Cologne. (1910). Photo in Rheinische Mus. Deutz. Siegesstrasze.
32. Q. Metsys (style of), Hieronymus, Solitude ou Vie des Peres ermites et des anchoretes. (Jacques Honerougt, editor, Paris 1636). Coll. of 112 engraving. Four aged patriarchs in spectacles: Evagrius, Ammon, Palamon, Marinus. Mentioned by Bourgeois, to be found in Library of M. Wendling, sculptor of the Rheim Cathedral.
33. Lukas van Leyden, St. Mark (1494–1533). Musee royal d'Anvers. Musee des Beaux Arts. Cf. also engraving and copy, sale Barbier.
34. —
35. Nicolo Alunno da Foligno, Philip, James and Matthew in spect. School of Umbria? 1430–1502? Triptych Vatican. On the predella 3 figures in spectacles, the apostles Philip, James and Matthew, described by Victor Reis. Quelques observations oculistiques dans l'art Italien. Nouv. Iconogr. d.l. Salpetriere, 1906. Binocle articule, acc. to Bourgeois.
36. Anonymous, St. Luke in pinching-spectacles (15th. cent.). French Livre d'Heures. Miniatrue. (Forrer: Unedierte Miniaturen des Mittelalters. Straszburg 1907). Pict. XIX.
37. Anonymous, The Apostle Matthew. Miniature dei libri corali del convento di S. Marco a Firenze. On the table a pair of spec. of the type of "besicles clouants". Museum at Florence. Ment. in Ann. di Ottalm. e clinica oculistica. 1922. Giuseppe Ovio. Invenziane degli Occhiali.
38. Master of Grosz-Gmain, Patriarch in spectacles (1498). Mus. Hist. of Art. Vienna.
39. Israel van Meckenem, St. Matthew (abt. 1490). Coll. Domela Nieuwenhuis in Boymans Mus. Rotterdam.
40. Spanish School, St. Paul (early 16th. cent.). Painted altar-wing, Retable peint. The figures of the 12 Apostles. Musee de Cluny. No. 1687. (old cat.). The bow-spect. are probably a "restoration".

St. Augustine

1. Anonymous, St. Augustine (1510). Tyrolese repres. of the patriarchs. Pupil of Mantegna's. Published by Prof. Greeff.
2. Friedr. Walther from Dinkelsbuhl, St. Augustine (1470). Block-book Munchener Hof und Staatsbibliothek. Xyl. 34. (Defensiorum inviolatae Mariae virginis). Monogram F. W. Copy Prausnitz. The book was written by the Dominican friar Franc. von Retz, who died in 1425.
3. Studio Erasmus Grasser, St. Augustine (1502). Bust in wood from the series of apostles and patriarchs. Choir-stalls Frauenkirche Munich. Nat. Mus. Munich. Room 20.
4. Tirolese School, St. Augustine (abt. 1520). Part of larger series, probably from altar. Owner: J. Rosenthal, Munich.
5. Anonymous, St. Augustine (15th. cent.). St. Augustine on Hieronymus-altar from Minken near Ohlau. Diocesan Mus. at Breslau.
6. Master of Tucher-altar, St. Augustine (abt. 1450). Liebfrauenkirche et Nurnberg. (Gebhart, Die Anfang der Tafelmalerei in Nurnberg, Straszburg 1908).
7. Master of Mondsee, St. Augustine (15th. cent.). Kunsthist. Mus. Vienna.

St. Hieronymus

1. Rembrandt, St. Hieronymus (1648). Etching No. 74.
2. Antwerp School, St. Hieronymus (middle 16th. cent.). Private property at Basel. Copy at Hallauer's.
3. Anonymous, Antwerp School, St. Hieronymus (middle 16th. cent.). Replica of copy in Boymans Mus. Rotterdam. 80. Math. Lempertz Sale. Oct. 1904 at Cologne.
4. Adr. Isenbrandt, Flemish School, St. Hieronymus (1510–1533). Sale Coll. M. P. M. Paris. Hotel Drouot. May 8th. 1908. Cf. also "Exposition de la Toison d'Or (Exh. of the Golden Fleece). Bruges 1907. No. 214.
5. Joost van Cleve, Antwerp, St. Hieronymus (1511–1540). Catal. Col. Rich. von Kaufmann 1917. Cassierer and Helbing.
6. Anonymous, St. Hieronymus (1550). Gallery Dresden. Formerly ascribed to Durer. Copy at Prausnitz's. Probably German copy after Van der Goes.

7. Jan Mostaert (contemp. of), St. Hieronymus (abt. 1475–1555). Dutch School. Coll. Dorus Hermsen the Hague. No. 33 Catal.

8. Master of the Death of Mary. Cologne School, St. Hieronymus (active 1515–1535?). Joos van Cleve 1460–1519; or Joost van Calcar? Prov. Museum. Hannover. Almost completely identical with copy in Boymans Mus. Cf. also in "Joos van Cleve" by Ludwig Baldaas. Kristall Verlag. Vienna 1925.

9. Anonymous, South. Netherl., St. Hieronymus. Kunsthandel (art-shop); Brussels. Copy. Kunsthist. Inst. Utrecht.

10. Anonymous, South. Netherl., St. Hieronymus. Goedhart, Amsterdam. 1918. Photo in Kunsthist. Int. at Utrecht.

11. Anonymous, St. Hieronymus (abt. 1480). Wood-cut from West-Bavaria. Copied after pict. occurring in H. Bouchot: Deux-cents incunables. (200 incunabula). Fig. 62. 1 copy at Munich and 1 in Brit. Mus.

12. St. Hieronymus. Schrotblatt. Kunsthist. Inst. Utrecht. Schrotblatt 79. Einblattdrucke des XV. Jahrh., edit. by Paul Heitz. Vol. 43, Part. II. Meister der Metallschneidekunst. Kunsthist. Inst. Utrecht.

13. Poilly, St. Hieronymus (1623–1693). Paris. Etching repres. by Mrs. Heymann.

14. Niccolo Alunno, Niccolo di Liberatore, St. Hieronymus (1430–1502). School of Umbria. Rome Galeria Corsini. Copy at Mrs. Heymann's.

15. Bartolomeus Vermejo of Cordova, St. Hieronymus (1490). Cathedral at Barcelona. Spanish Primitive. Pieta between Hieronymus and Canon Lluis Despla. Under Flemish influence. Copy: La Revue de l'Art XX. Cf. Dr. Simon nail-spectacles.

16. Domenico Ghirlandajo, St. Hieronymus (1499–1498). Florence. Church: di Agnissanti. Copy at Bock and Greeff's.

17. Joos van Cleve, ascribed to; Antwerp School, St. Hieronymus (1511–1540). Sale Col. Chillingworth, Lucerne, Sept. 1922. Replicas Mus. Prague, dated 1541, in Brussels Mus. Cat. 1900. No. 218 as Hemmessen. dated 1542. Eco le Brabancon.

18. G. van Roemerswaal or Quinten Metsys, Ascribed to, St. Hieronymus (1466–1530). Sale Bonomi, Cereda Milan 1896. Cenre pict. Mus. Boymans and of picta from coll. Hoch, ascribed to Metsys, though probably older and certainly much better. Do. in Aartsbissch. Mus. Utrecht (as Roemerswael). Do. Coll. Dhilingworth. Cf. Cat. formerly ascribed to Civetta and before that to Patenier. Replica in Mus. de Bruxelles, as Hemmessen.

19. Jan Massys, St. Hieronymus (1509–1577). Date probably 1542. Great resemblance to, partly copy of painting in Antwerp, Mus. Boymans, Rotterdam, f. cat. Heinrich Theodor Koch, Munich. 1892.

20. Anonymous, St. Hieronymus (1540). Boymans Mus., Rotterdam. Repres. resembling this are ascribed to Quinten Metsys, Jan Massys, Hemmessen, Van Reymerswaele or Roemerswael, Joos van Cleve, etc.

21. Quinten Metsys, St. Hieronymus. Kon. Galerie, Berlin. Copy cf. The masterworks of Massys. Edit. Hols, the Hague. Spectacles cannot be seen on the pict. Ace to Greeff there are spect. on the copy in the K. Friedr. Mus.

22. Marinus van Roymerswale, St. Hieronymus (1520–1560). Madrid. Prado Mus. Copy: Kunstgeschichte in Bildern. Vol. IV. G. Dehio.

23. Quinten Metsys (School of), St. Hieronymus. Coll. v. Pflugk, Dresden.

24. Antwerp School (Pupils and imitators of Q. Metsys), St. Hieronymus. Coll. Senft, Berlin.

25. Van Hemmessen, St. Hieronymus (abt. 1550). Salzburg Museum.

26. Copy after Metsys, St. Hieronymus. Museo Civico at Venice.

27. George Pencz. Nurnberg, St. Hieronymus (1544). Copy after Q. Metsys. Germ. Mus.

28.—

29. Antwerp School. Jan Metsys?, St. Hieronymus. Coll. Dorus Hermsen; the Hague.

30. Metsijs (ascribed to), St. Hieronymus. Castle of Harff. (same type as in Mus. Boymans, etc.).

31. Jan Metsys. (son of Q.). (1509–1575), St. Hieronymus (1537). Mus. of Hist. of Art. Vienna. Cf. also Antwerp.

32. Q. Metsys. (School of), St. Hieronymus (1450–1530). Rheims.

33. Hemmessen, St. Hieronymus (16th. cent.). Mus. at Brussels.

34. Jose de Ribera. (Spagnoletto). (1588–1666), St. Hieronymus (1656). Spanish School, Velancia. Uffizien, Florence.

35. Michelangelo Anselmi, St. Hieronymus (1494–1544). Brera.

36. Carpaccio. (Vittore), Funeral of St. Hieronymus (1480–1519). Venetian School. Painting in Scuola de San Giorgio e Trifone at Venice. Bourgeois.

Death of Mary

1. Anonymous, Painter from Frankfurt?, Death of Mary (1492). Wing altar of St. Anne from Dominican church at Frankf. o.t. Main., now in Hist. Mus. at Frankf. Copy. Otto Laufer. Hessenkunst. Kalender fur alte u. neue Kunst 1911. Copy in Kunsthist. Inst. Utrecht. 3266. South Netherl. School or South German.
2. H. Holbein. The Elder, Death of Mary (1502). Alte Pinakothek at Munich. Wing of High-altar of the conventual church at Kaisheim.
3. Abraham Benson. (ascribed to), Death of Mary (abt. 1515). Flemish primitive. Copy of specimen ascribed to van der Goes in London, Nat. Gall. and in Berlin K. Friedr. Mus. Copy Cat. Sale Coll. Smallenburg van Stellendam. Fred. Muller, May 1913. Cf. also copy Cat. Sale Lepke, Berlin 1910.
4. H. van der Goes (after?), Death of Mary (1482). Nat. Gall. London. Cf. also A. Benson.
5. Martin Schongauer, Death of Mary (1470). Engraving. Copy Bock: Drie Brille usw. Prausnitz.
6. Hugo van der Goes, Death of Mary (abt. 1480). K. Frieder. Mus. Cf. also replica Nat. Gall. Copy at Prausnitz's. Cf. also Benson.
7. Meister von Soest, Death of Mary (1430). Old Westphalian School. Orig. from the St. Walburgis-convent at Soest. Landesmus. at Munster. (Westph. Kunstverein). Copy at Prausnitz's.
8. Joos van Cleve, Death of Mary (1550–1580). Antwerp School. Wallraf Mus. Cologne. No. 430. Copy: Kunstgesch. in Bilder, Vol. 8. C. Dehio.
9. Anonymous, Death of Mary (abt. 1400). Viennese School? Property of Schnackenberg. Georgenstr. 7, Munich. Now in Alte Pinakothek. Cf. copy Bruckner and Furchtmaier. Beitrage z. deutsch. Kuntgesch. I.
10. Rembrandt, Death of Mary (1637). Etching.
11. Hans Multscher, Death of Mary (1440–1476). Gemalde Galerie Karlsruhe. Copy at Prausnitz's. Old-Swabian painter, master of the Sterzinger Altar.
12. Martin Schongauer, Death of Mary (1445–1491). Triest. Copy: partly at Feldhaus's. Die Technik usw.
13. Jan Joost van Calcar, Death of Mary (1505–1508). Haarlem School. High-altar of the St. Nicolai-church. Calcar. Copy in coll. Kunsthist. Inst. Utrecht 6064 B.
14. Anonymous, Swabian-Tyrolese Master, Death of Mary (abt. 1500). One of the seven wings of a painted altar. Sale Heberle 16 Nov. 1909.
15. Hans Holbein, the Elder, Death of Mary (1490). Pinakothek at Munich or Off. Kunstsamml. Basel.
16. Anonymous, Death of Mary (abt. 1486). Painter from Burgundy or Lyon. Copy in "Le Musee de Lyon". Coll. Publiques de France. Cf. H. Bouchot. L'Exposition des Primitifs Francais.
17. Martin Schongauer, Death of Mary (1470). Mus. at Wiesbaden. Copy Mrs. Heymann: "Lunettes et lorgnettes de jadis".
18. Swabian School, Death of Mary (1470–1480 or 1490). From Dinkelsbuhl. Now in Germ. Mus. at Nurnberg. No. 232.
19. Anonymous, Death of Mary (15th. cent.). Quadro central del antic altar major del Reial monastir de Stes. Creus. Museo diosa de Tarragona. Beg. 15th. cent.
20. Hans Holbein, the Elder, Death of Mary (1502). Off. Kunstsamml. Basel.
21. Hans Holbein, the Elder, Death of Mary (1509). Cathedral of Chalons sur Marne, Bourgeois.
22. Castilian School, Death of Mary (15th. cent.). Le Prado, Madrid.
23. Anonymous, Death of Mary (15th. cent.). Viktorsdom at Xante. n Painting on glass.
24. Michel Wohlgemut, Death of Mary (abt. 1497). Wing of altar at Hersbruck.
25. Anonymous, Death of Mary (1494). Diptych in choir-ambulatory of the church of St. Mary at Lubeck. Westph. School.
26. Master of the Tucher-altar, Death of Mary (1438). Black-and-White drawing. Univ. Libr. at Erlangen.
27. Swabian School, Death of Mary. (15th. C.). Enamel on copper. Gall. of Sigmaringen.
28. Hans Holbein, the Elder, Death of Mary. Art-dealer Kleinberger at Paris.
29. Anonymous, Death of Mary. Prague. In possession of K. Andre.
30. Anonymous, Death of Mary (beg. 15th. cent.). Viennese artist. Museum of Stift, Klosterneuburg. (Dreschsler and Liszt, Tafelbilder aus dem Mus. des Stiftes Klosterneuburg. Vienna 1902).

31. German Master, Death of Mary (1480). Westph. Landesmus. Munster.
32. Swabian School, Death of Mary (1490). Kirchenmuseum des Maximilianeums at Augsburg.
33. Pacher, Death of Mary (1481). Pacher Altar. St. Wolfgang.
34. Martin Schaffner, Death of Mary (1508–1536). Coll. A. Prouvost. Sale Fred. Muller, Oct. '27, Copy cf. Cat.

Circumcision; Instruction in the Temple

1. Master of the Tucheraltar, Circumcision (1451–1460). Suermondt Mussuem, Aix-la-Chapelle.
2. Friedrich Herlin, Circumcision (1466). Altar St. Jacobskirche, Rothenburg.
3. Daniel Hopfer? active in Augsburg, Instruction or Circumcision in the Temple (1493–1536). One of 4 small altar-wings. Copy Sale Coll. Kaufmann 1917. Cassirer and Helbing; also in Klass. Bilderschatz as "Grunewald", afterw. ascribed to Cranach.
4. Anonymous, Circumcision (abt. 1450). Venetian woodcut. Germ. Mus. Nurnberg. Copy Kristeler: Veroffentlichung der Graphischen Gesellschaft IX; an imitation of Venetian woodcut from the 15th. cent. in possess. of the city of Nurnberg.
5. H. Goltzius. Dutch, Circumcision (1594). Copper-engraving. Mus. Civico; Venice. Cf. also: painting after this engraving in Leningrad. (mentioned by Waagen).
6. A. Durer, Refusal of the expiatory sacrifice. Woodcut from the life of the H. Virgin.
7. Pepersack, La Presentation (the Instr.) (1640). Tapistry of the Rheims Cathedral, (burned during the war). Copy cf. Bourgeois; Ces besicles de nos ancetres.
8.—
9. Cigoli. Cardi (Lodovico da), Circumcision (1539–1613). Florentine School. Church of San Francesco di Prato, near Florence. Mentioned by Pansier.
10. Glockendon. (Nicolo), Circumcision (16th. cent.). German School. Miniature. Manuscr. de la Vie de Jr. Chr. Libr. d'Este at Modena.
11. Glodkendon. (Nicolo), Circumcision (end 15th cent.). Church at Fromentieres (Marne).
12. Glockendon (Nicolo), La Presentation au Temple. (Instr. in T.) (15th C.). Altar-wing. Sculpture of the Reims; Mus. ment. by Bourgeois.
13. Jordaens, The circumcision, 17 ct. Boymans Museum, Rotterdam.
14. Joerg Ratgeb. (of Gmund), The circumcision (1519). Swabian School. High-altar of the Stiftkirche at Herrenberg.
15. Massolino, The circumcision (beg. 16th C.). Kunsthist. Samml. at Vienna.
16. Antwerp School, The circumcision (beg. 16th C.). Altar of Pailhe. Musee des Arts dec. et ind. Brussels.
17. Hausbuchmeister (Middle-Rhenisch), The circumcision. Altar-wing. St. Stephanskirche at Mainz. 1500. Copy at Prasunitz's.

Christ in the Temple at the Age of 12

1. Anonymous, Chr. in the Temple at the Age of 12 (1468). North Nether. Breviary 1468. Krakow Mus. Czartoryskich 3091. Fol. 51 etc. Copy cf. Byvanck and Hoogewerff. Pict. 73.
2. Israel van Meckene, Chr. in the Temple at the age of 12 (bef. 1503). Bocholt. Copper-engraving.
3. A. Durer, Chr. in the Temple at the age of 12 (abt. 1500). Woodcut.
4. Hans Fries of Freiburg, The child Jesus and the scribes (1512). Kunstsamml. Basel.
5. Anonymous, The child Jesus and the scribes (abt. 1500). Gobelintapestry. South German. Descr. and repr. by Prof. Fr. Witte. Museum Cologne.
6. Master of the Dying Cato. Dutch Hist. painter, The child Jesus and the scribes (16th C.). Worcester U.S.A. (v. Wurtzbach Niederl. Kunstlerlexicon. III. 200 and II. 665. H. Voss. Charakterkopfe des Seicento 1908. Monatshefte f. Kunstwissenschaft 1909).
7. Hausbuch-meister, Chr. at the age of 12 among the scribes (abt. 1500). Life of Mary. Bildergalerie at Mainz.
8. Durer (School of), Chr. teaching in the Temple (1506). Galerie Dresden. Formerly constituting part of an altar in the Wittenberg Schlosskirche. Copy: Les Saints Evangiles by the Abbot Glaire. Paris. Goupil and Co. 1899.
9. H.F.E. Monogramist, Chr. in the Temple at the age of 12 (16th C.). Engraving of Italian master after painting by Mazzolini da Ferrara in K. Fr. Mus. Berlin. Coll. Domela in Mus. Boymans, Rotterdam.

10. Giulio Campi, Chr. in the Temple at the age of 12 (1500–1572). Fresco-painting at Cremona in the Church di S. Marcherita. Copy in "The Gospels in Art". Shaw. 1904.
11. Frans Francken, The child J. and the scribes (1581–1642?). Antwerp Cathedral.
12. Pepersack, The child J. and the scribes (1640). Tapestry at the Reims Cathedral.
13. Salomon Koninck. The child J. and the scribes (1609–1656). Alte Pinakothek. Munich. Copy: Vienna Academy.
14. Jan Steen, Chr. at the age of 12 in the Temple (1626–1679). Mus. Basel.
15. Josef de Ribera (Spagnoletto) (1652?). 1588–1656. Mus. Vienna.
16. Thaddaus Stammel, Chr. teaching in the Temple (died 1765). Libr. Benedictine convent at Admont. (Steiermark).
17. J.B. Franck (1600–1653), The child Jesus and the scribes. Mus. Bruges.

St. Joseph and Other Members of the Holy Family in Spectacles

1. Joos van Cleve, The Holy Family. Paris. Coll. Spiridon. Copy. Cf. Ludwig Baldaas: Joos van Cleve. Krystall Verlag Vienna. 1925.
2. Joos van Cleve, The H. Family (16th C.). Krystall-Verlag. Vienna 1925. Ludwig Baldass: Joos van Cleve. (Werkstattarbeit). Frau E. Mauthner-Markhoff.
3. Joos van Beke, called Joos van Cleve, the Elder, The Holy Family (active 1510–1540). Nat. Gall. London. 2603. (probably Master of the Death of Mary).
4. Jan Provoost or Prevost. Flemish School, De Deipara Virgo, announced by prophets and sybils (1524). Ermitage, Leningrad. (There as Q. Metsys). Copy. cf. Kunst and Leven (Art and Life) 1902–1903. Jan Provost by G. Hulin. Acc. to Bourgeois binocle articule.
5. Master of the H. Blood, Bruges, The H. Family (abt. 1510). Coll. Chillingworth. Sale Lucerne. Sept. 1922.
6. Dutch painter (Italianizing), The H. Family (17th C.). Sale Coll. Grosskopf. Firm of Bangel. May 1925.
7. Master of the Death of Mary, The H. Family (1460–1519). Coll. Salting. London. (Bourgeois).
8. Van Orley, The H. Family (1490–1542). Sigmaringen.
9. Joos van Cleve, The H. Family (16th C.). Krystall-Verlag. Vienna 1925. Ludwig Baldass: Joos van Cleve. No. 36 H. Family. Nat. Gall. London. No. 34. Copy. (Werkstattarbeit). Frau E. Mauthner-Markhoff.
10. Flemish Anonymous, The H. Family (16th C.). Royal Mus. Antwerp (gift of the society of Artibus Patriae). Room I.
11. School of Milan, (or Florence?); School of Leonardo da Vinci; The H. Family (16th C.). Private poss. at Budapest. Dr. Goldzieher. Copy by Greeff. Also described by him in Zeitschrift f. Opth. Optik. Vol. I. Page 73. 1913.
12. Flemish Anonymous, The H. Family (beg. 16th C.). Wallraff-mus. Cologne No. 428. Cat. '15. Copy to be had at Kunstgewerbe Mus.
13. Ghent Primitive, La descendance de Sainte Anne. (2nd half 15th C.). Triptych from Ghent Mus. Repr. at Maeterlincks', "l'Enigme des primitifs francais." 1921, and: Une ecole primitive meconnue. Nabur Martins, or Master of Flemalle 1913.
14. Master of the Chapel of the H. Blood; of 1528, H. Family (1520). Triptych. Kunsthalle at Hamburg. Photo in Kunsthist. Inst. at Utrecht.
15. Bodensee School, La descendance de St. Anne (abt. 1470). Dutch Art-shop.
16. Geertgen tot St. Jansz, La descendance de St. Anne (abt. 1470), Rijksmuseum; Amsterdam.

Christ and the Tribute-Money
Christ and the Adulterous Woman

1. Titian (School of), Christ and the Tribute-money (bef. 1576). National Gallery in London.
2. Tiarini (Allesandro), Christ and the Tribute-money (1577–1668). Gemalde-galerie, Augsburg. (Influence of Titian).
3. Jean de Boullongue, dit le Valentin, Christ and the Tribute-money (1591–1634). Musee du Louvre. Mentioned by Mrs. Heymann.
4. Varotari. (Allesandro), dit le Padouan, The adulterous woman (1590–1650). Belvedere, Vienna. (Venetian School).
5. Gabriel Metsu, The adulterous woman (1630–1667). Louvre.
6. Bonifacio Veronese II, Christ and the adulterous woman (abt. 1540). Brera. Milan.

7. Lucas Cranach, Christ and the Tribute-money (abt. 1530). Formerly in Alte Pinakothek, Munich.
8. Corn. de Belliuer, Me elder Christ and the Tribute-money (1607–1671). Germaldegalerie, Braunschweig.

Vocation of St. Matthew

1. J. de Paraja. Pupil of Velasquez. (formerly his slave), The Vocation of St. Matthew (17th C.). Prado. Madrid. Copy cf. Kuhn. Allgem. Kunstgesch. Cf. also Max Rooses: De schilderkunst van 1400–1800. (The art of painting from 1400–1800; edit. Elsevier).
2. H. ter Brugghen, The Election of the Apostle (1588–1629). Munic, Museum at Utrecht.
3. Jan van Hemessen, active at Antwerp and Haarlem, Apostolic vocation of Matthew (1504–1575). Formerly Alte Pinakothek at Munich.
4. Ludovico Caraci, School of Bologna, Election of the Apostle Matthew (1555–1619). Pinakothek at Bologna.

Christ before Pilate. Ecce Homo

1. Jordaens, Christ before Pilate (1593–1678). Mus. Boymans. Rotterdam. Drawing and Museum Ghent (1910 A.C.)
2. Giordano, Luca, called Fa Presto, Naples, Ecce Homo (1632–1705). Coll. Messinger. Sale Helbing 1918. April 16th.
3. Johann Wirier, ct. Andreas Trost, Christ before Pilate (1679). Page 9 of Passionsbuchlein; Dominicae Passionis Icones. Engraving by Andreas Trost. Landschaftliches Mus. Rudolphinum at Laibach (Bourgeois).
4. Joh. van der Straet (Stradanus). Ecce Homo (1523–1605). Black-and-white drawing; Boymans Mus. Rotterdam.

Old Tobia's Eye-sight is Restored

1. Rembrandt v. Rijn, A whole series of etchings and drawings (17th C.). Described by Prof. Greeff and by Dr. de Lint; Black-and-white drawing, Albertina; Vienna.

Bethsabe after her Bath
(Bethsabe, femme d'Urie, sortant du bain)

1. Rembrandt van Rijn, Bethsabe (1632). Museum Rennes. (painting).
2. Rembrandt van Rijn, Bethsabe (1643). Former coll. Steengracht.
3. Moreau le Jeune, Bethsabe (1763). Engraving after earlier painting.
4. F. Verwilt, Bethsabe (17th C.). Copy. Cat. Fred. Muller. June 1920.
5. P. v. Lint, Bethsabe (1642). Brussels Mus. of ancant Painting.

Adoration of the Magi

1. Pieter Breughel, the Elder, Adoration of the Magi (1564). Nat. Gall. London.
2. French Anonymous, l'Adoration des Mages. (End of the 15th C.). Altar-wing Church of Fromentieres.
3. German School, Adoration of the Magi (1466). Woodcuts mentioned at Bock's.

Descent of the Holy Ghost (Whitsuntide)

1. Conrad von Soest, Descent of the H. Ghost (1404). Church at Niederwildungen.
2. Guillaume Ernest, Greve, Descent of the H. Ghost (before 1639). Church of St. Agricol d'Avignon.

Christ Chasing the Merchants from the Temple

1. Hier. Bosch, Chr. chasing the merchants from the temple (abt. 1500). Coll. Claude Philips, London.
2. Jordaens, Chr. chasing the merchants from the temple (17th C.) Louvre, Paris.

Further Anachronistic Representation with Spectacles

1. Jacob Corneliszoon van Oostzanen, Needlework copie (abt. 1520). Rijksmus. Amsterdam.
2. Vermeyen, Raising of Lazarus (1500–1559). Museum Brussels.
3. School of Aragon, Registering of St. John by his father Zacharias (abt. 1500).
4. Johannes Sadeler, after Jodocus de Winge, King David singing psalms of praise to the harp (17th C.). Rijksprentenkabinet, Amsterdam.
5. Jan Steen, The fallen Simson (17th C.). Wallraf Mus. Cologne.
6. Jan Steen, David conquerer greeted by Saul's daughter Michal (17th. C.). Museum. Copenhagen.
7. Jan Steen, hagar disowned by Abraham. Museum. Dresden.

8. French or Flemish Art, Assuerus revoquant son edit contre les juifs. (A. revoking his edict against the Jews). Gothic tapestry (15th C.). Museum Nancy.
9. Mainardi (Andrea), Le sauveur comprime sous un pressoir. (The Saviour pressed in a press) (16th C.). Church of S. Agostino. Cremona.
10. Glockendon (Nicolo), Judas betraying Christ (16th C.). Miniature from manuscr. de la Vie de J. Chr. Libr. d'Este, Modena.
11. J. van der Straet (Stradanus), Judas seeking out the Jews to deliver (16th C.). Copy in Theatrum bibl. hist. sacrae veteris et novi testamenti 1674 by Piscator.
12. J. van der Straet, St. Paul before the proconsul F. (16th C.). Copy in Theatrum bibl. hist. sacrae veteris et novi testamenti 1674 by Piscator.
13. J. van der Straet, St. Paul before the Conseil of the priests at J. (16th C.). Copy in Theatrum bibl. hist. sacrae veteris et novi testamenti 1674 by Piscator.
14. J. van der Straet, St. Peter at the centurion (16th C.). Copy in Theatrum bibl. hist. sacrae veteris et novi testamenti 1674 by Piscator.
15. Reveil, engraving after J. Jordaens, J. Chr. reproaching the Pharisees (17th C.). Private poss. mentioned by Bourgeois.
16. Rembrandt van Ryn, Hannah teaching Samuel, elsewhere called; Timothy and his grandmother (1605–1669). Hermitage, Leningrad.
17. Rembrandt van Rijn, Similar representation (1605–1669). Copy in Rembrandt-Bibel by E.W. Bredt. Edit. Hugo Schmidt, Munich.
18. Rubens, P.P., Jesus at Simon the Pharisee's (1615–1620). Hermitage, Leningrad.
19. Octave van Veen, Jesus at Simon the Pharisee's (1558–1629). Reflected image. Variation on number 18. Copy Cat. Coll. M.E. Fetis, at Le Roy, freres. Brussels 1909.

Spectacles for Animals
by
Prof. von Pflugk

Reproductions

1. Boden 1910 The determination of the refraction of the eyes and spectacles of a dog.
2. A monkey, operated upon for cataract, with spectacles.

The Spectacle-Dealer
by
Prof. Greeff

1. Hans Frank: A merchant. 1516 (Engraving after Prof. Hallauer).
2. Lunetiers ambulants (Epoque Louis XIII, 1610–1643), after Madame Heymann.
3. A. van Ostade: The spectacle-dealer (1610–1685). (Reproduction after original etching by himself).
4. J. Cassonville (b. 1619), the French Ostake: the spectacle-dealer.
5. Corneliszoon Droochsloot (1586–1666); Itinerant spectacle-dealer. (After Brettauer).
6. Andreas and Jan Both (1610–1651): the itinerant spectacle-dealer. (After Brettauer).
7. Jost Amman (1539–1591); The peddler, with poems by Hans Sachs. (1494–1576).
8. N. Glantschnig (1661–1722) (Tirol). An itinerant spectacle-dealer. After a picture in the Museum at Innsbruck.
9. Piece of work made by N.G. Dupuis (1696–1770). After a picture by Franz Eisen, father (1685–1775).
10. Picture, Dutch school, first half of the 17th. ct., private property of Prof. Greeff.
11. Marcellus Laroon the younger. (1679–1772): The spectacle-dealer on the fair. (After an original in the possession of Prof. Greeff.)
12. Jaques Buys: The spectacle-trader. Amsterdam, 1776.
13. Conspicilia. Vignette with spectacle-dealer. (After Mme. Heymann).
14. Matthias Scheits (1640–1700): the spectacle-dealer. (After an engraving in the possession of Prof. v. Pflugk). This is an engraving after the picture by Dassonville (see 4.).
15. Chr. E. Dietrich (1712–1774). Weimar, Dresden; Itinerant Spectacle-dealer.
16. P. Cramer (1726 in Kopenhagen): spectacle-pedlar.
17. 18. M. Engelbrecht (1672–1733): An optician and his wife. In recoco-style.
19. Bouchardon (1740): Pedlar and spectacle-dealer.
20. The oldest known reproduction of a female pedlar, selling spectacles by the side of needles and thimbles. Cologne wood-cut of 1589. Original in the Municipal Historical Museum, Cologne.

21. Pienze Tempert (b. 1650): The spectacle-dealer (English). From a series of 50 prints: London hawker, (Cries de London).
22. Poisson: Spectacle-and cake-dealer from the series: Les cris de Paris (Paris Hawkers).
23. Annibale Carracci. Rome 1646: Itinerant Italian Spectacle-dealer. Copper-engraving from one of the oldest-known editions of the "Hawkers".
24. Viennese itinerant "perspective-dealer". Copper-engraving after an example by the Dutch painter Stradanus (abt. 1605) by L. Schuytz. (1600).
25. Coloured print (German); Spectacle-dealer.
26. Johannes Scheffler, called Angelus Solesius as a spectacle-dealer. After a libel, directed against him: Welldeserved chapter. (1664). Original in Breslau.
27. Itinerant spectacle-dealer. Hand-painted copper-engraving from the book by C. Suhr: The pedlars at Hamburg. 1808.
28. Larmessin (17th. ct.): Habit de Marchand Miroitiers Lunettier, Engraving from the album of the metiers.
29. "Die Past". Sondermann pinxit Simon sculpsit. (Modern). In the spectacle-shop.
30. Spectacle-trade and manufacture in Nuremberg, 1568, after Joost Amman. From Garzonis Piazza Universale, German edition of 1658.
31. Spectacle-sale in Italy, about 1580. Engraving after Jan Stradanus by Adriaen Collaert. Original with Prof. v. Pflugk.
32. "The spectacle-maker" from "Human Doings" by Johannes and Caspaares Luiken. Amsterdam. 1694.
33. Officina Burlini. Title-head from Raccolte di Macchine ed Istrumenti d'Ottica by Biagio Burlini. Venice 1758. After Prof. v. Pflugk.

Guilds of Spectacle-Makers
Masterpieces
by
Prof. Greeff

1. Nurmberg master-spectacles of 1680 (with illustration).
2. Master-spectacles from the Statutes of the Regenburg spectacle-makers.
3. Two pair of spectacles from the Statutes of the Nurmberg spectacle-makers.
4. Facsimile-copy of the whole of the Statutes of the Regenburg Spectacle-makers from the Germanische Museum at Nurmberg (Illustrations and texts).

Spectacles in Paper-Watermarks (Wasserzeichen)
by
Dr. Simon

No. 1.
Watermarks on paper with monocular spectacles.
Bolonia 1318.
Spectacle-case for nail-spectacles.
Lucca 1452.

No. 2.
Watermarks on paper with angular nail-spectacles with straight sides, comprising the following (classified as to place and date where the paper was used).
Barcelona 1452.
Barcelona 1462.
Barcelona 1466.
Montpellier 1495.
Voltera 1522.

No. 3.
Watermarks on paper with angular nail-spectacles provided with slightly bowed temples, comprising the following kinds:
Barcelona 1454.
Originating from Italy 1452. (Collection of Dr. Simon).
Barcelona 1462.
Lucca 1467.

No. 4
Watermarks on paper with spectacles of the same kind.
Perpignan 1457.
Barcelona 1458.
Barcelona 1461.
Barcelona 1461.

No. 5.
Watermarks with angular nail-spectacles with curved temples and lower tongue, comprising the following kinds:

Udine 1423.
Barcelona 1431.
Barcelona 1434.
Naples 1451.

No. 6.
Watermarks with angular pressnail-spectacles.
In pressing-form: {Burger 1387.
{Venice 1481.
With a spring: {Venice 1491.
{Venice 1478.

No. 7.
Watermarks with spectacles in Gothic pointed form.
Catania 1431.

The Spectacles in the Marking-Irons for Horses
by
Dr. Simon

No. 1.
Mark of the breed of the Marques of Vico Puglia: Kingdom of Naples, 14th century.
Mark of the breed of the Count of Canossa, Verona (Veneto).
Mark of the breed of Josefa Gimenez, Coria (Sevilla).
Mark of the breed of Lucas Muruve, Los Palacios (Sevilla).
Mark of the breed of . . . . Romero, Higuera de Llerena (Badajoz).
Mark of the breed of Jose Antonio Ortiz, Aguaja (Badajoz).
Mark of the breed of Pedro Domingo, Alcantara, Brozas (Caceres).

No. 2.
Among the horse-marks with spectacles provided with a semicircular bridge:
Mark of the breed of Pedro Simonato, Aznolcollar (Sevilla).
Mark of the breed of Manuel Saavedra Samartin. Francisco Mansio (Badajoz).

Family Coats-of-Arms
The Spectacles Occuring in Heraldry
by
Dr. Simon

No. 1.
Object. Coat-of-arms of Gorg Ammon, master-spectacle-maker at Nurmberg.
Epoch 1581.
Place: Churchyard of St. John. Nurmberg.

No. 2.
Object. Coat-of-arms of the masters spectacle- and plate-glass makers of Nurmberg.
Epoch 1530.
Bibliography. Seyler Gustav A. Berufswappen. Table 31.

No. 3.
Object. Coats-of-arms of the masters spectacle and plate-glass makers of Nurmberg.
Epoch. 17th cent.
Bibliography. Seyler Gustav A. Berufwsappen. Table 31.

No. 4.
Object. Coat-of-arms of the masters lens-grinders of Nurmberg.
Epoch 1680.
The manuscript lies in the German Museum at Nurmberg.

No. 5.
Object. Coat-of-arms of the masters lens-grinders of Nurmberg.
Epoch 1591.
Bibliography. Martin Gerlach. Allegories et Emblemes. Vol. I. sec. partie, Lamine 29.

No. 6.
Object. Coat-of-arms of the masters lens-grinders of London.
Epoch 1750.
Bibliography. Seyler Gustav A. Berufswappen. Table 161.
So this blazon dates from the year 1629.

No. 7.
Object. Coat-of-arms of the masters lens-grinders of London.
Epoch 1629.
Bibliography. The book of Public Arms. Arthur Charles Fox-Davies. London 1915.

No. 8.
Object. Coat-of-arms of the masters spectacle-makers and plate-glass makers of Paris.
Epoch 1581.
Bibliography. Mrs. Heymann. Lunettes et lorgnettes de jadis.

No. 9.
Object. Coat-of-arms of the guild of the fine tanners of saddles of Paris.
Epoch 16th cent.
Bibliography. Mrs. Heymann. (do).

No. 10.
Object. Coat-of-arms of the guild of the fine tanners of Chateau-Contier.
Epoch 16th cent.
Bibliography. Mrs. Heymann. (do).

No. 11.
Object. Coat-of-arms of the family of Occhiali?
Epoch 16th cent.
Place. Museo Civico. Sulmona. (Italy).
Bibliography. Prof. G. Alberlotti. Noticelle giruardanti la storia degli Occhiali. Occhiali sculptiti. Clinica Oculistica. Palermo 1907.

No. 12.
Object. Coat-of-arms of the family of Brille, originating from Bois-de-Duc.
Epoch 18th cent.
Bibliography. J. B. Rietstap. Armorial general des familles nobles et patriciennes de l'Europe.

No. 13.
Object. Coat-of-arms of the Barons of Labes. Prussian family.
Epoch 1786.
Bibliography. Armorial general by Rietstap.

No. 14.
Object. Coat-of-arms of the family of Dacher de la Lorraine.
Epoch 1663.
Bibliography. Armorial general by Rietstap.

No. 15.
Object. Mark of the House of Goldhan. Saxon family.
Epoch 1556.
Place. Pauline Kocke. University of Leipsic.

No. 16.
Object. Coat-of-arms of Francois Ullman. Mentioned at Nurmberg.
Epoch. Cent.?
Bibliography. J. Siebmacher. Grosses and Allgemeines Wappenbuch, berlegt von Rawo Raspe i. Wurzberg. Vol. 7.

No. 17.
Object. Coat-of-arms from the "Codex memorial de la fe catolica." (Memorial of the Catholic faith).
Epoch 15th cent.
Place. Cathedral of Fortosa. (Spain).

No. 18.
Object. Coat-of-arms of the town of Oudernarde.
Epoch 16th cent.

The Spectacles Occurring on Seals
by
Dr. Simon

No. 1.
Object. Seal of Jacques Gallochau, Canon of the Cathedral of St. Martin of Tours. (France), with the dignity of Magister Scholae.
Epoch 15th cent.

No. 2.
Object. Seal of Jacques Gallochau, Canon of the Cathedral of St. Martin of the department of "Gard". (France). The latter two have a pair of spectacles as a solution of the former.
Epoch 16th cent.

The Spectacles Occurring in Emblems and in
Allegorical Representations
by
Dr. Simon

No. 1.
Spectacles as symbols of ridicule or jesting.
Object. Woodcut. The fool book-lover from the Opus of Sebastian Brand. Navis Sultifera. Bale.
Epoch 1494.

No. 2.
Spectacles as symbols of ridicule or jesting.
Object. Woodcut. The court-fool rendered by A. Gazeau in the "Narren". (Fools).

No. 3.
Spectacles as symbols of ridicule or jesting.
Object. German woodcut-engraving: a satyr pulling up a blind.
Epoch 18th cent.

No. 4.
Spectacles as symbols of ridicule or jesting.
Object. Comical or droll helmet of Will Summers, court-fool to King Henry VIII of England. Presented by the Emperor Maximilian the First.
Epoch 16th cent.
Place. Tower of London.

No. 5.
Spectacles as symbols of calumny.
Author. Hegelunds. (Kopenhagen).
Object. Woodcut. Calumny.
Epoch 1579.
Place. In "Bagtalelsens gudinde", reproduced by Prof. Lundsgaard Brillernes Historie. Page. 39.

No. 6.
Spectacles as symbols of second-sight.
Author. Pieter van Breughel, the Elder.
Object. The Procession of the Fools.
Epoch 1559.
Place. Bibliotheque Nationale at Paris.

No. 7.
Spectacles as symbols of second-sight.
Object. Woodcut-engraving from the Opus of Johann Arndt. Samtliche Bucher. Christentum.
Epoch 1743.
Picture, which was kindly given me by Prof. Greeff.

No. 8.
Spectacles as symbols of second-sight.
Author. Joost van Craesbeck.
Object. Game of hazard. Painting on canvas.
Epoch 17th cent.
Place. Picture (painting) from the Royal Museum of Fine Arts at Antwerp.

No. 9.
Spectacles as symbols of moderation or temperance in the 15th cent.
Manuscript. Ethics of Aristotle. Library at Rouen.
Manuscript of Jaques of Armagnac, Duke of Nemerous. Bibliotheque Nationale at Paris. In the retinue of the Seven Virtues by Pieter van Breughel, the Elder.
Fragment of the wall-paper design: Justice. Royal Palace at Madrid.
Fragment of the wall-paper design: Faith: Royal Palace at Madrid.

No. 10.
Spectacles as symbols of moderation or temperance.
Object. Temperance. Woodcut.
Epoch 1589.
Place. Jost Amman's Wappen und Stambuch. Frankfurt.

No. 11.
Spectacles as symbols of happiness.
Author. Otto Vaemio.
Object. Picture. Happiness.
Epoch 1624.
Place. Emblemata sive symbola et principibus.

No. 12.
Spectacles as symbols of age.
Author. Otto Vaemio.
Object. Engraving. Age.
Epoch 1624.
Place. Emblemata sive symbola et principibus.

Spectacles in Proverbs
by
Dr. Simon

No. 1.
Object. Picture. The Muse of Astronomy offers a pair of spectacles to Voltaire, who holds Newton upside down before him, to read it. Illustration of the French sayings: Mettez vos lunettes. (Put on your spectacles). Il fallait chausser mieux ses lunettes. (You ought to have put on your spectacles better).
Epoch 18th cent.
Place. Bibliotheque Nationale at Paris.

No. 2.
Author. Goya.
Object. Picture. Filiation., by which is illustrated the Castilian proverb: Si no veo por los ojos, veo por los anteojos; (i.e. If you cannot look through your eyes, look through spectacles.)
Epoch 18th cent.

No. 3.
Object. French picture in illustration of the (old-fashioned) proverb: Bonjour lunettes, adieu filettes. When one has to begin wearing spectacles, it means good-bye to young girls.
Epoch 17th cent.

No. 4.
Author.
Object. Picture in illustration of the same proverb.
Epoch 1517.
Place. The Brosulein of G. von Kayserberg, published by Prof. Halauer.

No. 5.
Author. Jean Sadeler.
Object. Picture, illustrating the French expressions: To take a narrow vieuw of things.
Voir les choses par le petit bout de la lunette. Voir les choses par le gros bout (de' la lunette). To take a wide view of things.
Epoch 18th cent.
Place. Library of Arts at Barcelona.

No. 6.
Author. Jan Steen.
Object. Dutch painting, in which an allusion is made to the Dutch proverb: Wat baeten kaers of bille, als de uil niet zien en wille. What is the good of candle or spectacles, if the owl refuses to see.
Epoch 17th cent.
Place. Rijksmuseum (National Museum) at Amsterdam.

No. 7.
Object. Engraving in illustration of the Latin proverb: Subscribe incognita nunquam, Ante probent oculi, chartam quam dextera tenet. Free translation: Never put your signature under some document or other, before your eyes have approved of the contents of the paper which your sight hand holds.

Spectacles on Miniatures, Woodcuts, Paintings, Graphica, Etc.
by
Prof. H. Weve

1. Ambrosio de Morales, (Spanish historian) (1513–1591). (End 17th. or beg. 18th. cent.). From the Dioptrique du Pere Cherubin, represented by Mrs. Heymann, who took it over. M. Joseph Rouyer: Coup d'oeil retrospectif sur la lunetterie. Engraving.
2. Pacheco, Spanish Nobleman (1591–1654). Copy. Mrs. Heymann. Balthazar del Aliasar.
3. H. David. (fec). Frenchman, often signed H.D.F., Capivaceo Patavinas Philos. et Medicinae Professor, died 1589 at Padua (1638–1670). Presumably after the engraving of Ammon in the Libr. Chalcogr. Volume III. 1652.

4. P. Simon, the Elder. Paris 1640–1710. Portrait-engraver, Ant. P. Alvarez Orosio d'Avila Astorga; Viceroy of Naples. After P. Ronche. Catal. Coll. Wid. N. van Willes-Janse van Zoutelande en Werendycke. Van Stockum's antiq. Oct. 1916.
5. Anonymous. Contemporary of Van Eyck, Cup-bearer with patron-saint on priedieu. Museum Brugge (Bruges).
6. Tomasso da Modena, Fresco of Cardinal Nicholas of Rouen (1352). Chapter-house Dominican convent at Treviso.
7. Jan van Eyck, Canon Joris van de Paele (1434–1436). Detail of Madonna with Saints. Municipal Museum at Bruges. Cf. Copy in the Antwerp Museum.
8. Cologne Master of the Holy Sippe, Celestial Vision with Saint and Founder (1492). Germ. Nat. Mus. at Nurmberg.
9. Flemish Anonymous, Portrait of a man (End 15th. cent.). Strassburg Museum. Cat. 54.
10. Tomaso da Modena, Cardinal Ugone di Provenza (1352). Chapter-house belonging to chapel of Domin. Convent at Treviso. Publ. by G. Albertotti; Intern. Ophthalm. Congr. at Lucerne. 1904.
11. Anonymous of the Dutch school, Jacob van Driebergen (1502). Central Museum at Utrecht. Spectacle-case of easily recognizable shape. Identical with that of Hieronymus from the Boymans Museum.
12. Dom. Theoscopuli, called el Greco or Theotocopuli, abt. 1547–1614. The Cardinal Inquisitor Nino de Guevara (1596–1598). 2 Copies. Bust and full-length. Copy Cf. Aug. Mayer; El Greco. 1916. Coll. Hevemeyer. New-York. Coll. Nemes, Budapest bust.
13. Simon Bening, Self-portrait (1550). Victoria and Albert Mus. London. Copy in Planches documentaires of Les heures de Notre Dame. (Miniaturist at Bruges). Cf. also copy in La Miniature fl. Flam. du Cte. P. Durrieu.
14. Jacob Backer. Pupil of Rembrandt's, Johannes Uyttenbogaert (1635). Amsterdam Remonstrant Church. Pict. No. 159. Monography by Kurt Bauch. 1926.
15. Jacob Backer, Lawyer Francois de Vroude (1643). No. 162. Bauch. Berlin. Kaidser Friedrich Museum.
16. Joh. Lutma Jr., Johannes Lutma, the goldsmith (1696). Engraving or etching. Rijksmuseum 883 K. Copy. Cover: Introduction to the History of Dutch Artistic Forging, by Carel J.A. Begeer.
17. Lambert Lombard. Liege, Self-portrait (1505–1566). Musee Communal; Liege. Copy Cat. Exhib. of Flemish and Belgian Art. 1300–1900. 1927. London.
18. Rembrandt, Dr. A. Tholini. Etching No. 188.
19. Q. Matsys, Antwerp. Formerly ascribed to Holbein, Etienne Gardener, Bishop of Winchester; Lord High Chancellor of England (1460–1531). Furstl. Lichtenstein Galerie.
20. Q. Matsys, The man in spectacles; presumably self-portrait (1466?). Stadelches Institut at Frankfurt on the M. Copy in Klassischer Bilder schatz No. 219.
21. Rembrandt, His brother Adriaan (1650). Copy Rembrandt in Klassiker der Kunst.
22. Rembrandt, Preacher: Jan Cornelius Sylvius (1645). Alte Pinakothek at Munich.
23. Roger van Brugge; (the master of Flemalle), "Pius Joachim" (1430–1460). Bust in Kunstamml. at Basel. Sometimes ascribed to the Nurnberg School. The name "Pius Joachim" is a later addition.
24. Hans Holbein; the Younger. Augsburg, Thomas Morus (1497–1543). Musee d'Aix en Provence. Copy at Mrs. Heymann's.
25. B.E. Murillo, Man in bow-spectacles with earloops (1618–1682). Property of the pictureshop of Dr. Benedict & Co. Berlin W. 9. Friedr. Ebertstr. 2.
26. Raffael Santi, Leo X. after 1516 (1483–1520). Palazzo Pitti; Florence.
27. Crayon-drawing after picture by A. Graffs von Arnold, Chodowiecki (abt 1780). From coll. M. Stechow. Berlin. Sale Boerner; Leipsic. Dec. 1919.
28. Sir Joshua Reynolds, Self-portrait (1723–1792). Kaiser Fridr. Museum; Berlin. Cf. copy 1637. Vollst. Beschr. Katal. 1911, as well as in die Meisterwerke des K.F.M. This picture is repeatedly found.
29. Goya, Self-portrait (1746–1828). Coll. Bonnat, Musee de Bayonne. Copy Gazette des Beaux Arts, 1903.
30. Fr. Pacheco. Sevilla, El Padre Luis del Alcacar (1599). Libro de Description de Verdaderos Retratas, de Illustres y Memorables varones. 1599. No. 31.
31. Fr. Pacheco. El Mo Frai Pedro de Valderrama (1599). Libro de Description de Verdaderos Retratas, de Illustres y Memorables varones, 1599. No. 211.

32. Velasquez 1599–1660, The poet Quevedo (abt. 1628). Copy in Velasquez Des Meisters Gemalde in 256 Abbildungen. Edit. Val. v. Loga. There is also an engraving of much later date, after this portrait, repres. in Allgemeines Historisches Portratwerk. Munich 1887.
33. Engraving by Corn. Mart. Vermeulen, after picture by C. de Croyer, Benedictus van Haeften (1632). Engraving in coll. de Lint. Only 3 copies of the painting are known.
34. Portrait-engraver Collier, Guillaume II (dit le religieux); Duke of Bavaria (abt. 1626). Gallerie Hist. de Versailles. Coll. Dr. de Lint.
35. Jacob Brill, Leiden. (1639–1700). Engraving in possession of Dr. de Lint.
36. Gerard Soeste, Sir Richard Rainsford. Cf. Connoisseur 1912. II. 150.
37. Daniel Chodowiecke. Drawing Museum Boymans No. 7.
38. Lawrence, J.J. Angerstein. Nat. Galery. No. 129. See Illustrations to the Catalogue. Vol. III.
39. Spanish School, Marquess d'Altamura (16th cent.). Pinakothekat Parma.
40. Theodore Bry, born at Liege; died at Frankfurt. 1505–1579, Hartungius (1528–1598). Bibliotheca Chalcographia.
41. Theodore Bry, born at Liege; died at Frankfurt. 1505–1579, B. Halerus. 1492–1536 (1528–1598). Bibliotheca Chalcographia.
42. Clement Ammonio. Bibliotheca Chalcographia.
43. Clement Ammonio. Capivaccius. Francfordy Anno MDCL. Title-page Volume II. Do. Vol. III. Frankfurt 1652.

Learned Men

1. Anonymous, Learned man in his library (1510). Woodcut; Copy at Mrs. Heymann's.
2. Geiler von Kaiserberg? Learned man (1445–1510). Woodcut from
"Brosamelein" 1517. Copy at Bock's. Xth. Intern. Ophth. Congr. Lucerne 1904.
3. Anonymous, Learned man writing on parchment-roll (1475). Woodcut from: Rudimentum Noviciorum. Lubeck, L. Brandis. Pict. 5. in Monogr. z. deutsch. Kulturgesch. Vol. VII. Also at Halauer's "The spectacles 100 years before and 100 years after the invention of printing".
4. Gerard Dou, Old man mending feather pen (1628–1631). Prov. Museum at Hannover; (oval). Coll. Dr. J. Simon, Berlin, Octagonal, Copy, cf. Martin.
5. David Terniers, The Astrologer (1652). Sale Rud. Lepke. Berlin 1910.
6. J. A. van Staveren, The Astronomer (died 1669). Sale Hugo Helbing 1925.
7. Jan Lievens, Learned old man (1607–1674). Coll. Holtzmann van Baarle van Romunde. Sale Roos 1905.
8. G. L. Keultjes, Old man reading. Water-colour after L. Bramer. Museum Boymans.
9. Sal. Koninck, Learned man in library (1609–1656). Rijksmuseum, Amsterdam. Nr. 1375.
10. Sal. Koninck, The Astronomer, Amsterdam School. Mun. Gall. at Dresden. Copy in Die Meisterwerke der Kgl. Gem. G. No. 1589 A.
11. G. Brekelenkamp, The Philosopher (1663). Etching J. de Frey, 1796. Coll. van Stolk.
12. Gerard Dou, The Astronomer (1645). Grossherz. Museum. Schwerin. Copy Martin.
13. Gerard Dou, The Astronomer (1650–1655). Vienna Gallery: Schonborn, Copy Martin.
14. Gerard Dou, Learned old man. Sold at Heberle's. Cologne. From coll. J. L. Menke in Antwerp 1890. Pict. Sale-catalogue.
15. Gerard Dou, The gold-weigher (1664). Paris. Louvre. Copy Martin.
16. Gerard Dou. (Attribuee), Learned man in his room. Coll. Barbier. Brussels. Sale June 1912.
17. Rembrandt van Rijn, Reading man. Black-and-white drawing from Albertina at Vienna. Copy Knackfusz. Kunstlermon.
18. Remb. v. Rijn, The money-changer (1627). Kaiser Friedrich Mus. Copy Knackfuss Kunstlermon 1924.
19. Gerard Dou, Rembrandt's father writing (1628–1631). London. Earl of Northbrook. Copy Martin.
20. A. Boonen, Hermit reading. Dresden Pict. Gall. Copy in Coll. Rijksmuseum, Prentenkabinet, Amsterdam.
21. J. de Herdt, The Antiquary. Pict. Gall. Karlsruhe. Copy in Coll. Rijkspretenkabinet.
22. Gerard Dou, The Village-notary (1670–1675). Lowther Castle. Earl of Lonsdaele. Copy Martin.

St. Bernardus and St. Bernardinus

1. Carlo Crivelli, St. Bernardinus of Sienna (1477). Louvre at Paris. Copy at Feldhaus's: Die Technik, etc.
2. Carlo Crivelli, St. Bernardinus of Sienna, painted between (1468–1493). R. Galleria di belli arti. Venice: (Academia).
3. Carlo Crivelli. St. Bern. of Sienna (1468–1493). Academia Florence. Copy at Greeff's. Kl. M. Aug. 1913. Also at Berlin and Milan. (Brera).
4. Giorlamo del Pacchia. Florentine School, St. Bern. of Sienna. St. B. of S (1477 after 1535. beg. 16th cent.). Alte Pinakothek at Munich. Coll. Leonce Rosenberg. Paris. Sale June 1920. Mak. Amsterdam. Bernardus of Sienna, Franciscan preacher, represented with radiating sun, on which I.H.S. in memory of his veneration of the Holy Name.
5. Cima. Giovanni Batista da Conegliano, called "Cima". The Descent from the Cross (abt. 1450–1517). Modena. Among the spectacles to the right St. Bernardinus carrying spectacle-case on his girdle. Copy Benezit I. page 753.
6. Pinturicchio, Glorification of St. Bern. of Sienna, between Ant. of Padua and St. Lewis of Anjou (1454–1513). Engraving of Simon after Fresco from the Life of St. Bernardinus; in the chapel of Bugalini at Santa Maria. Ara Coeli. Rome.

Hermit

1. Gerard Dou, Hermit (1650–1665). London Wallace Collection. Cf. Martin.
2. Leonhard Bramer, The Temptation of St. Anthony (1595–1674). Sale Coll. Kathe Lauber, Dorotheum, Vienna; 1910.
3. Gerard Dou, Rembrandt's father, reading Bible (1628–1631). Coll. Baron H. de Rothschild. Paris. Copy at Martin's.
4. Gerard Dou, Hermit reading (1665). Original disappeared. Etching by K. de Moor repres. in Martin: Gerard Dou.
5. Gerard Dou, The Hermit (1664). Ryksmuseum, Amsterdam. Copy, cf. Martin: Gerard Dou. Des Meisters Gemalde with 247 illustr. 1913. Copy: Les chefs d'oeuvre du musee, etc.

Doctor and Spectacles

1. Anonymous, Doctor looking through spectacles at a patient's fundament (1550). Kupfertichkabinet. Dresden.
2. Vinckebooms, Quack wearing spectacles (1578–1621). Kon. Mus. van Schoone Kunsten. Antwerp.
3. Anonymous, La Consultation (the consultation). Kunstbeilage 57 D.M. Wochenschrift 1910, No. 37.
4. Anonymous, Peasant at the quack's.
5. Corn. Saftleven, Shoulder-operation (1607–1681).
6. Pieter Jansz. Quast, Foot-operation (1605–1647). Mediz. Kunstkalender. Kruseman.
7. Bartolom. Sprangers, Satyr looking for thorns (1546–1625). Copy at Bock's.
8. Robert Nanteuill, The Parisian antimonial-struggle (1566–1666). Copy, cf. Hollander. Die Medizin usw. Fig. 209.
9. A. Durer, Caricature; doctor with urinal (1471–1528). Copy Hollander. E. Die Karikatur und Satire in der Medizin.
10. Jan van Bruggen, The village-chirurgeon (1649). Copy. Mediz. Kunstkalender. Kruseman. Copy in Spiegelbild by Lingelbach in Welcome Museum.
11. Lunders, Chirurgeon performing operation. Galerie Borghese; Rome.
12. Dutch Anonymous, The stone-cutter (16th cent.). Property of Dr. Nuyens; Amsterdam.
13. Jan van Heemessen, The stone-cutter (1550). Madrid. Copy cf. Hollander: Die Medizin etc. fig. 270.
14. Rombouts, The dentist (1660–1690). Prado Madrid. Copy Hollander. Die Medizin usw. Fig. 281.
15. Anonymous, Doctor Wurmbrandt (1648). From pamphlet 1648. Germ. Museum. Nurnberg.
16. Theodore de Bry, Emblemata Secularia (1594). Copy. Der Arzt und die Karikatur by C. Veth. Die Karikatur und Satire in der Medizin. 2nd Edit. Fig. 103. Holland.
17. Jan Steen, Stone-cutter (1660). Museum Boymans, Rotterdam.
18. Jan de Bray, Stone-cutter (1640). Museum Boymans, Rotterdam.
19. Anonymous, Medical consultation (1524). Painting on glass from the barbers' and hairdressers' club at Zurich. Property of Prof. Rud. Rahn. Zurich. Landes Museum Zurich. Copy at Hallauer's.
20. Anonymous, Heidelberg danse macabre (end 15th cent.). Woodcut. Copy: Der Arzt und die Karikatur by C. Veth. Cf. also Hollander E. Die Karik. und Satire in der Medizin. Fig. 24. 2nd edit.

21. Anonymous (Japanese). Doctor examining tongue of female patient. Copy at C. Veth's. Der Arzt und die Karikatur.
22. Anonymous, The Operation (17th cent.). English School. Copy. Kruseman Haag. Medizinische Kunstkalender. Orig. Welcome Hist. Mus. London?
23. De Bry, Interior of a barber's (1600). Kabinet Koburg.
24. G. M. Mitelli, Theriac-dealer with serpent (1634–1718). Copy at Bock's.

Alchemist

1. A. v. Ostade, The Alchemist. Nat. Gallery. No. 846.
2. David Terniers. Antwerp. (1610–1690). Coll. Goudstikker. Pict. No. 35, Cat. XXXV. No. 77. Cat. Exh. Rott. Art-circle. Dec. 1928.
3. Hans Burgkmair? Alchemist (1520). Woodcut from Peterarch's Mirror of Comfort. "Of the Alchemist's Folly."
4. Hans Burgkmair, Alchemist's Laboratory (1473–1531). Woodcut. Probably at Bock's.
5. Breughel. The Alchemist. Copy, cf. Kraemer: l'Univers et l'humanite.
6. Quinten Metsys, Alchemist. Castle on Isola Bella near Palanza.
7. Thomas Wyck, The Alchemist (1616–1677). Rijksmuseum, Amsterdam. No. 2727.
8. Mathan, Alchemist in spectacles (1600–1654). Black-and-white drawing on parchment. Rijksprentenkabinet. (Dr. Nuyens at Amsterdam).
9. Stradanus, Maker of gold and necromancer. Copper-engraving by Pr. Galle after Joh. Stradanus abt. 1570. Munich. Kupferstichkabinet.
10. David Teniers, The Alchemist (1610–1690). Rijksprentenkabinet, Amsterdam. Prob. Self-portrait. Copy. Medicinal Art-calendar. Kruseman. Formerly: Alte Pinakothek. Munich.

Handicraftsmen and Their Workshops

1. Jan Joseph Horemans, Shoemaker's workshop. Vienna. Gemaldegalerie No. 1232. Copy in coll. Rijksprentenkabinet.
2. J. Stradanus, Interior of a clockmaker's (abt. 1570). Copper-engraving by J. Collaert after Stradanus. Munich. Kupferstichkabinet. Copy Mummenhoff; Der Handwerker in der deutschen Vergangenheit.
3. Quirijn Brekelendam, Tailor's workshop (1620–1668). Sale coll. Jules Porges. Jos. Fievez, Brussels. 1919.
4. Quirijn Brekelendam, The shoemaker. Tableau de la civilisation. Orfevre excecutant un gobelet. (Picture of civilization. Goldsmith making a goblet). wears nail-spectacles 1523. (1620–1668 end 15th cent.) Sale Fred. Muller. Nov. 1910. Black-and-white drawing after original repres. by Mrs. Heymann. Goldsmith at work. Woodcut. Copy at Hallauer's.
5. Alessandro Fei, The Goldsmith's Workshop. Florence 16th century (Scala/Art Source).

Usurers

1. Mar. v. Rommerswael. Flemish School, Notary writing; in hinged spectacles (or usurer). Sale. 1895, at Heberle's, Cologne. Specimen resembling that of M. v. Rommersw. Presumably this is a later replica of a pair of hinged pinching-spectacles. Coll. Viscount Cobham, Stourbridge.
2. Jan Metsys, or van Reymerswaal, The Misers. l'Ermitage, Leningrad.
3. Mar. v. Reymersw., The money-changers. Royal Coll. Windsor Castle. (is looked upon as the original). De Witt Library showed the existence of 28 different versions. Copy. The Graphic Febr. '28. Hinge-spectacles.
4. Q. Metsys (or contemp. of his?), The money-changers. Col. Oppenheim. Sale March 19th. '28 at Rud. Lepke's Berlin. Literature cf. Art. Gemalde Stud. in the 2nd July number '19 of "Cicerone".
5. Mar. van Rommerswale, The money-changers (1497–1567). (later copy painted on wood). Here bow-spectacles. Probably this is the original after which the drawing from the coll. van Stolk was made, though here too, there are small differences. Sold by the Landes-museum, Darmstadt; Oct. 1920 at Lempertz's, Cologne. Completely identical copy in Cat. sale Kilner Kunst u. Auctionshaus 1919, where it was ascribed to Q. Metsys or Corn. van de Capelle, a pupil of Q.M.'s. Bird is lacking; for the rest copy of specimen in Royal Gallery of Windsor Castle. Q.M.
6. (after) Mar. van Reymerswaele, The usurers or pawn-brokers, also called the misers. Drawing after picture ascribed to Q. Metsys. The nail-spectacles of v. Rommerswale ahve here been changed into bow-spectacles. Atlas van Stolk. No. 297. Indication here: 1550–1600;

presumably much later, perhaps as late as beg. 19th cent. Painting from 18th or beg. 19th cent? Copy? In possession of art-shop Hugo Helbing at Munich. Original Royal Gall. of Windsor Castle.
7. v. Rommerswael, The misers. Museum Bologna.
8. v. Rommerswael (after) Q. Metsys? 1460–1530, The money-changer (active 1521–1528). Coll. Enea Lanfranconi. Presburg.

Miser and Death

1. Death and the Rich man (end 16th cent). English black-art picture after a German painting; end 16th cent. Copy cf. Hollander; Die Medizin in der klass. Malerei. 1923. Fig. 164.
2. Nic. Maes, The Miser and Death (17th cent.). Washed black-and-white drawing Sir Jos. Duveen. New-York. Copy Valentier.
3. Death of the Rich man (15th cent.). Gothic Gobelin tapestry. Hist. Mus. Basel. Repres. by Hallauer.

"Sight" from the Series "The Five Senses"

1. Gole, exc., Sight (1660–1737). Black-art pictures. Atlas van Stolk.
2. C. Dussart, inv., Sight. Atlas van Stolk.
3. I. Gole, fec. Van Tilborch, Sight. Museum Brussels.
4. Jan Fyt. 1611–1661 and Theod. Rombouts 1597–1637, Sight. Young man holding a pair of Nurnberg spectacles in front of an owl. Exh. Brussels 1910. Copy. Cat. coll. G. v. Gerhardt, Budapest. Sale Lepke Nov. 1911.
5. "Sight"—From a series of the Five Senses, Meissen Factory, Germany.
6. The Eyeglass Peddler. Meissen Factory, Germany. 1756.

Schoolmaster

1. Jan Steen, Boys' and Girls' School. Lord Ellesmere.
2. Quiringh Gerritsz. Brekelenkamp. The schoolmaster waling about (1651). Under the influence of Dou. Copy. Cat. Sale Coll. Jansen at Muller's Amsterdam 1927. Other copy Provinzial Museum, Bonn.
3. Jan Steen, The schoolmaster (1663). Copy. Cat. Sale. Coll. Janssen.
4. Q. Brekelenkamp, Writing-lesson. Muller, Amsterdam 1927.

5. A. de Bosse, Engraving of a school (F. de Wit, exudit, 1649). Atlas van Stolk.
6. Gerard Dou, The old Schoolmaster (1671). Dresden. Gemalde Gal. Copy at Martin's.
7. Hans Burgkmair, Woodcut. School. Teacher with fool's head and lute (15th cent.). Copy. Kulturgeschichtliches Bilderbuch. Georg Hirth. Munich 1913.

Spectacles in Still-Life Art

1. Vincent Laurensz. van der Vinne, Still-life with spectacles (17th cent.). Frans Hals Museum, Haarlem.

Sources Consulted for Appendix 5

Prof. Dr. Greeff (Berlin)
Prof. Dr. O. Hallauer (Basel)
Prof. Dr. Lundsgaard (Copenhagen)
Prof. Dr. v. Pflugk (Dresden)
Dr. W. Reis Dozent (Lwów)
Dr. Simon (Barcelona)
Prof. Dr. Weve (Utrecht)
Katalog Einer Bilderausstellung zur Geschichte der Brille (Amsterdam, 1929).

Appendix 6

Great Ophthalmological Collections of Vision Aids around the World

1. The American Academy of Ophthalmology Foundation Museum. San Francisco, USA.
2. The Zeiss Optical Museum. Oberkochen, Germany.
3. The Zeiss Optical Museum. Jena, Germany.
4. The Smithsonian's American Museum of History and Technology. Washington, D.C., USA.
5. The Pierre Marley Collection. Paris, France.
6. The Otto Hallauer Collection. University of Bern, Switzerland.
7. The Wellcome Collection. Museum of Science. London, England.
8. The American Optical Company Museum. Southbridge, MA, USA.
9. The Jonas W. Rosenthal, M.D. Ophthalmology Museum. Tulane University Medical School. New Orleans, LA, USA.
10. The British Optical Association Foundation Museum. London, England.
11. The H.S. Raybauld Collection, Natal Museum. Pietermaritzburg, South Africa.
12. The American Optometric Association Museum. St. Louis, MO, USA.
13. Bernard Becker Ophthalmology Library. St. Louis, MO, USA.
14. Museum of Spectacles. Piere di Cadore, Italy.
15. Rottesmuller Luxottica Collection. Agordo, Italy.
16. Kees Kortland Collection. Rotterdam, Holland.
17. Lancaster and Thorpe Museum. Derby, England.
18. Keeler Museum of Windsor. England.
19. Anglo-American Optical Company. London, England.
20. Dollond and Aitchison Museum. London, England.
21. Dixey Optical Company. London, England.
22. University of Waterloo Optometric Museum. Waterloo, Ontario, Canada.
23. Optical Museum. Hannibal, MO, USA.
24. Udo Timm Optical Museum. Podbielskistrasse, Hanover, Germany.
25. Church, Monastery and Museum of the Cloisters. Wienhausen, Germany.
26. Rathenow Museum. Rathenow, Germany.
27. Museum of Antique Glasses (Murai Company). Fukui City, Japan.
28. Jersey Museum. St. Helier, Channel Islands.

29. Musée de l'instrumentation optique. Biesheim, France.
30. Dr. and Mrs. Walter H. Marshall Exhibit. Gainesville, FL, USA.
31. Dr. and Mrs. J. William Rosenthal Collection. New Orleans, LA, USA.
32. Dr. Charles Letocha. York, PA, USA.
33. Dr. and Mrs. John Tull Collection. York, PA, USA.
34. Dr. Spencer Sherman Collection. New York, NY, USA.
35. Dr. Norman Medow Collection. New York, NY, USA.
36. Mütter Museum. Philadelphia, PA, USA.
37. Rosalind Berman Exhibit. Philadelphia, PA, USA.
38. Samuel Yale Cutter Collection. Philadelphia, PA, USA.
39. Teunisson Collection. Einthoven, Amsterdam.
40. Bascolm Palmer Library. Miami, FL, USA.
41. James Leeds Library. University of Indiana Optometry School, Indianapolis, IN, USA.
42. Frank Devlyn Collection. Devlyn Optical Company. Mexico City.
43. Museum of the Hospital de la Luz. Mexico City.
44. Dr. Jay Galst Collection. New York, NY, USA.
45. New York Academy of Medicine. New York, NY, USA.
46. Connecticut Medical Society Museum. Hartford, CT, USA.
47. Jeremy Norman and Company. San Francisco, CA, USA.
48. Boerhaave Museum. Leiden, The Netherlands.
49. Univerity Museum. Utrecht, The Netherlands.
50. Kees Kortland Collection. Rotterdam, The Netherlands.
51. Paul Aangenendt Collection. Waalre, Eindhoven, The Netherlands.
52. Museum of Optics and Eyewear. Stockholm, Sweden.
53. Nordic Museum. Stockholm, Sweden.
54. Private Ophthalmic Collection. Uppsala, Sweden.

Appendix 7

Concise Instruction in Grinding Lenses and Fitting Telescopes

By Gottlieb Christian Hilscher

Translated by Margaret F. Davison, Ph.D.

The author is indebted to Margaret F. Davison, Ph.D. for her translation from the German version. Dr. Davison states: "I have sought throughout to render a translation which is comfortably readable without, however, sacrificing too much of the style and manner of the early eighteenth-century original. Some passages, therefore, remain awkward. Still some others ambiguous. This is unavoidable given the orthographical inconsistencies typical of the period, as well as the stylistic, syntactic and semantic differences from contemporary Modern high German. One can easily determine from this description that these were not crude efforts, but were efforts based on mathematically and geometrically balanced formulas."

Hilscher's book contained three sections. Following are translations of the two sections relevant to the material covered in this book.

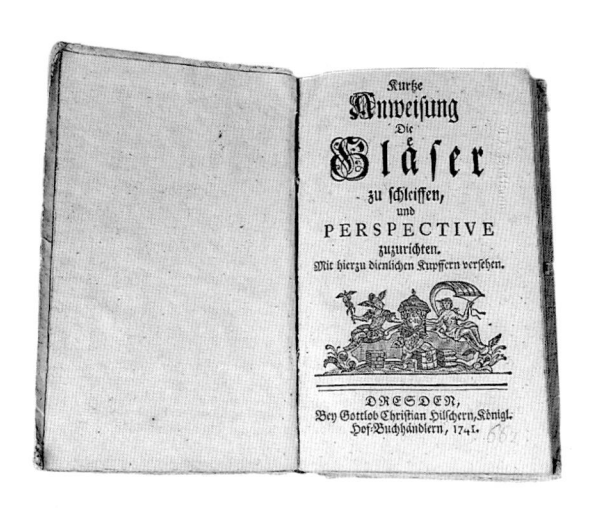

Figure 758. Title page of *Concise Instruction in Grinding Lenses and Fitting Telescopes*.

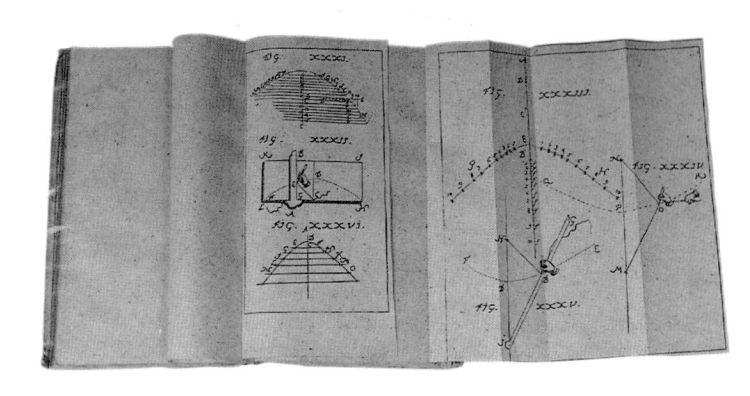

Figures 759–761. Steel engravings illustrating methods of lens grinding.

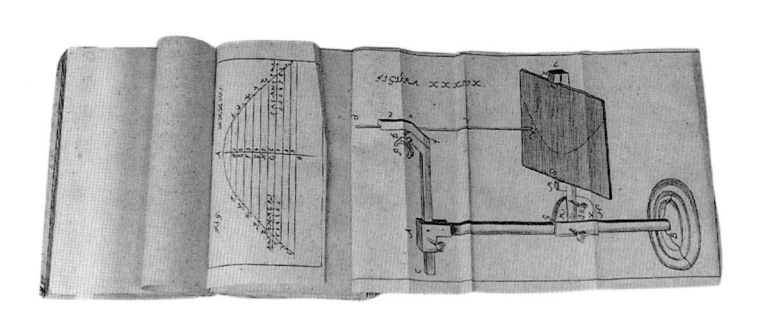

Figure 760.

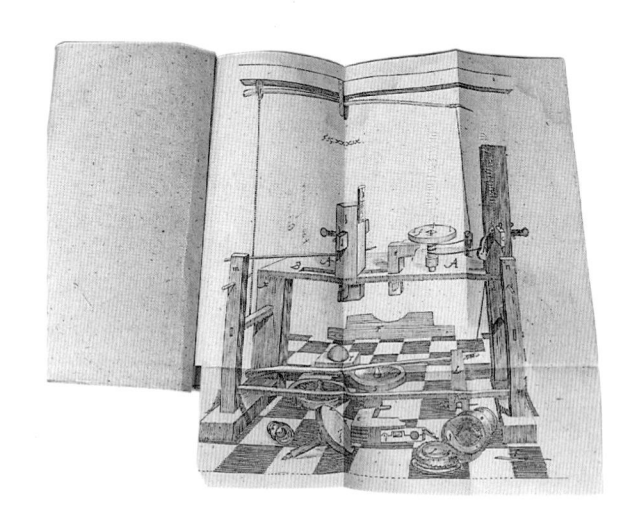

Figure 761.

468   APPENDIX 7

Concise Instruction in Grinding Lenses and Fitting Telescopes

Illustrated with Hereto Useful Copperplates

Dresden
By Gottlieb Christian Hilscher,
Imperial Court Booksellers,
1741

[Chapter I
Concerning Those Principles from Geometry Necessary for This Purpose]

Chapter II
On Conic Sections

In order to proceed to the purpose intended herein and to the so-called conic sections, it is necessary to know that we designate a cone, that which below is round and above tapers off to a point which, however, like a sugar cone, gradually loses its thickness; three features in particular of this form are to be observed in Figure 15: first the apex *a*, then the round base *bdklir,* then the axis *ac.*

From this round apex of the cone originate three graphic lines or strokes: an ellipse, otherwise called the small conic line or oval, herinafter designated with *ef;* the other, the hyperbola, the bent middle concave line ni, makes like-running or parallel lines with the axis *ae;* the third, the parabola or caustic line *ok,* runs parallel with *ab.*

Albrecht Dürer instructs in subsequent figures how to design this indicated cone as follows. First, for the ellipse, assume the cone *abd* and its base *bcde,* in Figure 16; from the *a,* he draws a vertical line down whose bad section is on the cone above at *f,* below at *g,* this section *fg* he divides with eleven points into twelve portions designated by *abcdefghikl.* Under this cone he then draws his base, whose center is *a,* and whose span around is *bcde,* and because a perpendicular has been dropped from the apex *A* to the center *A,* perpendiculars likewise fall from all divisions of the bad section to the base. When this has occurred, a compass foot is set within the cone into the perpendicular, at the height of the bad section *fg* of the point *a,* and at this height the compass is set with the other foot out on the line *ad;* this width is carried to the dropped base, and one compass foot is set into the center *a,* and the other into the extended line *a* and one draws base outwards toward the *d,* back to the line *a.* Thereafter the compass is set with one foot in the cone on the vertical line a, at the height of point *c* of the section *fg;* the other foot is set into the line *ad* and this same width is carried back to the base, and one foot of the compass is set into the center *a,* and the other onto the straight line *b* and one draws from there around toward the *d,* until again on the straight line *b.* One continues in this manner forth until at *d.* Then the compass is turned to the letter e, with one foot on the line ab, and one carries this down and draws in the base out of the center *a* around from the extended *e* towards the *d* until again at the line *e.* Thus one does through all marks and carries all things out of the upper cone into the base. Thereafter I make out of this base the plain line ellipse in this manner: I draw the length of the section *fg* vertically, as it then is divided with its eleven points into twelve equal planes, and I draw through all points eleven transverse parallels, thereafter I take the widths from the base onto the straight line *a,* and punctuate the widths at both sides, I do the same also through all letters. When these points are thus made all the way around, one then draws the oval ellipse, as it is designed on the side in Figure 16.

The parabola is to be made in the same manner, in as much as one draws the cone *abcd,* and therein the vertical line *a,* and cuts the parabola from the top downwards, until through the side *ab;* And this section shall be *f* above and *gh* below, as can be seen in Figure 17. I divide this line with eleven points into twelve equal planes, and cut transverse lines from all points in *fgh.* These same transverse lines I draw from the vertical line *a,* to the conic line or side *ad,* but those on the other side must stand; these I draw from the vertical line *a* to the lateral line of the cone *ab.* Thereafter I make the base of the cone under the cone, whose center is *a* and compass trace/circle (out)line is *acdf,* thereafter I have perpendiculars fall from all points through the round base, and designate them with their letters, as indicated with the ellipse. Then I take all widths in the cone, from the vertical line *a* to the two sides at all levels of the digits and letters, and carry them down to the base, and set the compass with one foot into the center *a,* and the other foot onto the straight line *a,* and draw out around towards the *d* until again at the line *a.* I do this on all marked lines, until I come completely to *gh.* Thus one has before one's eyes from this moment on the section of the parabola in the dropped base. In order that everything is finished, I make the line of the parabola or caustic line out of this base as follows: I cut a transverse line, place thereupon upright the height of the parabola marked with its transverse lines, thereafter I take out of the base the width *gh,* place this onto the transverse line, in such a manner that the vertical *f* stands in the middle, and I label these two points with *gh;* thereafter I carry from the base all widths through the mark of all straight lines, which are cut off by the compass trace/circle (out)line, to the vertical line *f* and punctuate them on both sides on all transverse lines so that the perpendicular *f* remains in the middle at all times. Then one draws the parabola or caustic curve from point to point, as it is designed in Figure 17.

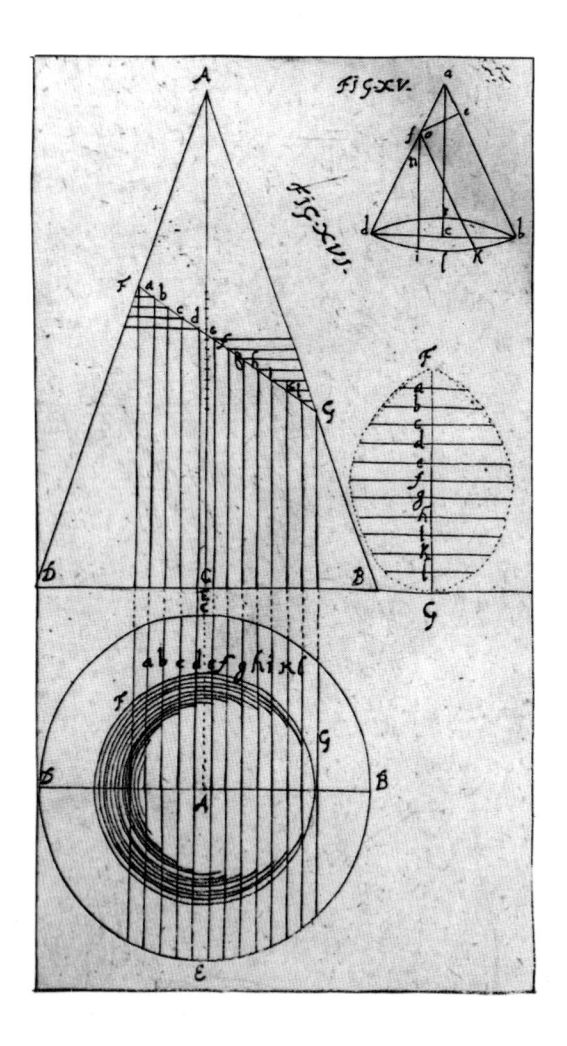

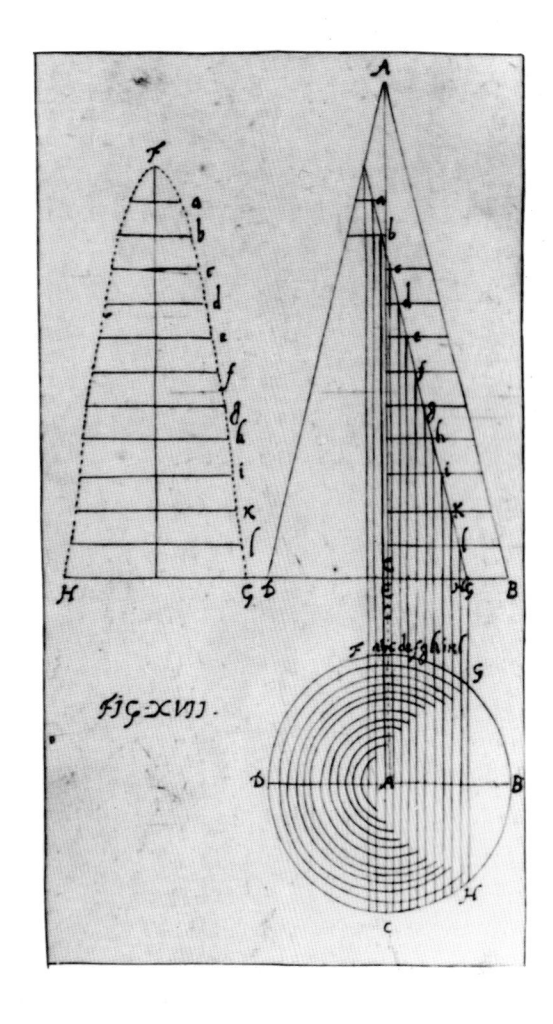

Mr. Albrecht Dürer proceeds no differently with the hyperbola, because again he draws the cone *abcde*, and in such line [he drops] the perpendicualr out of the point *a*; towards this [he draws] the hyperbolic line *FGH*, with which the side *D* is cut off; this is divided with eleven points into twelve portions, perpendiculars are drawn down, and again in the erected hyperbolic line *F* eleven transverse lines [are drawn], parallel and everywhere executed as already advised above.

(Mr.) Albrecht Dürer shows another way of designing the ellipse or oval, which is somewhat more general, and we therefore reasonably had misgivings about conveying it. Make a straight transverse line, let the beginning be *a* and the end *b*. Divide this with nine points into ten equal portions.

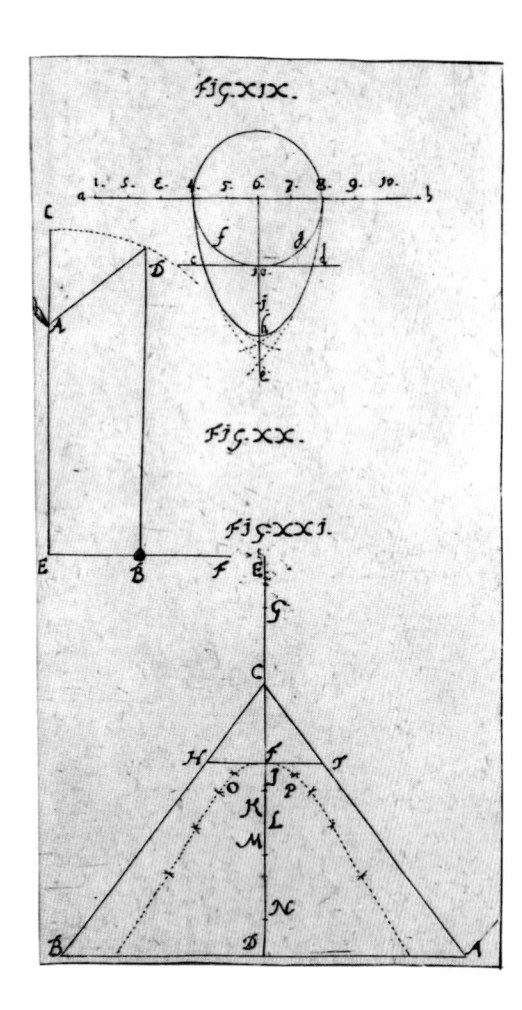

Thereafter place a compass with one foot in the middle of the line in point *5*, and with the other foot in point *7*, [and draw] around above and below. Thereafter place a compass with one foot in point *b* and with the other in point *3*, and from there draw around downward. Thereafter set the compass with one foot in point *a* and with the other in point *7*, and draw also from there downwards. Where the two round designs join, place an *e*. Thereafter draw under the transverse line a transverse parallel line towards the upper *ab*, and where the transverse line is intersected by the long round designs, in these same points place a *c* under point *3* and a *d* under point *7*. Thereafter draw a transverse line out of point *5* into the angle *e*, and where it intersects the transverse line *cd*, there one should see *10*. Thereafter divide the distance between *3* and *10* with a point *f* in the middle; thereafter divide the other distance between *10* and *7*, also in the middle with a little dot *g*. Then set a compass with one foot in the point *f* and with the other foot in point *d*, and draw down around through the vertical line *5e*. Thereafter set the compass with one foot in the other side in point *g* and the other foot in point *c* and draw down from there. Where the two curved lines connect on the vertical *5e*, there place an *h*. Then divide *h 10* into two equal planes with a point *i*, and set the compass with one foot in point *i* and the other in the compass trace/circle line *ch* on the shortest point so that you can reach it, and draw from there around until at the other section *hd*, as seen in Figure 19.

In continuation of the *Schwenterian Hours of Recreation*, (Mr.) Georg Phillip Haarsdörffer shows how to draw the parabola or caustic curve with a thread. in the 27th exercise in the second part of his *Continuation*, as can be seen in Number 20. Given that *A* is the focal point, *c* the depth, it can be assumed at one's discretion that *Ac* is the axis. Thus I can draw this line *AC* as far out as I want, and the basis of the same shall be *EF* [or: ..., and for the same reason there is line *EF*]. Now I secure in *A* the thread, which is as long as *AC, CE*. The other end of the thread *G* with the plumb bob I have running equal with *CE* at all times, and I begin at *C* with the graver, find the line *CD*, and continue this same line so it becomes the parabola or caustic curve. This is best done on a wall, since the plumb bob unimpeded indicates the perpendicular line of rest parallel with *CD*.

Just as the preceding can occur in many ways, thus also can, as in Figure 21, the hyperbola or concave line be determined in several ways, and taken shallower or deeper according to the nature of use. *ABC* make a triangle as desired, which is bisected by *ED*. Then set whatever depth you desire in *F*, and draw the line *HFT*, then set up *CH*, and determine *EC*, [come] back down again, and mark *CI*, likewise also *CF*, and determine the point *G*. From this point *G* all little transverse lines are measured, and drawn from point[s] *E* and *I*, and in this manner *OP* and all other little intersections are determined. Take points *LM* the same as *FH*.

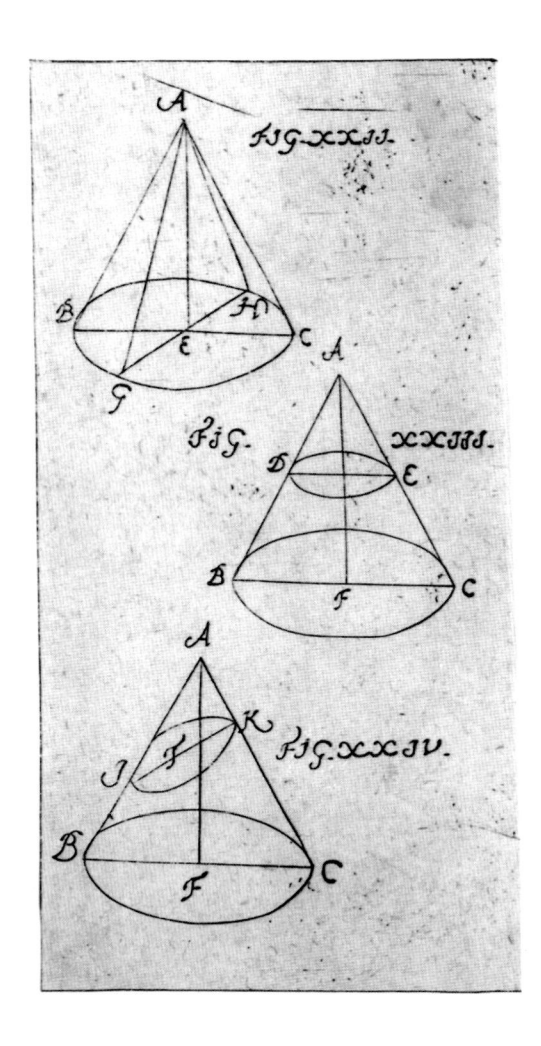

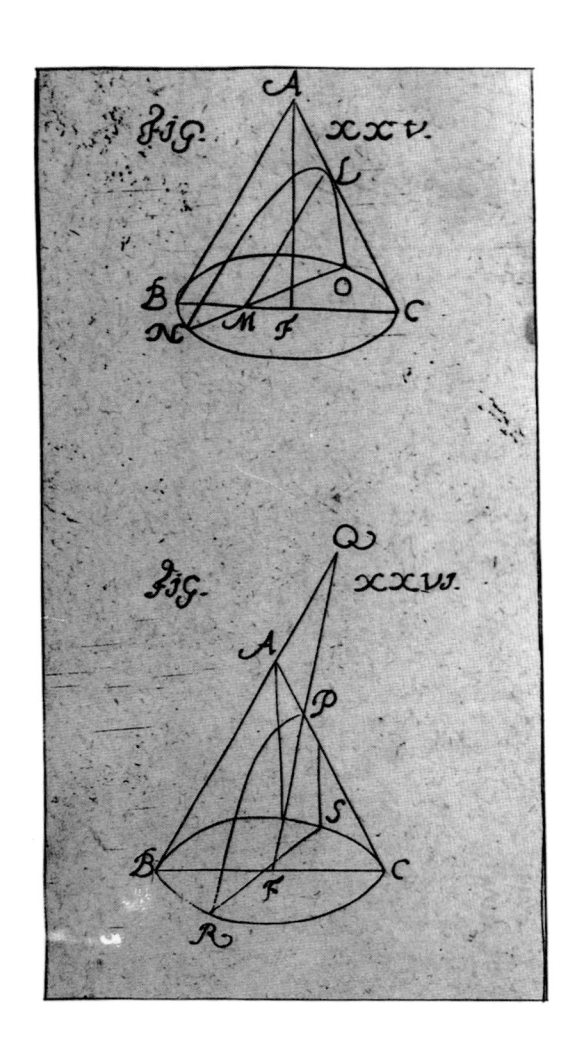

Father Traber, in his *Nervus Opticus*, Book 3, Chapter 25, divides conic sections in the following manner: A section, he says, is triangular, when the cone is cut from above to below, as to be seen in Figure 22, *ABC, AGH*. [The section is] a round circle, when, as seen in Figure 23, the cone *ABC* is cut by/at *DE* parallel to the base *BC*. He shows the ellipse in Figure 24 when the diameter *ITK* of the cone *ABC* makes the ellipse *IK* on the side *AB* as well as *AC* through the axis *AF* under the apex *A*, and is in no way parallel to the base. The parabola [results] in Figure 25, since the diameter *LM* intersects the side *AC* through the axis *AF*, and is parallel to side *AB*. The hyperbola [results] in Figure 26, since the diameter of the conic section *PF* intersects the side of the triangle *AC*, also the axis *af* extends the side of the triangle *AB* out to *Q*.

The rather famous Father Traber shows in the 3rd book of his *Nervus Opticus,* Chapter 25, Proposition 2, p. 205 and following, different manners of forming the ellipse; if the larger diameter of the ellipse is *AB,* and the smaller radius is *CD,* then the center can be found for both parts in *E* and *F,* insofar as the larger semidiameter *AG* or *BG* is permuted out

GRINDING LENSES AND FITTING TELESCOPES 473

E and *F*, then also the remaining *i h g s*, when they are permuted out of *E* and *F* into *OPQR*, will mark such points, and through such intersections the ellipse can thus be guided quite easily.

Some also draw the ellipse with a string or firm thread, because after the large radius *FD* and the small *FC* are marked, then they take the aperture of the larger radius, and bring such [the string?] to both sides out of *C* into *A* and *B*, this is secured with little nails, and with the graver *E*, in Figure 28, the string is directed around and around up to the circumference of the ellipse *DCEG*.

Others do it nearly more adeptly through an equal-angled cross-ruler *ABCD*, whose arms are long or short according to the size of the ellipse one wants to mark. For small figures a pasteboard is sufficient, the length of any half shoe, in the middle of such arms is a slit lengthwise, in order that the two sliders *EF* cannot deflect or, moved to and fro, cannot fall out/ be omitted, as seen in Figure 30. In order that the ruler *GH* be well secured, two rings are necessary, according to the size of the ruler, which are square and affixed above. When this is done, direct the ruler around, and in this manner the ellipse is marked, which is more dull or pointed according to whether the sliders are closer to or farther from each other.

In the third Proposition said Father Traber also instructs how to define the parabola in the following manner: For the axis of the parabola, take the perpendicular designated with *e* in Figure 31 [?], whose middlepoint is *B*; divide this same above in the direction of the apex into equal portions, for example eight, however should a larger segment be desired, take the remaining half from *B* to *c* as well, and divide it also into eight equal portions; through these sixteen points parallel lines are drawn, as the figure indicates. When this is done, I take the uppermost half towards the apex, permute this out of *b* into *d* and remaining points up to *E*; I then draw *D* out of *B* to the apex *A*, again out of *B* I draw out of Nr. 1 next to *D* again to *E* [*F*?] and so further, out of Nr. 2 into *G* & *c*, all these sections show how to form the parabola. However, because eight points still remain for the other part, I continue with one compass foot in *B* and mark with the other *OPQR*, until sixteen points are finished.

Figure 32 shows how to accomplish this mechanically as well. Assume a panel *HIKL* whose side *KL*, like the straight-

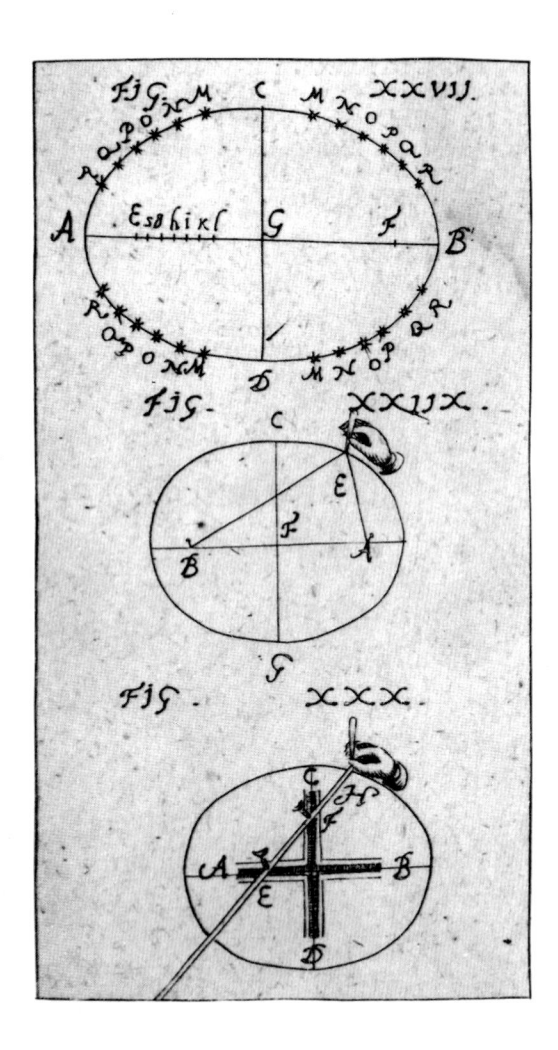

of the point *C* in(to) *E* and *F*, out of which one must draw all points because of the span around the ellipse; thus namely in the larger radius between *E* and *G* as desired the points g *h i k l* are drawn, the more of these there are however, the more exactly the ellipsis can be drawn. After this the aperture *AI* is taken out of the center *E* and *F* and carried toward *M* to the four points above and below, the same [for] the opening *BI* out of the center *EF*, thus are the preceding points in *M* intersected crosswise. If one takes of this figure at the points and intersections at *N* the apertures *BK* and *AK* out of the center

474   APPENDIX 7

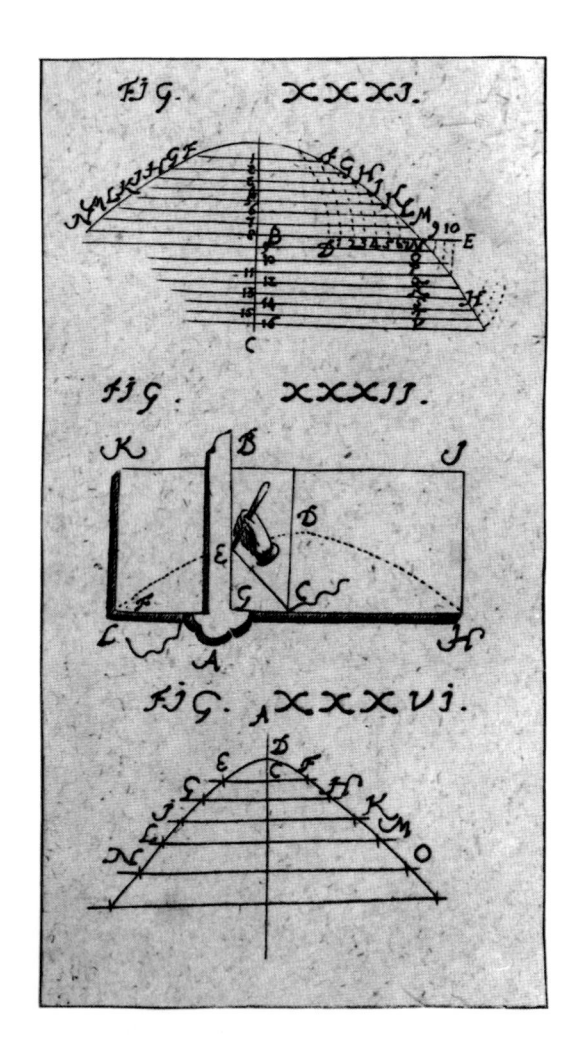

edge *AB* makes a correct perpendicular, so that also *BGL* is a straight angle; in addition one would need a string *CEG,* which is secured at *c*[*e*] and at the point of the straightedge *G* in such a manner, that it would touch the tip *D* doubled, one directs this string then in this manner further around, as shown in Figure 28 with the ellipse.

(Mr.) Caspar Schott, in the 7th book of his *Magia Optica* in the 2nd chapter, also points out the following method of marking the parabola: One draws, as seen in Figure 36, the straight line *A* down perpendicularly, takes thereon the middlepoint *c* of the reflection at a distance from *A* as desired. However, the further *c* is from *A*, the farther the mirror will reflect, one divides the section *Ac* in *D*, which becomes the apex of the parabola. Underneath *c* one draws straight lines, as many and as far apart from one another as one desires, but which after the perpendicular *A* make equal angles, for example *e, f, g, h, i, k, l, m, n, o*, and so forth. The closer these straight lines are to one another, however, the easier and better and also preciser the caustic line can be made. Take the size *A* with the compass, and set its foot in *e* and mark with the other foot here and there two points *G H*, and proceed in this manner to mark other points *IK, lM, NO*. Hereafter draw at both sides through these dots a curved line, thus is the parabola more finished.

Said (Mr.) Schott includes yet another method: Again the straight line *AB* is drawn, Figure 37, and it is divided at will into equal portions; the bigger these are, the bigger will be the caustic line as well, but the smaller they are, the more precise but also smaller the caustic line will fall. Through all these points straight lines are drawn, which, however, also fall perpendicular calculated against line(s) *AB,* and places numbers as desired. One foot of the compass is set in point *C* so that the end is on the perpendicular *AB* of the sixth portion; the other is set in *A*, and on both sides in *i*, again out of *I* on both sides in *P*, in this manner the planes will be equal to the little plane *CA*, between *CI* as well as between *IP*. Divide the little plane *IP* into six portions, which are equal to the portions of the straight line *CA*, and mark them with numbers, as these are seen in the Figure. And when one foot of the compass is set in *C*, then place the other in the point *K*, and in the first aligned, and draw on both sides two points *TT;* and in turn when one foot is set in *C,* then extend the other into the other dot *L* and draw the dots *uu*. In the same manner, when one compass foot is set *in M*, draw *xx* on both sides. *yy* is drawn out of *N*, and out of *O* the points *zz*, the points *PP* have already been drawn. Hereafter when one compass foot is set in *C*, then turn the other one in *Q*, and draw at Nr. 7 the dots *aa*, and out of the point *R* mark the points *bb,* and continue at will thus further through the apex *A*, and each of the points ordered on both sides, the parabola or caustic line is then drawn. To mark the hyperbola, however, Father Traber teaches in Proposition 4, here Figure 33, in the following manner: Take on line *AB* the middle *C* above and below, according to how pointed or broad the hyperbola should fall, take the points *D* and *E* in the same aperture, so that they then also are equally distant from *C*, just like the points *A* and *B*; then take yet other points as desired, as here at *f*, however [in such a manner] that these narrow together after the apex, and downwards stand farther apart from one another. Then take one or, to proceed more quickly, two compasses, of which one is set in *D*, the other in *E*, the two other feet come together in the point *f*. In the same aperture set one one compass foot in *A*, the other in *B*, so that both feet come together in *GH*, at the very place where little crosses/intersections are made for the remaining rendered sections. I take further the points *AB* out of *D* and *B* toward *f*, and this so often until the points of the hyperbola are sufficiently drawn. Others make a hyperbola, as shown in Figure 34, with the help of a string, or silk thread, or doubled smooth little cord, according to whether the hyperbola should fall larger, whose end is secured at *N* and *M*, and joined together at *P*, and held together with the help of a needle-eyelet; when the needle *O* is now drawn out of *P* back to *R*, *PR is* drawn on one side of the hyperbola. One does the same as well at *PQ* on the other side.

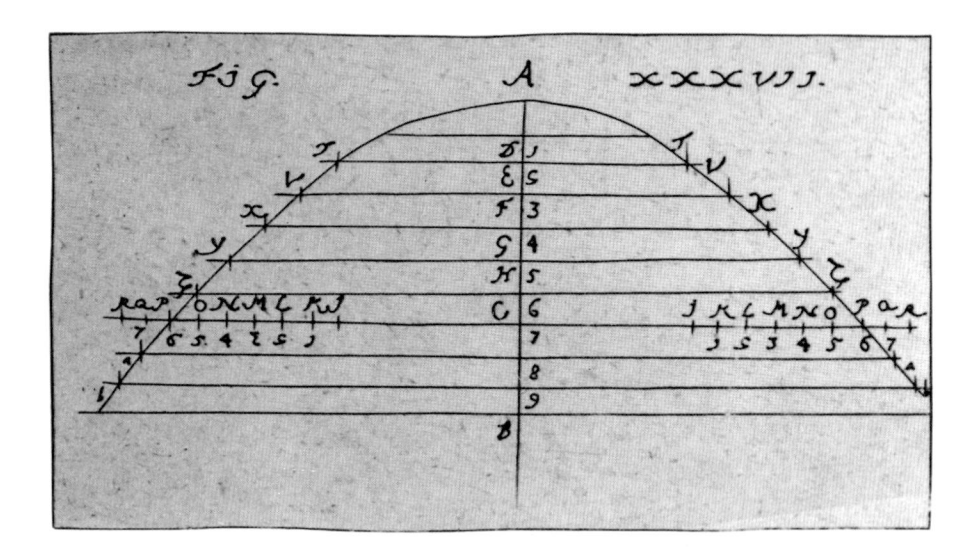

Some do this more adeptly with the help of a rule. The line *HI* is first made, as indicated in Figure 35, according to whether the hyperbola should be more pointed or broad; at *H* a string is attached, and at *I* the rule [is attached]. When the string touches the apex of the hyperbola at *e* [*c*?], and the remaining section of the same secured at *G*, with the graver the string held secure to the rule at *B*, and directed toward *E*, so will occur the drawn hyperbola.

Lastly, Father Traber also mentions an instrument, Figure 38, which he has made in Vienna, to draw all conic sections. For such a square rule *AB* is first necessary, at which part *A* there is yet another piece of wood, also square, yet attached generally/radically at both sides, so that the other rule *CD* can be held [?] and moved, finally at *D* another piece of wood is attached, to which that at *FU* is suited, then joined together with *P*. In the hole *EU* again an engraving is made, at/with which lastly a pencil [is] to draw the figures. In the middle of the rule *AB* a square piece of wood is attached in a way that it can be slid upwards and downwards, at whose inner part *I* the half compass is attached, on which another square ruler *KL is* attached at *K*, and secured at *X* in such a manner that it can be moved compasslike; on this last rule are the two small

GRINDING LENSES AND FITTING TELESCOPES 477

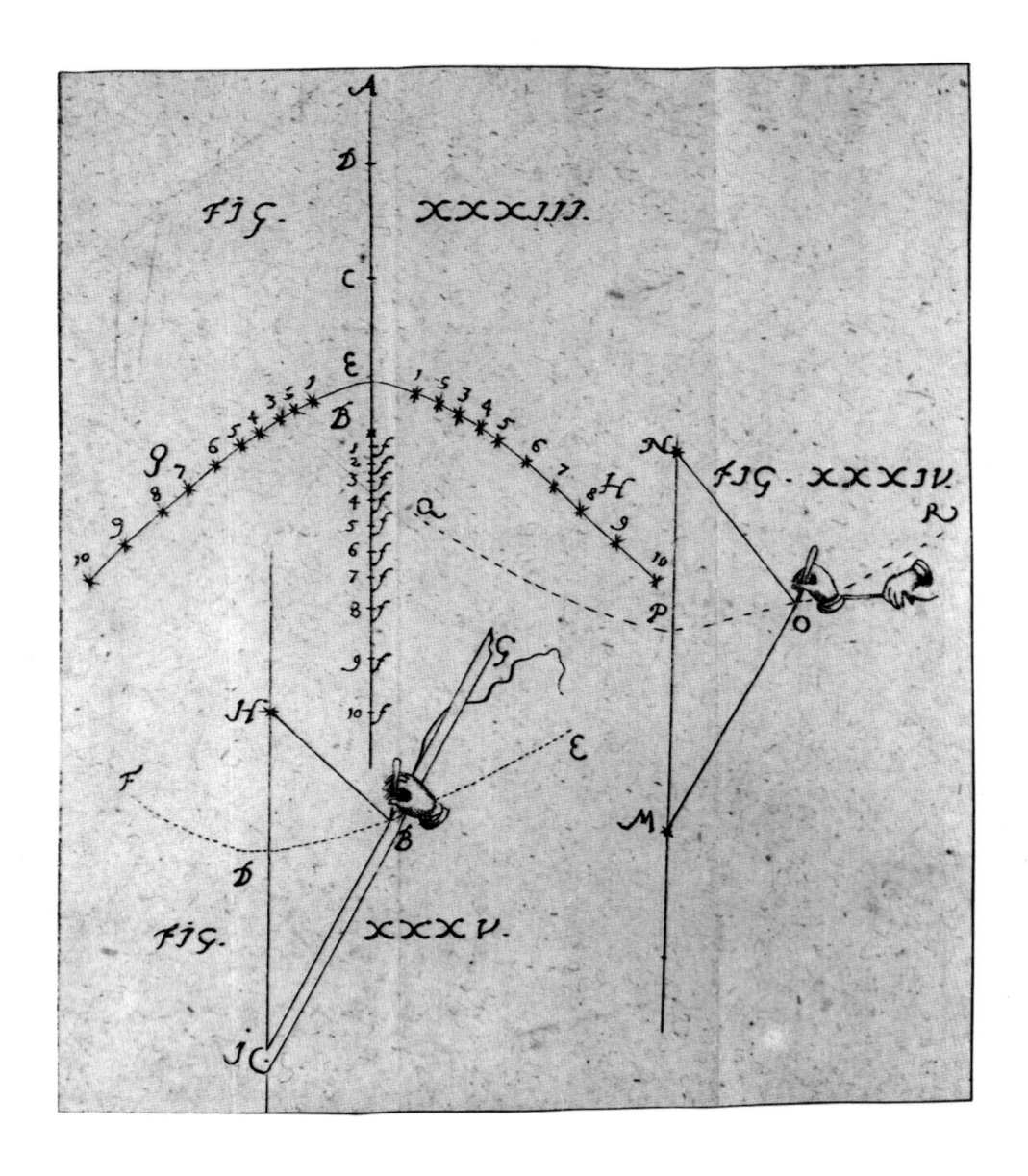

pieces of wood *MN,* which contain a board resembling a square. When now the pieces are well put together, and the board *ST* is well secured, then the rule *CD* can be slid in at *A* long or short as desired, and so directed/joined, that the conic section can be drafted with the part *QR* on the designated board.

Chapter III

On Options for Grinding, Polishing, and on Seating of Lenses in Telescopes

Venetian glass is best for this work, particularly the clear white, free of granules, bubbles and flaws, although it causes no real problem if the glass is somewhat green. One can use the pieces of the very well polished mirrors, which are very clear and translucent and without streaks, that which is well suited to rubbing and grinding is better than that [which] cuts well, such as can be obtained in Regensburg, even though Venetian glass is the best. Concerning the external form, the so-called lens-shaped glasses are equally level either on both sides, or only on one, with the other side either convex or concave. Some are convex or concave on both sides; some are convex on one side, concave on the other, and these in either spherical, elliptical, parabolical or hyperbolical manner. Lastly, according to their convex or concave form, some result from one type of section-cut on one side, from another section on the other. [Translator's note: This last sentence reads in the original, *Letztlich auch nach ihrer bauchigten oder eingehöhlten Form einerseits aus einem solchen, anderseits wfederum aus einem anderen Schnitt.* The terms *einerseits* and *anderseits* render the sentence, indeed the paragraph, ambiguous. *Einerseits-anderseits* normally denote "on the one hand-on the other hand," meanings which make little sense in this context, particularly as juxtaposed with the term *wiederum,* which can mean "on the other hand." Therefore, the translation "on one side-on the other side" seems more appropriate, even though in this paragraph and elswhere "on one side-on the other side" is written more normally as separate words, e.g.: *an einer Seiten.* Thus, this paragraph seems to be describing both converging and diverging meniscus lenses.]

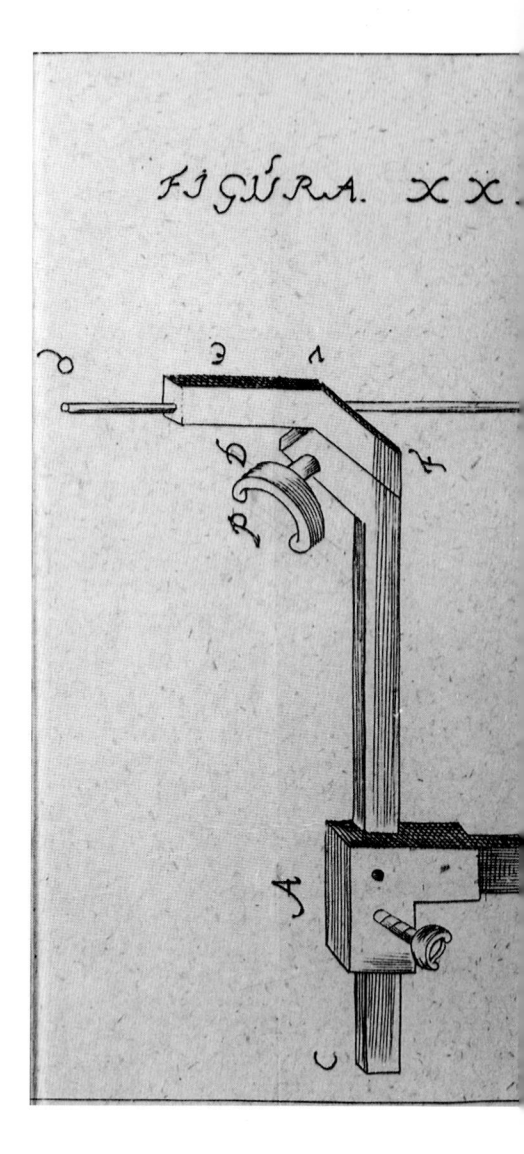

478   APPENDIX 7

GRINDING LENSES AND FITTING TELESCOPES 479

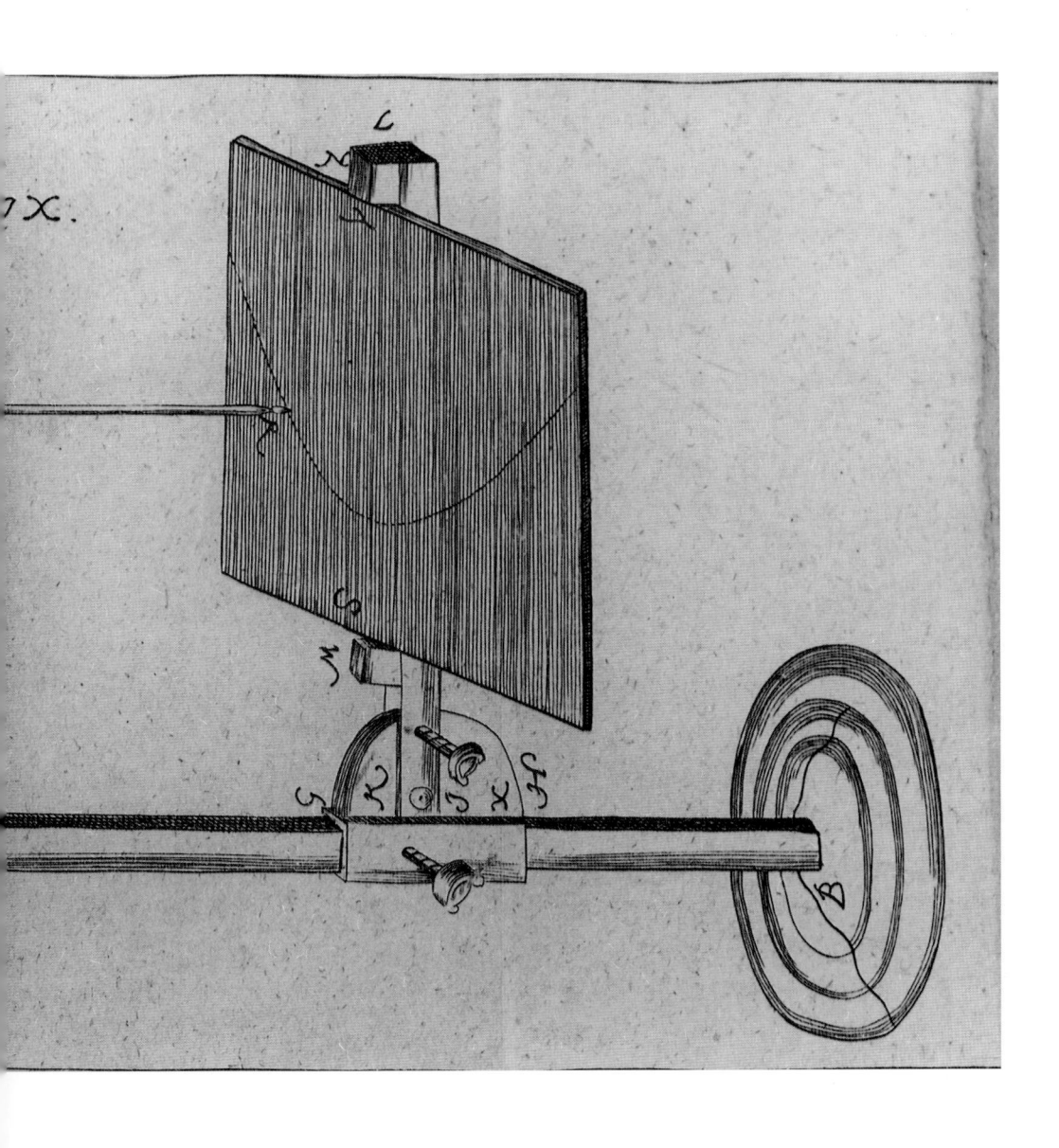

The size, width and breadth of such lens-glasses are taken from the circle, which is the base of all such forms, whose size is displayed by the diameter or middle intersection at both sides. The height [is] the perpendicular from the middlepoint to the circle. The thickness is [determined] by the greater or lesser height. The surface [is determined] according to the radius, from which the lens is a particular section. The roundness [is determined] by the relationship of the diameter and the radius to the circle. One lens may well be thicker than the other, but not therefore rounder, because the sections of small circles are rounder than that of larger.

Lenses which are equal and level on both sides are best for maintaining and strengthening the sight of young people, because the eyeglasses that enlarge are not always the best for sight, and one should therefore not begin using eyeglasses without great need. The other concave and convex glasses serve not only for old people, but for telescopes and reflectors as well. Concave lenses make distant objects clear to see; convex presents those closer. With concave lenses one can see clearly even the smallest thing, with convex however it seems larger but hazy. When one combines both, then one can see distant as well as close things clearly. There is also a difference in the concave lenses themselves: the less round and the larger the section, the shorter the distance one can see; on the other hand, the rounder they are and the smaller the section, the keener the sight.

The beginning of lens grinding is the preparation of the little dishes in which they will be formed through grinding; these are made out of lead, tin, copper, brass, iron or steel with a tin founder or red brass [brass and bronze] founder, or they are made mechanically. The former take on the forms more exactly, the latter retain them longer, and these are then either flat, or they are spherical, concave, or convex, elliptical, hyperbolic or parabolic. If the surface of such type of metal is prepared to some degree, then one can determine what is still lacking by means of a fine rule, and the two surfaces resemble one another so closely, that neither is much lacking of anything; if one rubs them both over with emery, as one hand washes the other, then they bring themselves during this manner of rubbing to the proper completeness. If one has a level whetstone, it will also be helpful to grind one after the other on it. For the concave dishes it is first of all particularly necessary that the section (according to which they are made) has its circle/roundness accurate, for if this is not the case, considerable trouble will later arise; Thereafter have a round concave and convex form made by a turner out of a good piece of hard wood, in such a manner that a hole is retained through which to pour some such material as is added with steel mirrors, and joins such together. The material for the steel mirrors, however, as far as this work is concerned, can be this: a half pound [250g] English tin, a quarter pound *Wissant* [?bismuth?] or marcasite, and a quarter pound saltpeter, melted together. With the convex dish one proceeds also in this manner. Some make the desired section with the instrument illustrated in Figure 44, out of paperboard or wood, more durably however out of tin-plate, which, when actually cut through, yields the concave as well as the convex form. Then prepare a viscous glue out of potter's clay, weak beer, horse manure, calf's hair and eggwhite, which is all well kneaded together, and make with both tinplates the concave and convex forms, and pour into them whatever metal you wish, this will subsequently be better finished with all manner of fine files, such as noted in Figures 42, 45, 46 and 47, as can be read in (Mr.) P. Schott, Book 10, Article 4, Chapter 1, pages 496 and following in the German edition, the same in (Mr.) P. Traber, Book 3, Chapter 24, Annotation 3. (Mr.) P. Schott teaches in the location just mentioned how to make a four-cornered box, without roof or floor however, so large that it will hold the wooden plate within it, as seen in Figure 43; one places this box over a board, which will serve in place of a bottom, and yet can be removed at will, and places thereupon, according to the measurement of curve *CD* in Figure 42, the concave wooden plate filed with the curved-file, in such a manner that the plate ascends in the box four fingers high over the plate(s). When this is done, sifted wet ashes are thrown into the box and plates until the box is filled to the top, and when the ashes have settled well, the box is covered with another board and turned upside down, the first board is removed, and the wooden plate is removed with the gently inserted tip of a knife; thus there will be in the ashes a convex model of striking likeness for a future pouring usable plate.

The wood in which the lens is held, must agree exactly in circumference and center with the circumference and center of the lens. The material, however, with which one putties, is the following: Take yellow pitch/cobbler's wax, resin and chalk, the former in equal parts, the latter half as much; let the resin and pitch melt in a brass/bronze pot, but over a medium flame; when it is hot add to that the finely grated chalk, and mix well; hereafter it is the custom to pour in also some Rhenish spirits [schnapps or brandy from the Rhineland], (some also mix in with the chalk half a walnut shell full of Venetian glass), when this is all well mixed, one pours it into a wooden vat which has been filled with fresh springwater, and lets it cool, then one pours the water off and it is then ready.

Concerning the turning lathes on which the glasses are turned and, in turning, ground, we have shown three such here. The one in Figure 41 is a small hand instrument of a renowned Jesuit, which is finely made out of hard metal to screw onto tables while traveling: stones can also be ground with this easily and practically; above at the tip the dishes are attached, and puttied on, the glass is also securely puttied onto a piece of wood and then turned. This figure is so clearly drawn that it requires no further description. The turning lathe in Figure 40 is also for such glass-grinders, and although the drawing is not of the best proportions, the figure is nonetheless clear and shows how this turning lathe is peddled in the manner of a spinning wheel, and thus the lenses are ground in a manner as one now and then encounters at turners. The turning lathe in [Figure] No. 39 is that of the renowned Hevelii, whose words we print here from his *Selenographia*, because it is rather garbled and confused by Kohlhansio in his *Tractatu Optica* page 352 :

[Latin, pp. 31–32]

P. Traber shows how better to prepare the convex lenses in *Dioptr.*, Book 3, Chapter 24, VII, as illustrated in Figure 48: secure to a table the board *ABcd*, on the side of which rod *f, g*, has been attached perpendicularly (it can also be fastened above on the cover *G*), in the middle of board *K* is attached a well-prepared dish, above the center of which [is] a rod with a steel pin, which can be revolved. Thereafter, *L* and *M* are joined together, and the lens is thoroughly shaped by the pin. To prepare the concave lenses, however, [Traber] instructs in Annotation XI, p. 201, as Figure 49 shows, that the glass be secured to a table or board and should be hollowed out with the instrument *DB*, onto which for this purpose a round ball,

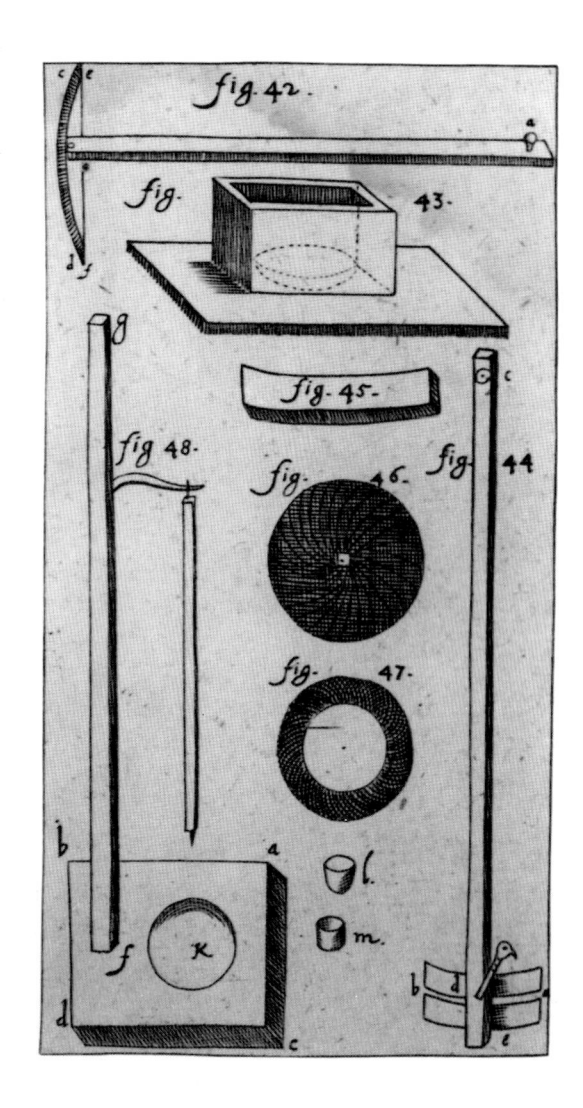

482   APPENDIX 7

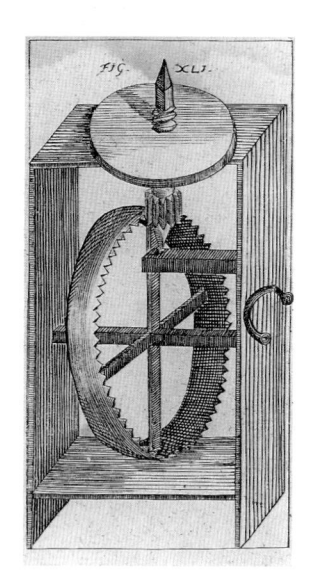

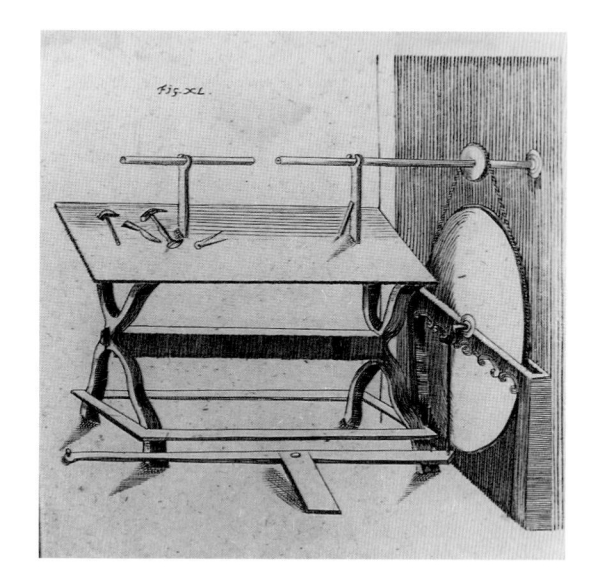

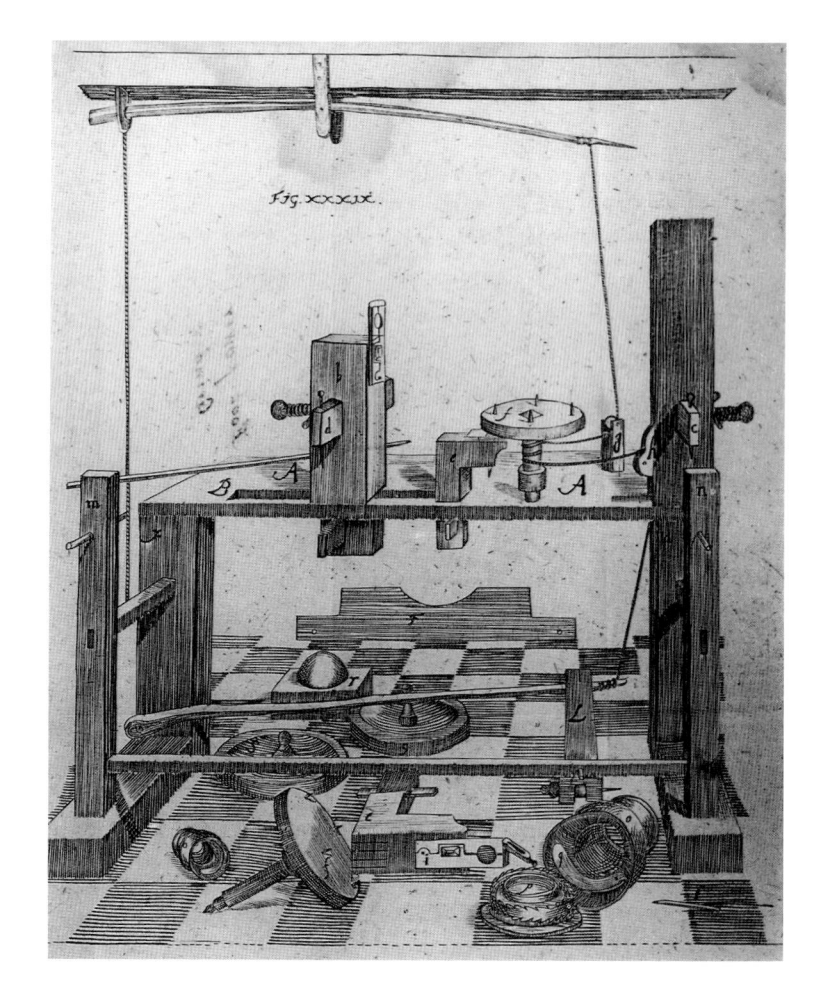

The grinding occurs with either sand or emery. The emery is well-washed and cleaned. Buy such emery as the stone cutters had and used, then fill two vessels half full with clear water, and then put into one of them as much emery as estimated to be enough. When one person now stirs the water continuously until the emery is completely wet and the finest of it rises, another shall with an appropriate vessel draw off the water with the rising fine and thin emery, [and] let it stand and settle until the coarser sinks to the bottom and the finer is toward the top. When the emery has been thus floated off into the fourth or, depending on the nature of the emery, the fifth vessel, then it is suitable and usable for grinding; the standing water is poured off and the emery is somewhat dried off.

Such moistened emery, even though it may look like gruel/mash, is put into the dish in which one intends to grind the lens. If it becomes somewhat dry during grinding, it is wet a bit again, though should there be too much water, more emery can be added as judged.

Antonius Schirlæus de Rheita and also P. Traber use instead of the emery the well and finely sifted sand, which they put dry into the dish; and when subsequently the glass takes the shape of the dish, then (Mr.) Rheita takes the same sand and moistens it if has become finer during grinding.

(Mr.) P. Traber, however, uses the red moistened sand [rouge] from the hourglasses or clocks, and grinds both until no more sound is made and the sand has become black.

One must be careful, however, not to heat the lens too much during grinding, since it can be cooled with water, or set it aside as one works meanwhile on something else, or one waits; although one would hope the heat will not so easily damage the putty described above. One polishes generally with rottenstone, which is somewhat better for this purpose than the tin-ashes. Test whether the rottenstone is good with the tongue, whether it is rough like ashes or, rather, more like flour, because it is best that way; and because there are often hard grains in it, it is necessary to watch out for that; it is finely scraped off with a knife and moistened, and also guarded that nothing is added/that nothing gets in it. When the lens has been ground, it is dried with deerskin or felt, and polished over a secured piece of wood formed like the lens. Indeed, this is practically best done on a tin dish, because tin lends itself to

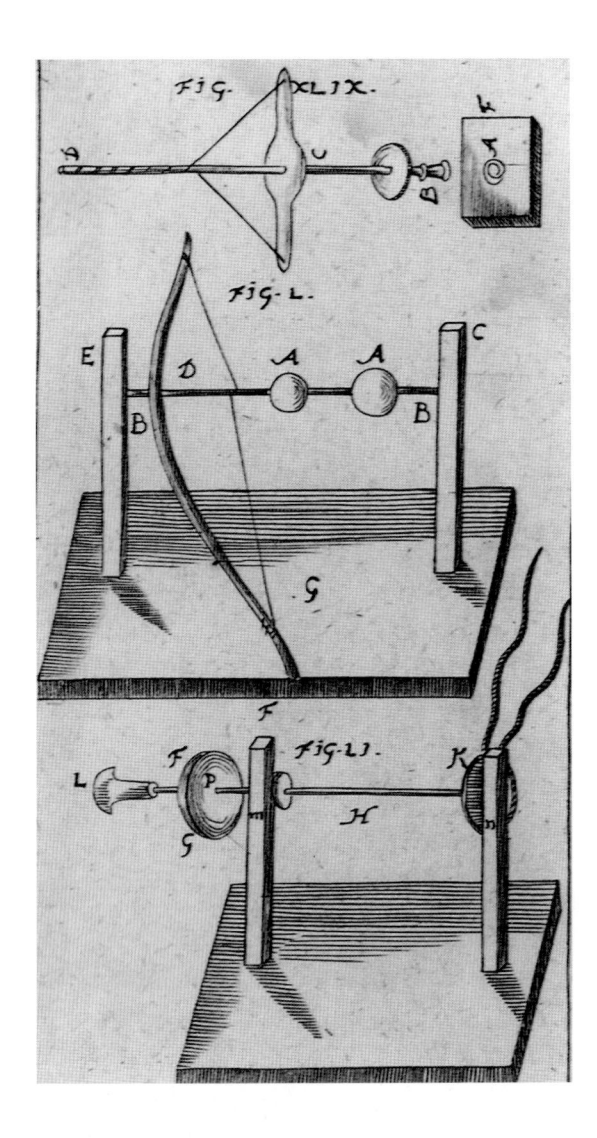

according to the size of the lens, is attached at *B*. He demonstrates a yet more convenient method of preparing this with an iron or metal ball *A*, in Figure 56, which is attached to the iron axis *B* and moved to and fro with a somewhat slack string *D*, that the glass is thereby hollowed out. Lastly, he considers it to be the best method to prepare this with a lead plate *FG*; in the shape of a spherical lens, and as large as the diameter, through which at *P* the iron rod *mn* goes to *HK*, and when this is turned around with the slack string described above, it will give the lens the best form.

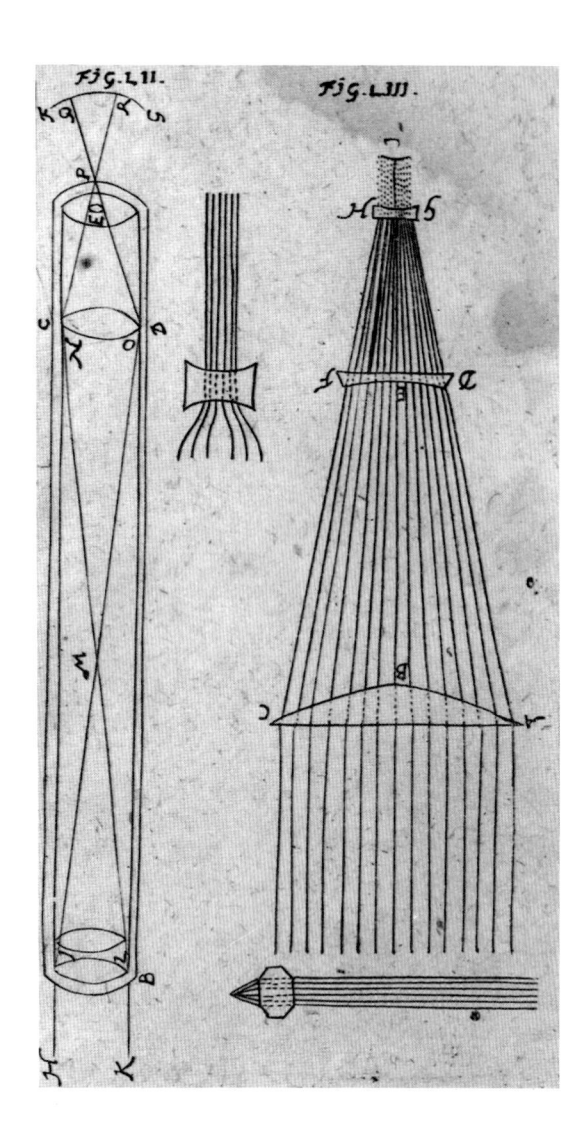

polishing by nature. The concave lens is polished on the turning lathe, or with a sphere prepared according to its form. For grinding some praise also the *fuliginem tartari*, willow or juniper ashes, but one is free to have a preference.

The telescopes with which one can observe the planets are made thus, see Figure 53. If *ABC is* the largest lens, flat on top and ground according to the elliptica underneath, hereby the rays are collected in great number, and held apart by/from the lens *AEF* as well by/from the third lens *GH*, until they are ultimately driven together in the center of the eye *I*, whose tube is not larger than the eyeball. One can arrange even more of these lenses in such a manner and lengthen the tube to 30 or 40 shoes. The curved-in glass collects the rays, the uncurved one distributes them. P. Traber represents this in the following figures for Figure 52.

[Description of telescopes in Figure 52, followed by the procedure for placing lenses in the telescope body, pp. 32–39.]

Three-Part Appendix

To conclude these instructions in lens grinding, we wanted to add as a three-part appendix this description of the following instruments.

The first [description] is of an instrument, as illustrated in Figure 57, which a well-known painter in a famous princely residence presented as his own brand-new invention, for which he claimed great advantages, and from which he further looked to profit greatly; until he was confronted with it by a certain person, not only in [the works] of Schwenter, Schott and Kircher, but also from the works and drawings of Albrecht Dürer, and thus [was] he rather shamed before art lovers.

The instrument consists, however, of the following: A clear mirror-glass is slid into the frame *abcd*, and this is placed securely onto the foot/base *ef*, hereafter a four-cornered piece of wood is slid in under *g*, into which in turn another is brought under *i*, and on this at *k* a sight with a small hole through it is fixed. Behind this pane one sets, as seen in *Lit. I*, the piece one wishes to paint, and looks through the aforementioned sight where everything is presented on the glass. In order that one might write on this with a finely ground red-chalk pencil, it is well brushed with thin rubber-water using a small brush, and then allowed to dry.

It also possible to brush it with vinegar or a good malty and rich beer.

If one wants to draw a geometric base or outline of a building, or anything else perspective, then one lays at *Lit. I* the geometric outline behind the glass, and it can be traced larger or smaller onto the glass according to how far or close behind the glass it is, or how far or near to the pane the wood *i* has been slid, and if one slides the wood *i* higher up and again traces the geometric outline, the perspective projection is made at the same time.

As much noise as this painter made about his borrowed

GRINDING LENSES AND FITTING TELESCOPES   485

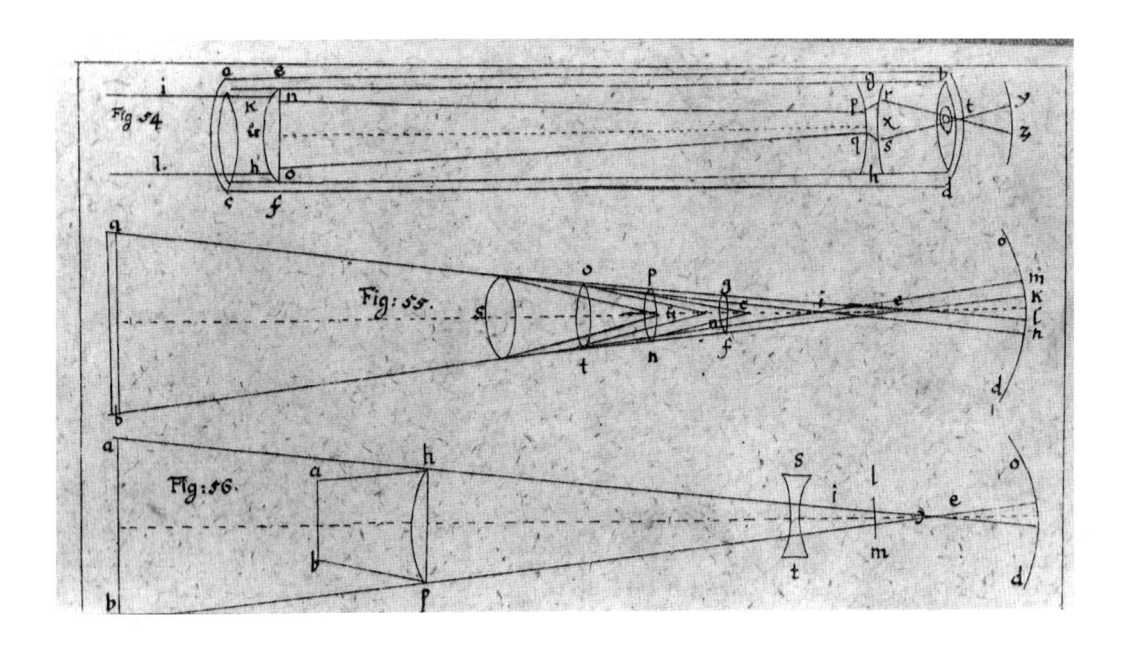

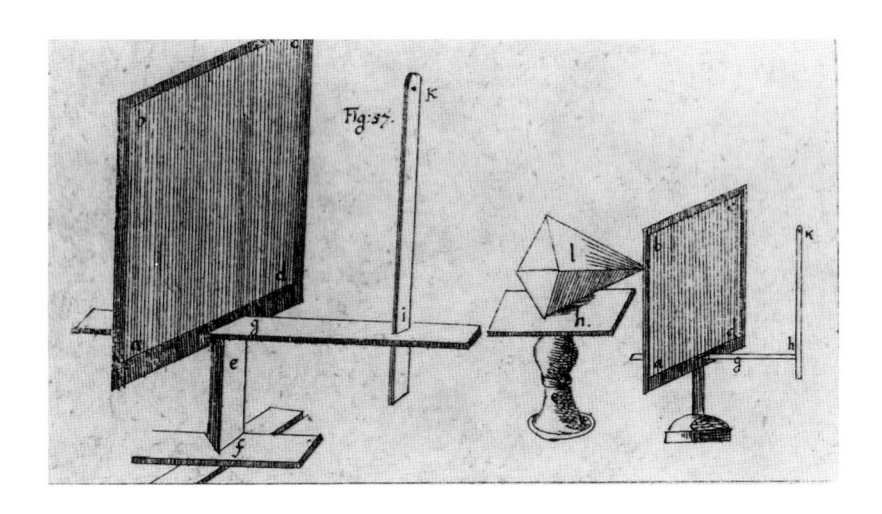

Fig. 58.

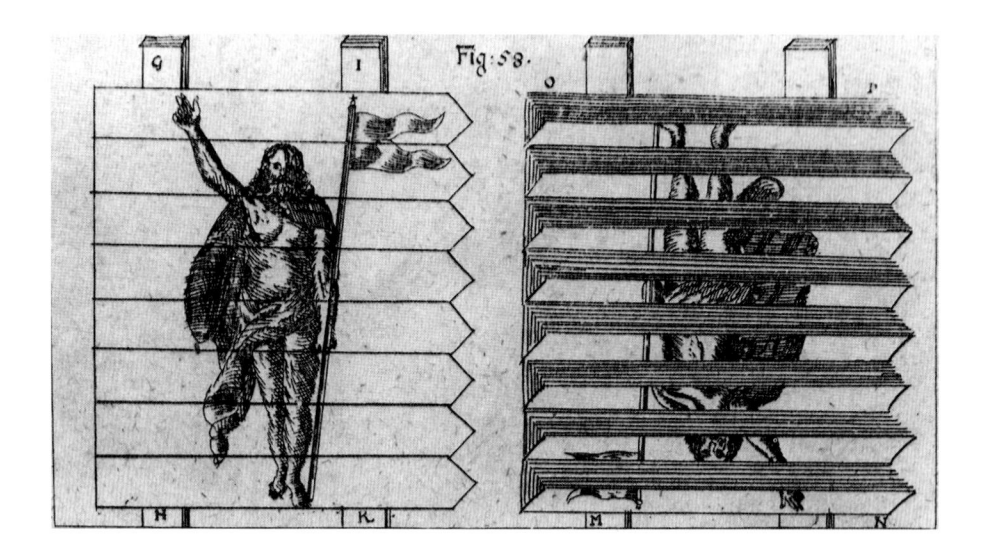

invention, he was ignorant of the proper use of it as given here; considering that his lack of knowledge and understanding has fairly well come to light, he must learn accordingly the great difference there is between himself and an honestly studied and knowledgeable painter, who thoroughly understands geometry as well as the proper placement and shadows from the perspective. Arrogance and bragging, however, are sure signs of a foolhardy and rash imprudence and this one would have done better had he remained with his supposed invention at home with the uninformed.

Figure 58 Illustrates How to Paint a Concealed Picture on Several Woods.

Make equal-sided triangular pieces of wood, which are of a size according to the size of the figure. Such triangles must be laid onto two equal pieces of wood and secured to them, (which the Figure shows clearly enough).

From *OP* one will not see the picture, depending on how one is placed or stands, but from *MN* [one can] see and recognize [it] clearly.

As concerns the mirror and how one is to proceed, one can read in the renowned (Mr.) Harsdörffer's third part and [in] the *Continuation* of the *Schwenterian Hours of Recreation*, pp. 256 and following. The remaining three Figures show:

How the Distorted Perspective Paintings Are Supposed to Be Made

The painting is placed in an equally divided square, and each field is designated with numbers. Then a straight line *e* is drawn, as seen in Figure 60, and line *I* is directed to/at equal angles. Whatever height for this is desired, the face/sight must be held accordingly away from the perspective figure. A diagonal line is drawn from *L* to *Q*, where it first intersects the line at *Lit. M*, the line *MQ* is made, [and] at *N, O, P, Q* in turn the transverse lines which represent the fields in the perspective figure from the square. Now whatever stood in each field in Figure 59 is brought according to proportion [in] Figure 60 into precisely that field designated by number, and the figure, as Nr. 61 has already shown, [is] drawn, and has its completed form, and greatly amazes the inexperienced.

GRINDING LENSES AND FITTING TELESCOPES 487

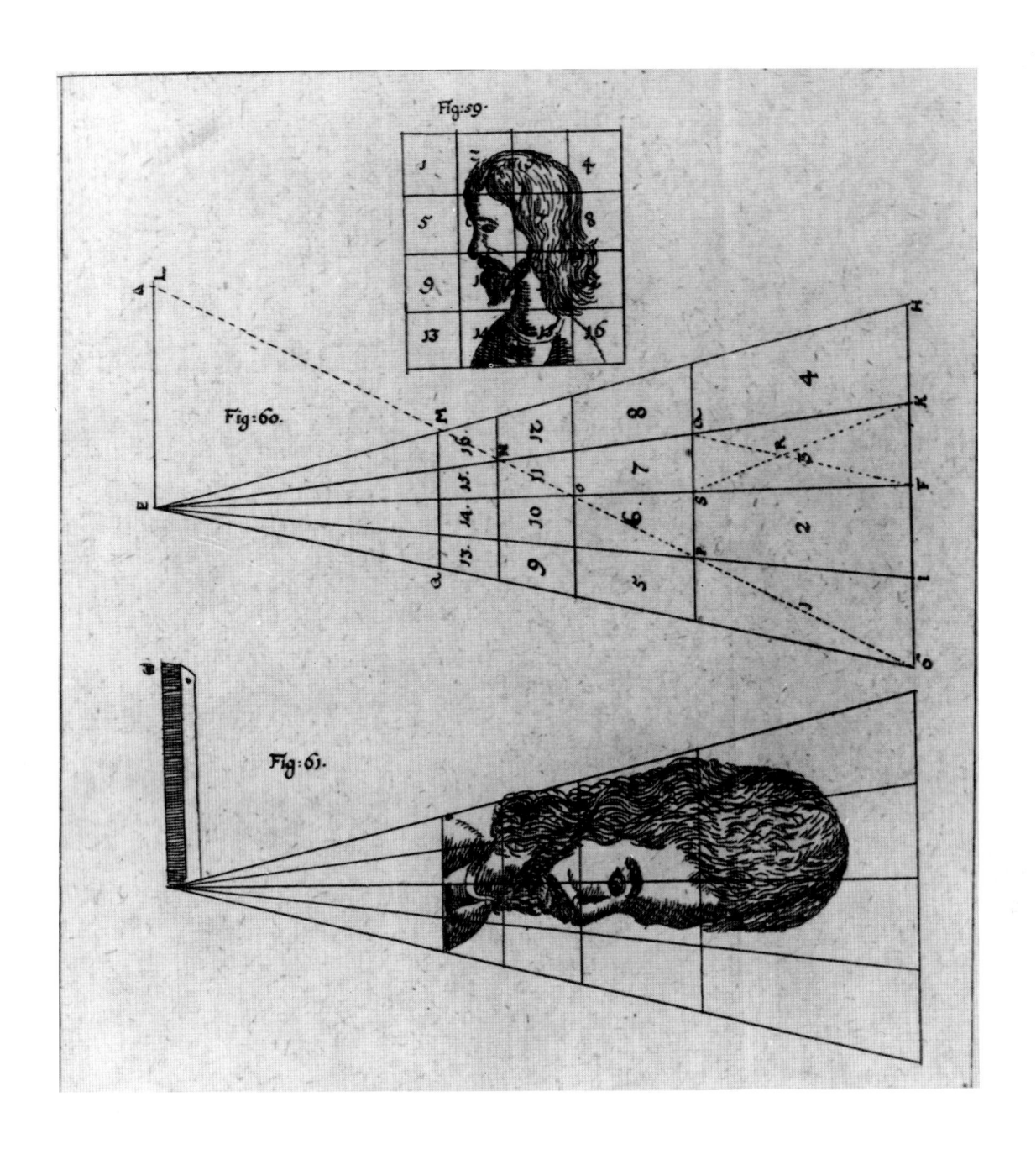

Appendix 8

Outline on the Early History of Spectacles

The following outline on the early history of spectacles was taken from the accompanying notes to an exhibit at the Washington Armed Forces Medical Library, Reference Division, 1956. This outline is illustrative of what may be found in various places where the history of spectacles is discussed. Although some of the material has been covered previously in the text, some is original and informative.

Early History of Spectacles*
by Justine Randers-Pehrson

Spectacles are the composite invention of many of the most brilliant men in the history of science. Philosophers, monks, mathematicians, physicists, microscopists, astronomers, and chemists all played vital roles in developing this instrument which we today take so much for granted.

Magnifying and burning glasses were known to the ancients, but the use of the lens as a corrective instrument was unknown.

Undoubtedly a magnifying glass was used in pre-spectacles times for the deciphering of manuscripts. A convex lens of rock crystal or quartz would be pushed from word to word across the parchment.

No one knows who first mounted a lens that could be held near the anterior focus of the eye. Spectacles of some sort began to be used in Europe, perhaps first in Italy, not long before the middle of the thirteenth century, when Venetian glass manufacture began.

Francecso Redi (1626–1698) had in his library an old manuscript, written circa 1299, in which the author speaks of wearing "okiali" which had been "recently invented for the sake of old men whose eyesight had begun to fail." This is purported to be the earliest reference to spectacles.

Redi seems to have distorted deliberately another document, to the effect that the monk Alessandro della Spina of Pisa was the actual inventor of spectacles. Other historians interpret the document, which quotes a sermon of Giordano da Rivalto, circa 1305, to mean that Spina had seen spectacles made by someone else and had thereupon proceeded to manufacture others. Spina is sometimes referred to as the "rediscoverer" of spectacles.

The problem of identification of the inventor of spectacles was attacked by Domenico Manni, who dedicated his *Degli ochiali da naso* (1738) to his hero, Salvino degli Armati of Florence, a friend of Spina's. Armati was supposed to have invented spectacles in 1285, but there is little to substantiate the claim.

---

* Mr. Milton A. Murayama's translation of the Chinese and Japanese material is acknowledged with thanks.

Armati's restored tomb in Florence bears the following inscription: "Here lies Salvino degli Armati of Florence, inventor of spectacles. May God pardon him his sins. 1317."

The oldest known pictorial representation of spectacles, a fresco painted by Tommaso Barisino of Modena in 1352, shows Cardinal Ugone da Provenza wearing "rivet" glasses. This form merely perched on the nose, or was held at the rivet with the thumb and forefinger.

The early spectacles were prized possessions of rich scholars and churchmen and are mentioned frequently in wills and other documents. A letter circa 1415 from the monk Johannes Hildebrand in Ostergotland to Bishop Knut Bosson Natt och Dag of Linkoping says, "Holy Father, I beg you to return the spectacles I gave you, since they have been broken. I will not fail to send others in return."

The first book on spectacles was written by Cardinal Nicolaus Cusanus (1401–1464). *De Beryllo*, which contains the earliest record of mounted lenses as eyeglasses, includes remarks on concave lenses, which must have been decidedly uncommon at the time the book was written. This book probably fixed *brille* as the German word for glasses. Beryl was one of the original materials used for lenses, probably because of its property of cleavage into layers suitable for polishing.

The first modern-language book on spectacles was the *Uso de los ojos*, written by Daca de Valdez, a notary of the Spanish Inquisition, in 1623. This practical volume contains accurate information about ametropia and presbyopia, as well as the corrective properties of spectacles.

An interesting feature of the work is the system of designating the refractive power of glasses by measuring the apparent enlargement by convex lenses or reduction by concave lenses of a circle of known dimensions.

The AFML [Armed Forces Medical Library] copy of this rare volume is one of the treasures of the literature of optics.

Spectacles were not immediately accepted by the medical profession. Bernard de Gordon (died circa 1308) according to his Lilium medica apparently preferred salves to spectacles. "Hoc collirium est tante virtutis quod decrepitum facent legere literas minutas sine oculo berillino."

Guy de Chauliac (1300–1370) the most famous surgeon of his time, wrote "If this collyrium does not help, one must have recourse to spectacles of glass or crystal."

Physicians in general persisted in their distrust of spectacles. Georg Bartisch (1535–1606) wrote "Aber es sey inm wie ihmwolle, so ist es nicht eine gute gewonheit, und ist viel besser und nutzlicher das man den Brillen nicht bedarff."

Spectacles caught the popular imagination. The fact that they were associated with scholars and with wisdom is reflected in works of art. Saints and patriarchs were anachronistically depicted wearing them.

Saint Jerome (331–420) is only occasionally shown with spectacles, in spite of the legend that he invented them. He was regarded as a patron saint by Venetian spectacle makers.

Guirlandaio's portrait shows spectacles at the side of the writing desk.

Since spectacles symbolized wisdom to the simple-minded, it was natural that charlatans should adopt them. The "Theriakhandler" almost invariably wore them.

Hawkers sold spectacles in the streets. The purchaser tried on various pairs and selected the one of his preference.

John Lydgate's London Lackpenny, circa 1400, contains a street cry:

"Master what will ye copen or buy?
Fyne felt hattes, or spectacles to rede?"
"Povert a spectacle is, as thinketh me,
Through which he may his verray frendes see."
  "The Wife of Bath" in Chaucer's *Canterbury Tales*

Panurge "took four French ells of a coarse brown russet cloth, and therein appareling himself as with a long, plain-seamed and single-stitched gown, left off the wearing of his breeches, and tied a pair of spectacles to his cap."
  Rabelais

"I lost fair England's view
And bid mine eyes be packing with my heart,
And called them blind and dusky spectacles
For losing ken of Albion's wished coast."
  Queen Margaret in Shakespeare's *Henry VI part 2*

"Spectacles are for Sight, and not for Shew,
Necessity doth Spectacles commend,
Was't not for need, there is but very few,
That would for wearing Spectacles contend."
  Bunyan's *Book for boys and girls, or Country rhymes for children.*

Spectacles appear in the armorial bearings of noble families and of towns, on coins, in ecclesiastical sculpture, and in stained glass (circa 1500 from the Netherlands).

That spectacles were at one time all the rage in the more frivolous ranks of society is indicated by a letter by Madame de Mothe, dated 1679.

The invention of spectacles implies a combination of optical knowledge and technical skill that would have been impossible before the thirteenth century. Even then, as Sarton says, the invention was premature because some of the problems involved could not have been formulated. Neither the nature of light nor the function of the crystalline lens and retina was understood.

At the end of the twelfth century, the first Latin translation of Ibn al-Haitham's *Optics* appeared, stirring the imagination of European scholars.

Witelo, the Polish physicist (1220–1280) was the first European scientist of any stature to write on vision. His *Optics*, composed between 1270 and 1278, was derived in large part from Ibn al-Haitham's work and constitutes an important link in the transmission of Arabic knowledge to Europe.

There is no reference to spectacles in this comprehensive study.

Though Witelo's work was almost entirely derivative, his fame was so enduring that Kepler, writing on optics in 1604, entitled his book *Ad Vitellionem paralipomena*.

It has been conjectured that spectacles were invented by Roger Bacon (1214–1294). The principal evidence in Bacon's favor is contained in his *Opus Majus*, but the passage on the convex lens refers to the holding of it above letters to magnify them.

The lurid tale of his flight from England and his stealthy communication of the art of spectacle–making to a go–between who carried the information to Italy is now known to be an elaborate hoax.

Bacon did actually experiment with burning glasses, and vaguely foresaw the wave theory of light.

It is interesting to observe that Bacon was largely neglected by scholars before the sixteenth century. His most important work was printed for the first time in 1733.

Some historians feel that Bacon alone had the requisite knowledge for the invention of spectacles. However, Robert Grosseteste, Bacon's teacher, was the first medieval writer to discuss the properties of mirrors and lenses systematically.

Grosseteste, who had one of the most scintillating minds of his age, held that the laws of optics were basic to the explanation of all natural phenomena.

Archbishop John de Peckham of Canterbury (circa 1240–1294) was another contemporary of Roger Bacon whose knowledge of optics was comprehensive. His pioneer volume on optics in English contains a summary of the theory of convex and concave lenses. The 1504 edition of his *Perspective* contains what is probably the oldest printed diagram of the eye.

A stumbling block was the lack of understanding of the way in which the eye forms an image. Witelo, Bacon, and Peckham, following Ibn al-Haitham, had recognized the function of the crystalline lens as a focusing organ, but all supposed it to be also photosensitive.

Francesco Maurolico of Messina (1494–1575) was the first to show correctly how the crystalline lens focused the rays onto the retina. As a result, he was able to explain far and near sightedness and the use of corrective lenses. He was baffled, however, by the inverted retinal image.

Giambattista della Porta (circa 1535–1615) thought that the visual image was formed on the surface of the crystalline lens and that the retina acted as a concave reflector. He is considered to be one of the founders of modern optics because of his work with the camera obscura. He discussed convex and concave lenses in his *De refractione*, explaining the use of the concave in myopia.

Felix Platter (1536–1614) was first to recognize the function of the retina and to describe the crystalline lens as solely a dioptric instrument.

Johannes Kepler (1571–1610) observed that the retina is essential to vision, forming a real inverted image. He took the preliminary steps in the formulation of the law of refraction when he showed that the angle of refraction for small angles is proportional to the angle of incidence.

Kepler's work on the retina had been theoretical. Father Christopher Scheiner (1579–1650) made a practical demonstration by removing a portion of the opaque outer layers at the back of the eyeball and making the retinal image directly visible.

Scheiner also did pioneer work in deducing that the crystalline lens altered its refractive power when the eyes were turned from a distant point to a point nearby.

Willebrod Snell (1591–1626), professor of mechanics at Leyden, was the formulator of the sine–law of refraction. Snell's unpublished calculations are generally considered to have antedated those of Descartes.

Early artisans were incapable of producing flawless optical glass, accurately ground as we expect it to be today. Spectacle-makers selected pieces of glass that they considered suitable from lots intended for ornamental creations. Even as late as 1770, Deshais-Gendron complained of spectacles that "They are badly polished, which affects their transparency, there is never the same thickness in the two glasses, their material is usually thready, filled with bubbles and other imperfections. . . ."

Glassmaking is an ancient art that consists essentially of melting certain ingredients at a temperature high enough to produce a fluid mass that permits the escape of any bubbles forming in it.

Historians assume that the first spectacles were made of Muranese glass. Venice was ideally situated, having easy access to vast supplies of wood from Yugoslavia for the furnaces, with the sand of the Lido and Verona close by, and with a fine clay for crucibles available at Vicenza. Salt could be taken from the sea, and soda of finest quality could be brought in ships from Egypt.

In 1224 there were 19 persons listed in Venice as *friolari*, and in the same century, codes of trade regulations were drawn up. In 1268 the glassworkers became an incorporated body, and shortly afterwards the entire industry was transferred to the island of Murano, apparently as a safeguard against fire.

Georg Agricola in his *De re metallica* (1556) described in detail the processes of glassmaking that he had observed in Italy. The furnace shown is three-chambered, being fired from below.

There was little change in the procedures of optical glassmaking until the eighteenth century. John Dollond in the *Philosophical Transactions* of 1758 presented his "Account of some experiments concerning the different refrangibility of light," reporting his discovery of a means of making achromatic lenses by combining crown and flint glass.

Flint glass obtains its name from the fact that when lead glass was first made, flints were used as a source of the silica in its composition.

The expression "crown" appears to have been applied originally to the type of window glass made in the shape of discs, the center of which formed a bullion such as may still be seen in the windows of early colonial houses.

Joseph Fraunhofer (1787–1826) originally worked with Pierre Guinand who was the first to advocate the stirring of molten glass to overcome the lack of homogeneity. Fraunhofer, who was a brilliant self-taught mathematician, originated the specification of refraction and dispersion of glass in terms of certain lines of the spectrum discovered by him and subsequently named Fraunhofer lines. He invented grinding and polishing machines and methods of testing by means of Newton's rings.

The process of grinding and polishing was for centuries carried on by hand. The discs of glass were brought to the proper form by being rubbed upon appropriately shaped "tools." Convex lenses were ground in a concave copper dish called a lanx, while concave lenses were shaped by rubbing the glass on a metal tool formed like a part of a sphere.

One grade of moist emery was usually used throughout the process, and final polishing was done with a cloth impregnated with putty powder or tripoli.

Various mechanical contrivances were devised for grinding and polishing. These machines were often the invention of leading scientists whose interest was lens making for microscopy or for telescopes.

Hevelius, the Danzig astronomer, invented a mechanical grinder.

Christopher Wren (1632–1723), who was an anatomist, microscopist, and astronomer as well as architect, contrived an "engin" for shaping hyperbolic lenses. He made a further contribution to the development of corrective spectacles by measuring and drawing the spheres of the humors of the eye.

Wren's friend Robert Hooke (1635–1703), like Wren a man of extraordinarily diversified interests, as Curator of Experiments of the Royal Society tested and invented much apparatus for perfecting lenses. He also constructed an artificial eye for the study of optics. Hooke's *Micrographia* is a classic, containing the original formulation of the wave theory of light.

Christian Huygens (1629–1695), the celebrated Dutch astronomer and mathematician, is best known for his investigations on the wave theory of light. His interest in optics led him to devise methods for grinding and polishing lenses which he described in his *De vitris figurandis*.

The illustration shows stages of making a "tool" for final polishing invented by Huygens and perfected by Molyneux. This tool was a thick plate of cast brass that was ground with emery and two flat polishing stones. It was polished by coating one stone with pitch and feeding emery between the metal and pitch under considerable pressure. The glass blank was placed in a concave depression to correspond to the finished lens.

Most of the early works on lens-making are addressed by scientists to others with similar interests. Cherubin d'Orleans wrote his *Dioptrique oculaire* (1671) with the apprentice in mind. This how-to book contains the first description of polishing machinery.

With the basic problems of optics and technology solved, the correction of specific difficulties of vision became possible.

In the Bakerian lecture for 1801, Thomas Young presented the first description of astigmatism, analyzing his own defective vision. He attributed the condition to an obliquity of the crystalline lens in relation to the visual axis.

Young did not realize the importance of his discovery. The term *astigmatism* was not suggested by him, but later by William Whewell, Master of Trinity College.

Astigmatism is probably the most common of ocular defects, being present in almost all eyes to some extent. Rays of light are not brought to sharp points on the retina but from short lines (our stars are not seen as dots: we seem to see light radiating from them).

Sir George Biddle Airy, Astronomer Royal, discovered astigmatism in his left eye about 1825. He calculated the focal powers needed for correction and had Fuller of Ipswich grind a sphero-cylindrical lens for him. This was the first time that a cylindrical lens was used in correction.

Airy wrote with satisfaction, "I have found that the eye which I once feared would become quite useless can now be used in almost every respect as well as the other."

Isaac Hays, surgeon at Wills Eye Hospital, Philadelphia, reported the fifth case of astigmatism in the entire world in 1834.

The spectacles prescribed by Hays were ground by the McAllisters in Philadelphia, one of the earliest optical establishments in the country. The McAllisters were first to grind cylindrical lenses in the United States.

Benjamin Franklin is generally credited with the invention of bifocal lenses. The Franklin type was made by halving lenses of differing powers and cementing the segments together with a straight line across the middle.

Franklin's bifocals were probably made by Peter Dollond of London. Thomas Jefferson had similar glasses made to his specifications by the McAllisters of Philadelphia.

The form of lenses engaged the attention of the physicist, William Hyde Wollaston (1766–1828). He experimented with meniscus lenses (their curve had suggested the "moon" designation) and in 1804 published an article in the *Philosophical Magazine* "On an improvement in the Form of Spectacle Glasses."

Wollaston commented that while the crossed lens of Huygens gave minimum spherical aberration for direct axial pencils and could therefore be used for microscope objectives, it gave mediocre results when used as a spectacle lens.

"The more nearly any spectacle glass can be made to surround the eye...the more nearly will every part of it be at right angles to the line of sight...lenses should be more convex on their exterior surface, and concave within."

The sole manufacture and sale under patent was given to Peter Dollond.

In steel frames, the periscopic spectacles cost 10s 6d a pair, compared to the usual 3s 6d for similar frames with flat lenses.

When Dollond's patent ran out in 1818, competition set in. Periscopic lenses were then manufactured on the continent in Germany.

Pastor Johann Heinrich Duncker (1767–1843) is noteworthy as the founder of the Rathenower Optische Industrieanstalt (1801) in which disabled soldiers, as well as orphans of soldiers, were employed. In the interests of this rehabilitation project, Duncker devised and patented a lens-grinding apparatus.

Prismatic lenses are usually considered to be the invention of Donders, but the principle had been set down in 1792 by the American-born physician, William Charles Wells (1757–1817) of Charleston, South Carolina. Wells, the son of a Tory

Scotsman, moved to Britain at the time of the American Revolution.

In his "Essay upon single vision with two eyes," he says, "If flat-sided prisms were fixed in spectacle frames with their refracting angles towards each other, they would assist the long-sighted somewhat, without producing the evil which is said to arise from the convexity of glasses, and spectacles of this kind with more property than any others be called preservers."

A few remarks on the gilds: It is possible that the first spectacles industry outside of Italy was in the Netherlands. One of the Merry Pranks of Till Eulenspiegel says that he told the Bishop of Trier, "Gnadige Herr, ich bin ein Brillenmacher und komme aus Brabant." (Gracious Sir, I am a spectacle maker and come from Brabant.) Eulenspiegel died in 1350, and the Pranks appeared in 1483.

The year 1535 is considered to be the birthdate of the German spectacles industry. In that year the regulations of the Nurnberg spectacle makers' gild were formulated.

Up to 1500, twelve spectacle makers in Nurnberg are known by name. The first ones were independent, but in 1530 they had banded together and adopted an emblem.

The ordinance of the Regensburg spectacle makers is of a somewhat later date than its Nurnberg counterpart. At the peak period of the Regensburg trade, requirements for the mastership were extremely severe. Ten masterpieces were required, as well as the making of all kinds of implements and iron tools for manufacturing spectacles. One month was the working period stipulated for the making of the masterpieces.

In 1465 there was a procession through the streets of Paris of 80,000 merchants and artisans, passing in review before Louis XI. The spectacle makers marched under 49 banners, together with the shopkeepers and carpet makers. The device shown dates from 1575 or later: at that time the spectacle makers joined the mirror makers in one gild.

In 1628 eleven London opticians and their legal advisors met to consider putting their craft on an official basis. King Charles I granted a charter in 1629. This document is the only one of the gild's records that survived the Great Fire.

Apparently the company was a sizeable one. It is known that at the start they had a master, two wardens, eight assistants, and a clerk.

Although ancient figurines give evidence that eye protectors were used in the Orient in the Stone Age, the lenses described in legends of Cho-Tso, the patron of opticians, and in the annals of the T'ang Dynasty (618–906) probably were not ground for optical purposes. Apparently they were burning glasses known as "fire pearls," which were imported into China either from Kashmir or from the vicinity of Java.

In the Tung tien ch'ing lu, written by Chao Hsi-kung of the Sung Dynasty (960–1278) there is said to be a character "ai-tai," which means spectacles. The meaning given for the character is, "Old men were unable to distinguish minute writing. Hence they covered this over their eyes and writing became clear." Certain etymologists feel that "ai-tai" was an expression that originated beyond the borders of Western China.

Although glass manufacture was introduced into China before the Anterior Han Dynasty of the Five Dynasties period (907–960) it is unlikely that there is any substance to the unverified report that Marco Polo found spectacle wearers in China.

There is general agreement among historians that spectacles were not a Chinese invention but were introduced by early missionaries, possibly by the Spanish Jesuits in 1583. There is a striking similarity between the thread attachments of the Spanish models of that period and those of Chinese models drawn in the eighteenth century.

Early Chinese glasses were large and round. They were used not only for failing sight but also as a sign of dignity, and sometimes as a remedy for diseased eyes. They were generally plano-convex, made of tinted rock crystal or topaz. The character shown means "tea stone."

Frames were of horn, tortoiseshell, or paper mache, with brass or white alloy bridges.

Convex spectacles were numbered according to age.

Powers for concave spectacles were named after animals, ranging from pig (the weakest) through intermediate strengths dog, cock, monkey, sheep, snake, dragon, rabbit, tiger, and ox up to the strongest, i.e., rat.

The rivet glasses of the Orient closely resemble their European predecessors.

Some historians believe that the Chinese invented the hinged frame. Others attribute this invention to the London optician James Ayscough (1719–1762). There is a remote possibility that Ayscough might have seen and copied Chinese models, but in all likelihood the Ayscough models made their way to China and were copied there.

Spectacles were an importation in Japan, since the Japanese had no independent study of optics. A foreign missionary is reported to have given a pair to Yoshitaka Ouchi, circa 1532.

There are spectacles preserved in the Buddhist temple in Kunoyama in Shizuoka that are supposed to have been used by Ieyasu Tokugawa (1542–1616). These are the Spanish thread type.

The Kaikoku shidan (Maritime histories) states that Gobei Hamada of Nagasaki went to countries south of Japan in 1632 and learned how to make spectacles. Hamada returned to Japan and taught the art to Fujiyoshi Ikushima.

The nose support is typical of Japanese spectacle frames. This post attached to the bridge was designed to keep the lenses from contact with the eyes of persons with low nose bridges.

Bibliography

Agarwal, Rishi Kumar. *The Optician,* September 14, 1962, p. 250; November 20, 1964, p. 512.

Ahlstrom, Otto. "Edward Scarlett's Focus Marks." *The Optician* July 15, 1951.

Aitken, M. J. and S. J. Fleming, S. J. *Authenticity Tests by Thermoluminescence.* Research Laboratory for Archaelogy, February, 1971.

American Optical Company. "The Story in a Pair of Spectacles." Reprinted from *The Book of Wonders,* 2d ed. 1921.

American Optical Company. *Spectacles, Eyeglasses, Lenses.* Southbridge, Mass. (circa 1933).

American Optical Company Catalog, 1924, pp. 230–259.

American Optical News. Vol. 5, No. 5, 1968.

Anderson, A. M. *Technique of Fitting Contact Lenses.* 1944. McGill Lithograph.

Anonymous. *Amer. J. Ophthal.* 32(1949):1064.

Anonymous. *The Optician.* December 30, 1960.

Anonymous. *The Optician.* July 15, 1960, p. 3.

Anonymous. *Minerva Med.*, Tor. (It.) 48:(82)(1957):1648–53.

Anonymous. *Policlinico.* (Prat) (It.) 67(1960):1425–26.

Anonymous. *The Optician.* 142(1961):611–616.

Anonymous. *Ophthal. Antiques Int'l. Collectors' Club Newsletter,* September 1982, p. 8, and July 1994.

Anonymous. *History of Spectacles in Japan.* Osaka, 1989.

Appuhn, Horst. *Spectacles.* Publisher, Carl Zeiss, Oberkochen/Wurtt. No. 27, p. 1.

Arrington. *A History of Ophthalmology.* New York: M.D. Publications, 1959.

Bannister, Judith. *English Silver Hallmarks.* London: W. Foulsham and Co., 1983.

Barck, C. *The Optician.* 139(1960):457–463. Reprinted from *Open Court* 21(1907):206–226.

Bartisch, George. *Augendienst.* Dresden, 1583. Facsimile: Hanover: Th. Schäfer GmbH, 1983.

Bausch and Lomb Company. *Ophthalmic Lenses.* Rochester, N.Y., 1935.

Bausch and Lomb Optical Company. "The Theory and Design of Orthogon Lenses." *Scientific Technical Pub.* #17. Rochester, N.Y., 1937.

Bayefsky's Spectacles. Canadian Portofolio Editions. Toronto, Canada, 1980.

Beacher, L. Lester. *Contact Lens Technique.* New York Contact Lens Research Lab, New York, 1944.

Beck, Richard. *A Treatise on the Construction, Proper Use, and Capabilities of Smith, Beck, and Beck's Achromatic Microscopes.* John Van Voorst, Paternoster Row Pub., London: circa 1865.

Benedictine Convent of Perpetual Adoration, Article S43.

Bennett, A.G. *The Optician.* July 21, 1972, pp. 6–11.

Bennion, Elisabeth. *Antique Medical Instruments.* University of California Press, 1979, pp. 148, 227, 236.

Bentzon, M., and A. H. Emerson. "Improvements in Bi-focal Lenses and Their Manufacture, and in Apparatus to Be Employed in the Said Manufacture," Brit. Pat. 28,823 (1904).

Bier, N. *Contact Lens Routine and Practice.* London: Butterworth's, C.V. Mosby, 1953.

Blodi, Fred C. "Ophthalmology and Philately." *Hist. Oph. Intern.* 1(1979):201–208.

Bock, Emile. *Die Brille.* Vienna, 1903.

Bronson, L.D. *Early American Specs.* Glendale, Calif.: Occidental, 1974.

Bryden, D. J. and D. L. Simms. "Spectacles Improved to Perfection and Approved of by the Royal Society." *Annals of Science,* 50(1993):1–32.

Bucklin, C.A. *Visual Imperfections and Test Type.* New York: Spencer Opt. Co., 1881.

Bugbee, L.W., Jr. and Sr. *Bifocals.* Indianapolis, Ind.: One Piece Bifocal Lens Company (Pub.), 1921.

Bull, Edward C., O.D. *American Optometric Association.* San Francisco, 1926.

Bull, G. J. *Lunettes et pince-nez.* Paris: S. Masson, 1889, p. 65.

Cadore, Pieve di. *Il Museo dell'Occhiale.* Gruppo Editoriale Fabbri, Bompiani, Sonzogo, Etas S.p.A.—Milano, 1990, p. 99.

Carter, R. B. *Good and Bad Eyesight.* Philadelphia: P. Blakiston & Co., 1882.

Cashell, G. T. W. "A Short History of Spectacles." *Proc. Royal Soc. Med.* 64 (October 1971).

Chamblant, M. *Nouveaux verres d'optique, Aux Surfaces de cylindre.* Brevet pour l'exécution, rue Basse-porte-St. Dénis, No. 26. Chamblant, Paris.

Chan, Eugene and Winfred Mao. "The History of Spectacles in China." *Proceedings of the XXVth International Congress of Ophthalmology,* Rome, May 4–10, 1986, pp. 731–734.

Charles, A. M., M. Callender, and T. Grosvenor. "Efficacy of Chemical Ascepticizing System for Soft Contact Lenses." *Amer. J. Optom.* 50(1973):. 777–781.

Chiu Kai Ming. *Harvard Journal of Asiatic Studies.* July 1936, pp. 186–193.

Comstock's Philosophy. New York: Pratt, Woodford & Co., 1850.

Corson, Richard. *Fashions in Eyeglasses.* London: Peter Owen, Ltd., 1967 and 1980.

Courmettes, H. A., "Bifocal Lens and Method for Making the Same," US Pat. 1,160,383 (1915).

Davidson, D. C. *Spectacles, Lorgnettes and Monocles.* Bucks, UK: Pub. Aylesburg, 1989.

Davis, Audrey B. and Mark S. Dreyfuss. *The Finest Instruments Ever Made.* Arlington, Mass.: Med. Hist. Pub. Assn. 1986.

DeCarle, J. "Bifocal Lenses" in J. Stone, and A.J. Phillips, *Contact Lenses* 2nd ed. 1981, pp. 571–573.

Denviendt, Jean Marie. *Theaterverrekijkers.* Ostende: Published by the author, 1995.

Devlyn, Frank. "The History of Eyewear in Mexico." *Ophthal. Antiques Int'l. Collectors' Club Newsletter,* October 1994.

Diamandopoulou-Drummond, Ann H. "Society and Optical Aids." Doctoral thesis.

Dickinson, F. "A Report on a New Contact Lens." *Optician* 118(1949):141.

Doesschate, G. Ten. *Brit. J. Ophthal.* 30(1946):660–664.

Dollond, P. and J. *Periscopic Spectacles.* London: Dollond, 1804.

Donders, F. C. *On the Anomalies and Accommodations and Refraction of the Eye.* London: New Sydenham Society, 1864.

Drake, S. *Isis* 52(1961):95–96.

Duke-Elder. *System of Ophthalmology.* Vol. XIV & V. St. Louis: C.V. Mosby & Co., 1972.

Emerson, S. A., "Some Recent Improvements in Modern Ophthalmic Lenses," *Trans. Opt. Soc.* 27(1925/6):1–8.

Enoch, J. "Descartes Contact Lens." *Amer. J. Optom.* 33(1956):77–85.

Feinbloom, W. "A Plastic Contact Lens." *Amer. J. Optom.* 14(1937):41–49.

Feinbloom, W. "The Tangent Cone Contact Lens Series. *Optom. Weekly.* 36(1945):1159–1161.

Ferry, Andrew. "Vignette." *Argus*. San Francisco, 1990.

Fick, A. E. "A Contact Lens." *Arch. Ophthal.* 17(1888):215–226. English translation of "Eine Contactbrille."*Archiv f. Augenheilkunde.* 18:279–289.

Fischer-Hamberger, Esther. *Geschichte der Medizin*. Berlin: Springer, 1975.

Fisher, E. J. "Hydrophilic Contact Lenses." *Can. J. Optom.* 29(4)(1968):139–144.

Fisher, W. B. *The Genopthalmic Refractor*. Mt. Vernon, NY: General Optical Co., Inc., 1922.

Fleischman, W. E. "The Single Vision Reading Contact Lens."*Amer. J. Optom. Arch. Am. Acad. Opt.* 45(6)(1968): 408–409.

Fox, Samuel L. *Highlights in the History of Spectacles*. Baltimore, MD.

Franklin, Benjamin. *Survey Ophthal.* 4(1959):683–686.

Freedman, M. *Ophthal. Optician* 2(1962):435–436, 445.

Fryor, Colin B. "History of Spectacles." *The Optician* October 1988, November 1988, February 1989, April 1989. Surrey, England.

Fukushima, G. *J. Clin. Ophthal.* 16(1962):730–732 (Tokyo).

Gannon, Fred A. *Optical Journal Review*, January 15, 1941, p. 180.

Garzoni, Tomaso. *La Piazza Universale*. Venice, 1585.

Gasson, Walter. *The Optician*, April 23, 1971, p. 14.

Glancey, A. E. *Amer. J. Physiol. Optics* 6(1925):393–402.

Gorin, George. *History of Ophthalmology*. Wilmington, Dela.: Publish or Perish, Inc., 1982.

Graham, R. "Evolution of Corneal Contact Lenses." *Amer. J.Optom.* 36(1959):55–59.

Greeff, Prof. Dr. (Berlin). *Katalog Einer Bilderausstellung zur Geschichte der Brille*. Amsterdam, 1929.

Grossmann, T. *Klin. Mol. Augenh.* 129(4)(1956):559–561 (Ger.).

Grosvenor, T., A. M. Charles, and M. Callender. "Soft Contact Lens Bacteriological Study." *Can. J. Optom.* 34(1)(1972):11–18.

Gyorffy, S. *Transactions of the International Ophthalmic Optical Congress (1961)*. London: C. Crosby Lockwood & Son, Ltd., 1962, pp. 266–267.

Hakushima, G. *Amer. J. Ophthal.* 55(1963):612–613.

Hardy, S. *The Optician* 148(1964):566.

Hardy, W. E., "John Hamer Sutcliffe, A Great Champion of Ophthalmics," *The Optician* 141(1961):33–34.

Hartridge, G. *The Refraction of the Eye*. Chicago: W. P. Deim & Co., 1895.

Heitz, R. F. *History of Contact Lenses 1984*. (*Contact Lenses: The CLAO Guide to Basic Sciences and Clinical Practice*, ed. O.H. Dabezies).

Herschel, J.F.W. *Encyclopedia Metripolitania*, 1845. 4.396–404. (Cited in J. Stone and A. J. Phillips, *Contact Lenses*, 1980.)

Hertel, Christian G. *Vollstandize Anweisung zum Glas*. Schleiffen, 1716.

Hill, Emory. *American Encyclopedia of Ophthalmology*. Vol. 7. Chicago, Cleveland Press, 1915, pp. 4894–4953.

Hilsdem, G. L. *A Short Work on Glazing*. Dresden, 1741.

Hirschberg, Julius. *History of Ophthalmology*. Vol. 2. Bonn: Wayenborgh, 1985, pp. 266–273.

Hofstetter, H. W., and R. Graham. "Leonardo and Contact Lenses." *Amer. J. Optom.* 30(1)(1953):41–44.

Holtmann, H.W. "A Short History of Spectacles in Hirschberg. *History of Ophthalmology* Bonn: Wayenborgh, 1982.

Horne, Richard. *Fraser's Magazine*. England, 1876.

Hudson, J. T. *Useful Remarks upon Spectacles, Lenses, and Opera-Glasses; with Hints to Spectacle Wearers and Others.*... London: Joseph Thomas, Finch-Lane, Cornhill, 1840.

Hudson, J. T. "On the Best Materials for Spectacle Lenses," in *Useful Remarks upon Spectacles, Lenses, and Opera-Glasses; with Hints to Spectacle Wearers and* Others. . . . London: Joseph Thomas, Finch-Lane, Cornhill, 1840, pp. 16–17.

Hudson, M. T. *On Coloured Shades and Lenses*. Chap. V., p. 25.

Hukushima, M.D. "Giiti." *Amer. J. Ophthal.*, 1963.

Hunt, G. D., F.S.M.C. *The Optician*. February 22, 1963, p. 168.

Hutten, E. P. *Optical Journal Review*. January 15, 1941, p. 97.

Il Museo dell'Occhiale Verona, pp. 73–83.

Inns, H. D. E. "The Griffin Lens." *Amer. J. Optom.* (1973):977–983.

Jackson, Edward. *Amer. J. Ophthal.* 10(1927):606.

Javal, Emile. *Annales d' oculistique.* Volume 55, 9th pub., Volume 5, 3d & 4th issues, March 31 & April 30, 1966. Translated by Mrs. Linda L. McDonald in the December 10, 1970, issue of *Optometric Weekly*, p. 23.

Jenkins, L. "The Development of the Modern Contact Lens." *The Optician* 141(3660)(1961):541–547.

Jockel, Nils. *Vor Augen Formen, Geschichte und Wirkungen der Brille.* Hamburg: Museum für Kunst und Gewerbe, 1986.

Jordan, Robert T. *Stechert-Hafner Book News.* 18(8)(1964): 97–100, (9):113–117.

Jugler, J. H. *Bibliothecae Ophthalmicae.* Hamburg, 1783. (The first bibliography and history of ophthalmology.)

Katz, Sylvia. *Early Plastics.* Bucks, UK: Shire Publishers, Ltd. Cromwell House, Aylesbury, 1986.

Kelly, Gary. "Hornucopia." *Blade,* August 1993, p. 12.

Kirsch, H. *Klin. Monatsbl. Augenh.* 115(1949):109–111 (Ger.).

Knoll, Henry A. *J. Amer. Optom. Assn.* 38(1967):946–948.

Korb, D.R. *Clinical Observations on Current Microscopic Corneal Lens Perforations.* 1950c. Author's Publication.

Kortland, Kees. *Het Oog Wilook Wat.* Rotterdam, 1990.

Kuisle, Anita. *Brillen.* Munich:Deutches Museum, 1985, pp. 56–60.

La Lente, *Collection of Fritz Rathschuller.* Genova: Edizioni Culturali Internazionali, 1988, pp. 180–185.

Law, F. W. *Ann. Oculist.* 199(1966):143–154 (Fr.).

Law, Frank W. *The Worshipful Company of Spectacle Makers,* 1978.

Leiss, C. *Die Optischen Instruments.* Leipzig, 1899.

Leonardo da Vinci. *Leonardo on the Eye.* New York, 1979.

Letocha, Charles E., M.D. "The Invention and Early Manufacture of Bifocals." *Survey of Ophthalmology,* 35(3), November/December 1990.

Levene, John R., *Clinical Refraction and Visual Science.* Boston: Butterworth's, 1977.

Li, Raymond. *A Glossary of Chinese Snuff Bottles Rebus.* Kowloon, Hong Kong: Nine Dragons Publishers, 1976, p. 18.

Lloyd, Ralph I. *Guildcraft* 16(1), June/July, 1942, pp. 34–50.

MacGregor, R. J. S. *Collecting Ophthalmic Antiques.* Ayrshire, UK: Ophthalmic Antiques International Collectors' Club, 1992, p. 36.

MacGregor, R. J. S. *Restoring Ophthalmic Antiques.* Ayrshire, UK: Ophthalmic Antiques International Collectors' Club, 1990.

Maddox. *The Clinical Use of Prisms.* London, 1893.

Magne, C. *Hygiène de la vue.* Paris, 1847.

Manni, D. M. Degli *Occhiali da Naso Inventati da Salvino Armati.* Florence, 1738.

Marley, Pierre. *Spectacles.* France: Hachette/Marsin, 1980.

Marley, Pierre. *Spectacles and Spyglasses.* Paris: Hoebeke, 1988.

Martens, T. G. *Proc. Mayo Clin.* 35(1960):217–222.

Mauzini, G. *L'Occhiale all'occhio.* Bologna, 1660. (The second book on the making of spectacles.)

McAllister, Francis W. *The Optical Journal,* March 15, 1917, p. 761.

McAllister, Wm. Y. *Optical Catalogue.* Philadelphia, 1870.

Milburn, John R. *Benjamin Martin.* Leyden: Nordhoff Int'l. Publishing, 1976.

Milburn, John R. *Retailer of the Sciences.* London: Vade-Mecum Press, 1986, pp. 13, 18, 56.

Monnerel, J. *Le Lunetier-Opticien.* 2d ed. L. Eyrolles, editor. Paris, 1890.

Morrison, R. J. "Hydrophilic Contact Lenses." *J. Amer. Optom. Assn.* 37(3)(1966):211–218.

Mueller, K. *Klin. Mol. Augenh.* 137(1960):104–107. (Ger.).

Mueller-Welt, A. "The Mueller-Welt Fluidless Contact Lens." *Optom. Weekly* 41(1950):831–834.

Muggeridge, J. F. C. "The Discovery of Spectacles." *Royal Soc. Health J.* August 1982.

Muller, F. A. and A. C. Muller. *The Artificial Eye.* 1910 (cited by J. DeCarle. "Who Fitted the First Contact Lens?" *The Optician* [1988, supp. 4]).

Nagaoka, Dr. Hiroo. *History of Spectacles in Japan.*

Neaman, Judith S. "The Mystery of the Ghent Bird and the Invention of Spectacles." *Viator.* Los Angeles: University of California Press, 1993, vol. 24

Needham, N.J.T.M. *Science and Civilization in China*. Vol. 4, Part 1, Cambridge, 1962, pp. 118–122.

Nerney, George. "Developments in Metal Frame and Mounting Manufacture." *Optical Journal Review*, January 15, 1941.

Newbold, H., and W. R. Williams, "Improvements in Bifocal Lenses and Apparatus for Their Manufacture," Brit. Pat. 5,441 (1912).

Newbold, Stanley. *The Optician*. April 1961.

Newton, I. *Opticks*. London, 1704.

Obrig, T. *Contact Lenses*. New York: Obrig Laboratories, 1942.

Obrig, Theo E. *Modern Ophthalmic Lenses and Optical Glass*. New York: The Chilton Co., 1935, pp. 1–11.

Obstfeld, Henri. *Int'l. Coll. Club Newsletter*. October 1991.

O'Driscoll, K. F. "Polymeric Aspects of Soft Contact Lenses." In A.R. Gasset and H. E. Kaufman, *Soft Contact Lenses*, St. Louis: Mosby, 1972.

Oliver, G. H. *Brit. Med. J.* October 25, 1913, pp. 1049–1054.

Orford, H., and A. Lockett. *Lens-Work for Amateurs*. London: Pitman, 1938.

Orr, Hugh. *Illustrated History of Early Antique Spectacles*. Kent, England: Hugh Orr, 1985, p. 84.

Panoptik Primer. Panoptik Co., 1935.

Pascal, J. "The Origins and Development of Contact Lenses." *Opt. J. and Rev. Opt.* 78(2)(1941):57–61.

Percival, MacIver. *The Fan Book*. London: T. Fisher Unwin Ltd., 1920, pp. 169–175.

Phillips, R. J. *Spectacles and Eyeglasses*. Philadelphia: Blakiston, 1902.

Pike's Scientific and Medical Instruments. Vol. I & II, pp. 193, 373.

Pointer, Jonathan. "Markings on Antique Spectacles." *Ophthalmic and Physiological Optics* 15(4)(1995).

Poulet, W. *Art and Spectacles*. Vol. 2. Berlin: Wayenborgh (Pub), 1935.

Poulet, W. *Atlas on the History of Spectacles*. Translated by Frederick Blodi, M.D., Badgodesberg, West Germany: Wayenborgh Publishers, 1978.

Powell, Lyle S., M.D. *The Eye Ear Nose and Throat Monthly*. Lawrence, Kansas. March, 1930.

Rakusen, C. P. *Chinese Medical Journal*. 53(3)(1938):379–390 (Peking).

Randers-Pehrson, Justine. Notes to accompany an exhibit on the early history of spectacles at the Armed Forces Medical Library/Reference Section—Washington, July–August 1956.

Rare Visual Aids. Woodside, N.Y.: The Kono Manufacturing Company, 1952.

Rasmussen, O. D. *Chinese Eyesight and Spectacles*. Tonbridge, England: Tonbridge Free Press, Ltd., 1925.

Rasmussen, O. D. *History of Chinese Spectacles*. Hankow, China, 1915.

Rasmussen, O. D. *The Optician*. 139(1960):569–570.

Redi, Francesco. *Lettera intorno all'invenzione degli occhiali*. Florence: F. Onofini, 1678.

Reetz, Hans. *Bildnis und Brille*. Oberkocken: Carl Zeiss, 1957.

Reynolds, C. P. "Benjamin Franklin." *Gourmet Magazine*, April 1990, p. 100.

Rienitz, Sammlung. *Kulturgeschichte des Fernrohrs*. Tubingen, 1985.

Robb, C. J. *The Optician*. 141(1961):526.

Rosen, E. *Isis*. (Cambridge, Mass.) June 1953, pp. 135–136.

Rosen, E. *Arch. int. d'histoire des sciences*. 7(1954):1–15.

Rosen, E. *J. Hist. Med.* 11(1956):13–46, 183–218.

Rosenthal, J. Wm. *A History of Spectacles*. AAO Museum Pamphlet, 1991.

Rosenthal, J. Wm. *Lorgnettes*. Cecil O'Brien Lectureship. Tulane University, New Orleans, 1991.

Rossi, Frank. *Die Brille*. Edition. Leipzig, 1990.

Rucker, C. W. *Proc. Mayo Clin.* 35(1960):209–216.

Rucker, C. W. *Curr. Med. Digest* 29(1962):51–57.

Sabell, T. "The Early Years." *The Optician* (1988 supp.): 6–21.

Salt, John Dixon. "Optical Patron Saints." *Ophthal. Antiques International Collectors' Club Newsletter*, October 1994.

Sarcey, Francisque. *Mind Your Eyes*. Translated by Henry Bruns. New Orleans, 1886.

Schiffler, Herman. *Theory of Ocular Defects and Spectacles*. London: Longmans, Green & Co., 1869.

Scott, W. F. *The Optician.* 140(1960):269–72.

Scrini & Fortin. *Manuel pratique pour le choix des verres de lunettes et l'examen de la vision.* Paris, 1906. First Edition.

Shastid, Thomas. *Encyclopedia of Ophthalmology.* In Casey Wood, *The American Encyclopedia and Dictionary of Ophthalmology.* Chicago: Cleveland Press, 1915, p. 8525.

Shirayama, Sekiya. "The Introduction of Spectacles into Japan." *Oph. Antiques Int'l. Collectors' Club Newsletter,* April 1991.

Shirayama, Sekiya. *Ophthal. Antiques Int'l. Collectors' Club Newsletter,* July 1991.

Sichel, Dr Jules. *Les Lunettes.* Paris, 1848.

Sichel, Dr. Jules. *Spectacles.* Boston, 1850.

Siebel, J. *Spectacles, Their Uses and Abuses.* Boston, 1850.

Sines, G. and Y. A. Sakellararkis. "Lenses in Antiquity." *Amer. J. Archaeology* 91(1987):191.

Smith, E. T. *Med. J. Australia.* 2(19328):578–587.

Snyder, C. *Arch. Ophthal.* 55(1956):397–407.

Snyder, Charles. *Our Ophthalmic Heritage.* Boston: Little, Brown, & Co., 1967.

Sorsby, Arnold. *A Short History of Ophthalmology.* London and New York, 1948.

Speel, Erika. "Enamelled Opera Glasses." *The Antique Collector.* December 1989.

Spencer Optical Company. Catalog #17, 1914, pp. 79, 86.

Strajduhr, J. *Lijecnicki Vjesnik* March–April 1952, pp. 70–71 (Zagreb, Yugoslavia).

Strong, D. S. *Leonardo on the Eye.* New York: Garland, 1979.

Sutcliffe, J. H. "Improvements in and Relating to Lenses for Spectacles or Eyeglasses and in Methods of an Apparatus for Manufacturing the Same." Brit. Pat. 6,263 (1900).

Tabacchi, V. et al, *Il Museo dell'occhiale* (at Pieve di Cadore, Belluno) (Milan: Del Gruppo Editoriale Fabbri, 1990), 197.

Tato-Guerra, T. "Benito Daca de Valdes." *J.A.O.A.*, February 1961, p. 541.

Teng Tak. *Fine Arts.* Kowloon, Hong Kong, 1992.

Thompson, C. J. S. *The Connoisseur.* 94(1934):231–239 (London).

Trevor-Roper, P. D. *Med. Illust. Lond.* 6(7)(1952):359–368.

Tse, C. Y. Personal communication. Hong Kong, 1992.

Turner, G. L. E. *A Spectacle of Spectacles.* London: Druckerei Fortshritt Erfurt, 1988.

United Kingdom Optical Company, Limited., E. Culver, and F. B. Watson. "Improvements to Fused Bifocal Lenses," Brit. Pat. 255,941 (1926).

Valdes, Daza (Daca) de. *Uso de los Antoios.* Seville, 1623.

Von Rohr, Dr. M. *Eyes and Spectacles.* London: The Hatton Press, Limited, 1912.

Warner, Deborah Jean. *Antiques,* p. 158.

Warner, Deborah Jean. *OHS Proceedings,* Southbridge, Mass., 1984.

Wells, Edwin P. *The Optical Journal,* p. 26.

Wells, G.W. Quinebaug Historical Society Leaflets, American Optical Co., Part 3, pp. 191–192.

Wells, J. S. *The Scientific Use of Spectacles.* London, 1862.

Wells, Ruth Dyer. *The Wells Family.* Privately printed, 1979, Southbridge, Mass.

Wichterle, O. and D. Lim. "Hydrophilic Gels for Biological Use." *Nature* 185(1960):117.

Wilbur, C. Keith. *Antique Medical Instruments.* Westchester, Pa.: C. Keith Wilbur, 1987.

William, H. A. *Aesthet. Med.* 13(1964):1–15 (Berlin).

Williams, C. A. S. *Outlines of Chinese Symbolism and Art Motives.* New York: Dover Pub., 1976.

Winkler, Wolf. *A Spectacle of Spectacles.* Jena: Carl Zeiss Edition Leipzig, 1988.

Woglom, Wm. H., M.D. *Discoverers for Medicine.* Chapter VIII. New Haven: Yale University Press, 1949.

Wollaston, W. H. *Periscopic Spectacles.* London, 1804.

Won, Shi-hwan. *History of Eyeglasses in Korea.* Seoul, Korea: Opticians Association of Korea, 1986.

Wood, Casey A., M.D. *The American Encyclopedia and Dictionary of Ophthalmology.* Chicago: Cleveland Press, 1915.

Wood, Casey A., M.D. "The First Scientific Work on Spectacles." *Annals of Medical History,* p. 150.

Wyler, Seymour. *Old Silver.* New York: Crown Publishers, 1937.

Young, John M. *The History of Eyewear.* Southbridge, Massachusetts: Optical Heritage Museum, 1985, pp. 71–82.

Young, T. "On the Mechanism of the Eye." *Phil. Trans. R. Soc.* 16(1801):23–88 (cited by M.B. Alpern, *Amer. J. Optom.* 25(1948):198).

Zeiss, Carl. *History of Spectacles.* Oberkochen: Zeiss Optical Company, 1958.

Index of Names

[Note: This index includes the names of individuals, companies, institutions, or organizations. Page numbers for figures, photographs, or illustrations are followed by *f*. Page numbers for tables are followed by *t*. There is a separate Subject Index.]

A. A. Webster & Co. (Brooklyn, NY), 186, 203
A. B. Griswold & Co. (New Orleans, LA), 199, 201
A. J. Stark and Co. (Denver, CO), 193
A. L. & Co., 429
A. L. J. C., 429
A. Meulemans Opticien (Brussels), 193
A. O. (1869), 429
A. Perain Optician (Paris), 192, 202
A. Stowell & Co. (Boston, MA), 183, 193, 203
Abbe, Ernst (Jena, Germany), 140, 371
Abelstrom, 31
Ackley, E., 429
Adams, George (London), 42–43, 44*t*–45*t*, 46, 115, 118, 276
Adams, Henry (Elmira, NY), 429
Adler, Coleman E. (New Orleans, LA), 198, 200
Aehle (of Whelan-Aehle-Hutchinson Jewelry Co.), St. Louis, MO, 186, 203

Aelfric, Abbott, 37
Ahlers, Henry C. (San Jose, CA), 175, 200
Aitken, M. J., 281
Alberone, Francesco, 357
Alhazen, 27
Allen, Alden, 52
Allen, Josiah Bennett, 52
American Academy of Ophthalmology Foundation Museum (San Francisco, CA), 20, 278, 309, 465
American Optical Company (Southbridge, MA), 29
  activities of, 52–60 passim, 65, 97
  advertisements of, 243
  Catalogs, various titles, 356
  development of, overview, 61*t*
  founders of, 54–57, 429
  Museum, 284, 465
  opera glasses, prices of, 163
  spectacles of, 236, 237*f*, 252, 254, 273, 293*f*, 314*f*, 384
  sunglasses, 273
  trial lens sets, 308, 315, 316
American Optician (Paris), 191
American Optometric Association Museum (St. Louis, MO), 465
American Optometric Society, 8
American Society of Appraisers, 166
Ammidown & Company, 55*f*, 61*t*
Ammidown & Putney, 61*t*
Ammidown & Son, 61*t*

Ammidown, Hanna, 54
Ammidown, Henry C., 56
Ammidown, Holdridge, 54, 55, 61, 61*t*
Ammidown, Lucius, 54, 55, 55*f*, 56, 61*t*
Ammidown (Southbridge, MA), 429
Anderson & Randolph (San Francisco, CA), 177, 200
Anderson, A. M., 374
Anderson Bros. (Camaguey, Cuba), 252
Andrew J. Lloyd & Co. (Boston, MA), 176, 184, 185, 191, 192, 202
Anglo-American Optical Company (London), 465
  Catalog, 356
Ann de Beaupre, Saint, 344
The Antiquarian Scientist (Dracut, MA), Catalog, 356
Antique Scientifica (Charleston, IL), Catalog, 357
The Antique Trader (Dubuque, IA), 356
Archbull, J. (London), 356
Archbull, W. E. (London), 356
Archer, J. E., 375
Archimeder Deposse, 167, 172
Aristophanes, 25
Armati, Amato degli, 35
Armati, Salvino, 395–428, 397*f*
Armiger, Jas. R. (Baltimore, MD), 184, 200
Arnhold Opticien (Paris), 193, 200
Arnold, M. (Ann Arbor, MI), 186
Artes, Chas. F. (Evansville, IL), 183, 200

Asprey (London), 192, 200
Aucott, Jarius, 271
Audemaire (Paris), 167, 172–173
Audomarus, Saint, 347
Austin Motor Company, 329
Ayscough, James, 21, 41–42

B & C (spectacles maker), 429
B & L Rootenberg Fine Books, Catalog, 357
B & McC (Butler & McCarthy), Philadelphia, PA, 429
B. H. Stief Jewelry Co. (Nashville, TN), 186, 203
B. Kahn & Son (NY), Catalog, 357
Bach, L. (Munich), 198
Bacon Bros. (Lowell, MA), 185, 200
Bacon, Roger, 27, 35
Badger, F. W. (Beaumont, TX), 182, 200
Bailey, Banks & Biddle Co. (Philadelphia, PA), 173, 183, 195, 200
Bailey, E. E. (Portland, ME; Claremont, NH), 429
Ball, Black & Co. (New York, NY), 190, 200, 429
Banks (of Bailey, Banks & Biddle Co.), Philadelphia, PA, 173, 183, 195, 200
Barber, W. (Philadelphia, PA), 429
Bardou, A. (Paris), 200
Barnes, William C., 57
Barry Dock (Cardiff, England), 194, 201
Bartou306, A., 167, 173
Bascolm Palmer Library (Miami, FL), 466
Bassoli, F. (Milan), Catalog, 357
Batchelder, J. W. (Buffalo, NY), 192, 200
Bate, Robert Betell, 118
Bates, Joel H., 174
Bauch, John J., 10, 51
Baumann, A. (New Orleans, LA), 199, 200
Bausch and Lomb Optical Company (Rochester, NY)
    contact lenses, 379
    history of, 21, 60–61, 251
    Ophthalmic Lens Catalog, 356
    sunglasses, 273
    trial lens sets, 315, 316
Bausch, E. (Rochester, NY), 183, 200
Bausch, George (Syracuse, NY), 186, 200, 243
Bay State Opt. (BSO) Co., 429
Beck, Richard, 342

Becker, Bernard (St. Louis, MO), 8
    Collection in Ophthalmology Catalog, 356
    Ophthalmology Library, 465
Beecher & Cole, 56*f*, 61*t*
Beecher, Hannah Jane, 54
Beecher, Jane Elizabeth, 54
Beecher, Nancy Ellen, 54
Beecher, Smith, 54
Beecher, William (Southbridge, MA), 3, 54, 55*f*, 56, 56*f*, 61*t*, 429
Beecher, William Ammidown, 54
Beethoven, 230
Benjamin, B., 429
Benjamin Pike, Jr. (NY), 163, 276
Bennett, A. G., 370
Benson, John, 50
Benz (spectacles maker), 429
Berman, Rosalind (Philadelphia, PA), Rosalind Berman Exhibit, 466
Bernard Becker Ophthalmology Library (St. Louis, MO), 8, 465
Bernhard, F. (Carlsbad), 198
Bertier, M. (Paris), 167, 173, 191
Besthoff (New York, NY), 193, 200
Beveridge, Martha, 395
BH & Co. B & L (after 1851), 429
Biddle (of Bailey, Banks & Biddle Co.), Philadelphia, PA, 173, 183, 195, 200
Bier, Norman (London), 375–376, 377
Birely & Son (Oshkosh, WI), 200
Bismarck, 230
Black (of Ball, Black & Co.), New York, NY, 190, 200
Blair, H. J. (Bristol), 182, 200
Blanchard Optical Company, 57, 58
Blodi, Frederick C., 26
Boekhandel, B. C. (Amsterdam), 356, 357
Boggs, John, 52
Bogleston, Edward (Stockbridge, MA), 429
Bohli (spectacles maker), 429
Boilly, 230
Bolles & Day (Hartford, CT), 429
Bonaparte, Napoleon, 115
Bontemps, 21
Borhek & Son Opticians (Philadelphia, PA), 184, 200, 429
Borsch, John L., Jr., 263
Borsch, John L. (Philadelphia, PA), 263
Boss (spectacles maker), 429
Boston Optical Works, 53–54
Bowers, Philip, 51

Bowles, H., 429
Brachet, 273
Braff, Solon (Los Angeles, CA), 375–377
Brewer (spectacles maker), 429
Brewster, Sir David, 53
Briely & Son (Oshkosh, WI), 172
Brieux, Alain (Paris), Catalog, 356
Briggs (spectacles maker), 429
British Optical Association (London)
    Foundation Museum, 465
    Museum and Library Catalog, 356
Brown & Kirby (New Haven, CT), 429
Brown, D. V., 43
Brown (of Williams, Brown & Earle), Philadelphia, PA, 185, 203
Browning, John, 284
Broy, 191
Bryden, D. J., 27, 29
BSO (Bay State Opt.) Co., 429
Bugbee, B. L., 57, 58
Bugbee, Benajah V., 57
Bugbee, L. W., 57–58
Bugbee, Willis, 58
Bull, G. J., 32, 33, 33*f*
Burnet, John, 276
Burt, John, 53
Burt, M. (Cleveland, OH), 196, 200
Busch (A-G), Emile (Brussels; Rathenow, Germany), 167, 173, 180, 189, 197, 200
Busch (Jena, Germany), 167
    See also La Princesse
Busch Multinee D.R.C.M., 173, 202
Busch, Multinett, 198
Butler & McCarthy (B & McC), Philadelphia, PA, 429
Butlon, E. W. (Bridgeport, CT), 172, 200

C & M Devel Teague, 193
C & R (spectacles maker), 429
C. C. & S. (spectacles maker), 429
C. D. (opera glass manufacturer), 167
C. F. (spectacles maker), 429
C. R. Co. (spectacles maker), 429
C. Ulrich Opticien (Nice; Paris; Vichy), 176, 203
Cadman, 43
Cadwell (spectacles maker), 429
Caldwell, J. E. (Paris; Philadelphia, PA), 167, 173, 182, 186, 200
Cardoni, Richard, 395
Carl Zeiss Company (Jena, Germany), 149, 172
Caron, J. A., 58

Caron, Leon, 58
Carpentier (Paris), 167, 173
Cass, N. W., 429
Central Mills Company, 59
Central Optical Company, 57, 58
Chaille' Jamison, 199
Challoner & Mitchell (Victoria, B.C., Canada), 193, 200
Champs Glass Works (Birmingham, England), 21
Chan, Eugene, 63
Chandler & Darrow (NY), 430
Chandler, Diamont (NY), 429
Chang Ching Chih, 63
Chao I Ou Pei, 63
Charles II, 7
Chavance & Co. (Paris), 167, 173
Chavance & Co. (Pittsburgh, PA), 201
Chavonnoz Ingenileer Opticien (Cours de L'Intendance), 187, 201
Cheney, A. M., 56, 61*t*
Cherdin, 99
Chevalier, 150*f*
Chevalier, Arthur, 30
Chevalier, Charles, 30
Chevalier, Guy (Paris), 168
Chevalier, Opticien (Paris), 173, 174, 201
Chevallier (of Maison de Guy Chevallier Opt.), Paris, 175
Chicago Optical Supply Company, Catalog, 356
Chin Shih, Emperor, 77
Chodowiecki (Chodofeeki), Daniel, 99
Christie's (South Kensington, London), Catalog, 356
Church, Monastery and Museum of the Cloisters (Wienhausen), 465
Ciba Vision, 379
Ciba-Geigy, 379
Cicero, 24
Cijuge Cissot Opticien (Paris), 180
Clark, Alvan, 53
Claudel, E & L (New Orleans, LA), 199, 201
Clay, Henry, 12
Clegg, James (Buffalo, NY), 179, 201
Clichy Glass Factory (France), 18
Cobb, G. E., 430
Codman & Shurteff (Boston, MA), *Eye Instruments* Catalog, 356
Cohen, Gilbert Blass, 278, 365*f*
Cole, E. Merritt, 56, 61*t*
Cole, Ella, 56

Cole, Robert H., 54, 55, 56–57, 61*t*
Collection in Ophthalmology, Bernard Becker (St. Louis, MO), 8, 356
Collins, 183
Colmont Bro. (Paris), 163, 164, 165, 176, 183
Colmont, Marguerite, 176
Colmont (of Geivoc & Colmont), Paris, 168
Colmont (Paris), 168, 175–176, 199, 200
Colton, I. [?], 430
Confucius, 23, 26, 63
Connecticut Medical Society Museum (Hartford, CT), 466
Continental Optical Company, 58
Cooke, L. J. (Findlay, OH), 181, 201
Cooper, G., 430
Cornichon (Paris), 193, 201
Corson, Richard, 41, 174, 230
Cottet, Jules (Morez-du-Jurain), 252
Coup, Elias (Bridgeport, CT), 430
Court, 40
Covent Garden Theater, 149
Cow (spectacles maker), 430
Crasset, Jean, 96
Cravel, Diplom-Optiker (Bremerhaven), 192, 201
Crescent (Paris), 168, 176
Cresco (Paris), 168, 176, 201
Cromwell (spectacles maker), 430
Crookes, Sir William, 273, 384
Cross (Paris), 168, 176
Crosthwaite, Peter, 276
Cuignet, 31
Curley & Bro. (New York, NY), 201
Curley, J. (NY), 182
Curtis & Stills (Woodbury, CT), 430
Cutter, Samuel Yale (Philadelphia, PA), Samuel Yale Cutter Collection, 466

da Vinci, Leonardo, 284, 369
Daca (Daza) de Valdes, Benito, 32, 40, 271, 354, 355*f*
Dachtera Bros. (New York, NY), 183, 201
Daguerre, Louis Jacques Mandé, 53
Dallos, Josef (Budapest), 372–374
d'Armato, Salvino. *See* Armati
Darrow (of Chandler & Darrow), New York, 430
Daviel, Jacques, 316
Davison, Margaret F., 467
Dawson, Steward (London), 193, 201
Day (of Bolles & Day), Hartford, CT, 429

de la Hire, Phillipe, 369–370
Debutant (Paris), 168, 176
DeCarle, John (London), 381
Decelles, M. Ernest, 58
Delany, 59
della Spina, Alessandro, 38, 395
Deposse, Archimeder, 167, 172
Deraisme (Paris), 168, 176, 177, 205
Derepas (Palais Royal, France), 168, 177, 183, 201
Derress (opera glass manufacturer), 194
Descartes, René, 369
Desroisier, E. D., 58
Devlyn, Frank (Mexico City), Frank Devlyn Collection, Devlyn Optical Company, 466
Diamanta (spectacles maker), 430
Dickens, Charles, 234
Dickinson, Frank, 377
Diplom-Optiker Cravel (Bremerhaven), 192, 201
Dixey Optical Company (London), 465
Dixon and Hampenstall (Dublin), 193, 201
Dobler, J. H. (Berlin), 230
Dollard (London), 168, 177, 201
Dollond and Aitchison Museum (London), 465
Dollond, J., 21, 29, 30, 141
Dollond (London), 168, 201
Dollond, P., 30
Dominelli, H. (France), 168, 177
Dominelli, V. (France), 168, 177
Donders, F. C., 31, 308
Dorner (spectacles maker), 430
Doster, M. (Philadelphia, PA), 430
Driefus, 379
Drury Lane Royal Theater, 149
Duchesse, 168, 177, 200
Duchesse, Jumelle, 171, 172, 187, 190
Dudgeon, R. E., 289
Duke-Elder, S., 369, 370
DuPaul Central Optical Company, 58
DuPaul, George, 58
DuPaul, Joseph M., 58
DuPaul Lockart (lens plant), 58
DuPaul Young Optical Company, 57, 58
Durand (Paris), 168, 177
Dürer, 239
Dwelle (spectacles maker), 430
Dyer, 30

E & L Claudel (New Orleans, LA), 199, 201

E. B. (Edward Bogleston[?]), Stockbridge, MA, 429
E. Bausch & Son (Rochester, NY), 183, 200
E. Borhek & Son Opticians (Philadelphia, PA), 184, 200
E. Edmonds & Son, 56, 58
E. Gome Optician (Paris), 201
E. Gome Opticien (Paris), 192
E. Krauss & Cie. (Leipzig, London, Milan, Paris, St. Petersburg), 178, 201
E. W. Butlon & Co. (Bridgeport, CT), 172, 200
Eagle, Theo (St. Louis, MO), 186, 201
Earle (of Williams, Brown & Earle), Philadelphia, PA, 185, 203
Eastern Optical Company, 58
Eaton, Mrs. Ruth (Beecher), 54
Eccel Rest Guard Company, 58
Edmonds, C. S., 56
Edmonds, E., 56, 58
Eldridge, E., 430
Elite (Paris), 167, 168, 177, 191
Ellis Island Museum, 180
Eltonhead (Baltimore, MD), 430
Emile Busch (A-G) (Brussels; Rathenow, Germany), 167, 173, 200
Enoch, J., 369
Entrement (Paris), 168, 177
Estberg & Sons (Waukesha, WI), 191, 200
Evans, Sir Arthur, 24
Evans (spectacles maker), 430

F. & Co., 430
F. E. C. N. (spectacles maker), 430
F. W. McAllister Co. (Baltimore, MD), 182, 202
Fabergé, 153
Fairfield (of Hight & Fairfield), Butte, MO, 195
Fairford, Alan, 276
Fargier, Leon, 273
Farr, J. C. (Philadelphia, PA), 430
Farriday, 21
Faye, I. A. (Hot Springs, AR), 201
Feinbloom, William (NY), 375, 380
Fenno, John, 258
Fick, Adolph Eugene, 370–371, 376
Field (of Hammersmith & Field), San Francisco, CA, 191, 201
Fieuzel (Paris), 273
Firce (spectacles maker), 430
Fisher (Philadelphia, PA), 430

Fitz, Henry, 52
Flammarion, Jelle (Paris), 169, 177, 201
Fleming, Robert J., 245, 252
Fleming, S. J., 281
Fleurigny (Paris), 168, 177, 201
Fontaine (Paris), 168, 177
Food and Drug Administration, U.S., 378, 379
Fortin, 37
Foster, N., 430
Foster, T., 430
Fowlers (Chicago, IL), 168, 191, 201
Fox, Edward, 43
Fox, G., 430
Foye, I. A. (Hot Springs, AR), 167, 188
Franklin & Co. (Washington, D.C.), 175, 201
Franklin, Benjamin, 29, 99, 258–259
Franklin Institute, 52
Franklin (Washington, D.C.), 430
Frantz & Opitz (New Orleans, LA), 199, 201
Frantz, Chas. S. (Lancaster, MO), 172, 201
Fraunhofer, 21
Freeman, J. J. (Toledo, OH), 193, 201
Fridolin, Saint, 35
Frigerio (New Orleans, LA), 199, 201
Fritsch, A. (Graz, Austria), 168, 178
Frois, Louis, 96
Fronmuller, George, 308
Frontier Contact Lens Laboratory (Buffalo, NY), 379
Fuller, 30
Fulton, Robert, 284

G. B., 430
G. Santi Opticien (Marseilles), 192
G. T. (spectacles maker), 430
G. W. Jewelry Co. (Peoria, IL), 191, 201
G. W. Wells Foundation, 57
Galileo, 21, 138
Galipeau, Alfred, 58
Galst, Jay (New York, NY), Dr. Jay Galst Collection, 466
Garrett, P., 430
Garzoni, Tomaso, 32
Gatenaux, Felix, 58
Geivroc & Colmont (Paris), 168
Gemmary (Redondo Beach, CA), Catalog, 356
Geneva Optical Company (Chicago, IL), 163
    Catalog, 356

Genossen. *See* Institute of Schott and Genossen
Genroz & Colmont, 168, 178
Geo. C. Shreve & Co. (San Francisco, CA), 183
Geo. Elliot, & Company (NY), *Our Eyes, Spectacles* Catalog, 356
Geoffrey & Co. (New York, NY), 254
George C. Shreve & Co. (San Francisco, CA), 203
George Tiemann & Company (NY), Catalog, 357
George I, King, 14, 14f
George II, King, 14–15, 14f
George IV, King, 271
Gerhardt, William, 51
Gesell, 273
Giamanta (spectacles maker), 430
Giegrist (Switzerland), 369
Gilpin, William, 276
Gilsey, James, 358, 359f
Giordano, Friar, 38
Giordano, R. V., 356
Godchaux, Joseph (Paris), 193, 201
Goethe, 115
Gold (of Stevens & Gold), 432
Goldsmith & Son (Washington, D.C.), 191, 201
Gome, E. (Paris), 192, 201
Good (spectacles maker), 430
Goodrich (of Hyde & Goodrich), New Orleans, LA, 200, 201
Goodthein (of Platt and Goodthein), Cincinnati, OH, 187, 202
Gould, George M., 253, 261
Graff, Anton, 99
Graffe, H. C. (Fort Wayne, IN), 190, 201
Graham, R., 377
Gravière (Paris), 180
Gray, N. C., 430
Gray, Thomas, 275–276
Grey (Paris), 201
Griffin Laboratories (Toronto, Canada), 379
Griswold, A. B. (New Orleans, LA), 201
Griswoll, G., 430
Grube, 37
Gscheidel, F. (Koenigsberg), 193, 201
Guild of St. Odilia (Consulting Opticians), 347
Guilmette, Ronaldo, 58
Guinaud, P. L., 21
Guy Chevalier (Paris), 167, 174–175

H & H (Hall & Hewson), Albany, NY, 430
H. C. Ammidown & Co., 56
H. C. Warner (Fresno, CA), 182, 203
H. Lamay (Paris), 169, 179
H. (M & deer), 430
H. Murr's & Sons (Philadelphia, PA), 196, 202
H. S. Raybauld Collection, Natal Museum (Pietermaritzburg, South Africa), 465
Habermeier (spectacles maker), 114, 430
Hadley, John, 32
Hall & Hewson (H & H), Albany, NY, 430
Hall, Frederic, 51
Hall, M. B., 430
Hallauer, Otto (Bern), 273, 357
  Otto Hallauer Collection, University of Bern, 465
Hamblin, T. H., 316, 317f, 373
Hammersmith & Field (San Francisco, CA), 191, 201
Hammon, J. H., 263
Hampenstall (of Dixon and Hampenstall), Dublin, 193, 201
Hardin, Jack (Chicago, IL), 252
Hardy, 59, 192, 201
Hardy & Hayes (Pittsburg, PA), 192, 201
Hardy Optical (Chicago, IL), 252
Harris & Co. (Washington, D.C.), 184
Harris, H. M. (France), 201
Harris, M. H., 192
Harris, R. (Washington, D.C.), 201
Harrison, Charles C., 53
Harvard University, 63
Harvey Lewis Co. (USA), 187, 202
Harwood Brothers, 430
Hasert, Bruno, 51
Hassler, M., 52, 53
Hauserman's (Patterson, NJ), 193, 201
Hawkins, 264
Hayes Brothers, 194
Hayes (of Hardy & Hayes), Pittsburgh, PA, 192, 201
Hazebroucq Opticien, 157
Heinrich Rath, Hof-Optiker (Munich), 192
Heitz, R. F., 370
Helmholz, 31
Hemmingway, William, 252
Henry Adams & James Peters (Philadelphia, PA), 429

Henry Kahn & Co. (San Francisco, CA), 182, 201
Herbert, Pitt, 233
Herschel, Sir John F. W., 370, 373
Herve, Saint, 347
Hewson (of Hall & Hewson), Albany, NY, 430
Hieronymus, Sofronuis Eusebius, 35
Higgins (spectacles maker), 430
Hight & Fairfield (Butte, MT), 195
Hill, A. M. (New Orleans, LA), 200, 201
Hillner (spectacles maker), 430
Hilscher, Gottlieb Christian, 29, 32
  Concise Instruction in Grinding Lenses and Fitting Telescopes (English translation), 467–487, 468f
Himmler, Otto (Berlin), 371
Hiroo Nagaoka, 97
Hirsch & Kaiser (San Francisco, CA), 191, 201
Hirschberg, Julius, 26, 35, 37
Hirth, Fr., 27
Hixson, W. T. (El Paso, TX), 183, 201
Hobron, A., 430
Hoen, J. (Lyon, France), 193
Hoffman (Columbus, OH), 167, 194, 201, 430
Hogarth, 363f
Holcomb, Amasa, 52
Holtman, W. H., 62, 230
Hooper, W. (Point Portsmouth), 198
Hopkins, 43
Horne, Richard, 220
Howell, John, Catalog (San Francisco, CA), 357
Hoya (Japan), 379
Hudson, J. T., 22, 32, 149
Hugh of St. Cher [Cardinal Ugone], 35
Hughes, E., 430
Hunt, Robert, 271
Hutchinson (of Whelan-Aehle-Hutchinson Jewelry Co.), St. Louis, MO, 186, 203
Hutten, E. P., 254
Hyde & Goodrich (New Orleans, LA), 200, 201
Hyde, B., 430
Hyde, James (New Orleans, LA), 430
Hyde (spectacles maker), 430
Hydron, 379

IDA (Paris), 169, 178, 205
Ilikit (spectacles maker), 430
Imperial Optical Co. (Paris), 198, 201

Independent Optical Company, 58
Ingenileer, Chavonnoz (Cours de L'Intendance), 187, 201
Institute of Macro-molecular Chemistry (Prague), 379
Institute of Schott and Genossen, 21, 22
Iris (Paris), 169, 178
Isa, Ali B., 27
Isen, Allen (Buffalo, NY), 379
Israel, B. M. (Amsterdam), 356, 357

J. & H. T. (England), 430
J. & J. R. (spectacles maker), 430
J. A. Hill, Bookseller, Catalog (NY), 357
J. A. (spectacles maker), 429
J. and W. E. Archbull (London), Catalogue and Price List, 356
J. Curley & Bro. (NY), 182
J. E. Caldwell & Co. (Paris, Philadelphia, PA), 167, 173, 182, 186, 200
J. E. Milch (Mielck), St. Petersburg; Moscow, 171
J. E. S. & Co., 431
J. H. Johnson and Co. (New York, NY), 192, 201
J. Hoen Optn (Lyon, France), 193
J. K. (spectacles maker), 430
J. Robinson Optician (NY), 183, 202
J. S. & Co., 175
J. W. (Philadelphia, PA), 182, 183, 201
J. Waldstein, Optikea (Vienna), 190
J. Winreurgh and Son (Utica, NY), 185, 203
J. Wiss & Son (Newark, NJ), 192, 203
Jaccard (of Mermod and Jaccard Jewelry Co.), 185, 202
Jaeger Bros. (Portland, OR), 196, 201
James McCreery & Co. (New York, NY), 191, 202
James Prentice & Son, 185
James Sinclair Co. Ltd. (London), 197, 203
James W. Queen, and Company (NY), *Optical Instruments* Catalog, 357
James Willmott & Sons Company, 329–330
Jansen, L. (New Orleans, LA), 200, 201
Janssen, Zach, 138
Jas. R. Reed & Co. (Pittsburgh, PA), 173, 202
Javal, Emile, 30, 31
  History and Bibliography of Astigmatism (English translation), 433–436
Jelle Flammarion (Paris), 169, 178

Jenkins, L., 370
Jeremy Norman and Company (San Francisco, CA), 466
   Medicine and the Life Sciences Catalog, 357
Jersey Museum (St. Helier, Channel Islands), 465
Jessen, George (Chicago, IL), 377–378
Jobe Rose Jewelry Co. (Birmingham, AL), 182, 202
Jockey Club (Paris), 169, 181
John Weiss & Son (London), *Catalogue of Ophthalmic Instruments and Apparatus,* 357
Johnson, A. B. (Hill, NH), 430
Johnson and Johnson, 380
Johnson, J. H. (New York, NY), 201
Johnson, Samuel, 103
Johnston, J. H. (NY), 192
Jonas W. Rosenthal M.D. Ophthalmology Museum, Tulane University Medical School (New Orleans, LA), 465
Jos Linz and Bros. (Dallas, TX), 185, 202
Joseph Godchaux Optician (Paris), 193, 201
Joslin & Park (Salt Lake City, UT), 184, 201
Julius King Opt. Co., 198
Jumelle De Tir, 178
Jumelle, Duchesse, 171, 190
Jumelle Elliptique Brevetée S.G.D.G., 195
Jumelle (France), 169, 178, 197, 198

Kahn, B. (NY), 357
Kahn, Henry (San Francisco, CA), 182, 201
Kai Ming Chiu, 63–64
Kaiser (of Hirsch & Kaiser), San Francisco, CA, 191, 201
Kalt, Eugen (Paris), 372
Kang-hsi, Emperor, 37
Katalog-Einer Bilderaustellung zur Geschichte der Brille, Drs. Greeff, Hallauer, Lundsgaard, Pflugk, Reiss, Simon, und Weve (Amsterdam), 357
Keeler, 316
Keeler Museum of Windsor (England), 465
Keeler Ophthalmic Equipment (London), Catalog, 357
Keith, T. (Worcester, MA), 430
Keith, W. (Worcester, MA), 430
Kelley, Gary, 11

Kempston, Peter (England), 430
Kendall, W. B., 430
Kendrick, Wm. (Louisville, KY), 167, 191, 201
Kent, J., 430
Kern (spectacles maker), 430
Kikeriki, 230
Kiltner (spectacles maker), 430
King, Julius (Cleveland, OH), 430
King (St. Louis, MO), 202
Kippen (spectacles maker), 430
Kirby (of Brown & Kirby), New Haven, CT, 429
Klein Dezso (Budapest), 198
Knight and Son (North Hampton), 196
Koller, Karl, 370
Kornblum (Pittsburgh, PA), 175, 193, 201
Krauss, E. (Leipzig; London; Milan; Paris; St. Petersburg), 169, 178, 201
Kriegsman Brothers, 52
Kublai Khan, 26

L & H (spectacles maker), 431
L & R (opera glass manufacturer), 169, 178
L. Ulrich Opticien (Nice, France), 191, 203
L B & Co. (Paris), 169, 178, 202, 431
La Belle (Paris), 169, 179
La Corona (Paris), 167, 169, 179, 191
La Dauphine (Paris), 169, 179
La Favorite (Paris), 169, 179
La Fontaine (France), 169
La Gorona (Paris), 169
La Heijnen, LaHaye, 191
La Heynen, 202
La Merveilleuse (Paris), 179
La Mier (Lamier), Paris, 169
La Mignonne Gravière (Paris), 180, 202
La Mons (France), 169, 180
La Monte (Paris), 169, 180
La Princesse (Jena, Germany), 169, 180
   See also Busch
La Princesse (Paris), 170
La Reine (Paris), 170, 180
La Roque (Paris), 170, 180
La Touraine (Paris), 163, 170, 181, 191
La Vil (Lavel), Paris, 170, 181
LaBelle (Paris), 179
LaFontaine Optn (Paris), 179
Lafontine Optn (Paris), 169
Lago, Inc. (Paris), Catalog, 357
Laine (Paris), 202

LaLente, Fritz Rathschuler, Catalog (Genova), 357
Lamaier (Paris), 179
Lamaire (Paris), 179
Lamarye (Paris), 187
Lamay, H. (Paris), 169, 179
Lamayre (Paris), 169, 179
Lambe (spectacles maker), 431
Lamier (La Mier), Paris, 169, 179–180
Lamier (Paris), 179
L'Amour (Paris), 169, 180
Lamy, H. (Paris), 21, 180
LAMY (Paris), 169, 180
Lan, Martayan (NY), Catalog, 357
Lance, L. (Paris), 193, 202
Lang Ying, 64
Lange and Lange (Dubuque, IA), 193, 202
LaPierre, Alfred, 58
Laronde Philippe Voir & Cie (Paris), Catalog, 357
Latimer, Darsie, 276
Latour (France), 170, 180–181
Laval (opera glass manufacturer), 170, 181
Lavel (La Vil), Paris, 170
Lavel (Paris), 170, 181
Lavière (Paris), 170
Lavil (Paris), 202
Laville (Paris), 181
Lavoice, Wilfrid, 58
Lazarus & Morris, 431
Le Clair (Paris), 170, 181
Le Fils (Paris), 170, 181, 199
Le Jeune (Paris), 170
Le Jockey Club (Paris), 169, 181
Le Maire, 163
Le Maître (Paris), 170, 187
Le Mieux (Paris), 170, 187
Le Miux (Paris), 170, 187
Le Père (Paris), 170
Le Prince (France), 170, 187
Le Roi (Paris), 170, 187, 191
Le Roque (Memphis, TN; Paris), 167, 170, 187, 191
LeClaire, Edward, 58
LeClaire, Hector M., 58
LeClaire, P. N., 58
LeClare (Paris), 181
Leeds, James, 8
   James Leeds Library, University of Indiana Optometry School, 466
Lefevre, A. (Paris), 197
Lefils (Paris), 181
Leglaire, 170, 181

Lehmann, Caspar, 20
LeJeune (Paris), 181
Lemaire, 162f, 164, 165, 180, 204–205
Lemaire (Paris), 153, 155f, 166, 170, 182–187, 198, 199, 200
Lemière, 170
Lemiere (Paris), 187
Lensdale Company (MA), 57
Leo X, Pope, 220, 230
Lepage, Anne Marie, 143
LePage, M. Zepherin, 58
Letocha, Charles (York, PA), 258, 466
Levene, John R. (Memphis, TN), 258
Lewenberg, Leon, 51
Lewis, A., 431
Lewis, Harvey (USA), 187, 202
Librairie Thomas-Scheler (Paris), *Livres Anciens d'Ophthalmologie*, Catalog, 357
Library of Congress, 8
Ligtmeyer, Archie (Milwaukee, WI), 182, 202
Lim, 379
Linz, Jos. (Dallas, TX), 185, 202
Lippershey, Johannes, 138
Liu An, 63
Lloyd, Andrew J. (Boston, MA), 176, 184, 185, 191, 192, 202, 431
Lloyd, Harold, 384
Lloyd (spectacles maker), 431
LO N.Y. (spectacles maker), 431
Lock, W., 431
Lockett, A., 60
Loehr (of Scribner and Loehr Co.), Cleveland, OH, 175, 202
Loewenstein, H. Y. (St. Louis, MO), 181
Lohnstein (Berlin), 369
Lomb, 51
London Company of Virginia (Jamestown), 21
Lorraine, Claude, 274–277
Louchet (Paris), 170, 188, 204
Louis XVI, King, 145
Lover, Mary, 106
Lowenstein, H. Y. (St. Louis, MO), 202
LSF & S (spectacles maker), 431
Lucia, Saint. *See* Lucy, Saint
Lucy, Saint, 5, 6f, 7, 35, 344–347, 345f, 347f
Lumière of Paris, 149, 161, 170, 180
Lundsgaard, 357
Lynch, T. H. (Union Square), 187
Lyon, T., 431

M&R Industries, 57
M. Burt and Co. Jewelers (Cleveland, OH), 196, 200
M. Hassler & Co. (Philadelphia, PA), 52, 53
M (M & deer), 430
Mac Keown, S. C. (Lawrence, KS), 184, 202
Mac Naught (of White & Mac Naught), Minneapolis, MN, 184, 203
MacGregor, Ronald J. S., 4
Magne, 233
Maison de Guy Chevallier Opt. (Paris), 175
Makepeace, F. A., 355f
Mallowan, M. E. L., 18
Mannerbruk, Wm. (Reading, PA), 431
Manni, Domenico Maria, 395
    About Eyeglasses for the Nose Invented by Salvino Armati Florentine Gentleman (English translation), 398–428
Mao, Winifred, 63
Mar Neil (Paris), 171, 188, 202
Marchand (Paris), 170, 188, 200
Marco Polo. *See* Polo, Marco
Marcon (Paris), 171, 188, 202
Marley, Pierre, 138
    Pierre Marley Collection (Paris), 465
Marquisette (Paris), 188
Marshall, John, 27, 29
Marshall, W. H., 309
Marshall, Walter H. (Gainesville, FL), Dr. and Mrs. Walter H. Marshall Exhibit, 466
Martayan Lan (NY), Catalog, 357
Martin, Benjamin, 42, 43, 106–110, 354
    New Elements of Optics—A Catalogue of W. & S. Jones (London), 357
Martin, John, 106
Martin, Joshua Lover, 106
Marvo Spelio Cemetary, 24
Mason, William, 275
Maurolycus, Franciscus, 31
Max Meyer & Bro. (Omaha, NE), 182, 202
McAllister, 30, 36f, 51
McAllister & Brothers (Philadelphia, PA), Catalog, 357
McAllister, F. W. (Baltimore, MD), 182, 202
McAllister Opt. Co. (Philadelphia, PA), 176, 202

McAllister, W. Y. (Philadelphia, PA), *Optical and Mathematical Instruments* Catalog, 357
McAllister, William Y. (Philadelphia, PA), 163, 354, 355f, 431
McCarthy (of Butler & McCarthy), Philadelphia, PA, 429
McCreery & Co. (New York, NY), 202
McCreery, James (New York, NY), 191
McDonald, Linda L., 433
McDougal, 254
McIntyre, Isadora F., 190
McKinstry, C. B., 57
McLean, Thomas, 230
McMaster, Robert W., 54, 59
Medow, Norman (New York, NY), Dr. Norman Medow Collection, 466
Meissonnier (Paris), 171, 188
Mercier, 143
Mermod and Jaccard Jewelry Co.(Paris; St. Louis, MO), 185
Mermod Jaccard & King Co. (NY; St. Louis, MO), 191, 202
Merriman (spectacles maker), 431
Merry Optical Company (Kansas City, MO), 163
    Catalog, 357
Merveille et Cie (Paris), 167, 171, 188
Metius, 138
Meulemans, A. (Brussels), 193, 202
Meyer, Max (Omaha, NE), 182, 202
Meyrowitz Bros. (Albany, NY), 175, 192, 202
Meyrowitz, E. B., 43
Meyrowitz, E. B. (New York, NY), 202
Meyrowitz, E. B. (NY), 175, 182, 191
    Ophthalmic Apparatus Catalog, 357
Meyrowitz, E. B. (Paris), 175, 182
Meyrowitz, Paul A., 196
Mezi, 63
Mielck (Milch), J. E. (Moscow; Paris; St. Petersburg), 167, 171, 188, 202
Miles, John, 174
Miller, Pardon (Providence, RI), 431
Mitchell (of Challoner & Mitchell), Victoria, B.C., Canada, 193, 200
Modena, Tommaso da, 35
Monoyer, 32
Monroy (Paris), 171, 188, 202
Monseret, 149
Moody, Daniel D. (Monson, MA), 431
Moore, Thomas, 230
Morck, August, 261

Morris (of Lazarus & Morris), 431
Morrison, Robert (Harrisburg), 379
Moses, 35
Mourlon (Paris), 171, 188
Mulford (Memphis, TN), 191–192, 202
Muller, A. C., 370
Muller, August (Gladbach), 370–371
Muller, C. (San Francisco, CA), 192, 202
Muller Company (Weisbaden), 372
Muller, Friedrich A. (Weisbaden), 370–371
Multinee, Bush, 202
Munroe, M., 431
Murr, H. (Philadelphia, PA), 196, 202
Musée de la Lunetterie (Morez, France), Catalog, 357
Musée de l'instrumentation optique (Biesheim, France), 466
Museo dell' Occhiale (Verona: Pieve di Codore), Catalog, 357
Museum of Antique Glasses (Murai Company), Fukui City, Japan, 465
Museum of Science (London), Wellcome Collection, 465
Museum of Spectacles (Piere di Cadore, Italy), 465
Museum of the Hospital de la Luz (Mexico City), 466
Mütter Museum (Philadelphia, PA), 466

N. & T. Foster, 430
Nagel, 32
Nagel, William (Paducah, KY), 192, 202
Narcissus (Paris), 171, 188
Natal Museum, H. S. Raybauld Collection (Pietermaritzburg, South Africa), 465
National Health Service (Great Britain), 329–330
National Library of Medicine, National Institute of Health, Catalog (Bethesda, MD), 357
National Museum of American History, 50
National Museum of History and Technology, 275
National Patent Development Corporation (NY), 379
Negretti & Zambra Opticians (Holborn), 192, 202
Neill, John (Philadelphia, Pa), 377
Neitz Company (Japan), 316, 317f
Nepos, Cornelius, 24
Nerdi (Paris), 202

Nerney, Peter, 47
Nero, Emperor, 24, 270
New Era Optical Company, Catalog (New Orleans, LA), 357
New Era Optical Company (Chicago, IL), 163
New York Academy of Medicine (New York, NY), 466
Newberry & Co. (Brooklyn, NY), 431
Newbury, Edwin (Brooklyn, CT), 431
Newbury (Philadelphia, PA), 431
Nicole, Leon (Lyon, France), Catalog, 357
Nie Chong Hou, 63
Nissel, George, 373
Nitsche & Gunther, Hauptkatalog (Rathenow, Germany), 357
Noack, Chas. J. (Sacramento, CA), 174, 193, 202
Noël (Paris), 171, 188
Nomar Optical Company, 58
Nordlinger, S. (Los Angeles, CA), 175, 202
Norman, Jeremy (San Francisco, CA), 466
  Jeremy Norman and Company *Medicine and the Life Sciences* Catalog, 357
Nuremberg Museum, 35

OB & T (NY), 196, 202
Obrig Laboratories, 377
Obrig, Theo. E., 25, 370–377 passim
Occhiali Italiani (Milan), Catalog, 357
Ochs (of Wall and Ochs), Philadelphia, PA, 197, 203
O'Dell, Lawrence (New York, NY), 431
Odilia, Saint, 346–347
O'Driscoll, K. F., 379
Oerte, C. E. (Philadelphia, PA), 431
Okihiro Nishi, 98
Olbricht, B. (Brooklyn, NY), 183, 202
Old Sturbridge Village (Museum), 57
Olmsted, Nathaniel (Farmington; New Haven, CT), 431
Ophthalmic Antiques International Collectors' Club, 4, 329, 346
Ophthalmic Museum, University of Bern Medical School, 273
Opitz (New Orleans, LA), 201
Optical House of M. H. Harris, 192
Optical Institute (New York, NY), 51
Optical Institute (Paris), 191, 202
Optical Museum (Hannibal, MO), 465

Optical Specialty Company, 58
Optical Works (North Oxford, MA), 53
Optico Utrecht (Netherlands), Catalog, 357
Optic-Oculistic Institute (Leipsig), 52
Optisches Museum (Oberkochen), *Die Brille* Catalog, 357
Orford, H., 60
Orr, F. H., 58
Orr, Hugh, 337
Ostwalt, 31
Otto Hallauer Collection, University of Bern (Switzerland), 465
Ouimet, Joseph, 58
Owen, J.[?] (Philadelphia, PA), 431

P. L. Taylor & Co. (Brooklyn, NY), 432
P. Miller & G. U. Wright, 431
Paine, Charles M., 53
Paine, George, 53
Paine, Henry M., 53
Paine, John P., 53
Park (of Joslin & Park), Salt Lake City, UT, 184, 201
Parker, C., 105
Parker (spectacles maker), 431
Pascal, J., 370
Pauthier, 37
Payton, E. L., 329
Peacock, C. D. (Chicago, IL), 175, 182, 184, 197, 202
Peale, Rembrandt, 99, 102f
Peck, A. G. (Osterbrooke, OH), 431
Peck, Alex (Charleston, IL), *Antique Scientifica* Catalog, 357
Peirce (Philadelphia, PA; Boston, MA), 431
Perain, A. (Paris), 202
Percival, MacIver, 31, 228
Peters, G. (Philadelphia, PA), 431
Peters, James (Philadelphia, PA), 429, 431
Peters (spectacles maker), 431
Pflugk, 357
Philip, Trevor (London), 357
Phillips, Nigel (London), *Medicine* Catalog, 357
Pierce, John (Boston, MA), 431
Pierre Marley Collection (Paris), 465
Pierson, Richard, 271
Pike, Benjamin Jr. (NY), 163, 276
Pinchbeck, Christopher, 12
Pitkin, J. O. (Hartford, CT), 431
Pitkin, O., 431
Pitkin, W., 431

Platt and Goodthein (Cincinnati, OH), 187, 202
Platt (spectacles maker), 431
Pleasanton, A. J. (Philadelphia, PA), 271
Pliny the Younger, 17, 24, 27, 37
Polo, Marco, 26, 35, 37, 62–63, 64, 270
Polymer Technology Corporation, 380
Porter, L. C. (Hartford, CT), 431
Porterfield, William, 308
Poulet, W., 62, 299, 358
Praecedo, 171, 189
Precioptic Levallois, 171, 189
Premier (Paris), 171, 189
Prentice, C. F., 31
Prentice, James, 185
Price, J., 431
Prince, Abraham, 52
The Printer's Devil (Decatur, GA), Ophthalmic List Catalog, 357
Prism Optics, 196
Prosper Bunoust Ingr Opticien (Paris), 194, 202
Prussen, E., 51
Pryor-Ingopt, G. E. (Paris), 191, 202
Ptolemy, Claudius, 27
Pugh (spectacles maker), 431
Putney, Jairus, 55, 61t

Quality Lens Company, 58
Queen & Co. (Philadelphia, PA), 189, 202, 431
Queen, James W., 357

R. Harris & Co. (Washington, D.C.), 184, 201
Randolph (of Anderson & Randolph), San Francisco, CA, 200
Raphael, Saint, Archangel
Rasmussen, Otto Durham, 26, 62, 63, 68, 77, 87, 270
Rath, Heinrich (Munich), 192, 202
Rathenow Museum (Rathenow, Germany), 465
Ravenscroft, 7, 20, 21
Raybauld, H. S., 465
Reed, Jas. R. (Pittsburgh, PA), 173
Reich (spectacles maker), 431
Reiss, 357
Research Laboratory for Archaeology and the History of Art, 281
Revlon, 306
Ribright, 145
Richard, Karl, 62
Richards, Stephen, 58
Richardson, John, 259

Richter, F. W. (Dresden), 191, 202
Riggs Optical Company, Ophthalmic Instruments and Equipment Catalog, 357
Rittenhouse, David, 50
Rivera (France), 171, 189
Roach, John, 52
Robert H. Cole & Company, 56, 61t
Roberts, F. (Philadelphia, PA), 431
Robinson, J. (NY), 183, 202, 431
Rodenstock, Josef, Optiker (Berlin; Charlottenburg; Munich), 171, 189, 202, 205
Rootenberg, B., 357
Rootenberg, L., 357
Rose & Co. (London), 203
Rose, Jobe (Birmingham, AL), 182, 202
Rosen, Edward, 395
Rosenberg, H. (Canon City, CO), 195
Rosenthal, Bertha, 364f
Rosenthal, Jacques, 35
Rosenthal, Jonas William (New Orleans, LA)
    Dr. and Mrs. J. William Rosenthal Collection, 466
    Jonas W. Rosenthal M.D. Ophthalmology Museum, Tulane University Medical School, 465
Ross & Co. (London), 186, 202
Ross (London), 171, 189, 194
Rottesmuller Luxottica Collection (Agordo, Italy), 465
Rowley, William, 308
Royal Astronomical Society of London, 21
Royal Society, 27, 29
Rumse, C., 431
Rushmer Jewelry Co. (Pueblo), 185

S. F. & Co., 431
S. G. N.Y. (spectacles maker), 431
S. Nordlinger & Son (Los Angeles, CA), 175, 202
S.T.D.C. (spectacles maker), 431
Sabell, Tony, 371
Saemisch, E. T. (Bonn), 370–371, 381
Sakellarakis, Yannis A., 25
Salvatori, Phillip, 374
Santa Maria Majore Church (Florence), 396f–397f
Santi, G. (Marseilles), 192, 202
Santi, Raphael (Orbino), 220, 230
Sargeant, J. (Hartford, CT), 431
Scarlett, Edward, 32, 41, 99, 111
Schaer, Paul (Brussels), 171, 189, 202
Schauz (Dresden), 273

Scheidig (spectacles maker), 431
Schild (spectacles maker), 431
Schildknecht (spectacles maker), 114, 431
Schmura (Budapest), 198
Schmutz, E., 191, 202
Schnaitman, Charles, 53, 114
Schnaitman, Isaac, 51, 431
Schneider (spectacles maker), 431
Schneider, Ulz, 21
Schneirer (spectacles maker), 431
Schneizer (spectacles maker), 431
Scholetzer, Edward, 52
Schott. See Institute of Schott and Genossen
Schreiber (spectacles maker), 431
Schubert, Franz, 364f
Schumacher & Toreman (Baltimore, MD), 191, 203
Schweizer (spectacles maker), 431
Scientia (Arlington, MA), Historic Medicine Catalog, 357
Scientific Instrument Society Bulletin (London), 357
Scooler, M. (New Orleans, LA), 200, 203
Scott, Sir Walter, 276
Scribner and Loehr Co. (Cleveland, OH), 175, 202
Scrini, 37
Segttz, K., 431
Sekiya Shirayama, 96
Selfridge (London), 197
Semmons Wien (Vienna), 171, 192, 203
Seneca, Lucius Annaeus, the younger, 24, 27
Senter, Wm. (Portland, ME), 191, 203
Shaws, E., 431
Shen Kuo, 63
Sherman, Spencer (New York, NY), Dr. Spencer Sherman Collection, 466
Shih Hong, 63–64
Shih Tsung, Emperor, 97
Short, Mace, 47
Shreve & Co. (San Francisco, CA), 188, 203
Shreve, George C. (San Francisco, CA), 183, 203
Shrisheim, Louis, 53
Shuan Tsung, Emperor, 63, 97
Shuron Continental Company, 57, 58
Shuron (spectacles maker), 431
Shuron Standard Company, 58
Shurteff (of Codman & Shurteff), Boston, MA, Eye Instruments Catalog, 356

Shurtleff, Louis E. (New Bedford, MA), 172, 203
Sichel, Jules 31
Silliman, Benjamin, 52
Simmons Bros. (Columbus, OH), 175, 203
Simms, D. L., 27, 29
Simon, 357
Simon Bros. (Columbus, OH), 203
Sinclair, James (London), 197, 203
Sines, George, 25
Singer, Martin, 273
Sirturus, 27
Sleulen (London), 192, 203
Slofman (spectacles maker), 431
Smith & Still, 431
Smith, Addison, 29, 42
Smith, J. L., 431
Smith, John, 52
Smithsonian Institution (Washington, D.C.), 20
   American Museum of History and Technology, 465
   Press Catalog, 357
Smyth & Co. (Birmingham), 329
Snell, Willebord, 32
Snyder, Charles, 258
Société des Lunetiers (Paris), 355f
   Catalog, 357
Société d'Optique (Paris), 171, 189
Sohnges, Willie (Munich), 377
Solex Laboratories, 377
Solomons, A., 431
Solomons, Elias, 271
Solomons, George, 271
Sommer, Balthasar, 50
Sotheby's (NY), Catalog, 357
South Toric Lens Company, 58
Southbridge Historical Society (MA), 54
Southbridge Optical Company (MA), 57–58
Southbridge Optical Supply Company (MA), 58
Southbridge Spectacle Manufacturing Company (MA), 58
Southbridge Toric Lens Company (MA), 58
Spaulding and Co. (Paris), 185
Spec Shop (Southbridge, MA), 57, 58, 59
Spectacles makers' Company, 29
Spectacles makers' Guild, 39, 42
Speel, Erika, 153, 157
Spencer, Charles A., 52, 53

Sportière (Paris), 171, 189
Sporting Club (Paris), 198, 205
Sportreil (Paris), 171, 189
St. Louis (France) Glass Factory, 18
St. Marco Monastery (Florence), 118
Stanton, Wm. P. (Providence; Nantucket, RI), 431
Staples, C., 431
Stark, A. J. (Denver, CO), 193, 203
Starr, Theodore B. (New York, NY), 193, 197, 203
Stearns, Oakman, Rev., 54
Steinbach, John A. (San Francisco, CA), 182, 203
Steiner, J. P. (Philadelphia, PA), 431
Stenre (Paris), 171, 190
Stern Opt. Co., 431
Stevens & Co., 432
Stevens & Gold, 432
Steward Dawson and Co., Ltd. (London), 193, 201
Stief, B. H. (Nashville, TN), 186, 203
Stiegel, Henry W., 21
Still (of Smith & Still), 431
Stills (of Curtis & Stills), Woodbury, CT, 430
Stockhausen (Dresden), 273
Stokes, 21
Storer, William, 42
Stowell, A. (Boston, MA), 183, 193, 203
Strauss (spectacles maker), 432
Stridiron, Ester Ann, 54
Suetonius, 24
Superior Glasses, 177, 198
Suspice, 30

T. Lyon & Bro., 431
Taine (Paris), 175
Taylor, P. L. (Brooklyn, NY), 432
Taylor, W. S. (Utica, NY), 182, 203
Tesseract (Hastings-on-Hudson), Catalog, 357
Tetreault, François, 58
Teunissen, 40
Teunisson Collection (Einthoven, Amsterdam), 466
Thacher, Hester Billings, 54
Therbusch, Anna Dorethea, 230
Thézard (Paris), 171, 190, 203
Thomas, Edward, 52
Thomin, 41, 99, 141
Thompson, G. R. (USA), 191, 203
Thompson Jeweler, 191

Thompson, William (Philadelphia, PA), 273
Thomson, Elihu, 51
Thutmose II, 17
Tiemann, George (NY), 357
Tiffany & Co. (New York, NY), 196, 203
Tillyer, 384
Tokugawa Shogunate Ieyasu Tokugawa Memorial Museum, 97
Tolles, Robert, 53–54
Topocon, 314f, 315
Toreman (of Schumacher & Toreman), Baltimore, MD, 191, 203
Toshisada Naba, 63
Traub & Co. (Detroit, MI), 176, 203
Traub Bros. & Co. (Detroit, MI), 204
Trevor Philip & Son, Ltd. (London), Catalog, 357
Trotting Hill Park Antiquarian Booksellers (Springfield, MA), Catalog, 357
Tscherning, 31
Tsung Po, 63
Tu Long, 64
Tulane University Medical School, Jonas W. Rosenthal M.D. Ophthalmology Museum, 465
Tull, John (York, PA), 352
   Dr. and Mrs. John Tull Collection, 466
Tumelle Duchesse, 172
Tuohy, Kevin, 377
Tuthill, George P. (St. Paul, MN), 183, 203

Udo Timm Optical Museum (Hanover), 465
Ulrich, C. (Nice; Paris; Vichy, France), 176, 203
Ulrich, L. (Nice, France), 191, 203
Ungar, 119
Unite, Geo. (Birmingham), 432
United States Optical Company, 58
University of Bern (Switzerland) Medical School, 273
   Otto Hallauer Collection, 465
University of Iowa Medical Museum (Iowa City), *In the Eye of the Beholder* Catalog, 357
University of Waterloo Optometric Museum (Waterloo, Ontario, Canada), 465
Usener, Charles, 51
Uzanne, 228, 229

V & H Dominelli, Frères (France), 168, 177
van Straet, Jan, 289
Vendôme (Paris), 190, 203
Verdi (Paris), 172, 190
Verne (Paris), 190
Vertier (Paris), 190
Victoria, Queen, 14, 15
Villanova, Arnaldo de, 38
Vinton and Jacobs Spectacle Shop, 57
Voelk (spectacles maker), 431
Voigtlander, Johann Friedrich (Vienna), 47, 149, 231
Von Augen Museum für Kunstund Gewefe (Hamburg), Catalog, 357
von Graefe, Albert, 316
von Greeff, Karl, 24, 115, 358
von Greeff, R., 46, 97, 357
von Pflugk, Albert, 115
von Rohr, Moritz, 40, 42, 60, 231
Von Stosch, Baron Phillip, 46, 231

W. H. Walmsley Company (Philadelphia, PA), *Illustrated Catalogue of Spectacles, Eyeglasses, etc.,* 357
W. S. Taylor & Son (Utica, NY), 182, 203
W. T. Hixson Co. (El Paso, TX), 183, 201
Wagner, Anton, 31
Wagner, Fred (Cincinnati, OH), 184, 203
Walburga, Saint
Waldstein, J., Optikea (Vienna), 47, 172, 190, 203
Wall and Ochs (Philadelphia, PA), 197, 203
Walmsley, W. H. (Philadelphia, PA), 357
Wanamaker, John (New York, NY), 186, 203
Warner, Deborah Jean, 50, 275
Warner, H. C. (Fresno, CA), 182, 203
Warner-Lambert, 57
Washington, George, 50, 115
Washington, Martha, 36f
Waterer, 39
Waterman, Trevor, 29
Watson, J. (Philadelphia, PA), 432
Watt, Madge Robinson, 193
Wattenbach, Wilhelm, 37
Webb, J. W. (Dallas, TX), 182, 203
Webster, A. A. (Brooklyn, NY), 182, 186, 203
Weinfurter (New Orleans, LA), 200, 203
Weiss, John (London), 357

Wellcome Collection, Museum of Science (London), 8
Wells, Albert, 57
Wells, Albert B., 57
Wells, Channing McGregory, 57
Wells, Cheney, 57
Wells Foundation (G. W. Wells), 57
Wells, G. W., 56–57, 59
Wells, George B., 57
Wells, George W., 59, 61t, 261
Wells, H. C., 56
Wells, Hiram, 56
Wells, John, 57
Wells, L., 432
Wells, McGregory, 57
Wells, Turner, 57
Wesley, Newton (Chicago, IL), 377–378, 380–381
Wesley-Jessen Laboratory (Chicago, IL), 377–378
Wessex (Portsmouth), Catalog, 357
Weve, 357
Whatley, George, 258
Wheeler, A. W., 57
Whelan-Aehle-Hutchinson Jewelry Co. (St. Louis, MO), 186, 203
White & Mac Naught (Minneapolis, MN), 184, 203
White, W. B. (Quincy, MA), Illustrated Catalog, 357
Whitney, Thomas, 51
Wichterle, 379
Wilcox, Alvan (New Haven, CT), 432
Wildnecht, Jos., 432
Wilfred, Saint, 38
Wilfrid of York, 37–38
Willard, William, 53
William IV, King, 15
Williams, Brown & Earle (Philadelphia, PA), 185, 203
Willmore (England), 432
Willmott, Fred, 329–330
Willmott, James, 329–330
Willmotts North Works, 329
Wilson, Ruth E., 183
Wilson, T. A., 273
Wilson, Woodrow, 364f
Winreurgh, J. (Utica, NY), 185, 203
Wirth, Adolph, 51
Wise, M. (New York, NY), 432
Wiss, J. (Newark, NJ), 192, 203
Wistar, Casper, 21
Wm. Kendrick & Sons (Louisville, KY), 167, 191, 201

Wm. Senter & Co. (Portland, ME), 191, 203
Wolfe, John George, 51
Wollaston, William Hyde, 29–30, 29f, 53, 354
Wollensak, B.L. (Rochester, NY), 172, 190, 203
Wood, Casey, 30, 43
Wright Bros., 432
Wright, G. U. (of P. Miller & G. U. Wright), 431
Wu-Ti, 18

Xavier, Francisco, Saint, 96–97

Yoshiharu Ashikaga (Shogun), 96–97, 97
Yoshimasa Ashikaga (Shogun), 96
Yoshitaka Ohuchi, 96–97
Young, Jacob (New Orleans, LA), 203
Young, John M., 251
Young, Leon, 58
Young, Thomas, 30, 31, 370

Zambra (of Negretti & Zambra), Holborn, London, 192, 202
Zeiss, Carl (Jena, Germany), 172
Zeiss Company (Jena, Germany), 316, 317f, 372
Zeiss Optical Museum (Jena; Oberkochen, Germany), 465
Zeiss Optical Works (Jena, Germany), 371
Zentmayer, Joseph, 51
Zhao Hsi Hou, 63
Zhao O Bei, 64
Zhu Mu, 64

Index of Subjects

[Note: Page numbers for figures, photographs, or illustrations are followed by *f*. Page numbers for tables are followed by *t*. There is a separate Name Index.]

Abalone
    opera glasses, 154*f*, 174, 178, 188, 191, 194, 195, 211*f*, 213*f*, 216*f*
    spectacle cases, 323, 327, 329, 335*f*
About Eyeglasses for the Nose Invented by Salvino Armati Florentine Gentleman; Historical Treatise (Manni), 398–428
Accession numbers, for collection artifacts, 2
The Account of Yoshitaka Ohushi, 96
Achilles mounting, for pince-nez, 245
Achromatic lenses, 21, 29, 51, 141, 342–343
Adaptation spectacles, 300
Advertisements
    American advertising card, 366*f*
    commercial catalogs as, 354, 355*f*
    of early opticians, 29–30, 29*f*, 30*f*, 31*f*, 50–54, 78, 86*f*, 217*f*
    on spectacle cases, 323, 324*f*
    See also Markings on spectacles
Affluence, spectacles as sign of, 64–65, 65*f*, 78
Agate monoculars, 141
Ai tai (*Ai Dai*) teastone spectacles, 7, 7*f*, 18, 19*f*, 62, 63–64, 270

Ai-tai-king, 37
Airy's spherocylindrical lens, 30
Albex/Wilson/American Optical goggles, 288*f*
Alexandria, Turkey, 18
Algae, as an optical molding compound, 374
Alloy metals, 12, 68, 68*f*, 71*f*, 85*f*, 103, 105, 384, 388
Aluminum
    opera glasses, 158*f*, 160*f*, 172–175, 177, 179–180, 182–183, 186–187, 189–193, 195–199, 206*f*
    oxide, added to optical glass manufacture, 21
    pince-nez, 253
    spectacle cases, 95*f*, 255, 256*f*, 327, 327*f*
Amber-colored lenses, 271, 272*f*, 295, 296*f*, 297*f*, 298*f*
The American Encyclopedia and Dictionary of Ophthalmology (Wood), 30–31, 43
American Institute Fair, 51, 52
American Journal of Science, 52
American Optical Company. *See* Name Index
American Society of Appraisers, 166
American spectacles
    bifocals, 29, 97, 258–259, 260*f*, 323, 326*f*, 327*f*
    cases, 323, 326*f*, 327*f*, 333*f*, 335
    early contact lenses in, 372

    examples of, 15*f*, 30*f*, 47*f*, 54, 55*f*, 56*f*, 385*f*, 386*f*, 387*f*
    first American optician, 50
    frames, 385*f*, 386*f*, 387*f*
    goggles, 288*f*, 293*f*
    hallmarks on, 14
    lorgnettes, 119, 127*f*, 128*f*, 129*f*, 132, 132*f*
    manufacturing of. *See* Optical manufacturing
    opera glasses, 163, 166, 167, 168
    pince-nez, 248*f*, 485*f*
    shooting glasses, 295, 297*f*
    sunglasses, 387, 387*f*
    See also specific companies or manufacturers in Name Index
Amethyst lenses, 68, 273
Ametropia, 369, 370
    half-glasses for, 302
Amulets, 7
Anatolia, Russia, 24
Anesthetics, topical, and early contact lenses, 370–371, 372
Animal horn. *See* Horn
Aniseikonic lenses, 302
Anti-glare spectacles, 287*f*, 292*f*
    See also Sunglasses
Antique vision aids
    collecting of. *See* Management of historical collections
    optical history landmarks (timetable), 389–393

Antiquity, optical landmarks during, 389–393
Appraisals, of historical collections, 2
Aquamarines, 38
Arabia, 27, 62
Argentina, Cordova del Tucuman glass factory, 21
Armorials, 42, 269
Arnotto, 12
Art & Spectacles (Poulet), 358
The Art of Preserving Sight Unimpaired to an Extreme Old Age, 220
Art, spectacles depicted in. See Spectacles in art
Artifacts, collecting. See Management of historical collections
Artificial eyes, 370, 372
Arundel lenses, pink, 273
Asthenopia (atonia), 26–27
Astigmatic clip, 246, 246f, 247f
Astigmatism
 history and bibliography of, 433–436
 pinhole spectacles for, 63
 Thomas Young's research on, 30, 31, 370, 433–436
 trial lenses for, 312f, 313
Astronomy instruments, 50
 See also Telescopes
Atonia (asthenopia), 26–27
Aus Der Geshichte Der Brille (Greeff), 97
Australia, pince-nez, 245
Austria, 21
 opera glasses from, 153, 155f
Authenticity Tests by Thermoluminescence (Aiken), 281–282
Automobile driving goggles, 58, 284, 287f–288f
Aviator goggles, 284, 286f, 287f, 300

Babylonia, 17
Baccarat (France) glass factory, 18
Bakelite opera glasses, 191
Balearic Islands, 21
Baleen
 bridges, 41, 41f
 defined, 11, 11f
 Eskimo eyeshades, 279f
 frames, 11
 pince-nez, 236, 238f, 239
Ball drop test, for safety glass lenses, 291
Bamboo spectacle cases, 84f, 89, 91f, 335
Bar springs, for pince-nez, 246, 246f, 247f
Barium, 21

Barometers, 51
Baseball bifocal/trifocal lenses, 264
Bat sign, on Chinese spectacles, 69, 69f
Bavaria, 21
Belgium
 fine glass from, 21
 lorgnettes, 129f
 opera glasses, 167, 172, 207f
 pince-nez, 239, 240f
 spectacle cases from, 323, 325f
Beliefs
 about spectacles, 35, 66, 68, 270–271, 304
 See also Fashion; Social customs
Belus River, 17
Benedictine Convent of Perpetual Adoration, 346
Beryllium aluminum silicate (beryl) lenses, 38, 99
Besicles, 99
Bezels, for glass filters, 274, 275f
Biblical references, to vision aids, 27, 35
Biconcave lenses, 53
Biconvex lenses, 27, 53, 107
Bifocal lenses, 29, 50, 51, 57, 60, 97, 258–265
 American, examples of, 260f, 261
 antecedents to, 259, 259f
 August Morck's perfection bifocal, 261, 261f
 Benjamin Franklin's, 29, 97, 258–259, 260f
 Borsch's, 262f, 263
 cement bifocal, 261, 261f, 262f, 263
 cemented kryptok, 263, 384
 clip-on additions, 259f
 contact lenses, 380–381
 executive, 262f, 263, 264
 fused, 262f, 263
 Hammon's, 263
 hang-on additions, 259f
 hinged "near" glass, 259f
 invention of, 258–259
 invisible, 263–264
 kryptok, 57, 60, 261, 262f, 263, 384
 optifex, 263
 orthogon "D," 60
 Panoptic, 263
 perfection, 261, 261f
 progressive, 264
 Richardson's, 259, 259f
 Schnaitman's, 51
 Tillyer "D," 57

trifocals, 264, 264f
Ultex one-piece, 60, 263, 263f, 384
Binocular magnifiers, 342, 342f
Binoculars
 optometers, 309f
 origins of, 149
 prism, 149, 151f
 Stanhope, 349, 352f
 Black-lip pearl opera glasses, 153, 154f, 176–179, 186–187, 195, 198, 212f, 213f
Blowing, glass. See Glassblowing
Blue-colored lenses, 271, 272f, 273, 273f, 295, 296f
Blued-steel frames, 47, 47f, 99, 296f, 298
Bohemia, 20
Bone
 Eskimo eyeshades, 279f
 frames, 38, 39f
 lorgnettes, 119
 magnifying glass handles, 339f, 340
 opera glasses, 153, 153f, 192, 195, 211f
 pince-nez, 236
 quizzing glasses, 222
 slit, for bridges, 38, 39f, 46, 236
 whale jaw, 11
Bonnet straps, 99
Book of Rites, 63
Books, designed to store reading spectacles, 320
Boric acid, 21
Borneo, 10
Boston lens, 380
Boudoir-style hand mirror, with telescope, 143, 144f
Bows, 35
 extendable, 42–43
 riding, 43, 46, 244f
Boxwood spectacle cases, 86f
Brass
 as base, for vermeil process, 11–12
 bridges, 46
 cases, 320
 frames, 42, 68, 68f, 71f, 72f, 76f
 on invalid eyeshades, 266, 267f, 268f, 269
 opera glasses, 152f, 153, 172–200, 206f, 211f
 optometer, 309f
 pince-nez, 239
 rings, for opera glasses, 153, 154f
 temples, 41, 114
Brazil
 hard rubber from, 10

pebble glass from, 22, 32–33, 38, 42, 284, 285*f*
quartz from, 8
St. Lucy statue from, 346, 347*f*
Bridges
baleen, 41, 41*f*
bone, 38, 39*f*, 46, 236
brass, 46
copper, 46
crank, 46, 46*f*, 99, 102*f*, 295, 297*f*
C-shaped (English), 46, 46*f*, 99, 100*f*, 107, 108*f*, 111, 112*f*, 295, 297*f*, 302, 316
folding, for opera glasses, 149, 151*f*
glass, 47
gold, 12*f*, 15*f*, 46, 46*f*
hinged-spring, 40, 41*f*
identifying marks on, 15
K-shaped, 46, 99, 102*f*, 296*f*, 298
leather, 41, 41*f*, 46
lorgnettes, 118, 119, 132, 133*f*
modern, 384
on Chinese spectacles, 71*f*
original design of, 46
pince-nez, 36*f*, 46, 236
saddle, 46
slit, 36*f*, 38, 39*f*, 46, 236
steel, 46
tortoiseshell, 70*f*, 97
X-shaped, 46, 46*f*, 99, 101*f*, 111, 285*f*, 298, 298*f*
Z-shaped, for lorgnettes, 132, 134*f*
Brilliants (rhinestones), 119, 132*f*, 134*f*
British silver hallmarks, 5, 6*f*
Bronze
frames, 71*f*
mirrors, 27, 63
opera glasses, 176, 194, 198
Bull (animal) sign, on Chinese spectacles, 70*f*
Bull scale, of pouces, diopters, 33*f*
Burning glass, 25, 27, 33
Butterfly sign, on Chinese spectacles, 69, 69*f*

Cable temples, 15, 15*f*, 304, 304*f*, 384
Calligraphy, 77, 89
Camera lenses, 51, 53
Canes (walking), monoculars in, 146*f*, 147
Carbon dating, of artifacts, 281–283
Cardboard
barrels, for opera glasses, 153
cases, 165
monoculars, 141
telescopes, 42

Caricatures, illustrating spectacles, 358, 360*f*–361*f*
Cartouches, 118, 119, 125*f*, 126*f*, 323, 329
Carvings
on Chinese spectacles, 69, 69*f*–70*f*, 71, 78
on spectacle cases, 78, 79*f*, 81*f*–84*f*, 87, 87*f*, 89, 90*f*, 103, 103*f*
Casein (cellulose acetate), 10, 239, 291
Cases for spectacles, 234, 234*f*, 320–331
advertising the optician, 78, 86*f*
aluminum, 95*f*, 255, 256*f*, 327, 327*f*
American, examples of, 323, 326*f*, 327*f*
bamboo, 84*f*, 89, 91*f*, 335
Belgian, 323, 325*f*
boxwood, 86*f*
brass, 320
carved, 78, 79*f*, 81*f*–84*f*, 87, 87*f*, 89, 90*f*, 103, 103*f*
cetorhinus, 9, 89*f*
chatelaine, 322*f*, 323, 325*f*, 329
Chinese, 10, 10*f*, 11, 11*f*, 19*f*, 66*f*, 76*f*, 78, 79*f*–95*f*, 329, 329*f*, 332, 334*f*, 335
chinoiserie, 322*f*, 325*f*
clamshell, 95*f*, 103, 103*f*, 108*f*, 320, 321*f*, 327, 329
clay over wood, 87, 87*f*
cloisonne, 11, 11*f*, 89, 91*f*
coffin-shaped, 104*f*, 105
embossed, 13*f*, 323
embroidered, 80*f*, 87, 87*f*, 88*f*, 89, 92*f*, 93*f*, 94*f*, 335
English, examples of, 10*f*, 322*f*, 328*f*, 329
engraved, 13*f*
for evening wear, 327, 328*f*, 329
fenestrated wood, 82*f*, 119
flat, with slide insert, 89, 92*f*
flip-top, 107, 108*f*, 114, 114*f*, 322*f*, 323, 325*f*
for folding spectacles, 66, 67*f*, 81*f*, 83*f*, 85*f*, 86*f*, 87, 89*f*
gutta-percha, 10*f*, 84*f*
hammered, 13*f*
horn, 89, 92*f*, 320
incised with sayings, 86*f*, 90*f*
for industrial goggles/spectacles, 284, 286*f*, 287*f*
inlaid with stones, 82*f*, 89, 90*f*, 323
ivory, 85*f*, 89, 92*f*, 96, 323, 325*f*, 326*f*
Japanese, 96, 97, 98
for jealousy glasses, 140*f*
lacquer, 78, 79*f*, 84*f*, 89, 90*f*, 91*f*, 322*f*, 323, 323*f*, 324*f*, 325*f*, 334*f*, 335, 335*f*

leather, 66, 95, 105, 164*f*, 165, 255, 256*f*, 320, 323, 327, 327*f*, 334*f*, 335, 335*f*, 336*f*, 337
for lorgnettes, 118, 119, 123*f*, 127*f*
machine-made, 89, 93*f*
for magnifier, 40*f*
manufacturing of, 329–330
mother-of-pearl, 206*f*, 323, 327, 329
opera glasses, 164–165, 164*f*, 165*f*, 186–187, 190–193, 195, 197–198, 206*f*, 217*f*
pai-tung, 86*f*
papier mache, 13, 13*f*, 84*f*, 322*f*, 323, 323*f*
pince-nez, 47*f*, 237*f*, 239*f*, 250*f*, 255, 255*f*, 256*f*
plastic-covered metal, 95*f*
pressed, 13*f*, 95*f*
reed, 9
repousse, 12
sandalwood, 82*f*
sash weights for, 66*f*
sea snail, 327, 329
shagreen, 9, 9*f*, 66, 78, 80*f*, 85*f*, 87, 88*f*, 114, 165, 320, 323, 325*f*, 334*f*, 335, 336*f*, 337
silk, 80*f*, 164*f*, 165
silver, 10*f*, 89, 94*f*, 320, 323, 324*f*, 325*f*, 327*f*, 328*f*, 329, 334*f*, 335, 335*f*, 336*f*, 337
slip-top, 322*f*, 323
steel, 99, 100*f*, 103, 103*f*, 104*f*, 320, 321*f*, 323, 326*f*, 336*f*
tangerine-skin, 86*f*
tinplated, 104*f*, 105, 323, 326*f*
Tonbridgeware, 9
tortoiseshell, 10*f*, 72*f*, 89, 94*f*, 114, 320, 322*f*, 323, 324*f*, 329, 335, 335*f*, 339*f*
transfer-decorated lacquer, 89, 91*f*, 324*f*
wig spectacles, 113*f*, 114, 114*f*, 323, 324*f*, 325*f*
wooden, 9, 66, 78, 81*f*–84*f*, 87, 103, 103*f*, 165, 239*f*, 256*f*, 320, 321*f*
Catalogs
examples of, 355*f*
historical, usefulness to collector, 354
list of, 356–357
Cataract disease, 32, 63
postsurgical lenses for, 316, 387
Celluloid (plastic) spectacle frames, 9–10, 103
Cellulose acetate (casein), 10, 239
laminating lenses with, 291
Cellulose nitrate, 9–10
Cement bifocals, 261, 261*f*, 384
Centex lenses, 59
Ceramics, 197, 198

Cerium, for coloring lenses, 274
Cetorhinus spectacle cases, 9, 89f
Ceylon, 18
Charms (jewelry)
    miniature spectacles as, 349, 351f
    monoculars as, 147, 147f
Chatelaine spectacle cases, 332–337
    American, 333f, 335
    Chinese, 334f
    English, 322f, 323, 334f, 335, 335f
    for evening wear, 328f, 329
    French, 333f
    history of, 332, 333f
    Italian, 325f
    Japanese, 335
Chien Lung period, 18, 76f
China. *See* Chinese spectacles
Chinese Eyesight and Spectacles (Rasmussen), 26
Chinese spectacles
    ai tai lenses, 7, 7f, 18, 19f, 62, 63–64, 270–271, 271f
    beliefs about, 62, 68, 78, 270–271
    bridges, 71f
    carvings on, symbolism of, 69, 69f–70f, 71, 78
    cases for. *See* Cases for spectacles
    chatelaine-like cases for, 332, 334f, 335
    dating of, using historical contexts, 5, 7, 18, 19f, 77
    folding, 11, 64, 64f, 72f, 76f
    frames, 41, 66–68, 67f, 68f, 71f–76f
    glass lenses, 7, 7f, 19f, 68f
    half-eye, 68
    invention of, 62
    monoculars, 68
    optical knowledge and, 63–64
    plano lenses in, 270, 271f
    plastic imitations of, 21–22
    removing, to show respect, 68, 78
    rimless, 64, 64f, 74f
    rock crystal lenses, 33
    social customs and, 68, 78
    for sun or glare protection, 270–271, 271f
    sunglasses, 35, 36f
    superstitions about, 270–271
    tangerine-skin, 78, 86f
    teastone lenses in, 7, 7f, 18, 19f, 62, 63–64, 270–271, 271f
    techniques of wearing, 65–66, 65f, 66f, 332, 334f, 335
    temple strings/weights, 65–66, 65f, 66f
    tortoiseshell, 36f, 67f, 68f, 74f, 79f

variety of, 71f–77f
    See also Spectacles
Ching dynasty, 97
Chinoiserie, 5, 322f, 325f
Chrome oxide, for coloring lenses, 274
Chrome plating, on opera glasses, 173–174, 176–177, 180–199 passim
Chromium-plated frames, 99
Citrine decoration, on lorgnettes, 119
Civil War period, 47, 50, 53
Clamshell-type spectacle cases, 95f, 103, 103f, 108f, 320, 321f, 327, 329
Classic Me (Mezi), 63
Claude Lorraine
    glass, 276
    glass filters, 274–277, 275f, 277f
    landscape mirrors, 275–276
Clay spectacle cases, 87, 87f
Cleaning, of historical collections, 4
Clip-on spectacles
    for bifocals, 259f
    for near vision, 384, 385f
    for shooting, 298, 298f
Cloisonne
    cases, 89, 91f
    defined, 11, 11f, 77
    opera glasses, 191
Clothes-clip lorgnettes, 132, 134f, 135f
Clouté fan, 224, 225f
Cobalt oxide, for coloring lenses, 274
Cocaine, as topical anesthetic, 371, 372
Coin silver, 8
Collyria, 38
Color vision, 30
Colored lenses, 17, 18, 41, 42, 60, 63, 103, 111
    amber, 271, 272f, 295, 296f, 297f, 298f
    blue, 271, 272f, 273, 273f, 295, 296f
    for eye protection in factories, 289, 289f
    manufacturing process of, 274
    pink, 273, 274f
    for protection from sun or glare, 270–277, 271f–275f, 277f
    in protective goggles/spectacles, 284, 285f, 289f
    for shooting or hunting, 295–299
Compound lenses, 59, 60
Concave lenses, 26, 27, 30, 32, 52, 53, 57, 138
Concave mirrors, 27, 63
Concise Instruction in Grinding Lenses and Fitting Telescopes (Hilscher), 29
    English translation of, 467–487, 468f

Conjunctivitis, pince-nez sunshades to treat, 251
Conservation convex/concave glasses, 52
Contact lenses, 369–383
    Adolph Eugene Fick, as father of, 371
    antecedents to, 369–370
    bifocal, 380–381
    corneal, 377–378
    disposable, 380
    early plastic (Plexiglas), 372
    extended-wear, 380
    first clinical use of, 370–372
    first laboratory in America, 374
    first use of term, 371
    fitting of, by trial case method, 375–377
    Food and Drug Administration and, 378
    gas permeable, 380
    ground glass, 372
    hydrodiascope device, 369
    hydrophilic, 378–380
    laboratories to manufacture, 377–378
    Leonardo da Vinci's ideas on, 369
    molded glass, 372–373
    molded plastic, 373–377, 376f
    monovision procedure with, 380
    plastic, various types of, 374–380
    Poller's Negacoll and, 372–373, 374
    soft, 379
    Thomas Young's research on, 370
    topical anesthetics and, 370–371
    trial sets of, 372, 373
    Zeiss lenses, early, 371, 372, 373
Convex lenses, 25, 27, 30, 32, 53, 57, 107, 138, 220
    in wig spectacles, 111
Convex mirrors, 27, 63
Copper
    bridges, 46
    frames, 42
    opera glasses, 175, 181, 191, 195
    pince-nez, 239
    in Pinchbeck alloy spectacles, 12
    spectacle cases, 85f, 119
Cork pads, 46, 242f, 243
Corneal neutralization, contact lenses for, 369–370
Cosmetics, spectacles to use while applying, 306–307, 306f, 307f
Cost, of opera glasses, 163
Cow horn, 10
Craniofacial dysostosis, frames for, 304
Crank bridges, 46, 46f, 99, 102f, 295, 297f
Crete, 24–25

Crookes' sunglasses, 273, 384
Crossed eye, occlusion glasses for, 303
Crown glass, 21, 263
Crutch spectacles, to treat ptosis, 303
Cruxite (pink) lenses, 273, 274f
Crystal
   ai tai (teastone), 18, 19f, 270–271, 271f
   defined, 20
   lenses, 24, 27, 32–33, 68
   mirror, 33
   rock, 24, 25, 27, 33, 42, 68, 270–271
Crystalline, defined, 7, 20–21
C-shaped (English-style) bridges, 46, 46f, 99, 100f, 107, 108f, 111, 112f, 295, 297f, 302, 316
Customs, social. *See* Social customs
Cycloplegics, 30
Cylinder lenses, 57, 59
Cyprus, 24
Czechoslovakia, 21, 32
D lens, 103
Daguerreotypes, 51, 52, 358, 359f
Daisenin Temple, Kyoto, Japan, 96
Damascene, 9, 9f
Dating, of antique vision aids, 5–16
Decal (transfer) decoration, 5, 6f, 89, 91f, 323, 324f
Decalcomania, 323, 324f
Decorum glasses, 141
Diamonds
   for cutting glass or lenses, 20, 22, 32
   on lorgnettes, 119, 125f, 129f, 131f
   on monocles, 231
   on opera glasses, 196
Didymium, for coloring lenses, 274
Diopters, 8
   Bull table of, 33f
   defined, 32
   measurement system, 15, 32, 33f, 59
Dioptic Review, 345
Diplopia, 31
   occluder lenses for, 303
   opera glasses and, 149
Dissolving Scenes, 51
Diver's (underwater) goggles, 284, 289, 289f
Dong Tien Qing Lu (Zhao), 63–64
Double D-shaped lenses, 284
Dowels, 8, 9f, 109
Dragon's Blood, 12
Drawers, to house historical collections, 2
Drilling tools, ancient, 26, 26f
Driving goggles, 58, 284, 287f–288f, 300

Dry eye, spectacles for, 304
Duplicates, avoiding in historical collections, 2–3
Dutch spectacles, 21
   in art, 367f
   in Japanese writings, 97
   opera glasses, 153, 155f

Ear trumpets, lorgnettes and, 119, 127f
Eclipse viewing, with glass filters, 274
Edgers, lens, 20, 32
   See also Lens grinding
Edo period (Japan) spectacle shops, 97
Egypt, 7, 7f, 17, 18, 24–25
Electroplating, 11–12
Embossed spectacles
   cases, 13f, 323
   opera glasses, 152f, 174, 177, 180, 191, 195, 198, 212f
   process of, 13, 13f
Embroidered spectacle cases, 80f, 87, 87f, 88f, 89, 92f–94f, 334f, 335
Emeralds
   as early lenses, 38
   emerald-design opera glasses, 155f
   as viewing glasses, 24, 270
En plein method, 157
Enameled spectacles
   lorgnettes, 119, 128f, 129f, 130f
   monoculars, 141, 142f
   opera glasses, 153, 155f, 156f, 157, 158f, 173–200 passim, 209f
Encyclopedie von Diderot und d'Alembert, 29
England
   art of, depicting spectacles, 366f
   Birmingham, 21
   chatelaine spectacle cases, 322f, 323, 334f, 335, 335f
   Chiddingfold (Surrey), 20
   colored lenses used in, 271, 272f
   frames, 15f, 386f
   glass factories in, 20–21
   hallmarks of, 5, 6f, 14
   leather spectacles, 15f
   lorgnettes, 127f
   magnifying glasses, 343f
   monoculars, 13f, 139f, 142f, 146f, 147f, 234–235
   opera glasses from, compared to French, 149
   papier mache cases, 13f
   protective spectacles from, 285f
   quizzing glasses, 221f

   rubber products in, 10
   Sheffield, 14
   spectacle cases, 10f, 322f, 328f, 329–330
   trial lens/frame sets, 311f
   Tonbridge, 9
   Warrington, 20
English-style (C-shaped) bridges, 46, 46f, 99, 100f, 107, 108f, 111, 112f, 295, 297f, 302, 316
Engraving process, 13–14, 13f, 14f, 20
Entropion, crutch glasses for, 303
Ephesos, 24
Eridu, 17
Eshnuna, Babylonia, 17
Eskimo eyeshades, 11, 97, 278–283
   baleen, 279f
   bone, 279f
   dating ancient examples of, 281–283
   individual eye covers, 281, 281f
   inside of, 279f
   materials used, 278, 279f, 281, 281f
   need for, 278
   pinholes in, 270, 278
   to prevent snowblindness, 278
   slit in, 278, 280, 280f
   types of, 279f
   wooden, 279f, 280, 280f
Essay on Vision (Adams), 43, 43f
Etuis, 143f, 145, 146f
Eventail cocarde (flirtation fan), 224, 226f
Evil eye miniatures, 349, 353f
Examination of artifacts
   for condition, 13–15
   for historical context, 5–8
   for repairs, 13
   See also Management of historical collections
Executive lenses, 262f, 263, 264
Exhibiting historical collections, 2, 3
Exophthalmic patients, and pince-nez, 236, 237f
Expanding opera glasses, 159, 160f
Ex-votos, 7, 7f, 12f, 344–348, 345f, 347f, 348f
Eye diseases
   cataracts, 32, 63, 316, 387
   dry eye, 304
   entropion, 303
   exanthematous, 271
   eyeshades for, 266–269
   hemianopia, 300, 301f
   inflammatory, 266
   keratitis sicca, 304
   keratoconus, 63, 370, 371, 372, 376

muscular imbalances, 300, 301f
patron saints of. *See* Patron saints (optical)
ptosis, 303
retinal detachment, 298, 303, 303f
Soëgren's syndrome, 304
An Eye on the Monocle (Herbert), 233
Eye shields. *See* Eyeshades for invalids
Eyeglasses. *See* Spectacles
Eyeshade cases, leather, 266, 267f
Eyeshades for invalids, 266–269
bases for, 266, 267f
cases for, 266
lead, 63
permanent, 266, 267f, 269
portable, 266, 267f
pylon type, 266, 267f

Facial disfigurement, frames for, 304
The Fan Book (Percival), 228
Fang Chau Tsa Yen (Chang), 63
Fang Yu Sheng Lan (Zhu), 64
Fans
cockade, French, 225f
eventail cocarde, 224, 226f
"flirtation," 224, 226f
French brisé, 224, 225
lorgnettes in, 224, 228f
mirrors in, 224, 226f
monoculars in, 145, 145f
on eyeshades, 266–269, 267f, 268f
optical uses of, 224–229
peepholes in, 224, 227f
telescopes in, 224, 225f, 227f
Fashion
chatelaine spectacle cases and, 332–337, 333f–336f
fans, to conceal spying aids, 224–229
lorgnettes and, 118
monocles and, 230–231, 233, 234f
pince-nez and, 248f, 249, 249f, 251, 253f, 255f
quizzing glasses as, 220, 221f, 222–223, 222f
spectacle size, type, 40, 42, 65, 71f
sunglasses, 40–41
wig spectacles and, 111–114
See also Social customs
Feldspar, 18
Felt, for collection storage, 2
Fenestrated materials
opera glasses, 152f, 153
spectacle cases, 82f, 119
Fennel, 38

Ferrous iron oxide, for coloring lenses, 274
Fick's phenomenon, 371
Field glasses, 149, 151f, 176, 184, 195, 213f
leather, 151f
Filigree, 14, 14f
chatelaine cases, 336f
on opera glasses, 188, 197
on pince-nez, 253
Filters
for adaptation to darkness, 300
Claude Lorraine, 274–275, 275f, 277f
for viewing landscapes or sky, 274–277, 275f, 277f
Finger-piece eyeglasses, 252, 298
Fits-U model, of pince-nez, 236, 237f, 252, 384
Fitting of spectacles
pince-nez, 236, 237f, 245, 245f, 246f
trial lenses and frames, 308–315
Flash burns, spectacles to prevent, 289, 289f–290f, 300, 302f
Flint glass, 7, 20, 21, 22, 263
Flip-top spectacle cases, 107, 108f, 114, 114f, 320, 321f, 322f, 323, 325f
Foam, hazards of, in housing historical collections, 2
Focal length, markings for, 32, 59
Folders (pince-nez), 251
Folding spectacles, 11, 64, 64f, 66, 66f, 72f, 76f, 97
cases for, 66, 67f, 81f, 83f, 85f, 86f, 87, 89f, 328f, 336f, 337
opera glasses, 158f, 159, 159f, 206f, 210f, 213f
The Four Treasures of the Study (Tu), 64
Frames
American, examples of, 385f, 386f, 387f
baleen, 11
blued-steel, 47, 47f, 99
bone, 38, 39f
brass, 42, 68, 68f, 71f, 72f, 76f
bronze, 71f
Chinese, 66–68, 67f, 68f, 71f–76f
chromium-plated, 99
copper, 42
cosmetic or makeup, 306–307, 306f, 307f
evolution of, 1900 to present, 384–388, 385f–388f
focal marks on, 32, 59
gold, 42, 46–47, 107f, 384, 385f, 387f
horn, 11, 38, 41, 46, 67, 71f, 73f, 76f
ivory, 96

leather, 15, 15f, 38
metal, 38, 46, 68, 68f, 306f, 384, 388
modern, 384–388, 385–388f
nickel-plated, 99
oxhorn, 42
oxygen-administration spectacle, 300, 302, 302f
plastic, 9–11, 103, 307f, 384, 386f, 387
quizzing glass, 222
raffia, 66, 66f
reed, 9, 66, 66f, 76f
rhodium-coated, 99
sandalwood, 67
silver, 5, 6f, 14, 14f, 42, 56f, 76f, 107, 107f, 384, 385f
steel, 41, 47, 47f, 99, 100f–103f, 103, 295, 297f
tortoiseshell, 7f, 66, 67f, 72f, 73f, 103, 111
trial sets of, for fitting, 308–315
wooden, 8–9, 66, 67, 99, 103
See also Bridges; Spectacles; Temples
France
art of, depicting spectacles, 332
Baccarat, 18
chatelaine spectacle cases from, 333f
Clichy, 18
dating antiquities from, 5, 7, 7f
fans of, to conceal spying aids, 224, 225f, 226f
glass factories in, 18, 20, 21
hallmarks of, 14
lorgnettes, 119, 122f, 123f, 124f, 125f, 132f, 137f, 140f
miniatures, 143, 143f, 148f
monoculars, 139f, 140f, 141, 141f, 143f, 146f, 148f, 196, 231, 232f, 233, 233f, 234f
opera glasses, 149, 150f, 153, 155f, 156f, 157, 159, 159f, 161, 162f, 163–166, 209f, 210f, 213f
compared to English, 149
prospect glasses, 225f
protective spectacles, French X-bridge, 285f
quizzing glasses, 221f, 222f
St. Gobain, 21
St. Louis, 18
Val St. Lambert, 21
Franklin Institute Fair, 51, 53
Fraternal induction goggles, 304, 304f
Fraunhofer Lines, 21
Freedom sign, on Chinese spectacles, 69, 69f
Fronts, spectacle, 67–68, 118

Galleries (monocle), 231, 232f, 233, 233f, 234f
Galuchat. See Shagreen
Gambage, 12
Gas-mask spectacles, 305f
The Gazette of the United States, 258
Germany
  colored lenses in, 271, 273
  Euphos glass from, 273
  glass factories in, 21
  hallmarks of, 14
  Jena, 21–22, 167, 316, 371
  lorgnettes from, 123f
  Meissen, 5, 6f, 367f
  monoculars from, 231, 233–234
  opera glasses, 149, 167, 169, 171, 172
  opticians from, immigrating to America, 51–54
  pince-nez, 97, 239, 239f
  tin cases from, 287f
  trial lens sets, 308, 310f
  votive offerings, 344
Ghent Bird, 38
Gilding process, 11–12
Glare protective lenses. See Eskimo eyeshades; Sunglasses
Glass
  bridges, 47
  burning, 25, 27, 33
  colored, 17, 18, 41, 60, 63, 103, 111
  Crookes', 273
  crystalline, 7, 21
  diamond cutting of, 20, 22, 32
  filters for, 274–277, 275f, 277f
  flint, 7, 20, 21, 22
  history of, 17–23
  lead, 20, 21
  lenses, 7, 7f, 19f, 107, 111
  optical, in antiquity, 18, 19f, 24–25
  pebble, 22, 32–33, 38, 42, 107, 111, 284, 285f, 338
  plate, 21
  prospect, 40–41
  quizzing, 15
  soda, 7, 7f, 18, 20, 21
  teastone, 7, 7f, 19f, 24, 62, 63, 66–67, 74f, 76f
  thallium, 21
  Val St. Lambert type, 21
  Venetian, 20, 20f, 21, 33
  zinc crown, 21
  See also Lenses; Optical manufacturing

Glass factories
  Baccarat, France, 18
  Bausch and Lomb, Rochester, New York, 21, 60
  Champs Glass Works, Birmingham, 21
  Chiddingfold, England, 20
  in China, 18
  Clichy, France, 18
  Cordova del Tucuman, Argentina, 21
  London Company of Virginia, Jamestown, 21
  Manheim, Pennsylvania, 21
  Meissen, Germany, 5, 6f
  Murano, Italy, 20, 20f
  Perthshire, Scotland, 18
  Pueblo de los Angeles, Mexico, 21
  St. Gobain, France, 21
  St. Louis, France, 18
  Schott and Genossen Institute, Jena, Germany, 21–22
  Val St. Lambert, France, 21
  Venice, Italy, 20
  Warrington, England, 20
  See also Optical manufacturing
Glass filters, for viewing eclipses, landscapes, 274–277, 275f, 277f
Glassblowing
  antecedents to, 17, 18
  spectacles for, 300, 302f
Glasses, scissors. See Scissors glasses
Glassmaker guilds, 20
Glassworks. See Glass factories
Glazing, vitreous, 17
Goggles, 11, 58
  for adaptation to darkness, 300
  American, 288f, 293f
  Eskimo eyeshades, 278–283
  for fraternal induction, 304, 304f
  See also Protective spectacles
Gold
  bridges, 12f, 15f, 46, 46f
  cases, 89, 94f, 323
  filled, 12, 12f, 46, 57, 58
  frames, 42, 46–47, 107f, 384, 385f, 387f
  gilding, 11–12, 12f
  lorgnettes, 118, 119, 120f, 121f, 122f, 123f, 125f, 128f, 129f, 130f, 131f, 132, 133f, 137f
  Martin's Margins, 42f, 107, 107f, 320
  miniature spectacle pins, 350f, 351f, 352f
  monoculars, 141, 142f, 231, 232f, 233f
  on eyeshade cases, 266, 267f
  opera glasses, 153, 157, 159, 177, 180–181, 183, 185–186, 189–191, 194–196, 198, 207f, 208f

  pince-nez, 237f, 253f
  Pinchbeck alloy as imitation of, 12
  plated, 11–12, 12f, 15, 15f
  quizzing glasses, 221f, 222
  rolled, 12, 47
  temples, sliding extensions for, 41
Gold oxide, for coloring lenses, 274
Grab front additions, for near vision, 384, 385f
Great Britain. See England; Ireland; Scotland
Grecian curve spring, 43
Greece, 18, 24–27
Grinder's glasses, 292f
Grinding
  early tools for, 25, 26, 26f, 32
  hand, 15
  See also Lens grinding
Guilds, spectacle makers, applicants' miniatures, 349, 350f
Guilloche method, 153
Gunning glasses. See Shooting glasses
Gutta-percha, 10, 10f, 78, 84f

Hai Yu Cong Kao (Zhao), 64
Half-glasses
  Chinese "half-eye" spectacles, 68
  preacher's, 247f, 248f
  reverse, 302
  speaker's, 247f, 248f
Hallmarks
  American, 14
  coin silver, 8
  English, 5, 6f, 14, 14f
  British table of, 6f
  French, 14
  German, 14
  Russian, 14
  silver, 5, 6f, 8, 8f, 14, 14f
  sterling, 8, 8f
Hamblin loupe, 317f
Hammon patent, 60
Han dynasty, 18, 63
Hand-painted opera glasses, 153, 155f
Handled spectacles. See Lorgnettes
Handles, of opera glasses, 160f–162f, 161, 165, 213f, 214f, 216f, 217f
Hang-on additions, for near vision, 384, 385f
Hard rubber spectacles, 10, 10f
  magnifying glass covers, 340
  opera glass caps, 176, 197
  pince-nez, 239, 298

Hardy-Delaney patents, 59
Hawksbill (sea turtle) shells, 10–11, 10f
Healing powers, attributed to spectacles, 62, 65
Heat, protecting artifacts from, 2
Hemianopia, 300, 301f
Hinges
    double, 41–42, 99, 100f, 108f, 111, 113f
    for lorgnettes, 118, 119
    Martin's Margins, 108f, 109, 109f
    spring, 40, 41f
History and Bibliography of Astigmatism (Javal), 30
    English translation of, 433–436
The History of Ophthalmology (Hirschberg), 26–27, 35, 37
A History of Spectacles (Poulet), 62
Honcho Tsukan, 96
Hook-on additions, for near vision, 384, 385f
Horn
    bezels, 274
    cases, 89, 92f, 320
    covers, for lens set, 10f
    cow, 10
    defined, 11
    fans, 224, 225f
    frames, 38, 67, 71f, 73f, 76f, 89f
    inserts, 103, 107, 107f
    lorgnettes, 118, 119, 120f
    monocles, 231, 232f
    opera glasses, 161f, 192–195
    ox, 11, 42
    pads, 46, 66
    scissors glasses, 115, 117f
    temples, 41
    trial lens sets, 308, 310f
    water buffalo, 11
Horsehair, 68
Housing historical collections, 1–2
Hump bridges. *See* Crank bridges
Hun dynasty, 18
Hunting glasses. *See* Shooting glasses
Hutten Oxford eyeglasses, 254
Hyperopia, 30

Idaean Cave, Crete, 25
Illustrated Descriptive Catalogue (Pike), 276
Immigration, impact of, 50
India, 18, 36f
Industrial goggles/spectacles
    to prevent flash burns, 289, 289f, 300, 302f
    for welders, 289, 289f–290f, 292f, 300, 302f
    See also Protective spectacles
Industrial Revolution, 5, 8–9, 50, 99, 251
Inflammatory eye diseases, 266
Insects, protecting historical collection from, 2
Inserts, 99, 100f, 103, 107, 107f, 108f, 109, 109f
    See also Pads
Insignias, of opera glass manufacturers, 167–172
Insurance coverage, for historical collections, 2
Intelligence, spectacles as sign of, 64–65, 65f, 78
Invalids
    eyeshades for, 266–269, 267f, 268f
    reading prisms for, 300, 302f
Iraq, 27
Ireland, 52
Iridectomy, 316
Iron, 14, 266, 267f
Ironworkers, protective goggles for, 289
Italy, 18, 20, 20f, 21
    chatelaine spectacle cases, 325f
    miniatures, 323, 325f, 326f
    opera glasses, 169
    St. Marco Monastery, Florence, 118
    votive offerings, 344
Ivory
    cases, 85f, 89, 92f, 96, 323, 325f, 326f
    frames, 96
    identifying type of, 13
    lorgnettes, 119, 228
    magnifying glass handles, 339f, 340
    miniature spectacles, 352f
    monoculars, 13f, 139f, 141, 142f
    on Japanese spectacles, 97
    opera glasses, 151f, 153, 161f, 174, 177, 186, 188, 190, 192–196, 198, 214f
    pince-nez, 236
    prospect glass, 225f
    storing and protecting, in collections, 2

Jade, 18, 132f
Japan, 62, 78, 89
    chatelaine cases, 335
    chatelaine spectacle cases, 332–337
    contact lenses produced in, 379
    ivory spectacles, 97
    Kyoto, 9
    lorgnettes, 97
    Netsuke, 78, 360f
    opticians' shops, 98
    spectacle cases, 96, 97, 98
    spectacles from, 96–98
Japanning, 12
Jealousy glasses, 224
    cases for, 140f
    monoculars, 140f, 141
    wood, 225f
Jeweler's lens, 340, 341f
Jewelry, miniature spectacles as, 349, 350f, 351f
Jewels
    on lorgnettes, 2, 119, 123f, 125f, 131f, 131f–132f, 134f
    on magnifying glasses, 340, 341f
    on monoculars, 141, 143f, 144f, 148f
    on opera glasses, 154f, 197, 209f
    on quizzing glasses, 222
Jews, ancient, 24
Jockey goggles (horse racing), 284, 288f
Journal in the Lakes (Gray), 275
Jumellists, defined, 166

Kaleidoscopes, 224
Kai Yu Tsung Kao (Chao), 63
Kaolin, 18
Katalog Einer Bilderausstellung Zur Geschichte Der Brille (Greeff), 24–25
Keratitis sicca, 304
Keratoconus, 63, 370, 371, 372, 376
Knossos, Palace of (Crete), 24
Korean spectacles, 97
Kryptok bifocal lenses, 57, 60, 261, 262f, 384
K-shaped bridges, 46, 99, 102f, 296f, 298

Labeling, of historical collections, 2–3
Lacquer, 5, 12, 68, 76f
    cases, 78, 79f, 84f, 89, 90f, 91f, 322f, 323, 323f, 324f, 325f, 334f, 335, 335f
    opera glasses, 174, 184, 192, 194, 195
Lacrilens, 377
Lamination of lenses, 291, 291f
Landscape mirrors, 275–276
Lanstier (quizzing glass), 220
Lapel lorgnettes, 132, 134f, 135f
Lapidary instruments, 32
L'Art de l'Opticien (Chevalier), 30, 30f, 354, 356f, 397f
Latex rubber, 10, 10f
Le Livre de Marco Polo (Pauthier), 37
Le Lunetier-Opticien, 354, 355f
Lead eye shields, Tang dynasty, 63
Lead glass, 20, 21
    See also Flint glass

Leather
- bridges, 41, 41f, 46
- cases, 66, 95, 105, 164f, 165, 255, 256f, 320, 323, 327, 327f, 334f, 335, 335f, 336f, 337
- English, spectacle frames, 15f
- eyeshade cases, 266, 267f
- field glasses, 151f
- frames, 15, 15f, 38
- housing and protecting, 2
- monoculars, 141
- Moroccan, 266, 267f, 275
- opera glasses, 152f, 173–199 passim
- pince-nez, 236, 238f
- restoring, 4
- rims, 40
- spectacles, 35, 36f, 38, 39, 40, 42, 238f

Lens caps, of opera glasses, 152f, 166–167

Lens grinding
- edgers for, 20, 32
- history of
  - early methods, 24–26, 25f, 26f, 28f, 467–487, 468f
  - Hilscher's instructions on (English translation), 467–487
  - landmarks in (timetable), 389–393
  - in United States, 50–61
  - Marshall's process of, 27, 29
  - tools for, 26, 26f, 28f
- *See also* Glass; Grinding; Optical manufacturing

Lenses
- achromatic, 21, 29, 51, 141, 342–343
- in antiquity, 24–27
- bifocal. *See* Bifocal lenses
- Bull scale for, 33f
- colored. *See* Colored lenses
- compound, 59, 60
- concave, 26, 27, 30, 32, 52, 53, 57, 138
- contact. *See* Contact lenses
- convex, 25, 27, 30, 32, 52, 53, 57, 67, 107, 111, 138
- double, 99, 102f, 103
- drilling tools for, 26, 26f
- focal marks on, 32, 59
- glass, 7, 7f, 19f, 107, 111
- grinding. *See* Lens grinding
- meniscus, 29, 30, 30f, 31, 53, 60, 99, 384
- object glasses, 22, 51
- occlusive, 303
- pebble glass, 22, 32–33, 38, 42, 107, 111, 284, 285f, 338
- periscopic, 30, 31, 53, 57, 141, 224, 225f
- plastic, 388
- rock crystal, 24, 25, 27, 33, 42, 68, 270–271
- shapes of, 30, 57, 59, 65f, 67, 67f, 103, 103f, 111, 118
- size of. *See* Size of lenses
- strength of, methods of indicating, 31–32, 33f
- teastone glass. *See* Teastone glass (*ai tai*) lenses
- thickness of, 67, 67f
- trial lens sets, 308–315

Lensometers, 15
- to identify artifacts, 8

Lenticular lenses, 30

Les Lunettes (Sichel), 31

Lieou-li, 18

Lighting
- for collection displays, 2
- to examine artifacts, importance of, 13–15

Limoges-style opera glasses, 156f, 157

Lion passant, 14, 14f

Literature sources
- on history of spectacles, 40–41
- to identify artifacts, 8

Loans, of collection artifacts, 3–4

Lockets
- lorgnette, 119, 124f
- monocular, 144f

London Crystal Palace Exhibition, 51

Lorgnette poire, 141

Lorgnettes, 118–137
- American style, 119, 127f, 128f, 129f, 132, 132f
- Belgian, example of, 129f
- bone, 119
- bridges, 118, 119, 132, 133f
- cases for, 118
- classic (oxford) style, 132, 133f
- clothes-clip style, 132, 134f, 135f
- defined, 40–41, 46, 118–119
- diamond-studded, 119, 125f, 129f, 131f
- double-lens set, 137f
- dowager-duchess type, 119, 126f
- enameled, 119, 128f, 129f, 130f
- English, examples of, 127f
- in fans, 224, 228f
- forerunner of, 118
- French, examples of, 122f, 123f, 124f, 125f, 137f, 140f
- George Adams and, 118
- German, examples of, 123f
- gold, 118, 119, 120f, 121f, 122f, 123f, 125f, 128f, 129f, 130f, 131f, 132f, 133f, 137f
- ivory, 119, 228
- Japanese, 97
- jewel-encrusted, 2, 119, 123f, 125f, 131f, 132f, 134f
- long-handled, 119, 126f
- Louis spring, 118
- as magnifying glasses, 118
- marcasite, 119, 132f
- metal, 118, 119, 128f
- mother-of-pearl, 118, 119, 120f, 121f, 123f, 125f, 126f
- oxford (classic) style, 132, 133f
- plastic, 127f, 136, 136f
- prospect glasses compared to, 118
- Robert Betell Bate and, 118
- scissors glasses and, 115, 116f, 117f
- silver, 118, 119, 121f, 126f, 127f, 128f, 133f
- timepieces in, 119, 132, 135f
- tortoiseshell, 118, 119, 120f, 125f, 126f, 127f, 128f, 131f
- value of, 3
- *See also* Monoculars

Lorraine, Claude. *See* Claude Lorraine

Louis spring lorgnette, 118

Loupes, 316–319
- Beebe, 316, 318f, 319f
- Hamblin, 316, 317f
- headband style, 316, 319f
- Neitz, 316, 317f
- Zeiss, 316, 317f

Lucite plastic, 374

Lun Yu, 63

Magic Lanterns, 51

Magnesium, 21

Magnifying glasses, 338–343
- in antiquity, 24, 25, 27, 33
- binocular, 342, 342f
- covers for, 40f, 338, 339f, 340, 340f
- early lenses for, 338, 339f
- English, 343f
- handles, 339f, 340
- lorgnettes as, 118
- as low-vision aid, 340, 341f
- metal, 338, 340f
- mother-of-pearl, 338, 340, 340f
- pocket, 338, 339f, 340f
- silver, 340, 340f
- for special purposes, 340, 341f
- telescopic loupes, operating-room, 316, 317f–319f
- tortoiseshell, 338, 339f, 340, 340f
- varieties of, 40f, 339f
- wooden, 338, 339f, 343f

Mahogany, 9
Mahtsorf model, of pince-nez, 245
Makeup spectacles, 306–307, 306f, 307f
Malacca (Malaysia), 64
Malakka (Malaysia), 37
Malaysia, 10, 37, 64
Management of historical collections
   accession numbers and record
  keeping, 2
    appraisals, 2
    cabinets and drawers for, 1–2
    cataloging items in, 2–3
    cleaning, 4
    dating artifacts, 5–16, 281–283
    duplicates, how to avoid, 2–3
    establishing provenance, 2–3
    examining artifacts
     for condition, 13–15
     for historical context, 5–8
     magnification for, importance of, 13–15
     for repairs, 13
    exhibiting the collection, 2, 3
    insurance coverage, 2
    labeling items, 2–3
    lighting for displays, 2
    literature research, 4
    loaning items out, 3–4
    packing and transporting, 3–4
    pricing items, 3
    protecting from heat and insects, 2
    restorations, 4
    sales and swaps, 3
Marcasite lorgnettes, 119, 132f
Markings on spectacles
   focal lengths, 32, 59
   hallmarks, 5, 6f, 8, 8f, 14, 14f
   opera glasses, 163–164, 163f
   personal monograms, 15, 15f
Martin's Margins, 106–110
   cases for, 108f, 110
   examples of, 107f–109f
   gold, 42f, 107, 107f, 320
   history of, 42, 106–110
   pad inserts, 99, 100f, 103, 107, 107f, 108f, 109
    pince-nez as, 107
    silver, 107, 107f
    steel, 99, 107, 107f
    wig spectacles as, 109
Massachusetts Charitable Mechanics
   Association Fair, 52, 53
Mathematical instruments, 51
Medicine glasses, Chinese, 270–271
Mediterranean region, 17, 25

Meissen glass factory, Germany, 5, 6f
   Sight statue from, 367f
Meniscus lenses, 29, 30, 30f, 31, 53, 60, 99, 384
Mercury poisoning, from vermeil
   process, 12
Mesopotamia, 18
Metallic oxides, for coloring glass lenses, 274
Metals
   alloys, 12, 68, 71f, 85f, 103, 105, 384, 388
   frames, 38, 46, 68, 68f, 306f, 384, 388
   identifying grade of, 13–14
   lorgnettes, 118, 119, 128f
   magnifying glasses, 338, 340f
   monoculars, 139f
   opera glasses, 174, 180–182, 184, 186, 190, 193, 196–198, 210f
   pince-nez, 236
   quizzing glasses, 222
   restoring, 4
   See also specific metals
Mexico, 21
Mica stone, 63
Microscopes, 51, 52, 106
Middle East, 18, 24, 25
Ming dynasty, 26, 63, 64, 97
Miniatures
   evil eye, 349, 353f
   French monoculars, 143f, 148f
   of guild applicants, 349, 350f
   as jewelry, 349, 350f, 351f
   on Italian cases, 323, 325f, 326f
   of spectacles, 349–353, 350f–353f
   of Stanhopes, 349, 352f
   uses of, unusual, 353, 353f
Miocene period, 24
Mirrors, 24, 33, 50
   bronze, 27, 63
   Claude Lorraine, 275–276
   in fans, 224, 226f
   hand, with monocular telescope, 143, 144f
   landscape, 275–276
Moldite, for molding contact lenses, 374
Money sign, on Chinese spectacles, 69, 69f, 70f
Mongol dynasty, 26
Mongolia, 18, 270
Monocles. *See* Monoculars
Monoculars, 138–148, 230–235
   agate, 141
   to apply cosmetics, 307f
   in boudoir hand-mirrors, 143, 144f

   cardboard, 141
   cases for, 234, 234f
   as charms (jewelry), 147, 147f
   Chinese (yuan ching), 68
   defined, 40, 46, 138, 139f, 230
   developer of, 231–233
   diamonds on, 231
   disapproval of, by physicians, 233–234
   early, 138, 139f, 140f, 141
   enameled, 141, 142f
   English, 13f, 139f, 142f, 146f, 147f, 234–235
   examples of, 231f–234f
   in fans, 145, 145f
   French, 139f, 140f, 141, 141f, 143f, 146f, 148f, 196, 231
   galleries for, 231, 232f, 233, 233f, 234f
   German, 231, 233–234
   gold, 46f, 141, 142f, 231, 232f, 233f
   history of, 230–235
   ivory, 13f, 139f, 141, 142f
   jealousy glasses, 140f, 141
   jewels on, 141, 143f, 144f, 148f
   leather, 141
   materials for, 141, 141f–143f, 143
   metal, 139f
   mother-of-pearl, 143
   multiple-draw, 140f, 144f, 147f, 148f
   in parasol handles, 145
   parchment, 141
   in perfume flasks, 145, 145f
   pomponne, 141
   porcelain, 139f, 143
   quizzing glass known as, 220
   silver, 141, 231, 232f
   single-tube sliding, 139, 140f, 141
   synonyms for, 138
   tortoiseshell, 232f, 234f
   in walking canes, 146f, 147
   Wedgwood, 141
   wooden, 139f, 141, 141f
   See also Perspective glasses; Prospect glasses; Telescopes
Monograms, personal, on spectacles, 15, 15f
Moroccan leather cases, 266, 267f, 275
Motex lenses, 291
Mother-of-pearl
   cases, 206f, 323, 327, 329
   lorgnettes, 118, 119, 120f, 121f, 123f, 125f, 126f
   magnifying glasses, 338, 340, 340f
   monoculars, 143
   on papier mache, 12, 13f

opera glasses, 153, 154f, 155f, 164f, 172–200 passim, 207f, 208f, 213f, 216f
  pince-nez, 237f
  quizzing glasses, 222
  scissors glasses, 115, 116f
Mount Carmel, Syria, 17
Murano glass, 20, 20f, 21, 33
Museums, with ophthalmic collections, list of, 465–466
Musierwelle, 42, 239
Myopia, 27, 30
  de la Hire's theories on, 369–370
  half-glasses for, 302
  lenses to correct, 67, 68
  monocle to correct, 230f, 233–234
  quizzing glasses to correct, 220
  wig spectacles and, 111

Napoleonic era, 7, 7f
Nasal deformities, frames for, 304
Natron, 17
Neitz loupe, 317f
Netherlands. See Dutch spectacles
Netsuke (Japanese), 78, 360f
New York Daily Advertiser, 50
New York Gazette, 50
Newsletter, Ophthalmic Antiques International Collectors' Club, 346–347
Newtonian reflectors, 52
Nickel-plated spectacles
  frames, 99
  opera glasses, 176, 197
Niello-decorated lorgnettes, 131f
Nimrud (Middle East), 18
Nineveh, Iraq, 24–25, 27
Nitre, 27
Nokrome lenses, 60
Nola (United States), 25
Nose pads
  pince-nez, 239, 240f, 241, 242f, 243, 243f
  plastic, 384, 386f
Nounette du jalousie, 141
Nuremberg spectacles, 36f, 39, 39f, 41, 41f, 46, 97, 239, 239f, 320
  magnifying glasses, 338, 339f
Nylon, 10

Object glasses, 22, 51
Occlusive lenses, 303
Occupational spectacles, 302
  See also specific occupation
Octagonal lenses, 103
Ocular caps, defined, 163–164

Ocular muscles, 30
Ocular protection. *See* Eskimo eyeshades; Protective spectacles; Sunglasses
Oil of Brique, 22, 32
The Old Eyeglass Peddler, 5, 6f
Old Testament, 27
Onyx lorgnettes, 132f
Opera glasses, 149–218
  American, 163, 166, 167, 168
  Austrian, 153, 171, 172
  Belgian, 167, 171, 207f
  bone, 153, 153f, 192, 195, 211f
  boxes from initial sale of, 166, 217f
  bronze, 176, 194, 198
  cases for, 164–165, 164f, 165f, 186–187, 190–193, 195, 197–198, 217f
  chrome, 173–174, 176–177, 180–199 passim
  cloisonne, 191
  cost of, 163
  cylindrical-shaped, 211f
  demand for, 149, 153
  diamond-studded, 196
  Dutch, 153
  embellishments on, 153, 157, 159
  English, 149, 159, 168, 171, 172
    compared to French, 149
    examples of, 158f, 159f, 160f, 214f
  examples of, 206f–217f
  expanding, 159, 160f
  folding, 180, 189, 197, 206f, 210f, 213f
  French, 149, 153, 157, 159, 161, 163–166
    compared to English, 149
    examples of, 150f, 155f, 156f, 159f, 162f, 209f, 210f, 213f
  German, 149, 167, 169, 171, 172
  handles of, 160f–162f, 161, 172, 173, 213f, 214f, 216f, 217f
  hand-painted, 153, 155f
  history of, 149
  identifying marks on, 152f, 163–167, 163f, 204–205
  interpupillary distances and, 149
  Italian, 169
  ivory, 151f, 153, 161f, 174, 177, 186, 188, 190, 192–196, 198, 214f
  Japanese, 172
  lacquer, 174, 184, 192, 194, 195
  leather, 152f, 173–174, 176, 178, 180–199 passim
  lens caps, 152f
  manufacturers, list of, 167–198
  metal, 174, 180–182, 184, 186, 190, 193, 196–198, 210f

  mother-of-pearl, 153, 154f, 155f, 164f, 172–200 passim, 207f, 208f, 213f, 216f
  name for collectors of, 166
  New Orleans, descriptions of, 198–200
  nickel-plated, 176, 197
  novelties shaped as, 159, 160f
  ocular caps on, defined, 163–164
  oval-shaped lenses for, 149, 151f
  pebble glass for, 22
  pewter, 174, 189, 190, 211f, 212f
  platinum, 153
  porcelain, 153, 176, 190, 196, 209f
  reed, 172, 173, 187, 194, 199, 200
  retailers, list of, 200–203
  Russian, 169, 170, 172
  sea snail, 150f, 153, 154f, 172–200 passim, 212f, 213f
  shagreen, 153, 165, 187
  silver, 153, 157, 173, 180–181, 185–186, 190, 195–196, 198, 213f
  tortoiseshell, 150f, 153, 154f, 159f, 174, 177, 180, 186, 193, 195, 197, 198, 211f
  turquoise on, 192, 196, 197
  wood on, 153, 172, 193, 195
Operating room magnifying lenses, 316–319
Ophthalmic Antiques International Collectors' Club Magazine, 42
Ophthalmic Antiques International Collectors' Club Newsletter, 346–347
Ophthalmic lenses
  history of, 24–34
  landmarks in (timetable), 389–393
  scientific advances in, 31–32, 63–64
Ophthalmic miniatures. *See* Miniatures
Ophthalmometer, invention of, 31
Ophthalmoscope, invention of, 31
Optical filters, 274–277, 274f, 277f
Optical glass
  history of, 21–22, 389–393
  See also Glass; Lenses
Optical instruments/machines
  diopter, 8, 32, 33f, 39
  lensometer, 8, 15
  microscope, 51, 52, 106
  Musierwelle, 42, 239
  ophthalmometer, 31
  ophthalmoscope, 31
  optometer, 308, 309f
  phoropter, 313
  photographic, 51, 53
  retinoscope, 31
  sold by George Adams (in late 1700s), 44t–45t
  See also Spectacles; Telescopes

Optical Journal, 58, 161
Optical manufacturing
   competition in, 50, 53–54
   in Europe, 20–21
   first lenses made in U.S., 52
   frame-making, *versus* lens-grinding, 50, 53, 59
   grinding rooms, description of, 59
   impact of German immigration on, 51
   imports and, 50, 52
   industrialization and, 50, 52–54
   production expansion, late 1800s, 53–54
   production-line lenses, first, 59–60
   of scientific instruments, 52–53
   in Southbridge, MA, 54–60, 61*t*
   tariffs and, 50
   of telescopes, 52–53
   in United States, 50–61, 429–432
   See also under specific names in Name Index
Optical patron saints. *See* Patron saints (optical)
Optical Theraurus (Alhazen), 27
Opticians' shops, 31*f,* 41
   Japanese, 98
Optometer
   invention of, 308, 309*f*
   self-test, 308, 309*f*
Optometers, binocular, 309*f*
Optyl (plastic), 10
Opus Magnus (Bacon), 27, 35
Orthogon "D" bifocal lenses, 60
Orthogon lenses, 60
Orthoptic training, occlusion glasses for, 303
Orthoscopic spectacles, 300
Oval lenses, 103*f,* 111, 118
Oxford eyeglasses, 253–254, 253*f*
Oxhorn, 11, 42
Oxygen-administration glasses, 300, 302, 302*f*

Pacific cloth, 2
Packing and transporting, of historical collections, 3–4
Padouk wood, 9
Pads
   cork, 46, 242*f,* 243
   forehead, 66
   horn, 46, 66
   Martin's Margins, 99, 100*f,* 103, 107, 107*f,* 108*f,* 109
   pince-nez, 239, 240*f,* 241, 242*f,* 243, 243*f*
   plastic, 384, 386*f*
   for temples, 46, 99, 100*f,* 103, 107*f,* 108*f,* 109, 111, 113*f*
   tortoiseshell, 46
   in trial lens sets, 314*f,* 315
   of wig spectacles, 111, 113*f*
   See also Inserts
Pai-tung spectacle cases, 86*f*
Paillons (silver foil), on opera glasses, 157
Palace of Knossos (Crete), 24
Palaquium trees, 10, 10*f*
Pan ching (half-eye) Chinese spectacles, 68
Panoptik trifocal lenses, 262*f,* 263, 264, 264*f*
Paper pulp, 12–13
Papier mache
   cases, 13, 13*f,* 84*f,* 322*f,* 323, 323*f*
      English, example of, 13*f*
   defined, 12–13
   mother-of-pearl on, 12, 13*f*
   patent for, 12
   silver inlay on, 13
   wood for, 12
Parasol handles, monoculars in, 145
Parchment monoculars, 141
Patents
   biconvex-meniscus lenses, 53
   bifocal (improved), 51
   Bugbee, 58
   contact lenses, 377, 379, 380
   frames, 53
   Hammon, 60
   Hardy-Delaney, 59
   Hutten Oxford, 254
   internal screws, for opera glasses, 149, 150*f*
   papier mache, 12
   periscopic lenses, 30
   pince-nez, 236
   telescopes, 138
   tin spectacle cases, 105
Patron saints (optical), 344–348
   Sofronuis Eusebius Hieronymus, 35
   St. Audomarus, 347
   St. Fridolin, 35
   St. Herve, 347
   St. Lucy, 5, 6*f,* 7, 35, 344, 345*f,* 346, 347*f*
   St. Odilia, 346–347
   St. Raphael, 347
   St. Walburga, 348

Pearls
   (black lip) opera glasses, 153, 154*f,* 176–179, 186–187, 195, 198, 212*f,* 213*f*
   on quizzing glasses, 222
Pebble glass, 22, 32–33, 38, 42, 107, 111, 284, 285*f,* 338
Perfection bifocals, 261, 261*f*
Perfume flasks, monoculars in, 145, 145*f*
Perifocal spectacles, 53
Periscopic lenses, 30, 31, 53, 57, 141, 224, 225*f*
Personal monograms, on spectacles, 15, 15*f*
Perspective glasses, 40, 40*f*
   quizzing glasses known as, 220
   See also Monoculars
Perspex (plastic), 10
Petuntze, 18
Pewter opera glasses, 174, 189, 190, 211*f,* 212*f*
PHEMA (polyhydroxy ethyl methacrylate) plastic, 379
Philippines, 14
Phoenicians, 17, 27
Phoropters, 313, 315
Photographic lenses, 51, 53
Pike's Scientific and Medical Instruments, 274, 275, 277
Pince-nez, 236–257
   accessories to, 248*f,* 249, 249*f,* 251, 253*f,* 255*f*
   Achilles mounting for, 245
   amber-colored lenses for, 272*f*
   American, example of, 248*f,* 385*f*
   Australian model of, 245
   baleen, 236, 238*f,* 239
   bar springs for, 246, 246*f,* 247*f*
   Belgian, 239, 240*f*
   bone, 236
   bridges, 36*f,* 46, 236
   cases for, 237*f,* 239*f,* 250*f,* 255, 255*f,* 256*f*
   chain-reeling mechanism for, 249, 249*f*
   defined, 236
   development of, 236, 239, 241, 243, 245
   English, 238*f,* 245, 248*f*
   eye shields, 245, 245*f*
   finger-piece mountings for, 246, 252
   Fits-U model of, 236, 237*f,* 252, 384
   fitting difficulties of, 236, 237*f*
   fitting set, examples of, 245, 245*f,* 246*f*
   folding, 250*f,* 251*f*
   German, 97, 239, 239*f*
   hard-rubber frames for, 10*f*

Hutten Oxford model, 254
ivory, 236
leather, 236, 238f
leverage system of applying, 242f, 243
lorgnette, 132, 133f
Mahtsorf model of, 245
Martin's Margins as, 107
medical objections to, 253
metal, 236
mother-of-pearl, 237f
nose pads for, 239, 240f, 241, 242f, 243, 243f
Nuremberg-style, 97, 239, 239f
Oxford style, 253–254, 253f
preacher/speaker's half-glass style, 247f, 248f
replica of early, 237f
rimless, 47, 47f
shagreen, 243
shooting glasses, 297f, 298, 298f
snap-on temples for, 244f, 245
social customs and, 251–252
spring steel for, 239, 240f, 241
springs for, 242f, 243, 243f, 246, 246f, 247f, 298
sunshades, 250f, 251
tortoiseshell, 237f, 239, 239f, 241f, 248f, 250f, 253f
Pinchbeck alloy, 12
Pinhole spectacles, 63, 270, 278, 303
Pink arundel lenses, 273
Pivoted spectacles, 96
Plano lenses, in pince-nez, 251
Planoconcave lenses, 30
Planoconvex lenses, 25, 27, 30, 67
Planoconvex mirrors, 275–276
Planocylinder lenses, 30
Plastics
cases, 95f, 105
frames, 9–11, 103, 307f, 384, 386f, 387
in imitation Chinese spectacles, 21–22
lenses, 388
lorgnettes, 127f, 136, 136f
for magnifying glass covers, 340
nose pads, 384, 386f
PHEMA type, 379
Plexiglas, 372, 374
PMMA type, 374, 380
types of, 9–11, 372, 374, 379, 380
See also Contact lenses
Plate glass, 21
Plating process, 11–12
Platinum opera glasses, 153
Plexiglas plastic, 372, 374

PMMA (polymethyl methacrylate) plastic, 374, 380
Polaroid rotating lenses, 292f
Poller's Negacoll, for contact lenses, 372–373, 374
Polycarbonate lenses, 388
Polyhydroxy ethyl methacrylate (PHEMA) plastic, 379
Polymethyl methacrylate (PMMA) plastic, 374, 380
Pompeii, 25
Pomponne monoculars, 141
Pontocaine anaesthetic, 372
Porcelain
Chinese, 5, 6f, 18, 76f, 77
examination of, for repairs, 13
miniature spectacles, 350f
monoculars, 139f, 143
opera glasses, 153, 176, 190, 196, 209f
Pouces, 8, 33f
Preacher's half-glasses, 247f, 248f
Precious stones. See Jewels
Presbyopia, 26, 63
contact lenses and, 380–381
half-glasses for, 302
makeup spectacles and, 306–307
monocles to correct, 230–231
quizzing glasses to correct, 220
reversible glasses for, 302–303
Pricing, of collection artifacts, 3
Printing press
invention of, and demand for spectacles, 39
origins of, in China, 77
Prisms, 30–31, 50, 51
binocular, 149, 151f
diopters, 31
field glasses, 151f
for large-muscle imbalances, 300, 301f
for lens fitting, 308
for recumbent patients, 300, 302f
trial frames for, 314f, 315
Progressive bifocal/trifocal lenses, 264
Prospect glasses, 145, 147
French, 225f
quizzing glasses known as, 220
as small telescopes, 40–41, 118, 224, 225f
used to spy on others, 224
See also Monoculars
Protective spectacles, 284–294
for automobile drivers, 284, 287f–288f
aviator goggles, 284, 286f, 287f
cases for, 284, 286f, 287f

cobalt blue, for smelter workers, 289
with dark lenses, examples of, 289f, 291f
English X-bridge, 285f
French X-bridge, 285f
for ironworkers, 289
modern, examples of, 293f
to prevent flash burns, 289, 289f–290f, 300, 302f
for racing jockeys, 284, 288f
for railroad workers, 284, 285f
shatterproof glass as, 289, 290f, 291
for stone masons, 284, 286f
for underwater divers, 284, 289, 289f
U.S. Navy polaroid, 292f
variety of, 291f–293f
for welders, 289, 289f–290f, 292f, 300, 302f
See also Eskimo eyeshades; Eyeshades for invalids; Sunglasses
Provenance of artifacts
cataloging the, 2–3
researching, 4
and value of item, 3
Ptosis, crutch glasses for, 303
Punktal lenses, 60
Pupillary distance, trial lens and frame sets to measure, 313f, 315
Pylon eyeshade holders, 266, 267f, 268f

Qi Xiu Xu Gao (Lang), 64
Quartz, 8, 24, 38, 68
tea-colored (mica stone), 63
Quinebaug Historical Society Leaflets, 59
Quizzers. See Quizzing glasses
Quizzing glasses, 220–223
in cockade fan, 225f
defined, 220
English, examples of, 221f
fashion and, 220, 221f, 222–223, 222f
frames and handles, 222
French, examples of, 221f, 222f
lenses for, 220
materials for, 115, 116f, 221f, 222
for myopia, 220
shapes of, 222, 223f
uses of, 220

Racing (horse) goggles, 284, 288f
Raffia frames, 66, 66f
Railroad worker goggles, 284, 285f
Rare artifacts, value of, 3
Ray Ban lenses, 273
Ray skin. See Shagreen

Reading spectacles
    first reference to, 26
    quizzing glasses known as, 220
Redgauntlet (Scott), 276
Reed
    on opera glasses, 172, 173, 187, 194, 199, 200
    spectacles, 66, 66f, 76f
    types of, 9
Reflecting telescope, 52
Refraction, discovery of, 30–32
Religious artifacts, 5, 6f, 7
Repairs, examining for evidence of, 13
Repousse, defined, 12, 12f
Restoration, of artifacts, 4
Restoring Ophthalmic Antiques (MacGregor), 4
Retinal detachment, postsurgical spectacles for, 298, 298f, 303, 303f
Retinoscope, invention of, 31
Retinoscopy lens sets, 308, 310f
Reversible glasses, 302–303
Rhinestones (brilliants), 119, 132f, 134f
Rhinophyma, frames for, 304
Rhodium-coated frames, 99
Riding bows, 43, 46, 244f
Rimless spectacles, 47, 47f, 64, 64f, 74f, 384, 386f
Rims, 35, 103
    of horn, 11
    leather, 40
    steel, 40
    See also Frames; Lenses
Riveted spectacles, 38, 39f, 40, 46, 97, 99, 236, 237f, 320
    in artwork, 358, 359f
Rock crystal, 24, 25, 27, 33, 42, 68, 270–271
Rolled gold, 12, 47
Romans, ancient, 18, 24–27
Round lenses, 65f, 103f, 384, 385f
Roussette, 9
Rubber
    on spectacles, 10, 10f
    opera glass caps, 176, 197
Ruby glass, 89
Ruby-decorated lorgnettes, 131f
Russia, hallmarks of, 14

Saddle bridge, 46
Safety glass lenses, 291
Saffron, 12
Saghri. *See* Shagreen
Salvoc lenses, 291
Sales and swaps, of collection artifacts, 3

Salt and pepper shakers, shaped as opera glasses, 160f
Salt of tartar, 12
Sandalwood, 67, 82f
Sapphires, on lorgnettes, 119, 125f, 131f
Sash weights, 66f
Scandinavia, 21
Scrimshand decorations, on Eskimo eyeshades, 281
Scissors glasses, 115–117
    in art, 359f
    early, 38, 39f
    examples of, 116f–117f
    French, 12f, 116f
    history of, 115
    lorgnettes and, 115, 116f, 117f, 118
    Scotland, 18, 32
Screws
    opera glasses, 149, 150f
    spectacle, 99, 100f
Sea snail
    opera glasses, 150f, 153, 154f, 172–200 passim, 212f, 213f
    spectacle cases, 327, 329
Sea turtle shells, 10–11, 10f
Self-test optometer, 309f
Shadow boxes, 2
Shagreen
    cases, 9, 9f, 66, 78, 80f, 85f, 87, 88f, 114, 165, 320, 323, 325f, 334f, 335, 336f, 337
    defined, 9, 9f
    eye guards, for pince-nez, 243
    magnifying glass covers, 339f, 340
    opera glasses, 153, 165, 187
Shapes of lenses, 30, 57, 59, 65f, 67, 67f, 103, 103f, 111, 118
Sharkskin. *See* Shagreen
Sharpshooter glasses. *See* Shooting glasses
Shatterproof protective glasses, 289, 290f, 291
Shooting glasses, 295–299
    amber-colored lenses for, 295, 296f, 297f, 298f
    American style, 295, 297f
    pince-nez, 297f, 298, 298f
    target spectacles, 298f
    varieties of, 295, 296f–299f
Shops, opticians', 31f, 41
Shuron lenses, 384
Siberia, quartz from, 8
Sicily, 18
Side-pieces, spectacle. *See* Temples
Sight (Meissen statue), 5, 6f, 367f
Signeri apparatus, 51

Silk cases, 80f, 164f, 165
    for opera glasses, 164, 164f, 165
Silver
    base, for vermeil process, 11–12
    caring for, in historical collections, 2
    cases, 10f, 89, 94f, 320, 323, 324f, 325f, 327f, 328f, 329, 334f, 335, 335f, 336f, 337
    coin, 8
    filigree, 14, 14f
    frames, 5, 6f, 14, 14f, 42, 56f, 76f, 107, 107f, 384, 385f
    hallmarks, 5, 6f, 8, 8f, 14, 14f
    inlay, on papier mache, 13
    lorgnettes, 118, 119, 121f, 126f, 127f, 128f, 133f
    magnifying glasses, 340, 340f
    Martin's Margins, 107, 107f
    monoculars, 141, 231, 232f
    opera glasses, 153, 157, 173, 180–181, 185–186, 190, 195–196, 198, 213f
    pince-nez, 237f, 239
    quizzing glasses, 221f, 222
    spectacles, 55f, 56f, 272f
    sterling, 8, 8f
    temples, 15f, 41
    wig spectacles, 111
Size of lenses
    contrasted, 79f
    fashion and, 40, 42, 65, 71f
    larger, as sign of intelligence, 78
    lens thickness, 67, 67f
    social customs and, 65, 65f, 68, 71f, 384, 387f
Slip-top spectacle cases, 322f, 323
Slit bridges, 36f, 38, 39f, 46, 236
Snakeskin opera glasses, 194, 197
Snow eyeshades/goggles, Eskimo, 11, 97, 278–283
Social customs
    monocles and, 230–231, 233–234
    opera glasses and, 149
    pince-nez and, 251–252
    spectacles and, 62, 64–65, 68, 78, 118
    spying activities, 224–229
    See also Beliefs; Fashion; Status, social
Soda glass, 7, 7f, 18, 20, 21
Sodium carbonate, 17
Soëgren's syndrome, 304
Soflens contact lenses, 379
Softlite lenses, 273, 273f
Song dynasty, 63–64
The Southbridge Journal, 59, 60
Southbridge, MA, early spectacle makers of, 29, 54–59, 60

Spain, 9, 21
Spanish Inquisition, 40
Spatula temples, combined with cable, 304, 304f, 384
Speaces' achromatic object glasses, 51
Speaker's half-glasses, 247f, 248f
Specialized spectacles, 300–305
　See also under specific purpose or activity
Spectacles
　alternatives to, 40–41, 40f, 138
　American. *See* American spectacles
　in art. *See* Spectacles in art
　beliefs about, 35, 62, 65, 66, 68, 270–271, 304
　collecting historical. *See* Management of historical collections
　collections of, worldwide, list of, 465–466
　demand for, after printing press invention, 39
　description of early, 38–40, 39f, 40f
　English. *See* England
　fashion and. *See* Fashion
　frames for. *See* Frames
　handled, first patented, 118, 121f, 122f
　healing powers attributed to, 62, 65
　history of, 35–49
　Hilscher's treatise (1741), English translation, 467–487
　landmarks in (timetable), 389–393
　Manni's treatise (1738), English translation, 395–428
　identifying marks on, 5, 15, 32, 33, 36f, 53, 59, 107, 107f, 114
　invention of, 38, 62, 270
　made by Benjamin Martin. *See* Martin's Margins
　mass production of, early, 39
　meaning of term, 37
　miniatures of, 349–353, 350f–353f
　perspective. *See* Perspective glasses
　prospect. *See* Prospect glasses
　reversible, 302–303
　rimless, 47, 47f, 64, 64f, 74f, 384, 386f
　riveted. *See* Riveted spectacles
　as sign of intelligence, 64–65, 65f, 78
　specialized, 300–305
　as status symbol. *See* Status, social
　stored in book covers, 320
　techniques of wearing, 65–66, 65f, 66f
　using historical contexts to identify, 5–8
　See also Chinese spectacles; Lorgnettes; Monoculars; Protective spectacles; Scissors glasses; Sunglasses; Wig spectacles

Spectacles in art, 358–368
　caricatures, 358, 359f
　Danse Macabre, French illustration of, 332
　examples of, 359f–367f
　list of artworks depicting spectacles, 437–463
　"Old Pushpin," 358, 359f
　of riveted spectacles, 358, 359f
　Vanity Fair prints, 360f–361f
Speculums, telescope, 51
Spherocylindrical lenses, Airy's, 30
Splinternil lenses, 291
Sportsmen glasses. *See* Shooting glasses
Spring steel, for pince-nez, 239, 240f, 241
Spring temples, 243
Springs, 40, 41f, 43
　for lorgnettes, 118, 119, 122f, 132, 133f
　for pince-nez, 242f, 243, 243f, 246, 246f, 247f, 298
Spyglasses. *See* Monoculars
Spying (social), vision aids for, 224–229
Squint, 30
Stamp collector's lens, 340, 341f
Stanhope lenses, 52
　miniatures of, 349, 352f
Status, social
　cases as sign of, 320, 330, 330f–331f
　lorgnettes and, 119, 125f–126f
　spectacles as sign of, 64–65, 65f, 78, 78f, 97
Steel
　blued, 47, 47f, 99, 296f, 298
　bridges, 46
　cases, 99, 100f, 103, 103f, 104f, 320, 321f, 323, 326f, 336f
　detecting, in artifacts, 14
　frames, 41, 47, 47f, 99, 100f–103f, 103, 295, 297f
　Martin's Margins, 99, 107, 107f
　pince-nez, 239, 240f, 241
　quizzing glasses, 222
　rims, 40
　spectacles, 54, 57, 58
　spring, 239, 240f, 241
　temples, 41, 42f
Sterling silver, 8, 8f
Stone masons, protective spectacles for, 284, 286f
Stones, precious. *See* Jewels
Storage, of historical collections, 1–2
Sumatra, 10
Sunglasses, 24, 26, 62, 103
　American, examples of, 387, 387f

Chinese, examples of, 35, 36f
colored lenses for, 271–277, 272f, 273f, 274f, 275f, 277f
Crookes', 273, 384
Eskimo "snow shields," 270, 279f
fashion and, 40–41
pince-nez, 250f, 251
See also Eskimo eyeshades; Protective spectacles
Superstitions, about spectacles, 68, 270–271
Surgeon's telescopic loupes, 316, 317f–319f
Surveying instruments, 50, 51
Swaps and sales, of collection artifacts, 3
Swastika sign, on Chinese spectacles, 70f
Syllepsis glasses, 42
Syria, 17, 18

Tableaux de Paris (Mercier), 143, 145
Talmud, 27
Tang dynasty, 18
Tangerine-skin Chinese spectacles case, 78, 86f
Tanis, 25
Target spectacles. *See* Shooting glasses
Tcha-chi. See Ai tai (*Ai Dai*) teastone spectacles
Teastone glass (*ai tai*) lenses, 7, 7f, 19f, 24, 62, 63, 66–67, 74f, 76f, 270–271, 271f
Telescopes
　achromatic, 21, 51
　in antiquity, 24–25
　cardboard tube, 42
　demand for, 52
　discovery of, 138
　hand-held, 138
　in handles, 119, 196, 197
　history of lens-grinding methods for, 467–487
　lenses for, 33
　monocle known as, 231
　pebble glass and, 22
　prospect glass as, 40–41, 118, 224, 225f
　reflecting, 52
　See also Monoculars
Telescopic operating loupes, 316, 317f–319f
Temple of Artemis (Ephesos), 24
Temples
　cable, 15, 15f, 304, 304f, 384
　double-hinged, 41–42, 99, 100f, 108f, 111, 113f
　ends of, 99, 100f, 101f

extensions for, 41, 42f, 99, 101f, 111, 113f
inventor of, 111
markings on, 15, 15f, 33, 107, 107f, 114
Martin's Margins, 108f, 109
pads for, 46, 99, 100f, 103, 107f, 108f, 109, 111, 113f
personal monograms on, 15, 15f
reticulated, 70f
riding-bow, 43, 46, 244f
ring, 42f
silver, 15f, 41
sliding, 41, 42f, 99, 101f, 111
snap-on, 244f, 245
spatula, combined with cable, 304, 304f, 384
spring, 243
steel, 41, 42f
strings, 65–66, 65f, 66f, 89f
turn-pin, 42–43, 99, 100f, 111
weights for, 66f
of wig spectacles, 111, 113f
wire, 15, 15f, 384
See also Frames
Thallium glass, 21
Theater glasses. See Opera glasses
Thebes, 17
Thermoluminescence process, to date artifacts, 281–283
Thermometers, 51
Three Kingdoms, 78
Tillyer "D" bifocal lenses, 57
Tillyer hinge, 384
Tilting springs, 43
Timepieces, in lorgnettes, 119, 132, 135f
Tinplated spectacle cases, 12, 104f, 105, 323, 326f
Topaz lenses, 24, 68
Toric lenses, 30, 31, 57, 60, 384
Tortoiseshell
  bezels, 274
  bridges, 70f, 97
  carvings on, symbolism of, 69, 69f–70f, 71, 78
  cases, 10f, 72f, 89, 94f, 114, 320, 322f, 323, 324f, 329, 335, 335f, 339f
  Chinese spectacles, 36f, 67f, 68f, 74f, 79f
  defined, 10–11
  diving goggles, 284, 289, 289f
  fans, 228f
  frames, 7f, 66, 67f, 72f, 73f, 103, 111
  as good luck symbol, 66
  hawk's bill sea turtle, 10–11, 10f
  housing and protecting, 2
  inserts, 103, 107

lorgnettes, 118, 119, 120f, 125f, 126f, 127f, 128f, 131f
magnifying glasses, 338, 339f, 340, 340f
monoculars, 232f, 234f
opera glasses, 150f, 153, 154f, 159f, 174, 177, 180, 186, 193, 195, 197, 198, 211f
pads, 46
pince-nez, 237f, 239, 239f, 241f, 248f, 250f, 253f
quizzing glasses, 222
restoring, 4
sacredness of, to Chinese, 66
scissors glasses, 115, 116f
trial lens sets, 308, 310f
wig spectacles, 111, 112f
Touchmarks. See Hallmarks
Transfer (decal) decoration, 5, 6f, 89, 91f, 323, 324f
Transporting, of historical collections, 3–4
"Treading Through the Snow in Pursuit of the Plum Flower," 78
A Treatise on the Construction, Proper Use, and Capabilities of Smith, Beck, and Beck's Achromatic Microscopes (Beck), 342–343
Treviso, 35
Trial lenses and frames, 308–315
  cases for sets of, 311, 311f
  English, 311f
  frame sets, 308, 311f, 312f, 313, 313f, 314f, 315
  German, 308, 310f
  increments of measure on, 313, 313f
  lens sets, 308, 310f, 311, 311f
Trichromatism, 30
Trifocal lenses
  baseball type, 264
  executive style, 57, 302
  panoptik, 262f, 263, 264, 264f
  progressive, 264
  types available, 263, 264, 264f, 384
Triplex lenses, 291
Troy, 24–25
True-Color (grey) lenses, 273
T'u-schu-tsi-tsch'ong, 37
Tonbridgeware, 9
Turquoise
  on monoculars, 143f
  on opera glasses, 192, 196, 197
Tyre, 24–25

Ultex lenses, 261, 264, 384
Ultraviolet-absorbing lenses, 273, 300

Underwater divers, protective spectacles for, 284, 289, 289f
United States
  glass factories in, 21
  lens grinding in, history of, 50–61
  list of spectacle makers (1700-1850), 429–432
  Navy Polaroid glasses, 292f
  See also American spectacles
Univis lenses, 264
Uranium salts, to color glass, 273
Uso de los Antoios (Daca de Valdes), 40, 271, 354, 355f

Vanity Fair prints, depicting spectacles, 360f–361f
Venetian glass, 20, 20f, 21, 33, 42
Vermeil process, 11–12, 12f
  opera glasses, 195
Vertex refraction, 31
Vinaigrettes
  engraved English, 14f
  in lorgnettes, 119
Vision aids
  collecting and managing. See Management of historical collections
  ophthalmic collections of, worldwide, list of, 465–466
Vitreous glazing, 17
Vocational lenses, 302
  See also Bifocal lenses; Trifocal lenses
Votive offerings, 344–348
  Flemish, 344
  German, 344
  Italian, 344
  to optical patron saints, 7, 7f, 12f, 344, 345f, 346, 347f
  varieties of, 345f
Vulcanite orebonite, 10, 10f

Watches, in lorgnettes, 119, 132, 135f
Watchmaker's spectacles, 300, 301f
Water buffalo horn, 11
Wedgwood monoculars, 141
Welder's goggles, 289, 289f–290f, 292f, 300, 302f
Whale jaw bone, 11
Widesite lenses, 264
Wig spectacles, 111–114
  cases for, 113f, 114, 114f, 323, 324f, 325f
  Martin's Margins and, 109
  for rhinophyma patients, 304
  temples for, 111, 112f, 113f
Wilson/Albex/American Optical goggles, 288f, 293f

Wire frames, 15, 15f, 105, 239, 240f
Wire temples, 15, 15f, 384
Women opticians, 50
Wood
  boxwood, 86f
  cases, 9, 66, 78, 81f–84f, 87, 103, 103f, 165, 239f, 256f, 320, 321f
    Eskimo eyeshades, 279f, 280, 280f
    identifying types of, 8–9, 8f
    jealousy glasses, 225f
    magnifying glasses, 338, 339f, 343f
    mahogany, 9
    monoculars, 139f, 141, 141f
    on opera glasses, 153, 172, 193, 195
    optometers, 309f
    padouk, 9
    for papier mache, 12
    quizzing glasses, 222
    sandalwood, 67, 82f
Tonbridgeware, 9

X-shaped bridges, 46, 46f, 99, 101f, 111, 285f, 298, 298f
Xylonite (plastic), 9–10

Yoh shui (Chinese spirit force)
  in spectacles, 62
  in sunglasses, 35, 35f
Yoh-shui Yen-ching glasses, 270
Yuan ching (monocle) Chinese spectacles, 68

Zeiss loupes, 317f
Zhou dynasty, 63
Zinc, 12, 21
Z-shaped bridges, for lorgnettes, 132, 134f
Zyl, 253
Zylonite, 243

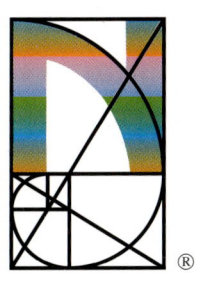

2500 copies of this work were printed in Hong Kong by Dai Nippon on acid-free 80-pound NPI paper using Iris Van ink. The book was designed by Steve Renick, Anselm Design. The photographs were taken by Strout Photographers, New Orleans. The text was set in Pagemaker by Paul Benkman of Tiki Bob Publishing & Design in San Francisco using Bodoni, Frutiger, Garamond, Garamond Expert, and Koch Antiqua, typefaces from Adobe Systems. Final text was output straight from disk to film by Dai Nippon in Hong Kong.

Members of the staff at Norman Publishing who participated in this project were Martha Nicholson Steele, Managing Editor; Jeremy M. Norman, Publisher; and Heather Austin, Editorial Assistant. The edition was completed in February 1996.